The Practice of Thoracic Anesthesia

EDITED BY

Edmond Cohen, MD

Associate Professor of Anesthesiology
Director of Thoracic Anesthesia
Department of Anesthesia
Mount Sinai School of Medicine
The Mount Sinai Medical Center
New York, New York

with 23 contributors

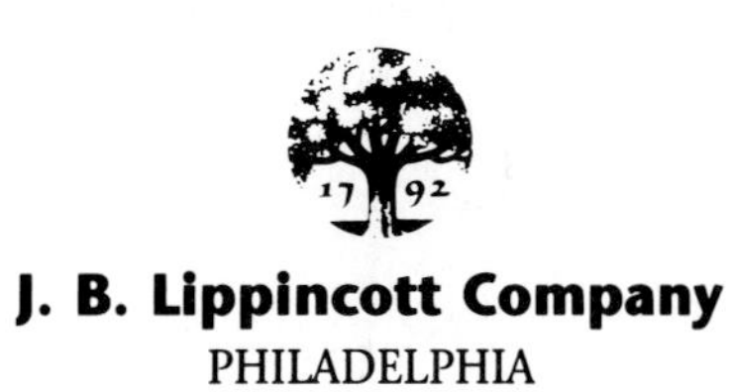

J. B. Lippincott Company
PHILADELPHIA

Acquisitions Editor: Mary K. Smith, Lisa McAllister
Indexer: Alphabyte, Inc.
Production Service: Textbook Writers Associates
Production Manager: Janet Greenwood
Production Coordinator: Mary Kinsella
Compositor: Circle Graphics
Printer/Binder: RR Donnelley & Sons Company, Crawfordsville

6 5 4 3 2 1

Library of Congress Cataloging in Publications Data

The practice of thoracic anesthesia / edited by Edmond Cohen ; with 23 contributors.
p. cm.
Includes bibliographical references and index.
ISBN 0-397-51078-0
1. Chest—Surgery. 2. Anesthesiology. I. Cohen, Edmond.
[DNLM: 1. Thoracic Surgery. 2. Anesthesia. 3. Lung—physiology.
WF 980 P896 1995]
RD536.P73 1995
617.9\6754—dc20
DNLM/DLC
for Library of Congress 94-32387
CIP

The authors and publisher have exerted every effort to ensure that drug selection and dosage set forth in this text are in accord with current recommendations and practice at the time of publication. However, in view of ongoing research, changes in government regulations, and the constant flow of information relating to drug therapy and drug reactions, the reader is urged to check the package insert for each drug for any change in indications and dosage and for added warnings and precautions. This is particularly important when the recommended agent is a new or infrequently employed drug.

To my beloved parents and family:
My wife, Myra,
and our children,
Jennifer and Adam

Contributors

Steven J. Barker, PhD, MD
Professor and Chairman
Department of Anesthesia
University of California
Irvine Medical Center
Orange, California

Elizabeth Behringer, MD
Assistant Professor of Anesthesiology
Department of Anesthesia
University of Pennsylvania School of Medicine
Philadelphia, Pennsylvania

Phillip O. Brindenbaugh, MD
Professor and Chairman
Department of Anesthesia
University of Cincinnati
College of Medicine
Cincinnati, Ohio

Jay B. Brodsky, MD
Professor of Anesthesiology
Department of Anesthesia
Stanford University Medical Center
Stanford, California

David Bronheim, MD
Assistant Professor of Anesthesiology
Director of Post Anesthesia Care Unit
Department of Anesthesia
Mount Sinai School of Medicine
The Mount Sinai Medical Center
New York, New York

Lee K. Brown, MD
Associate Professor of Clinical Medicine
University of Arizona
College of Medicine
Director, Pulmonary Function and Exercise Physiology Laboratory
Associate Program Director (Professional Services)
Department of Internal Medicine
St. Joseph's Hospital and Medical Center
Phoenix, Arizona

Linda Chen, MD
Associate Professor of Anesthesiology
Department of Anesthesia
Hospital of the University of Pennsylvania
Philadelphia, Pennsylvania

Edmond Cohen, MD
Associate Professor of Anesthesiology
Director of Thoracic Anesthesia
Department of Anesthesia
Mount Sinai School of Medicine
The Mount Sinai Medical Center
New York, New York

Andrew T. Costarino, Jr., MD
Assistant Professor of Anesthesiology and Pediatrics
University of Pennsylvania School of Medicine
Director, Fellowship in Pediatric Critical Care Medicine
Department of Anesthesiology and Critical Care Medicine

The Children's Hospital of Philadelphia
Philadelphia, Pennsylvania

James C. Crews, MD
Assistant Professor of Anesthesiology
Department of Anesthesia
University of Cincinnati College of Medicine
Cincinnati, Ohio

James B. Eisenkraft, MD, MRCP (UK), FRCA
Professor of Anesthesiology
Director of Anesthesia Research
Department of Anesthesia
Mount Sinai School of Medicine
The Mount Sinai Medical Center
New York, New York

Michael M. Hansen, MD
Assistant Professor of Anesthesiology
Head of Medical Critical Care Services
Director of Critical Care Education
Department of Critical Care Medicine
St. Francis Medical Center
Pittsburgh, Pennsylvania

John W. Hoyt, MD
Professor and Chairman
Department of Critical Care Medicine
St. Francis Medical Center
Pittsburgh, Pennsylvania

Paul A. Kirschner, MD
Professor of Surgery
Department of Cardiothoracic Surgery
Division of Thoracic Surgery
Mount Sinai School of Medicine
The Mount Sinai Medical Center
New York, New York

Robert Koorn, MD
Assistant Professor of Anesthesiology
Department of Anesthesia
St. Luke's-Roosevelt Hospital Center
Columbia University
College of Physicians and Surgeons
New York, New York

Bryan E. Marshall, MD
Horatio C. Wood Professor of Anesthesiology
Director for Center of Research and Anesthesia
Department of Anesthesia
University of Pennsylvania School of Medicine
Philadelphia, Pennsylvania

Steven M. Neustein, MD
Assistant Professor of Anesthesiology
Department of Anesthesia
Mount Sinai School of Medicine
The Mount Sinai Medical Center
New York, New York

David Reich, MD
Associate Professor of Anesthesiology
Co-Director of the Division of Cardiothoracic Anesthesiology
Department of Anesthesia
Mount Sinai School of Medicine
The Mount Sinai Medical Center
New York, New York

Theodore C. Smith, MD
Professor Emeritus of Anesthesiology
Department of Anesthesia
Loyola University Stritch School of Medicine
Maywood, Illinois

Daniel M. Thys, MD
Professor of Anesthesiology
Director, Department of Anesthesia
St. Luke's-Roosevelt Hospital Center
Columbia University
College of Physicians and Surgeons
New York, New York

Kevin K. Tremper, MD, PhD
Professor and Chairman
Department of Anesthesia
University of Michigan
Ann Arbor, Michigan

Charles B. Watson, MD
Associate Professor of Anesthesiology
Chairman, Department of Anesthesia
Bridgeport Hospital
Bridgeport, Connecticut

Leslie Weiss-Bloom, MD
Attending Anesthesiologist
Department of Anesthesia
Hackensack Medical Center
Hackensack, New Jersey

Roger S. Wilson, MD
Professor and Chairman
Department of Anesthesiology and Critical Care Medicine
Memorial Sloan-Kettering Cancer Center
Cornell University Medical College
New York, New York

Foreword

Anesthesiology continues to expand its base of clinical knowledge at a rapid rate. As a result, our training programs have been lengthened to 4 or even 5 years, and new subspecialities have been formed. Cardiothoracic anesthesia has been the largest and most attractive of these subspecialities due to the challenges presented by the pathophysiology, pharmacology, monitoring, and severe nature of the problems encountered. As thoracic surgery has continued to expand and develop new procedures such as videoassisted thorascopic surgery, which can be used in sicker and sicker patients, anesthesiologists have come to require even greater expertise in this field. Thus, the subspecialty of thoracic anesthesia has developed into a field of its own separate from cardiac anesthesia. Experts such as Dr. Cohen devote most of their time and energy to teaching, studying, and caring for particularly high-risk patients. To keep up with the rapidly evolving concepts and techniques, this subspecialty has generated the need for a single-author textbook and numerous multi-author reference books reviewing the subject matter in great detail. What has been missing up to now is a more practical, clinically oriented text designed for the resident or clinician who does not work in this field every day. *The Practice of Thoracic Anesthesia* is designed to provide the clinician with an approach to management of these difficult cases.

Thoracic anesthesia and surgery have come a long way since the late 1800s, when interest in intubation for lung inflation was combined with a bellows system for positive-pressure ventilation. This Fell-O'Dwyer apparatus was first used successfully in 1899 to remove a chest wall tumor. Intubation of the tracheobronchial tree has been advanced to a high art since the introduction of the double-lumen tube in the 1970s. Separation of the lungs and the management of one-lung ventilation have become the keys to understanding thoracic anesthesia. Prior to 1933, anesthetic agents used for thoracic surgery, such as ether, did not produce apnea and permit controlled ventilation; thus, surgeons still encountered many problems when working in an open chest. In 1934, Waters introduced cyclopropane, which induced apnea and permitted controlled respirations. Unfortunately, it was explosive and precluded use of the electrocautery. In the late 1950s, halothane came into widespread use, beginning the era of nonflammable inhalation anesthesia. Since then, numerous other inhaled agents and intravenous anesthetics have been introduced, and their effects during one-lung ventilation on hypoxic pulmonary ventilation have been widely studied. Anesthetic management of special thoracic diagnostic (eg, bronchoscopy) and therapeutic techniques (e.g., lung lavage) have always been a challenge. More recently, mediastinoscopy, lung transplantation, and tracheal resections have expanded the field. This book highlights all of these areas and makes the information available at a glance. It will be useful not only for the management of patients undergoing thoracic surgery, for whom it was primarily intended, but also for the patient with pulmonary disease undergoing other surgical procedures, as well as for all patients operated upon in the lateral position.

Thoracic anesthesia is now a full-time specialty. Those who do it well spend many hours reviewing the literature in the fields of anesthesiology, thoracic surgery, pulmonary physiology, and pulmonary medicine. They also learn the techniques of double-lumen tube insertion and positioning, fiberoptic bronchoscopy, invasive monitoring, postoperative pain management, and the intricacies of the latest ventilation equipment. For those anesthesiologists who have only occasional or brief exposure to this field (eg, thoracic approach to a hiatal hernia repair) the amount of information can be overwhelming. This concise text initiated by Dr. Cohen and his colleagues in the thoracic anesthesia group of the division of Cardiothoracic Anesthesia at The Mount Sinai Medical Center provides information on the most important techniques and procedures. Hopefully, it will also further contribute to the reduction of morbidity and mortality following thoracic surgery and improve care for all patients undergoing noncardiac thoracic procedures.

Joel A. Kaplan, M.D.
Horace W. Goldsmith Professor
and Chairman
Department of Anesthesia
Mount Sinai School of Medicine
The Mount Sinai Medical Center
New York, New York

Preface

When I began editing *The Practice of Thoracic Anesthesia,* many of my colleagues asked why I saw the need for such a book with others available. My thoughts then, as now, were not to replace any thoracic anesthesia books, but to offer something different in this critical and rapidly-expanding subspecialty of anesthetic practice.

I conceptualized a book that would be a true contribution to the field of anesthesia. It would appeal to the clinican who requires principles necessary to the modern practice of thoracic anesthesia. This book is not a comprehensive treatise covering the entire field of thoracic anesthesia. Specific topics, such as pediatric thoracic anesthesia, pacemakers, high frequency ventilation, laser surgery, and others, were not included.

The book is unique in that it reflects how we as anesthesiologists approach the patient. We discuss topics such as the preparation of the patient for thoracic surgery, intraoperative management, and postoperative care. The subjects are discussed linearly, just as we encounter these situations in a hospital environment.

The book is divided into five sections. The first addresses anatomy, lung physiology, pulmonary function tests, ventilation/perfusion distribution, hypoxic pulmonary vasoconstriction, and the physiology of one lung ventilation. The second section focuses solely on preoperative evaluation and patient preparation. The third section describes the special considerations of positioning and monitoring the patient during surgery. The fourth section pays particular attention to management of the immediate postoperative period. A final section discusses anesthetic management for special procedures such as bronchoscopy, resection of bullous emphysema, mediastinoscopy/mediastinal mass, and tracheal resection and reconstruction.

I thank the contributors for their fine work. They adhered to the goal of this book, namely, to confine their writing to topics of interest to practicing anesthesiologists. Although all are specialists in their own right, they have simplified difficult concepts in the somewhat complex subject of thoracic anesthesia. Each has succeeded admirably, and helped to produce what I hope will become a practical, clinical, and useful contribution to anestheiology.

The book was a long time in making, and would not have been possible without the support of many people. Most importantly, Dr. Joel A. Kaplan, an understanding, encouraging and supportive chairman, whose experience and valuable advice made this project possible; my editor at J.B. Lippincott, Mary K. Smith, and her assistant, Marybeth Meyer, who listened with infinite patience to my endless excuses and requests for extensions. I would like to thank and acknowledge the secretarial staff in our department, especially Helen Phillips, for their valuable assistance. Finally, to my wife Myra and my children Jennifer and Adam, who accepted this book at home as a part of the family rather than an intruder.

Edmond Cohen

Contents

SECTION

I

Pulmonary Physiology—The Lateral Position

CHAPTER

1

Anatomic Correlates of Physiologic Function

Theodore C. Smith

The respiratory and circulatory systems play a major role in the transportation of oxygen from the atmosphere to mitochondria and transportation of carbon dioxide from cells to the atmosphere. They accomplish these tasks by alternate steps of convection and diffusion. The respiratory system provides for the first two steps for oxygen, convection from the atmosphere and diffusion into the blood stream. Anatomic features are best understood by appreciation of their role in the several functions as outlined in Table 1-1. The structures includes an air-conditioning subsystem; a pump; and a marvelously fractile convective system, terminating in well-perfused, close-packed, polyhedral air spaces that ingeniously incorporate a very large area with the thinnest possible barrier between blood and gas, and an energy storage device to power the usually passive exhalation.

This chapter stresses that form and function are interrelated. Therefore it does not follow a distinctly anatomic organization.

The Muscle-Powered Air Pump

The work of breathing is supplied by two groups of muscles (three sets are inspiratory and three are expiratory) that act on skeletal and soft tissue structures of the trunk (chest plus abdomen or, in the classic Greek sense, the thorax). The thorax is bounded by the sternum, ribs, spine, intercostal muscles, abdominal wall muscles, clavicle and strap muscles superiorly, and the pelvic floor inferiorly. The actions of the muscles on the skeletal and soft tissue organs provide active inspiration, store energy in the parenchyma and thorax for passive exhalation, and, provide active exhalation when required Table 1-1).

The inspiratory muscles consist of the diaphragm; the external intercostals; and the so-called accessory muscles, including the strap muscles of the neck and the erector spini (Fig. 1-1).[1,2]

The diaphragm is a dome-shaped structure consisting of a central tendon with muscle fibers radiating outward to attach on the xiphoid, on the seventh to twelfth ribs, and on the vertebral bodies. Contraction under phrenic nerve control flattens the dome shape, increasing the cephalocaudad dimension (CC) of the lung. Simultaneously it displaces the liver, spleen, and stomach both anteriorly and laterally, increasing the anterior-posterior (AP) and the side-to-side or lateral dimension of the chest (S-S)

Table 1-1. Anatomy and Physiology Related to Pulmonary Function Tests

Major Function	Testable Physiology	Anatomic Feature	Applicable Tests
Ventilation	Pump	Skeleton	Inspection, radiography
		Muscles	PI_{max}, PE_{max}, vital capacity
	Conduits	Airways	Airway resistance, forced expiratory flow
		Small airways	Flow-volume loops
	Expandable tissue	Alveolar ducts	Lung compliance, Closing capacity
Perfusion	Pump	Right ventricle	Pre- and afterloads, ejection fraction, wall fraction, wall motion, cardiac output
Exchange	Distribution:		
	Gas	Alveolar interdependence	Chest radiograph
		Airways morphology	A-a differences/O_2, CO_2
	Blood	Hydrostatic gradient	DL carbon monoxide
		Vessel potency	
	Surface	Alveolar Facet	Capillary volume
			Inert gas ventilation-perfusion distribution
Defense	Filtering	Nose and pharynx	Inspection
	Humidification	Epithelium	Tantalum transport
	Mucociliary transport	Larynx	Cough reflex
	Separation from gut	Cell types	Bronchial brushing, lavage
	Immune mechanism		
Control	Sensors	Carotid body	Doxapram
		Aortic body	
		Medulla:	Ventilatory response:
		respiratory centers	to CO_2
		ventrolateral surface	to hypoxia
		Irritant and J Receptors	
	Reflexes	Vagus nerve	Breathing pattern
		Central connections	Response to loading

through passive movement of the rib cage (Fig. 1-2).

The rib cage volume is also increased by the action of the external (oblique) intercostal muscles. The fibers of these muscles run diagonally upward and backward from the top of one rib to the bottom of the next above. Three types of motion result from the slightly different articulation of (1) the first two or three ribs, (2) the middle ribs, and (3) the lowermost two pairs of ribs: pump handle, bucket handle, and caliper motion. The first three or four ribs lie in planes that slope primarily from back to front. When they move upward they increase the AP and CC diameters. This movement is like a pump handle. The next six or seven ribs lie in planes that are increasingly tilted to the side. When they move the S-S diameter increases by the bucket handle motion induced by the articulation of these ribs at the sternum as well as at the vertebral column. The eleventh and twelfth ribs move primarily outward, aided by pressure of the viscera, as well as upward, like the jaws of a caliper or tongs, primarily increasing the S-S diameter.[3]

Although the diaphragm or the external intercostals are independently able to supply the tidal volume and about half of the vital capacity, the accessory muscles most often play an accessory role. The paravertebral muscles can straighten the spinal kyphosis, and the strap muscles of the neck lift the thoracic inlet. The

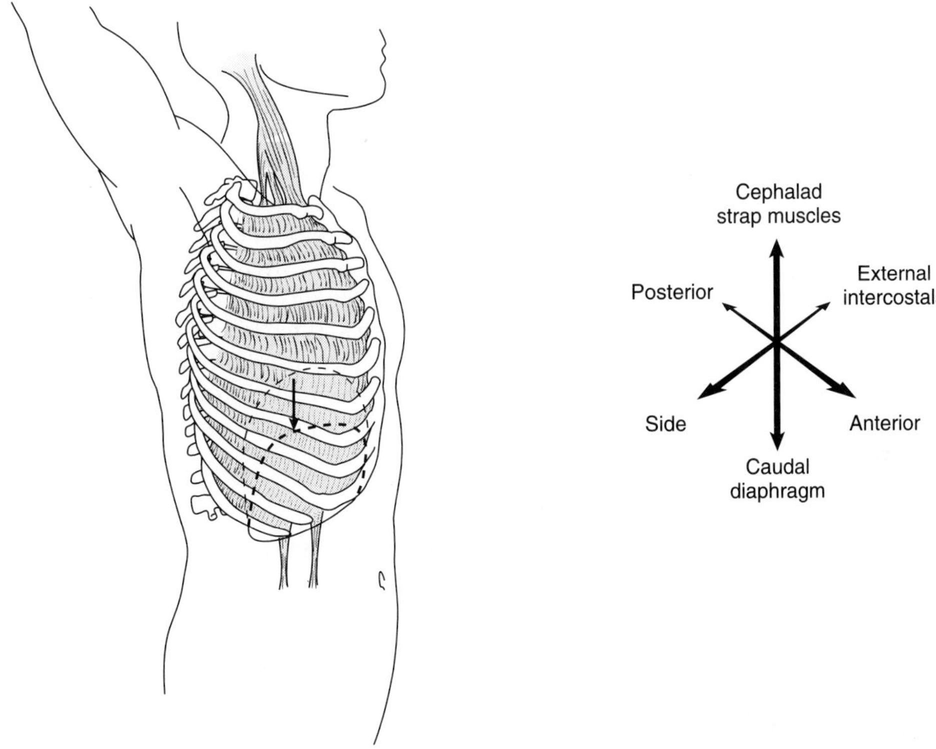

Figure 1-1. Inspiratory muscles. The major inspiratory muscles are the Diaphragm, the External intercostals, and, to a lesser extent, the strap muscles of the neck, particularly the Sternocleidomastoid and three Scalenes. Muscles of the shoulder girdle and spinal erectors may play a minor role at the end of a deep inspiration.

strap muscles of the neck, including most importantly the sternocleidomastoid, and also those muscles from tongue to hyoid to thyroid to cricoid to sternum, generally referred to as the accessory muscles of inspiration, are capable of adding perhaps 10% to the inspiratory capacity on their own. Normally, during inspiration, they have a phasic increase in tone with each breath (ie, isometric contraction), which serves to stabilize the thoracic inlet. This permits the external intercostals to increase the S-S diameter, each lifting the rib below. When the clavicle and first rib can be seen to move up and out, in either spontaneous or mechanical ventilation, one can be sure it represents an augmented tidal volume.[4]

The inspiratory muscles have expiratory functions as well. First, by stretching the expiratory muscles, they increase their contractility when activated. Second, they stretch the lung, and with large tidal volumes the rib cage as well, storing elastic energy for exhalation. Finally, their tone is decreased slowly and progressively during expiration, providing a braking effect on expiratory flow, minimizing expiratory flow problems, and tending to increase average lung volume (Fig. 1-3).

The expiratory muscles consist of the mus-

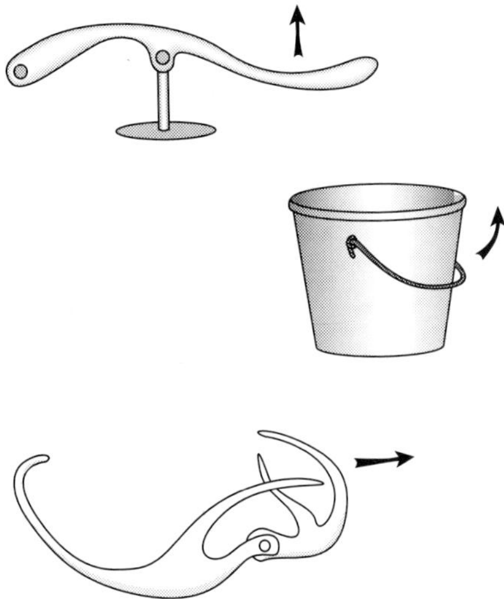

Figure 1-2. Motions of the ribs. The Scalene muscles, inserting on the first two ribs, the Sternocleidomastoid inserting on the sternum and clavicle, and the other strap muscles of the neck lift the thoracic inlet, expanding the craniocaudal diameter like a pump handle. External intercostal muscles lift the middle ribs like a bucket handle, expanding both the side-to-side and anterior-posterior diameters. Lower intercostals and the insertion of the diaphragm on the ribs lift the ribs and push them upward and outward, aided by pressure from the organs just below the diaphragm, notably the liver, stomach, and spleen.

cles of the abdominal wall, the internal intercostals muscles, and a number of other muscles of the upper limb and thorax. The expiratory muscles are not ordinarily involved in quiet expiration. They markedly increase expiratory flow in the sneeze or cough, and can decrease lung volume below functional residual capacity, to residual volume. The muscles involved in active expiration are, most importantly, those of the abdominal wall (external obliques, internal obliques, rectus abdominis, and transversus abdominis); the internal intercostals (whose fibers run more vertically than the External Obliques); and to a very small degree the muscles of the thoracic girdle and spine, which pull the shoulders forward and flex the vertebral column (and might be called the accessory muscles of expiration). These muscles ordinarily have little tone during anesthesia but come into play with cough. On emergence or in very light anesthesia the abdominal components may be activated at the end of expiration. This end-expiratory tightening of the oblique abdominals thrusts the abdominal wall forward and may be mistaken for an inspiratory effort. Attendants trying to assist breathing with resuscitation bags (Ambu-bags or equivalent) may thus be out of synchronization, and their efforts may be counterproductive.

Lung Volumes: Anatomic Determinants

The nomenclature of the lung volumes was originally based on four independent volumes: residual volume (RV) expiratory reserves volume (ERV), tidal volume (TV), and inspiratory reserve volume (IRV). A fifth, overlapping lung volume closing volume, (CV), has been added. Two or more volumes may be added to obtain a capacity.

(1-1)		
	Functional residual capacity (FRC)	= RV + ERV
	Inspiratory capacity (IC)	= TV + IRV
	Vital capacity (VC)	= ERV + TV + IRV
	Total lung capacity (TLC)	= RV + ERV + TV + IRV
	Closing capacity (CC)	= CV + RV

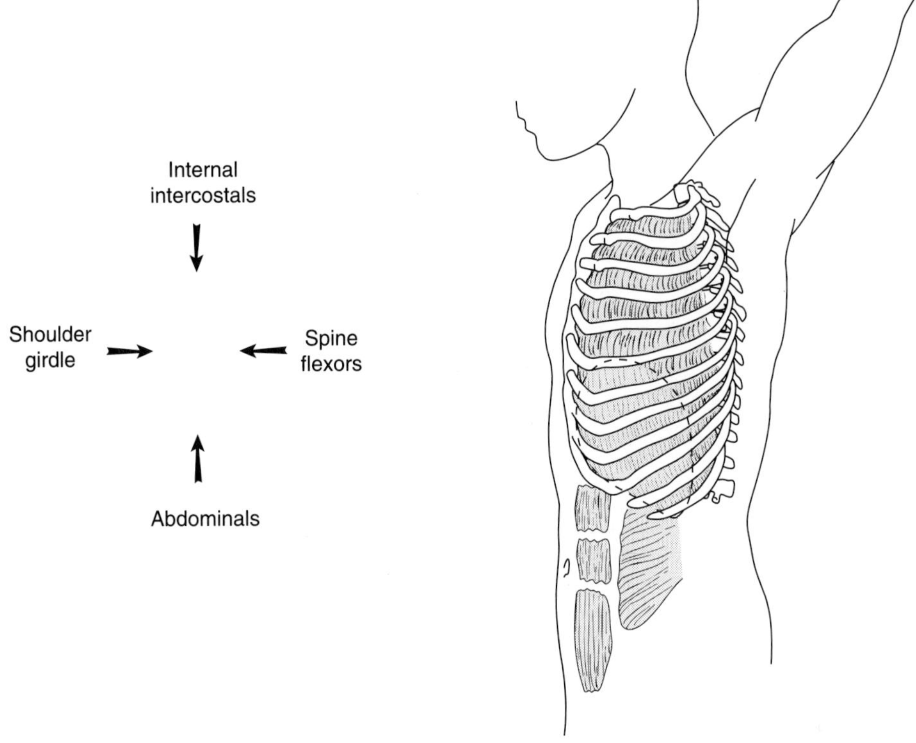

Figure 1-3. Expiratory muscles. The major expiratory muscles are the External intercostals which pull ribs down and in, the abdominal wall muscles which push viscera up against the diaphragm elevating it, and to a minor extent at the extreme of expiration, the shoulder girdle and spinal muscles which flex the spine. Elastic recoil energy stored during inspiratory muscle effort supplies a major portion of expiratory force.

When the lungs and viscera are removed from the body and all muscles are relaxed or paralyzed, the volume of the thoracic cage is several hundred milliliters larger than the functional residual capacity (FRC). Similarly, when the lungs are removed from the thoracic cavity and opened to the atmosphere, they decrease their volume by up to several hundred milliliters.

The resting position, the FRC, is set by equating the forces of the parenchyma to further collapse, with the force of the thorax tending to reexpand. At this point the expiratory muscles are stretched slightly beyond their rest length and can contract to decrease the gas volume in the chest from the FRC to the RV, but the limit of this contraction differs somewhat in children and youths from older adults (see below) (Fig. 1-4).

The VC is determined by the maximal excursion of the thoracic girdle, rib cage, spine, and diaphragm. From the FRC, the IC is limited by muscle shortening and rib excursion, not by lung compliance. The ERV and the RV are lim-

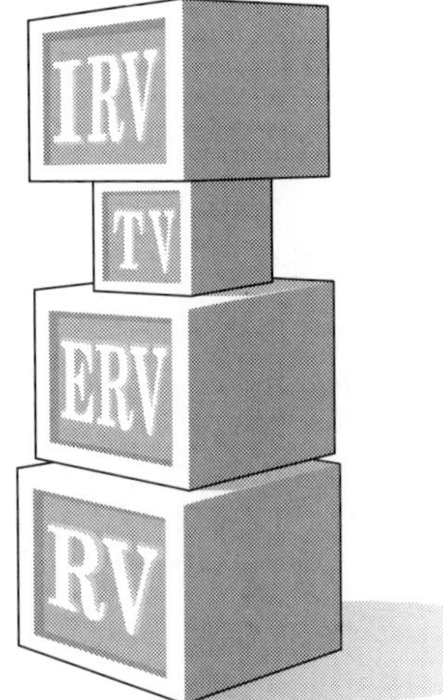

Approximate values for normal adults in liters

	Men	Women
IRV	2.5	2.0
TV	0.5	0.4
ERV	1.1	1.0
RV	2.0	1.5
TLC	6.1	4.9

Figure 1-4. The building blocks of lung volumes. The lung gas space is divided into four independent volumes: Residual volume (RV), Expiratory reserve volume (ERV), Tidal volume (TV), and Inspiratory reserve volume (IRV). A fifth volume, the Closing volume, is normally a portion of the ERV, but with age, recumbancy, and disease, may enlarge to include a portion of the TV. A Capacity is the sum of two or more volumes.

ited differently at different ages, however. In adults the RV represents the volume of gas in the lung when all small airways have closed due to loss of tethering effect (see below). In children the RV of the excised lung is somewhat smaller than the pleural cavity volume during maximum expiratory effort. Consequently the pleural pressure is always negative. With increasing age, the increase of the closing capacity of lung tissue makes it higher than the minimal volume of the bony thorax at maximum expiration. Now expiratory effort produces a positive pleural pressure.[5,6]

The Upper Airway

The conducting passages from the nares and lips to the larynx serve not only a simple conducting function but important defensive functions as well. They filter, warm, and humidify inspired gas and serve as a buffer against entry of irritating material to the more delicate lung parenchyma. During quiet breathing, maximal conservation of heat and humidity are obtained by nasal breathing. With hyperpnea, minimal work of breathing dictates mouth breathing, sacrificing supralaryngeal air conditioning. Bony, muscular, and mucosal structures provide for these optimalizations and for the switch-over.

The nasal portion of the airway has a framework of cartilage and bone covered internally with hair-bearing, squamous epithelium in the funnel-shaped vestibule and ciliated, pseudostratified respiratory epithelium in the deeper cavum. The entrance is a pair of oval openings framed by the alar cartilages and the anterior border of the septal cartilage. Hairs called vibrissae form a coarse net across the openings to filter large particles. They can elicit a sneeze when moved lightly. Slips of striated muscle (the nasalis muscle under facial, cranial nerve

VII control) dilate the entrance somewhat in hyperpnea. The nares can be narrowed, as in a sniff, when the decreasing pressure attendant on increased inspiratory air flow causes the lateral (cartilaginous) walls to move inward, narrowing the passageway and creating a jet directing the gas flow into the roof of the cavum in greater part. This has several functions: improving olfaction, clearing secretions into the pharynx, and directing dry cold gas over moist, warm surfaces (Fig. 1-5).

Beyond the vestibule the cavum opens up into two bilaterally symmetric chambers with a floor provided by the hard palate; a medial wall by the nasal septum; and a lateral wall by the maxilla with three curved, bony protuberances called turbinates or conchae. In the cavum the direction of the airstream is bent and the flow further broken up by the turbinates. The medial-lateral surfaces, about 150 square centimeters in area, are rarely more than a few millimeters apart, except along the floor of the cavum, where there may be as much a centimeter between medial, lateral, and inferior borders. Thus the floor is the obvious route of choice for advancing fiberoptic endoscopes and airways. The submucosa is so rich in blood vessels that it resembles erectile tissue. These vessels provide the heat and water necessary for the air-conditioning function of the nose. The nasolacrimal duct and orifices to the paranasal sinuses are found under the turbinates.

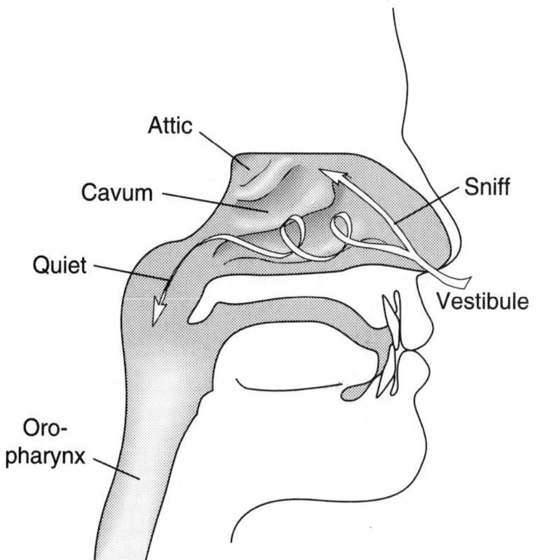

Figure 1-5. The nose. In quiet breathing the inspiratory air stream flows over and around the turbinates (promoting humidification), bends sharply at the pharynx (impacting large suspended particles on mucosa underlaid by lymphoid tissue of Waldeyer's ring), and enters the hypopharynx nearly fully humidified, at body temperature, and cleansed of large particulates. A sniff directs a jet of inspirate to the attic where olfactory nerves originate. The surface coiling attendant on inspiratory humidification promotes condensation of a major fraction of the humidity of alveolar expirate, thus conserving water.

Innervation for olfaction is provided in the attic of the cavum by bipolar neurons in the epithelium, whose axons pass through the cribriform plate to the olfactory bulb and synapse there with axons of the olfactory cranial nerve I. Sensation is provided by the first two branches of the trigeminal cranial nerve V, which have broadly arborized before entering the mucosa. Motor innervation for facial expression and emotion comes from the facial cranial nerve VII. Autonomic innervation comes from the cervical (sympathetic) ganglia following the arterial supply (branches of the external carotid and parasympathetics) from cranial nerve V. Through autonomic reflexes, cold, dry inspirate increases both the flow and volume of blood in the mucosa, supplying calories and water to the gas.

The nasopharynx begins at the posterior choanae with another sharp bend in the airstream. Inertia carries suspended particles into the posterior mucosal blanket where the rich supply of lymphoid tissue (Waldeyer's ring) promotes defense. The eustachian tubes draining the middle ear open into the lateral wall. The nasopharynx is bounded superiorly by the base of the skull and posteriorly by the vertebral column. When the soft palate and tongue are relaxed, the nasopharynx is a widely patent part of the airway with a cross-sectional area two to three times as large as the trachea.

The resistance to air flow provided by the nose is nearly half of the resting resistance of the total airway. Major components are the turbulent flow pattern and narrow spaces created by the conchae. Resistance provided by the vestibule is variable as noted above, however, with decreased air flow as the result of valving collapse of the lateral nasal cartilages during a sniff. Alar flaring opposes this collapse, decreasing resistance as well as conveying emotion. In contrast, the air flow resistance from the choanae through the nasopharynx is either negligible (nose breathing) or infinite (ie, closed). This valve-like function is due to the effect of the soft palate: when elevated it seals the nasopharynx, and gas transverses the oral cavity and pharynx with very little resistance to flow.

The oropharynx is simply the vertical continuation of the nasopharynx when the soft palate is relaxed in quiet breathing. With the switch to oral breathing and anterior movement of the base of the tongue, it becomes the segment of the airway with the lowest resistance and the largest cross-sectional area. It acts as a gentle curve directing gas flow into the larynx.

The hypopharynx consists of two funnel-shaped cavities, the pyriform sinuses, on either side of the larynx. The entrance to the esophagus is normally closed by the cricopharyngeus muscle. The superior laryngeal nerves are just submucosal in the anterolateral wall of the sinuses and may be blocked by two local anesthetic-soaked pledgets held at this spot. This is in contrast to the rest of the sensory innervation: no one other anatomically identifiable spot serves as a landmark for a nerve supplying a large area of mucosa. Hence topical anesthesia with several local anesthetic-soaked cotton swabs placed in the nose or throat do not produce satisfactorily topical anesthesia.[7]

Secondary functions of the nasal, oral, and pharyngeal anatomy are to give rich quality and variety to speech and song and to seal off the airway during deglutition. The details of these structure-function relations may be found elsewhere. With regret, the author notes that the newborn can do both simultaneously, that is, to suck and sing, or at least breathe and swallow. The neonate has a very curved and relatively long epiglottis that extends up to the soft palate to provide a sealed transit for gas to and from the nose through the oropharynx and to deflect liquid laterally around the larynx to the esophagus. This ability is lost in infancy. Worse still, throughout the rest of life the loss of those reflexes that make the separation of inspirate and alimentation less and less certain slowly accelerates (Fig. 1-6).

The functional anatomy up to this point may be diagrammed by a capital letter F in which are embedded four valves. The lateral alar cartilages move inward with increasing air flow through the nostrils to accelerate the airstream velocity and direct it upward in the nasal attic (V_1). This is partially prevented by the facial muscles, which stiffen and flare the external nares. The soft palate and base of the tongue, which move together to open the nasopharynx to breathing, move apart to promote oropharyngeal breathing (V_2). The lips and teeth govern the entrance to the mouth (V_3). The larynx is the fourth valve, which is described in the next section. These valves are the first line of pulmonary defenses.

The volume of this section of the airway is about 1 mL/kg during mouth breathing, and 1.5 mL/kg during nasal breathing. These numbers represent the reduction in dead space achieved by tracheostomy. The upper airway offers about one-half of the airway resistance at rest and one-third or less with hyperpnea and

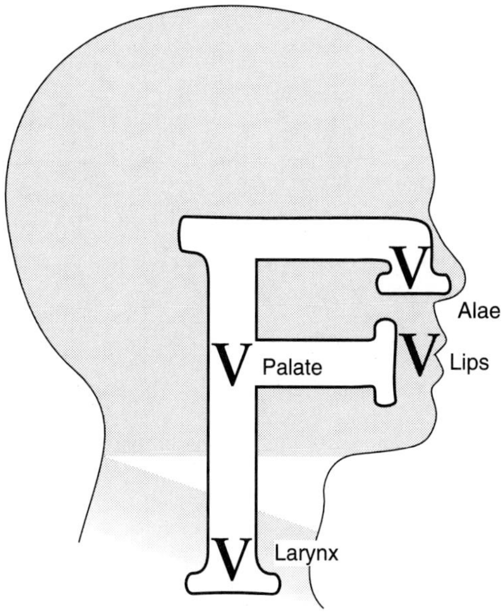

Figure 1-6. The airway valves. At four separate sites the airway can be narrowed or closed. At the nose, relaxation of the Dilator naris and aerodynamic force associated with rapid inspiratory flow narrow the aperture by inward movement of the alar cartilages. At the lips the orbicularis oris can close the mouth even with the mandible partly open. The soft palate can be elevated to seal off the nasopharynx (as when blowing up a closed balloon) or pulled down to seal off the oral cavity during nose breathing. The larynx is a complex valve with three separate mechanisms (see Fig. 1-7).

mouth breathing. Work of breathing overcoming this resistance normally represents about 1% of the basal metabolic oxygen demand. Bypassing the upper airway via tracheostomy or translaryngeal airways does not usually, by itself, provide an appreciable therapeutic effect. It does shift the burden of warming and humidifying the inspired gas and conserving calories and water on exhalation to another less elegantly designed site.

In summary, the upper airway is an active conduit with air-conditioning functions (heat, humidification, and filtration), defensive functions (coughing, sneezing, and swallowing), and certain advanced functions of civilization (including oration, singing, and emotional expressions like crying and laughing). It offers minor compensation for some disease processes. Paradoxically, it can increase airway resistance, thereby controlling lung volume and shifting the equal pressure point oral (pursed lip breathing). In the practice of thoracic anesthesia, understanding these anatomic correlates aids in the diagnosis and evaluation of dyspnea, in fiberoptic bronchoscopy for both diagnostic indications and as an aid in intubation, and in the management of emerging and postoperative patients.

The Larynx

Although it may be more common to view the rima glottidis as the dividing section between upper and lower airway, this chapter will consider the larynx as a whole as separating the upper and lower airway, and will include the hyoid as a laryngeal structures. The larynx is most simply a valve, which is open during respiration, closed during deglutition, and intermediate during phonation. It plays a minor but crucial role when increased intra-abdominal pressure is required (eg, defecating, lifting). Since this structure is required to move, to open and to close, it has the requisite structure and power. Most notably, it has three manners of closure, each more secure: The vocal cords close the larynx like a shutter, the epiglottis folds over the glottis, and the structures around the base of the epiglottis ball up and push the vestibular folds (false vocal cords) down onto the true vocal cords. This is rather like the box lock, the grille and the massive vault door in a safe deposit box facility.

The larynx consists of one bone, three unpaired and three paired cartilages, nine intrinsic muscles, a variety of extrinsic muscles whose number depends on just how far afield one goes, ligaments that interconnect these, and appropriate nerves and vessels. Its movement are both intrinsic (motion in respect to other parts of the larynx) and extrinsic (motion as a whole in relation to adjacent structures).

The hyoid bone is extrinsic to the usual description of the larynx. However it is as securely attached to the upper border of the thyroid cartilage as the cricoid is attached to the lower border by a tough membranous ligament. There is an aperture in each side, through which pass the superior laryngeal nerves and vessels. This provides a second site for neural blockade, a centimeter below and a centimeter anterior to the (posterior) greater corner of the hyoid, at a depth just subcutaneous. A tough ligament is perceived by an advancing needle at greater depths. Several muscles, extrinsic to the larynx, originate or insert on the hyoid, and are easily identified by the "hyo" in their name (eg, omohyoid, hyothyroid, etc). They are part of the accessory muscles of respiration and partake in the swallowing mechanism. There is also a small but constant ligament from the center of the hyoid to the center of the epiglottis. In some reconstructions it would seem to prevent the epiglottis from backward and downward rotation to cover the glottis, but it is either just long enough or just low enough to permit the epiglottis to fold over the larynx in one of the three mechanisms of laryngeal closure (Fig. 1-7).[8]

The epiglottis is a spoon-shaped cartilage of compound curvature, that is, it is concave inward in horizontal section and concave backward vertically. It is one of the three unpaired cartilages; the thyroid and cricoid are the other two. Fink has pointed out the action of extrinsic muscles on this compound curvature causes a folding motion, which brings the free top of the epiglottis down over the vestibule of the larynx like a hinged lid on a German beer stein.[9] This action is further promoted by the elevation of the larynx in the neck during swallowing, a motion that results from the collective effort of the strap muscles above the larynx (the genio-, glosso-, hyo-, stylo-, omothyroid and other thyroid muscles). Since these motions are programmed into the motor cortex as part of the swallowing action, they are a regular and reliable valving mechanism. With maximum voluntary effort they ball up tissue at the root of the epiglottis. This ball valve is the strongest of the three closing mechanisms. The inferior surface of the epiglottis is inverted by the vagus cranial nerve X, which also supplies muscles closing the glottis intrinsically by rotation of the aryteroids adducting the vocal cords (the least strong valve mechanism). The superior surface on the other hand is by innervated branches of the glossopharyngeal cranial nerve IX. Macintosh conjectured that stimulation of the inferior surface (X nerve) by a straight blade laryngoscope would be more likely to cause laryngospasm via motor fibers in the vagus than

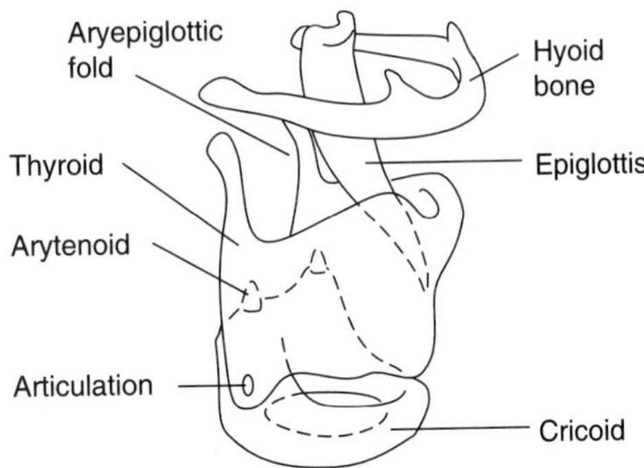

Figure 1-7. The laryngeal skeleton. The unpaired laryngeal cartilages (heavy outline) and hyoid bone provide support for the larynx. The glottis can be closed by (1) rotation of the arytenoid cartilages (dotted outline) adducting the vocal cords, by (2) folding of the epiglottis over the glottis, and by (3) forceful contraction of muscles in the neck which balls up tissue above and anterior to the epiglottis root. This pushes the vestibular folds onto the vocal cords.

stimulation of the hypopharyngeal mucosa innervated by the IX nerve). Anesthesia would more likely block a reflex that requires neuronal connection between two different cranial nuclei than a simple reflex involving one nucleus. This reasoning led to the design of the MacIntosh blade, but there are no published data confirming the conjecture.

The thyroid cartilage, the second of the unpaired cartilages, is a roughly hemicylindrical structure forming the major part of the anterior and lateral walls of the larynx. Its size and the prominent notch at the top front provide an easily observable or palpable landmark. The base of the epiglottis is tightly bound to its internal surface in the midline by a tough ligament just above the origin of the vocal cords from the midline of the thyroid cartilage. The thyroid is articulated to the cricoid by a paired set of true joints that permit rotation, rather like the visor of a medieval knight's headgear rotates on the helmet. This changes the tension on the cords and hence vocal pitch.[10]

The cricoid, the last unpaired cartilage, and the only completely circular cartilage in the airway. When its anterior arc (just below the thyroid) is identified and pressed posteriorly, the broad posterior arc compresses and seals the esophagus against the lower cervical vertebral bodies. Sellick demonstrated competency to over 100 mmHg pressure with this maneuver.

The cricothyroid membrane is a midline, nearly avascular fibrous layer between the thyroid above, the cricoid below, and the cricothyroid muscles laterally. It is rarely covered with thyroid tissue as may be found below the cricoid. Just subcutaneous, it is easily located by palpation of the thyroid notch and the rounded cricoid cartilage as landmarks. This membrane is useful for emergency surgical airway provision, jet ventilation, retrograde tracheal intubation techniques, and topical anesthesia of the larynx and trachea.

The Lower Airway

The trachea, bronchi, and bronchioles are primarily conducting passages that also serve as a backup heat and humidity exchanger (during hyperpnea or when tracheal intubation bypasses the upper airway) and as part of the pulmonary defense against inhaled particulates. Anatomic details contribute to its patency differently at different levels. Their design minimizes work of breathing. Recognition of certain features permits orientation of the image in bronchoscopy.

Patency of the trachea is primarily maintained by the C-shaped cartilaginous rings that resist most physiologic forces tending to collapse the extrathoracic trachea on inspiration and the intrathoracic trachea on forced expiration. The wall of the trachea is completed posteriorly by horizontally arranged smooth muscle, the cholinergically innervated trachealis muscle which is inserted not on the ends of the cartilages but higher up. When maximally contracted, the ends of the cartilage are pulled into a slightly overlapping arrangement. But when relaxed, the mucosa and trachealis can be pushed into the lumen of the intrathoracic trachea by a transtracheal pressure such as is generated just after the glottic opening of a hard cough. It moves inward not as a piston nor symmetrically, but more on one side than the other, producing a yin-yang-like figure that pushes any mucus and entrapped mucosal particulates into a glob, as does a squeegee. The combination of accelerating air flow and decreasing cross-sectional area creates sufficient aerodynamic force to lift balled up drops of mucus into the airstream and expel them. During quiet breathing, the coordinated action of cilia of the pseudostratified mucosa move the blanket of mucus and impacted debris toward the larynx at a rate of a few centimeters per hour. Inhalation anesthetics stop this action (Fig. 1-8).[11,12]

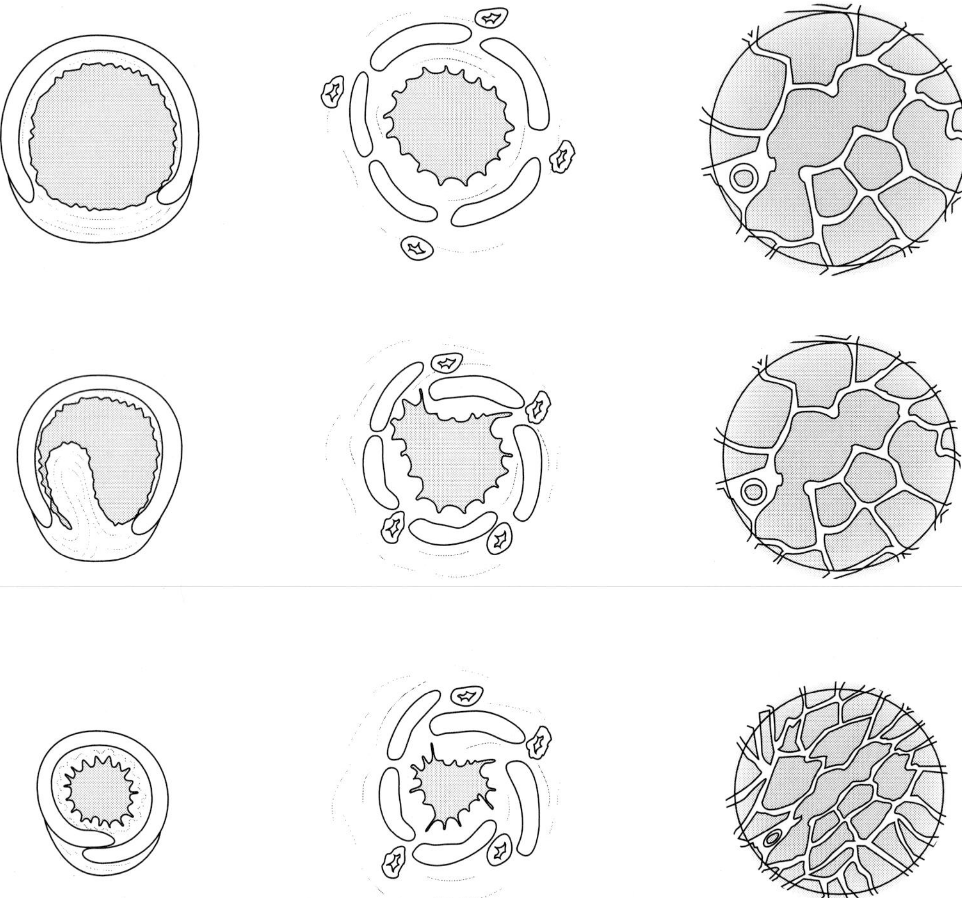

Figure 1-8. Schematic cross-section of the airway at rest (top row), during cough (middle row), and during bronchoconstriction (bottom row). The rows show, left to right, the trachea, a major bronchus, and alveolar duct, drawn to quite different scales! The tracheal lumen may be briefly invaginated by the trachealis muscle during the early moments of cough if the muscle is relatively flaccid. But, if constricted, the tracheal lumen becomes totally enclosed by its cartilage. In bronchi the plates of cartilage are normally separated but may partially overlap due to aerodynamic forces in coughing, or may be jammed close together in bronchoconstriction. The alveolar duct diameter is largely set by current lung volume, widely open at TLC by tethering action of adjacent alveolar facets, but capable of being pulled nearly closed by pneumoconstriction as with hypoxia or pulmonary emboli.

Patency of the bronchi is achieved by a combination of plates and arcs of cartilage that are connected by thicker encircling smooth muscle (as compared with the trachea). Although lying within the lung parenchyma, there is little or no connection of fibrous or elastic strands between lung tissue and bronchi. There is a network of lymph capillaries in the potential space around airways and vessels that may be compared to the network of vines encasing an oak in an old forest. As lymph moves from parenchyma toward the hilum, the total cross-sectional area of these capillaries decreases. As a result increased lymph flow meets an effective choke-point at the hilum. In the genesis of pulmonary edema, the first effect is distension of lymph vessels at or near the hilum producing perivascular and peribronchial cuffs of edema fluid. Transudation from the lymph capillaries begins at or near the hilum. Continued progression of the process causes an alveolar spread of irregular edema around the airway and vessels, both arterial and venous, with variable compression. The effect of airway compression is wheezing; the effect of vascular compression is spreading maldistribution of gas and blood.

Patency of bronchioles is maintained by anatomically different means. Bronchioles have no cartilage and less circular smooth muscle in their relatively thinner walls. There is no potential space around them, however. Fibers of collagen and elastin in the walls merge with the connective tissue of the parenchyma structure, alveolar ducts, and alveoli. These tissue strands are arranged radial to the bronchioles. They stretch as the lung gets larger and relax as the lung gets smaller. In fact, the closing capacity of a lung region is that volume where this radial tethering is so relaxed that there is no support to the thin bronchiole wall. The bronchioles then collapse (close) under small forces such as the decreased luminal pressure associated with air flow (Venturi effect) or positive pressure in adjacent alveoli.

Patency of the alveolar gas spaces is maintained by the normal recoil of the chest wall below FRC, by ventilation that brings more gas to the alveoli than the blood removes in uptake of oxygen and anesthetic agents, by the presence of inert gas such as nitrogen, and by the pull of adjacent air spaces in all directions. If the airway to a lung unit is closed (by collapse, tumor, secretion, or foreign body), continued perfusion of the distal air space continues to remove oxygen. Diffusion of carbon dioxide into the space stops when alveolar carbon dioxide tension equals that of mixed venous blood; this usually occurs within less than a minute of the cessation of ventilation. An inert gas such as nitrogen (or even nitrous oxide at a concentration equal to that in mixed venous blood) may slow the rate of collapse markedly, so that it takes many hours, but atelectasis is still the eventual outcome. High concentrations of oxygen and anesthetic gas, especially nitrous oxide at a partial pressure well above the concurrent mixed venous level, speed the rate of collapse. With 100% oxygen, total atelectasis occurs in eight to ten minutes. The pull of adjacent alveoli tending to hold lung air spaces open, which is analogous to stretching a spring, is called "interdependence." The total force applied to the spring is shared by each loop and is not concentrated near the end. Protection of the air spaces against flooding with fluid is described below. (Fig. 1-9).[13,14]

The airway design is basically dichotomous branching, although this sometimes varies. Not all of the branches are equal. At each branching the sum of the areas of the daughter limbs exceeds that of the parent, although together they conduct the same gas flow. Thus the linear speed of air flow decreases progressively from trachea to alveoli. From basic aerodynamic analysis, the least work of breathing results

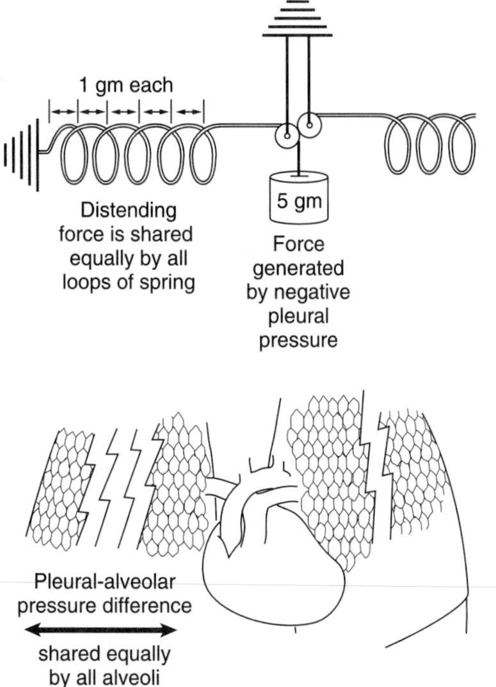

Figure 1-9. Pulmonary interdependence. The expansion of the lung is fairly uniform throughout the parenchyma even though the force is applied only at the pleural surfaces. It can be visualized as two springs stretched by forces analogous to the moving thoracic boundaries (diaphragm and rib cage). If the links are of uniform construction each will expand equally, distributing the distending force among all loops. Of course, if one loop is stiffer (analogous to local disease or scar) the equally-shared force would cause less expansion.

when the two branches of a parent airway are equal in size and branch at a 60-degree angle. If the two branches are unequal, however, the larger should be a more direct continuation of the parent axis. This relation is actually found, starting at the carina. The right bronchus is both larger and less angled from the tracheal axis (20–25 degrees away from the midline, as opposed to 40–50 degrees for the left-bronchus). The length of the bronchi is governed by the distance from the hilum of the gas spaces is supplies. The lower lobe bronchi, for example, give rise to a superior segmental bronchus almost immediately after the minor carina at the middle lobe (on the right) or upper lobe-cum-ligula (on the left). They then descend 4–6 cm to the basal segmental bronchi, which proliferate almost immediately in all directions. They give rise to subsegmental bronchi within a centimeter. Altogether there are about two dozen branch points from the major carina to the distal alveolar ducts, with an exponential increase in cross-sectional area and decrease in convective flow rate (Fig. 1-10).[15]

Thus the parenchyma of the lung can be divided into portions served by identifiable, named airways. The right and left lungs are served by main bronchi. Each side is divided into lobes: upper middle and lower lobes on the right, and upper and lower on the left (the lingula of the left upper lobe is analogous to the right middle lobe). The lobes are separated by complete or nearly complete fissures that are externally visible. This scheme varies considerably in other species. For example, in the dog there are usually four lobes on the right and two or three on the left depending on how completely the ligula is separated. This is of importance to anesthesiologists only if they practice bronchoscopy in an animal laboratory.

The lobes of the lung are divided into segments, each with a named (and often numbered) segmental bronchi. There are no fissures nor even fascial planes, however. Instead, the major venous drainage from two adjacent segments is the anatomic feature separating the segments. The surgeon follows these veins in segmental resection of the lung; this accounts for the usually higher blood loss and greater initial loss of lung function in these operations as opposed to lobar resections. The names and numbers of the segmental bronchi are given in Figure 1-10. Subsegmental bronchi may be identified and given a lower case letter to iden-

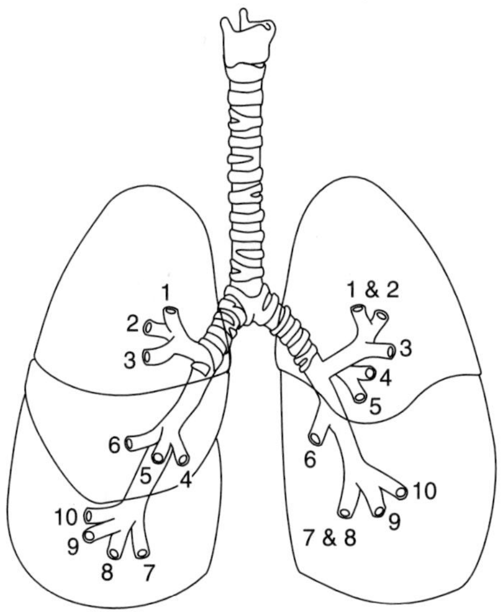

Figure 1-10. The tracheobronchial tree. The trachea divides into a right and left main bronchus, which further divide into upper lobes, a middle lobe on the right (for which the left lung has the analogous lingular portion of the upper lobe) and a lower lobe. Each lobe then divides into two or more segments with segmental bronchi that are numbered and named. Thus 1-apical, 2-posterior (usually fused with 1 on the left), and 3-anterior form the upper lobe. On the right 4-lateral, 5-medial form the middle lobe while in the left these are called superior and inferior lingular segments of the upper lobe. There is usually not a clear fissure separating the lingula from the rest of the left upper lobe. The lower lobe consists of a superior segment numbered 6, and medial, anterior, lateral and posterior segments labeled 7, 8, 9, and 10, on the right. On the left there is no clear 7-medial segment, the volume occupied by either expansion of 10 forward or 8 medially. Thus there are 18 segments, ten on the right and eight on the left (since 1 and 2, and 7 and 8 are fused on the left into one segment each).

tify them. Thus the three subsegmental bronchi to the posterior basal segment of the right lower lobe would be identified as rt B^{10}a, b, and c.

As the thoracic cage enlarges on inspiration, unfolding of the alveolar ducts accommodates most of the increased gas volume. Alveoli also increase in volume. Consequently there is little convective flow through distal alveolar ducts and into alveoli. The dimensions are so small (tens of microns), however, that the physical process of diffusion can mix the gas in the volume of alveolar ducts and alveoli that is distal to a single terminal bronchiole within the period of one breath. Phenomena of convection of gas and airway resistance are thus confined to the passages from terminal bronchioles to larger airways.

The Gas Spaces and Gas Exchange

Gas exchange begins at the respiratory bronchioles, daughters and granddaughters of a terminal bronchiole. They are lined with ciliated, pseudostratified columnar epithelium, mucus-secreting goblet cells, mucous, and Clara cells of unidentified function. Circular smooth muscle fibers are few. Bronchioles also have one or more true alveoli opening directly into the lumen. Distally, as each respiratory bronchiole branches into others, there are progressively more and more such openings into alveoli into further branchings of passages having alveolar walls for their boundaries. Eventually the openings are so numerous that there is no longer room for bronchial epithelium between them. These passages are termed alveolar ducts. The edges of alveolar facets bordering alveolar ducts have a few strands of smooth muscle encircling them as a geodesic framework. There is very scant intervention and little resting tone. However this three-dimensional cage of smooth muscle can contract, pull on the attached gossamer alveolar walls, reduce the cross-sectional area and compliance of the alveolar ducts, and hence reduce the gas volume and ventilation of air spaces beyond. Stimuli for such contraction include hypoxia, hypercarbia, cholinergic stimuli, aerosols, allergins, and hypoperfusion of the adjacent parenchyma (by an unsettled mechanism). Alkalosis blunts the response: a respiratory alkalosis of 7.6 cuts it in half (PCO_2 = 20), and 7.8 abolishes it entirely (PCO_2 = 10).

The alveoli are polygonal spaces with almost planar walls of (usually) five- to seven-sided facets. The walls are covered with very flattened cells called type I pneumocytes resting on a basement membrane. Typically each alveolar facet borders two adjacent alveoli. The epithelium sandwiches an interstitial space a few microns in width. This space contains a network of elastin and collagen fibers that give it its tensile strength but contribute little to elasticity. Woven into the network are the pulmonary capillaries, which scanning electron microscopy indicates occupy about half of the area of each facet. On cross section they appear to lie not symmetrically in the center of the interstitium but to weave from side-to-side and protrude somewhat into the alveolar spaces. The best analogy is a sort of three-dimensional fisherman's net, with long strands of kelp weaving in and out of the net (the capillaries). The entire "net" is covered with an attenuated film like a shrink-wrapped package of small items in a discount hardware display. This film is the lipid-lining layer of the lung, which when stretched by inspiration, stores most of the energy for exhalation as increased surface forces. The film contains degenerating lamellar bodies and their lipid content, produced by occasional type II pneumocytes among the type I cells.[16,17]

There is an important element of asymmetry in the alveolar wall, which is enhanced by a sharing of the basement membrane between the type I pneumocyte and the capillary endothelial cell where it bulges into the alveolar lumen. This is called the "thin side." The majority of gas exchange diffuses through this side (Fig. 1-11).

The other side of the capillary is within the interstitial space, where it has its own basement membrane separate from that of the alveolar pneumocyte on that side. In the interstitial space are found occasional wandering white blood cells, elastin and collagen fibers, and interstitial fluid. The latter derives in part from capillary endothelial cells by pinocytotic extrusion, in smaller part from leakage between the endothelial cells and their tight junctions, in part by diffusion of water through cells, and, in edema, from capillary leakage. The fluid flows along the interstitium on the thick side of the capillaries to the T- or Y-shaped mergers of alveolar walls that contain the smallest airways, arterioles, or venules. There, open-ended lymph capillaries are found that accompany the gas and blood conduits toward the hilum.

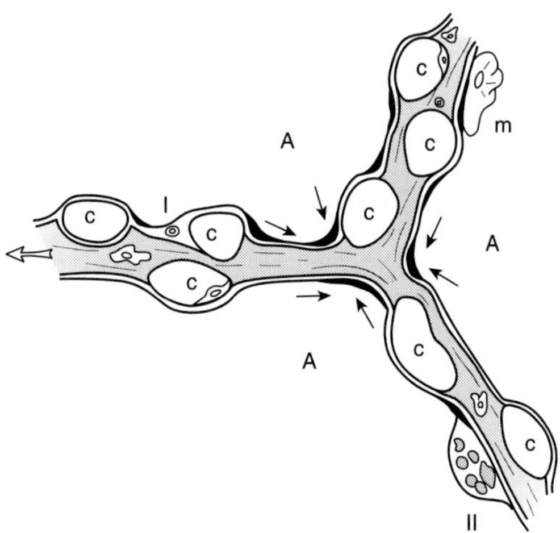

Figure 1-11. The junction of 3 alveolar facets in cross-section. The walls of the delicate alveolar membrane are composed of a core of elastin and collagen fibers with a few wandering white blood cells (m) supporting a mesh of capillaries (c) eccentric to the axis of the facets with very thin walls at the air spaces (A) for gas exchange, and thicker walls on their other side. Thin endothelial cells pave the capillary lumen, and equally thin type I alveolar epithelial cells pave the alveolar surface forcing the air space. These thinner cells share a common basement membrane. Type II pneumocytes produce a surface active material that causes retractile force at areas of curvature (arrows).

Although there are "elastic" fibers in the parenchyma, stretch of these fibers contributes little to elastic recoil of the lung except at very large lung volume. These fibers are quite stiff, and they unfold like a concertina more than stretch like a rubber band. A large part of the elastic recoil of the lung is attributable to the thin film of fluid, containing surface active molecules of a lipid called surfactant, which is primarily phosphatidyl inositol. Surfactant does lower the surface tension of the air-fluid interface, but it is more important to understand that surfactant produces a variable tension that is smaller at low lung volume. The lipid is produced by type II pneumocytes. Without it normal surface tension at the air-water (tissue) interface would cause the lung to retract to a very small volume and become atelectatic. Although this "lipid-lining layer of the lung" reduces the surface tension from 72 to 20 dyne-cm or less, it is still this surface tension of the curved surface where two alveolar facets meet that provides a major part of the elastic recoil of lung.

Pulmonary Vasculature

The lung has two entirely separate large vascular arborizations, the pulmonary arterial and pulmonary venous trees, and a third much smaller understory structure, the bronchial arterial circulation. There are no bronchial veins; bronchial capillary blood flows into pulmonary veins. Embryologically the lung bud begins as a ventral outpouching of the foregut epithelium; it is encased in mesenchymal tissue that derives from the sixth branchial arch and provides the bronchial arteries. It grows caudad into the thorax and splits into right-left buds along with the major vessel in the sixth arch, which eventually becomes the pulmonary artery. In contrast, the pulmonary veins arise from outpouching of the anlage of the cardiac atria as the primative ventral blood vessel folds into a S-shaped structure that becomes the heart.[18] The venous vasculature grows laterally into the thoracic portion of the lung bud, and eventually capillaries form to unite the disparate arterial and venous vessels. The result is a pairing of artery and airway, starting at the hilum, branching together as the three-dimensional fractal arborization proceeds distally, as in the mature lung. The veins take an entirely separate path to the gas exchange spaces. Only at the hilum are the triad of artery, vein, and airway seen. The surgeon uses the segmental veins as landmarks in dissection of segmental and subsegmental resections. Except at the lobar level, there are no clear fascial planes in the human lung.[19,20]

Although the pulmonary arteries do have thicker walls with more smooth muscle than the pulmonary veins, both are relatively amuscular and thin-walled compared to systemic vessels. Both are wrapped in a network of lymph vessels little bigger than capillaries. They are relatively free of collagenous attachment to the parenchyma through which they course, down to the primary lung unit level beyond terminal bronchioles.

Innervation

Somatic sensory, autonomic sympathetic, and parasympathetic innervation are all represented in the lung, but all three are relatively sparse. Somatic sensation is largely confined to the trachea and carina. Thus there is major retention of airway-clearing cough reflexes after bilateral, single-lung transplantation as two separate lungs as opposed to a two-lung-cum-tracheal transplant. Below lobar bronchi are few irritant receptor-mediating nerves in the mucosa. Few sympathetic nerves are traceable from the third and fourth segments of the cord through sympathetic ganglia. Alpha$_1$-adrenergic impulses do dilate smooth muscle of the tracheobronchial tree, but there is little demonstrable function of the sympathetic nerve in the vasculature. This is partly attributable to the relatively small amount of vascular smooth muscle.

The parasympathetic nervous system contains both efferent and afferent vagal fibers to the lung parenchyma; the latter predominate. Juxtacapillary receptors are responsive to both blood and airborne irritants as well as interstitial water volume. Both inflation (stretch) and deflation receptors, which fire synchronously with breathing, serve minor roles in modulating the pattern of breathing. There is little demonstrable central nervous system integration of these afferent activities in normal humans. Such reflexes (Hering-Breuer reflexes) are much more prominent in animals, especially rodents.

References

1. Agostini E. Kinematics. In: Campbell EJM, Davis JM. The respiratory muscles: mechanics and neural controls. London: WB Saunders, 1970:23.
2. Sharp JT. Organization of chest wall and diaphragm for coordinated interplay. In: Fishman AP, ed. Pulmonary diseases and disorders. New York: McGraw-Hill, 1980:1525.
3. Agostoni E, Mead J. Statics of the respiratory system. In: Ferin WO, Rahn H, eds. Handbook of physiology, Section 3. Respiration. Ferin WO, Rahn H, (eds.) Washington, DC: American Physiological Society, 1964:38.
4. Agostoni E, Hyatt RE. Static behavior of the respiratory system: Fishman AP, Macklem PT, Mead J, (eds.) In Handbook of physiology, Section 3. The respiratory System, volume 3: mechanics of breathing, part 1. Bethesda: American Physiological Society, 1986.
5. Miller A, ed. Pulmonary function tests in clinical and occupational lung disease New York: Grune & Stratton, 1986:15.
6. Wanner A. Interpretation of pulmonary function tests. In: Sackner MA, ed. Diagnostic techniques in pulmonary disease, Part I. New York: Marcel Dekker, 1980.
7. Ellis H, Feldman S. Anatomy for the Anaesthetists. 4th ed. Oxford: Blackwell Scientific Publications, 1983:16.
8. Fink BR. The human larynx: a functional study. New York: Raven Press, 1975.
9. Fink BR, Demarest RJ. Laryngeal biomechanics. Cambridge, MA: Harvard University Press, 1978.
10. Collins VJ. Endotracheal anesthesia: I. Basic considerations. In: Collins VJ. Principles of anesthesiology. Philadelphia: Lea & Febiger, 1976.
11. Staub NC. The interdependence of pulmonary structure and function. Anesthesiology 1963;24:831.
12. Staub NC. Basics of RD: lung structure and function. American Thoracic Society 1982;10:1.
13. Weibel ER. Functional morphology of lung parenchyma. In: Fishman AP, Macklem PT, Mead J, eds. Handbook of Physiology, Section 3: The respiratory system, Vol 3: mechanics of breathing, Bethesda: American Physiological Society, 1986.
14. Horsfield K, Cumming G. Angles of branching and diameters of branches in the human bronchial tree. Bull Math Biophys 1967;29:245.
15. Tompsett DH. The bronchopulmonary segments. Med Hist 1965;9:177.
16. Shields TW. Surgical anatomy of the lungs. In: Shields TW, ed. General thoracic surgery. 2nd ed. Philadelphia: Lea & Febiger, 1983:61.
17. Weibel ER. Anatomical distribution of air channels, blood vessels, and tissue in the lung. In: Arcangeli P, ed. Normal values for respiratory function in man. Milano, Italy: Panminerva Medica, 1970:242.
18. Fishman AP. Dynamics of the pulmonary circulation. In: Hamilton WF, ed. Handbook of physiology, Section 2. Circulation. Baltimore: Williams & Wilkins, 1963:1667.
19. Heath D, Smith P. The pulmonary endothelial cell. Thorax 1979;34:200.
20. Smith U, Ryan JW. Electron microscopy of endothelial components of the lungs: correlations of structure and function. Fed Proc 1973;32:1957.

CHAPTER

2

Pulmonary Physiology

Lee K. Brown

Mechanics of Breathing

According to the central concept of respiratory mechanics, the components of the respiratory system function as a pump, a machine that can be analyzed using the techniques of classical physics or engineering. Such analysis involves modeling the respiratory system as a combination of mechanical devices and writing a set of mathematical equations that define the movements of the machine in terms of the applied forces. Mead drew an analogy between a block attached to a fixed point by a spring sliding on a surface and a reciprocating bellows pump representing the lungs (Fig. 2-1).[1] To move the rectilinear system, a force must counter the three forces developed by the block:

1. A force proportional to displacement that is attributable to the elastic properties of the spring, defined by the linear elastance (K_m) of the spring.
2. A force proportional to the speed at which the block slides along the surface, defined by the frictional resistance (R_m).
3. A force proportional to the acceleration of the block, which is an effect of the inertia of the system, and is defined by the mass of the block (M).

When analyzed in terms of the bellows pump (respiratory system) in Figure 2-1, these forces become pressures. Displacement, speed, and acceleration are replaced by volume (V), flow ($\dot{V}$), and volume acceleration ($\ddot{V}$); and the proportionality constants become elastance (the reciprocal of compliance (C), or 1/C), flow resistance (R), and inertance (I). The final equation that relates these three forces is:

$$\text{(2-1)} \qquad Pa = (1/C)V + R(\dot{V}) + I(\ddot{V})$$

where Pa is the applied pressure.

Elastic and resistive forces generally far outweigh inertial effects, and the remainder of the section will concentrate on the mechanical parameters of compliance and resistance and related concepts of work of breathing.

Compliance

As implied in the previous discussion, compliance is a measure of the tendency of the respiratory system to return to a resting position after a volume change is imposed, ie, the "springi-

Rectilineal Mechanical (length-force; *l-f*)

Elements	*Equations of Motion*
R_m = frictional resistance (linear)	$f_a = K_m l + R_m \dot{l} + M \ddot{l}$
K_m = linear elastance	$f_a = K_m l + R_m v + Ma$
M = mass	

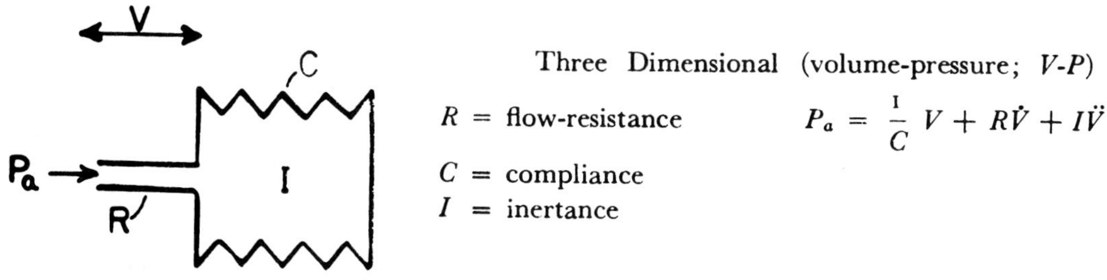

Figure 2-1. Linear and volumetric mechanical systems used to model the respiratory pump. See text for explanation. (Used with permission from Mead J. Mechanical properties of lungs. Physiol Rev 1961;41:286.)

ness" of the system. Older literature frequently makes reference to elastance rather than compliance. Elastance is merely the reciprocal of compliance: as elastance falls, the respiratory system is more easily expanded; as it rises, the respiratory system is stiffer and expands less readily. Compliance is measured in units of L/cm H_2O, thus representing the volume change produced by a unit change in pressure. When the respiratory system becomes more distensible, compliance increases, and when the system becomes stiffer, compliance decreases. Compliance may also be expressed in terms of the volume at which it is measured. This specific compliance (sC), measured in units of cm H_2O^{-1} compensates for lung size and is used to compare individuals who have widely different lung volumes.

Total respiratory system compliance (CRS) is a measure of distensibility of the entire system, including lungs and chest wall. CRS may be divided into two major components: lung compliance (CL) and chest wall compliance (CW). The measurement of CL is performed by computing the pressure change from alveolus to pleural space, whereas CW is computed using the pressure in the pleural space and atmospheric pressure. CL is thus a reflection of distensibility of the alveolar sacs, the walls of the conducting system, and the visceral pleura. The latter two factors add little to CL; the forces related to surface tension contribute most to alveolar distensibility.[1] CW is a measure of the elastic forces of the thoracic cage, chest wall soft tissues, and diaphragm. In addition, CW also reflects the elasticity of the abdominal wall and viscera because the abdomen must expand out of the way as the diaphragm descends.

CL and CW do not add in a straight algebraic manner to equal CRS. Rather, they add as reciprocals, thus:

$$C_{RS} = \frac{1}{\frac{1}{C_L} + \frac{1}{C_W}} \quad (2\text{-}2)$$

This is true wherever two compliances are placed in series. Parallel compliances, (eg, C_L for each lung), do add algebraically.

Figure 2-2 illustrates the typical relaxation-pressure versus volume curves for the chest wall and lungs, both individually and in combination. Distending pressure (abscissa) is measured at different volumes relative to vital capacity (ordinate) with the subject in a relaxed state, ie, not actively using any respiratory muscles. Note that at the end of a normal tidal breath (functional residual capacity or FRC), the tendency of the lungs to collapse (positive pressure), is exactly balanced by the tendency of the chest wall to spring outward (negative pressure). Thus no respiratory muscle activity is necessary to maintain this volume, and it has been called the "resting" lung volume. Because no effort is required, FRC is generally the measured value in tests of static lung volume (see below).

Figure 2-2. Relaxation-pressure versus volume curves for chest and lungs, individually (dashed lines) and combined (solid line). Note that at V_r (resting lung volume or FRC), the pressure needed to keep the chest wall from springing outward is equal and opposite to the pressure needed to keep the lungs from collapsing inward. (Used with permission from Rahn H, Otis AB, Chadwick LE, et al. The pressure-volume diagram of the thorax and lung. Am J Physiol 1946;146:170.)

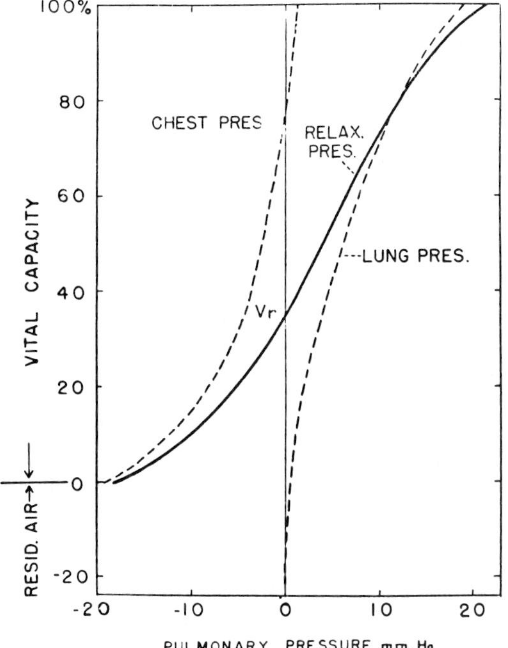

The determination of C_L requires the simultaneous measurement of the alveolar-pleural pressure gradient and relative lung volume. The latter is easily obtained using a spirometer, which is shown in Figure 2-3. Basically, a spirometer measures the volume of air introduced or withdrawn from the inverted bell by recording the height at which the bell floats in water. More modern devices use an elastic membrane rather than water to seal the volume-measuring element. Alternatively, a pneumotachograph may be used to measure flow at the mouth, and this signal may be electrically integrated to obtain volume. Most commonly, a pneumotachograph measures flow by monitoring the pressure drop across a very small resistance, such as a mesh screen (Fig. 2-4).

Pleural pressure is obtained by measuring esophageal pressure (P_{ES}) using an esophageal balloon (Fig. 2-5) attached to a strain-gauge pressure transducer and carrier amplifier. When placed in the lower esophagus (Fig. 2-6), esophageal balloon pressure correlates well with intrapleural pressure, especially in the upright subject.[2,3] Esophageal pressure is then referenced to atmospheric pressure, which is equivalent to alveolar pressure under static conditions, to obtain the transpulmonary pressure gradient.

In order for "static conditions" to be present, lung volume must remain constant (ie, flow is zero). This situation may be obtained by

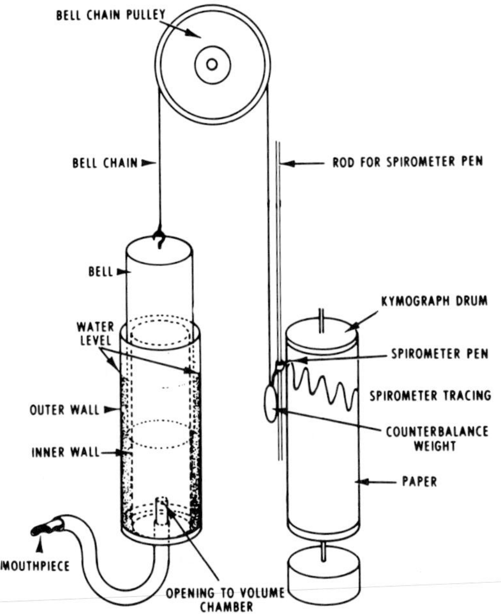

Figure 2-3. Typical water-sealed spirometer. The bell is suspended by the counterweighted chain in a container filled with water. A subject breathing on the mouthpiece introduces or removes air from the bell, thus changing its buoyancy and causing it to rise or fall a distance proportional to the volume change. A pen attached to the far end of the chain records the volume change on a kymograph drum and produces a spirogram. (Used with permission from Sackner MA. Gas volumes. In: Kline J, ed. Biological foundations of biomedical engineering. Boston: Little, Brown and Co., 1976:256.)

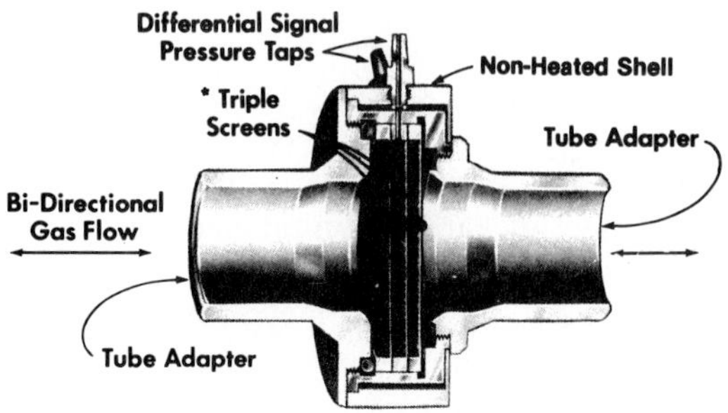

Figure 2-4. Pneumotachograph for measurement of airflow. The slight resistance to airflow caused by the three screens produces a pressure drop from one side of the apparatus to the other that is proportional to the flow. The differential pressure signal is converted by a pressure transducer to an electrical signal, which is amplified, scaled, and may then be integrated over time to produce a volume signal (spirogram). (Courtesy of Hans Rudolph, Inc., Kansas City, MO.)

having the patient hold his or her breath at the desired volume or by using a shutter to occlude the mouthpiece on which the patient is breathing.[4] Figure 2-7 illustrates the technique used to collect the data for the static pressure-volume curve during a series of slow exhalations from total lung capacity. CL is conventionally calculated from the ratio of volume change to pressure change between FRC and FRC + 0.5 liter. When calculated in this manner it is more precisely designated as "chord compliance."

Quasistatic (or dynamic) CL may also be measured during tidal breathing. Simultaneous flow, volume, and transpulmonary pressure tracings are collected (Fig. 2-8), and quasistatic conditions are obtained by measuring volume and pressure at points of zero flow. When obstructive airways disease is present, dynamic compliance (C_{dyn}) declines at higher respiratory rates, as poorly ventilated lung units cease to contribute to the measurement. Such a determination, which is known as frequency dependence of compliance, is the "gold-standard" measure of small airways obstruction.

Although CRS may be determined using a variety of techniques, it is most commonly measured by applying positive airway pressure, as in the case of an intubated patient who is mechanically ventilated and sedated or otherwise induced to cease voluntary respiratory efforts. The ventilator is then set to inflate to a given lung volume, and an inspiratory pause is used to obtain a static airway pressure. In a nonintubated patient, the technique of relaxation against a shutter at different lung volumes is used. Adequate voluntary relaxation of respiratory muscles is difficult to obtain in an un-

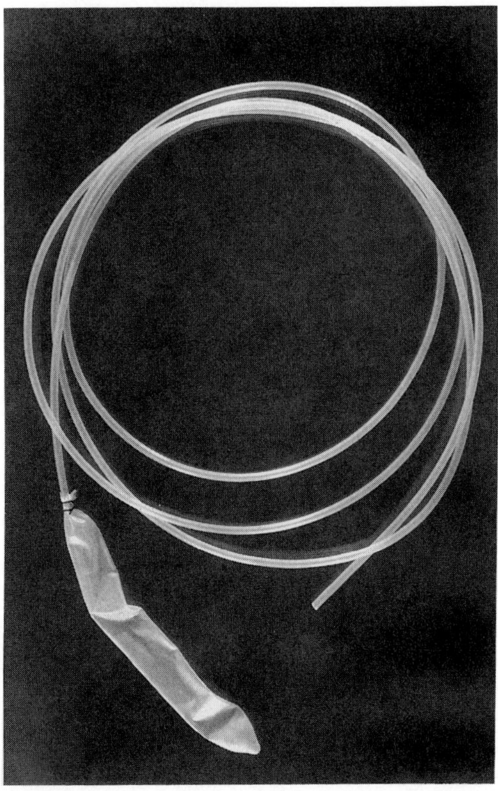

Figure 2-5. Esophageal balloon/catheter assembly for measurement of esophageal pressure. The thin-walled, latex balloon encloses a series of holes in the catheter. Suture material or cement secures the balloon to the catheter.

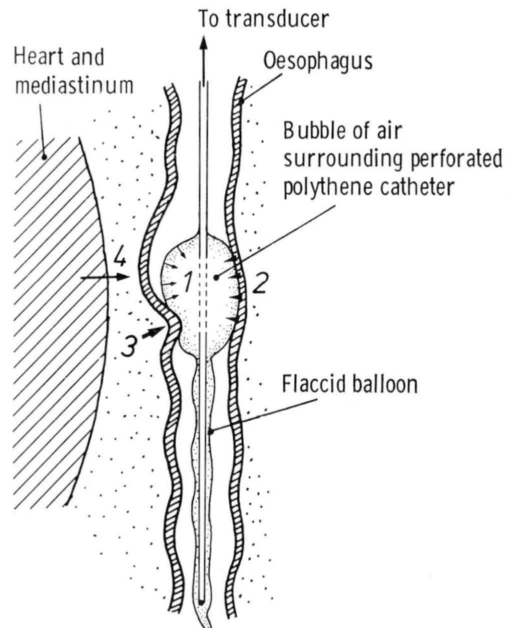

Figure 2-6. Schematic appearance of the balloon/catheter within the esophagus. A small amount of air in the balloon facilitates transmission of esophageal pressure to the transducer. The numbers indicate superimposed pressures that can lead to measurement artifacts: 1, balloon elastic recoil; 2, esophageal elastic recoil; 3, active esophageal contraction; and 4, pressure from surrounding mediastinal structures. (Used with permission from Gibson GJ, Pride NB. Lung distensibility. The static pressure-volume curve of the lungs and its use in clinical assessment. Br J Dis Chest 1976;70:146–147.)

trained subject; this severely limits the accuracy of this method.[5] CRS may also be determined using forced oscillation with random noise, in which a mixture of pressure waveforms of varying frequencies with very low tidal volumes is impressed on normal tidal breathing. A mathematical analysis is used to extract CRS (as well as resistance) from the pressure and flow waveforms.[6] At present this technique is of research interest only.

Reference values for compliance are not widely available. As a general rule, 0.2 L/cm H_2O is considered a normal value for CL, and 0.05 cm H_2O^{-1} a normal value for sCL.[7] Regression equations for CL based on sex, age, and height have been published by Begin et al, but the authors used a nonstandard method of calculating the chord compliance.[8]

The changes in CL associated with various diseases are summarized in Table 2-1, and the full pressure-volume (P-V) curves for some of these conditions are displayed in Figure 2-9. Generally, diseases that result in the destruction of lung elastic tissue (eg, pulmonary emphysema; α_1-antitrypsin deficiency) increase com-

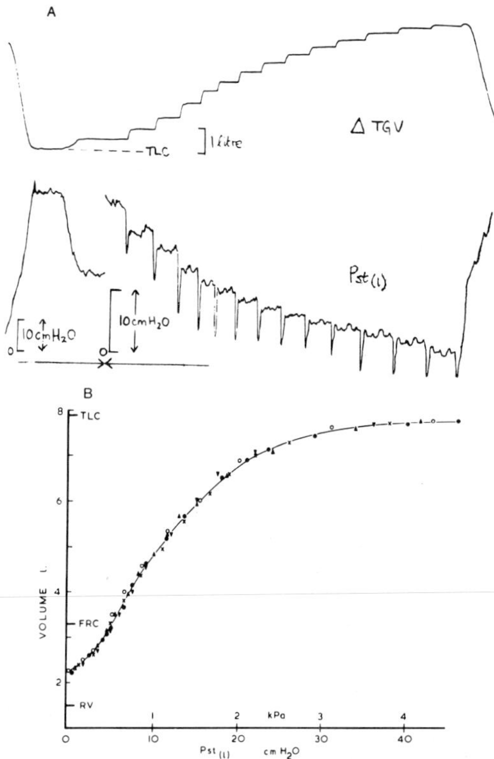

Figure 2-7. A, Lung volume (upper tracing) and esophageal pressure (referred to here as P_{ST}(l) or static lung recoil pressure) (lower tracing) versus time recorded during a slow exhalation from TLC. Expiration is interrupted by periodic shutter closures, at which time P_{ST}(l) is recorded to ensure static conditions; B, P_{ST}(l) and volume values obtained from multiple repetitions of the slow exhalation in A are plotted to obtain a lung compliance curve. Different symbols identify each trial. (Used with permission from Gibson GJ, Pride NB. Lung distensibility. The static pressure-volume curve of the lungs and its use in clinical assessment. Br J Dis Chest 1976;70:149.)

pliance and shift the P-V curve to the left.[9] Diseases that infiltrate the lung or increase lung connective tissue (eg, lymphangitic spread of carcinoma; pulmonary fibrosis) reduce compliance and shift the curve rightward.[10] Distension of the pulmonary interstitium or filling of alveoli with fluid, as in congestive heart failure or adult respiratory distress syndrome, also de-

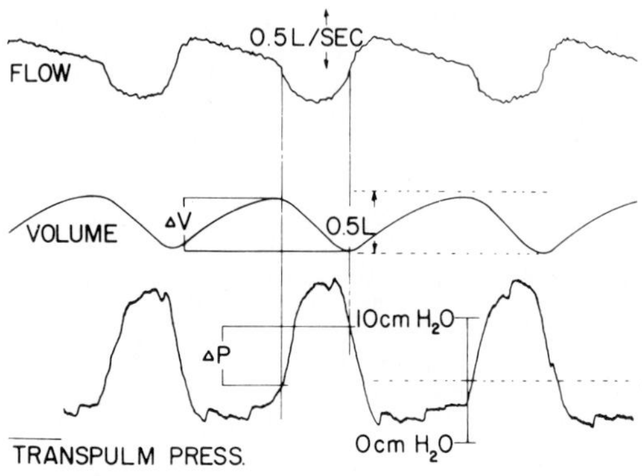

Figure 2-8. Calculation of dynamic lung compliance, Cdyn(l), by simultaneous recording of flow, volume, and transpulmonary pressure. Lines through zero flow identify points on the volume and pressure tracings simulating static conditions. ΔV and ΔP_{es} computed from successive zero-flow points are used to compute Cdyn(l). (Used with permission from Sackner MA, Landa J. Mechanics of breathing. In: Kline J, ed. Biological foundations of biomedical engineering. Boston: Little, Brown and Co., 1976:323.)

creases compliance. In exacerbations of bronchial asthma, CL remains normal or is slightly reduced, and the lung pressure-volume curve shifts to the left and upward. Any reduction in compliance probably represents airway closure to some lung units so that they do not contribute to the measured value.[11] The cause of the shift in the curve is less clear, but it may be related to a phenomenon known as stress relaxation.[12]

Resistance

Resistance (R) is a measure of the forces required during breathing to overcome friction in the respiratory system. It is expressed in cm $H_2O \cdot L^{-1} \cdot S^{-1}$ and represents the pressure generated in achieving a unit of flow. The reciprocal of resistance is conductance (G). Both R and G may be normalized to the lung volume at which they are measured (usually FRC). This is

Table 2-1. Lung Compliance in Pulmonary Disease*

Total Lung Capacity (TLC or FRC)	Functional Change	Example	Chord Compliance at FRC
Increased	Increased inspiratory muscle strength	Training	Normal
	Enlarged lungs and thoracic cage	Acromegaly	Increased
	Loss of lung recoil	Emphysema	Increased
	?Loss of lung recoil	Asthma	Normal or reduced
Normal	Loss of lung recoil and muscle strength	Aging	Slightly increased
Decreased	Alveolar stiffness	Pulmonary fibrosis	Reduced
	Reduced distension	Muscle weakness Thoracic deformity Pleural disease	Normal or reduced
	Vascular engorgement	Pulmonary venous congestion (early CHF)	Reduced
	Loss of alveolar units	Pulmonary edema (more severe CHF) Lung resection	Reduced

* FRC = functional residual capacity; CHF = congestive heart failure.
Adapted with permission from Gibson GJ, Pride NB. Lung distensibility. The static pressure-volume curve of the lungs and its use in clinical assessment. Br J Dis Chest 1976;70:179.

necessary because airway caliber (a determinant of resistance) varies with lung volume. Conductance is most frequently normalized in this way, with specific conductance (sG) computed as:

(2-3) $sG = G/FRC$

Just as CRS has several components, total respiratory system resistance (RRS) is divided into airway resistance (RAW), lung tissue resistance (RLT), and chest wall resistance (RW). RAW is produced by the friction of moving gas molecules against airway walls or each other. The use of resistance to describe this friction depends on a linear relationship between pressure and flow. Strictly speaking, this applies only in airways below a certain radius, depending on flow rate. This so-called laminar flow (Fig. 2-10) results in a resistance which varies directly with airway length and inversely with the fourth power of the radius. Turbulent flow occurs in larger airways, at higher flow rates, or in areas of irregularity or constriction (orifice flow). In such situations, pressure is proportional to the square of flow, and RAW is a linear approximation of a much more complex relationship.

RLT results from the friction between lung parenchymal structures as they slide past each other during lung expansion and contraction. RAW and RLT, when combined, are referred to as lung resistance (RL). RW is the resistance of chest wall tissues to movement. As resistances in series add algebraically, the relationship between these resistive components may be written:

(4) $R_{RS} = R_L + R_W = R_{AW} + R_{LT} + R_W$

Resistances are measured, as one might expect, by simultaneously determining flow and driving pressure. RAW, the most commonly used resistance in clinical evaluations, requires the measurement of mouth and alveolar pressure, and flow at the mouth. All are readily

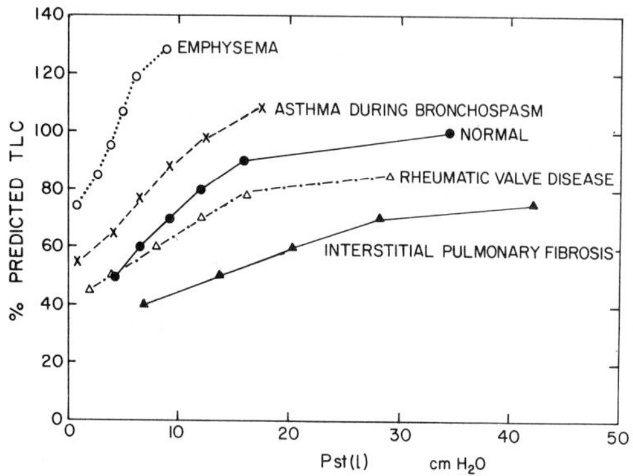

Figure 2-9. Static pressure-volume curves associated with various pulmonary disorders. (Used with permission from Bates DV. Respiratory function in disease. 3rd ed. Philadelphia: WB Saunders, 1989:30.)

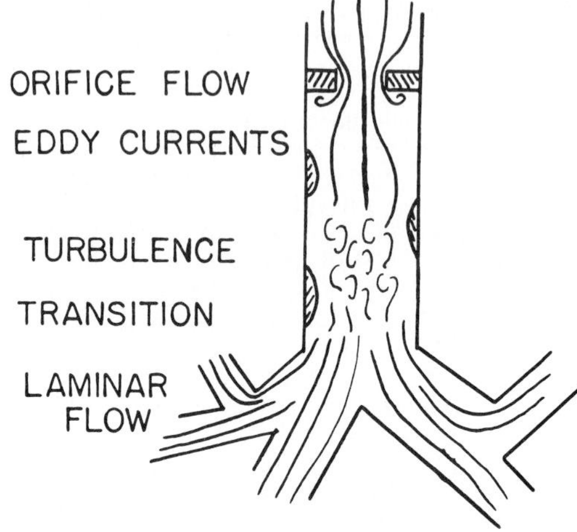

Figure 2-10. Different patterns of airflow present in the tracheobronchial tree. Turbulent flow and orifice flow result in a pressure drop proportional to the square of flow rate. Driving pressure is proportional directly to flow only under laminar conditions. (Used with permission from DuBois AB. Resistance to breathing. In: Fenn WO, Rahn H, eds. Handbook of physiology. Section 3: Respiration, Volume 1. Washington, DC: American Physiological Society, 1964:452.)

obtained except alveolar pressure. Earlier methods for measuring alveolar pressure (PA) relied on the interruptor technique, where airflow is abruptly terminated by occluding the mouthpiece; the mouth pressure (PM) immediately following the occlusion reflects PA. The equilibration between PA and PM under these conditions is often not rapid enough to provide sufficient accuracy, however, especially in subjects with airway disease. With the development of the body plethysmograph by DuBois and colleagues, rapid and accurate measurement of RAW became possible.[13]

An extensive description of body plethysmography is beyond the scope of this discussion. A working knowledge of the device is helpful in understanding several derived pulmonary function parameters, however, and the theory and use of this device is outlined both here and in the discussion of static lung volumes. Figure 2-11 represents a schematic form of the device, and Figure 2-12 shows a commercially available unit. A plethysmograph consists of a rigid, sealed box large enough for a seated subject. In the most commonly used system (a constant-volume device), a transducer samples

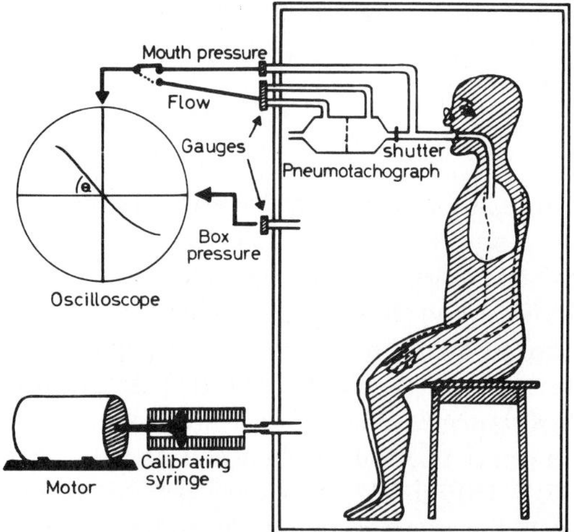

Figure 2-11. Schematic representation of a pressure (constant volume) body plethysmograph. (Used with permission from Cotes JE. Lung function. Oxford: Blackwell Scientific Publications, 1979:116.)

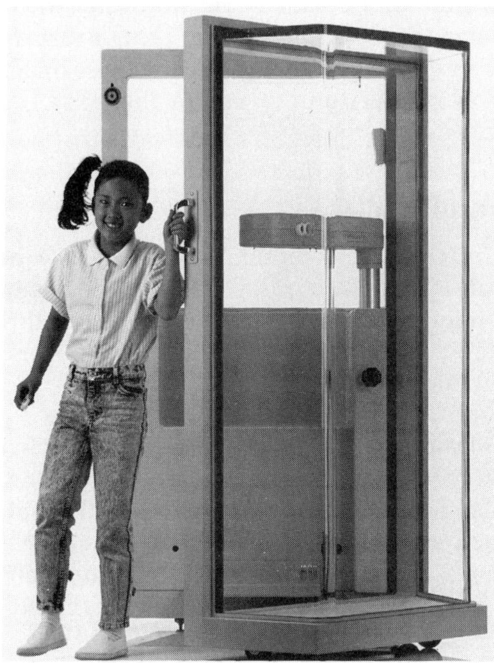

Figure 2-12. Commercially available body plethysmograph. (Courtesy of Medical Graphics Corporation, St Paul, MN.)

the pressure within the box (PBOX), which varies with the volume of any person or object contained in it. The subject breathes on a mouthpiece attached to a pneumotachograph for measurement of airflow. An additional transducer samples pressure at the mouthpiece (PM) and an electrically operated shutter between the mouthpiece and the pneumotachograph allows the airway to be occluded at will.

With a subject sealed within the body plethysmograph, inhalation reduces PA and increases PBOX producing the pressure gradient that drives air into the lungs: The reverse process occurs with exhalation as PA increases and PBOX is reduced. Therefore, a constant, inverse relationship exists between PBOX and PA. If the subject is then asked to breathe with the shutter closed, the same relationship between PA and PBOX persists, except now no airflow exists and mouth pressure (PM) also is equivalent to PA. (The patient does not breathe in the usual sense but expands or contracts the chest by rarification or compression of the air within it rather than moving air in or out of the mouth). Changes in PA, PBOX, and PM, with the shutter opened and closed, are interrelated in the following way:

$$\underset{\text{(shutter open)}}{\Delta P_A/\Delta P_{BOX}} \propto \underset{\text{(shutter closed)}}{\Delta P_M/\Delta P_{BOX}} \qquad (2\text{-}5)$$

The equation is written as a proportionality rather than an equality because the dividing point between gas in the body plethysmograph and gas in the lungs changes depending on whether the shutter is open or closed. With the shutter closed, this point is at the shutter. With the shutter open, this division occurs somewhere in the tracheobronchial tree. DuBois showed that a point halfway down the anatomic dead space is sufficient for this calculation for practical purposes.[13] Equation 5 then becomes:

$$\underset{\text{(shutter open)}}{\Delta P_A/\Delta P_{BOX}} = \underset{\text{(shutter closed)}}{\Delta P_M/\Delta P_{BOX}} \times (TGV + Vapp)/(TGV - Vd/2) \qquad (2\text{-}6)$$

where TGV is thoracic gas volume measured plethysmographically (see below), Vapp is the dead space of the breathing apparatus up to the shutter, and VD is the patient's anatomic dead space (may either be approximated at 200 cm^3, obtained from tables, or measured). A straightforward algebraic manipulation then allows the calculation of RAW from ΔPA/ΔPBOX (shutter closed) and $\dot{V}$/ΔPBOX (shutter open):

$$R_{AW} = \frac{\dfrac{\Delta P_M}{\Delta P_{BOX}} \times \dfrac{TGV + Vapp}{TGV - (V_D/2)}}{\dfrac{\dot{V}}{\Delta P_{BOX}}} - R_{app} \qquad (2\text{-}7)$$

where R_{app} is a correction factor for the resistance of the breathing circuit.

RL and RRS values are rarely obtained in the clinical laboratory. RL may be measured by passing an esophageal balloon, as in the determination of CL, and simultaneously measuring transpulmonary pressure ($P_M - P_{ES}$) and flow: the portion of $P_M - P_{ES}$ due to elastic forces must be subtracted.[14] RRS may be determined using the forced oscillation method, which also yields CRS, as described above.[6]

As is the case for CL, predicted values for RAW and specific conductance of the airway (sG_{aw}) are based on rather limited data, and regression equations are not available. Normally, RAW ranges between 0.6 and 2.4 cm $H_2O \cdot L^{-1} \cdot S^{-1}$ and sG_{aw} between 0.42 and 1.7 $S^{-1} \cdot cmH_2O^{-1}$.[7] Many laboratories use the relationship between FRC and RAW published by Briscoe to determine a reference value for RAW[15]:

(2-8) $$RAW = 4.2/FRC$$

RAW may be used to identify and quantitate obstructive impairment, although much simpler spirometric tests are more commonly used in this regard (see below). RAW and sG_{aw} are elevated during exacerbations of bronchial asthma,[16] and these values may be used in the assessment of the response to bronchodilators or in the conduct of bronchial challenge testing. Compared to spirometric indices, their somewhat greater variability requires a fairly substantial change before a positive response can be identified, however. For sG_{aw}, a change of 35% is generally acceptable. RAW is increased in chronic obstructive pulmonary disease where it may primarily reflect the degree of chronic obstructive bronchitis rather than morphologic pulmonary emphysema.[17] This may be a result of the way RAW is conventionally measured; it is determined during the inspiratory limb of a breath at low flow rates when dynamic collapse is unlikely to occur. RAW may also be elevated in conditions that cause upper airway obstruction (eg, lesions involving the trachea and larynx).[18]

Work of Breathing

No method for computing the total work of breathing is entirely satisfactory. The many techniques that have been developed for this purpose probably reflect this lack. These methods include:

1. Measurement of the work done by the respiratory system during spontaneous breathing.
2. Measurement of the work done on the respiratory system by a mechanical ventilator.
3. Measurement of oxygen consumption at different levels of ventilation to obtain the oxygen cost of breathing.
4. Theoretic calculation using measured mechanical constants and a mathematical model of the respiratory system.

Method 1 is referred to most commonly, and method 2 is of some interest in anesthesia practice. Both these techniques will be discussed in some detail. Methods 3 and 4 are primarily of research interest only.

A discussion of work of breathing may proceed from consideration of a simple rectilinear system that can then be expanded to represent a volumetric system. Figure 2-13 shows a block attached to a fixed point by a spring sliding on a surface, similar to that in Figure 2-1. By definition, work (W) is the integral of force × displacement:

(2-9) $$W = \int F dl$$

where W = work, F = force, and l = displacement. In Figure 2-13, three types of work are possible, analogous to the three forces devel-

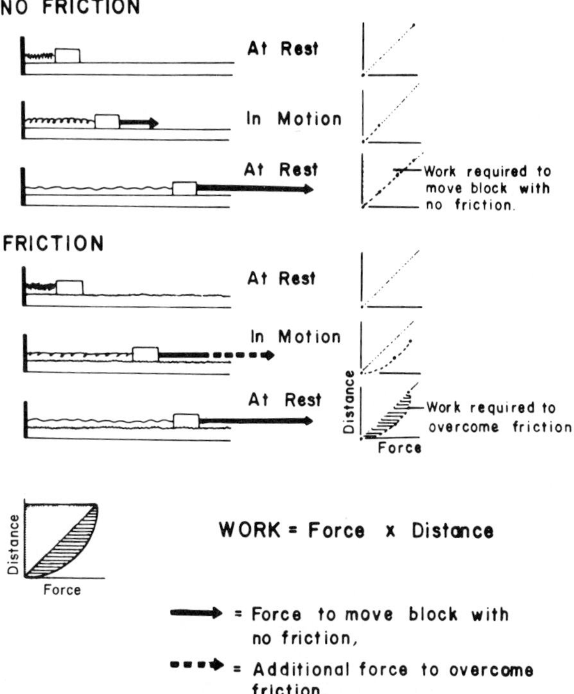

Figure 2-13. Calculation of work of breathing from consideration of a rectilinear model. The upper panel depicts elastic work, the middle panel frictional (resistive) work, and in the lower panel the two types of work are combined. (Modified, with permission, from Sackner MA, Landa J. Mechanics of breathing. In: Kline J, ed. Biological foundations of biomedical engineering. Boston: Little, Brown and Co., 1976:337.)

oped by the block: elastic work, resistive work, and inertial work. The upper panel depicts graphically how the elastic work (alone) is computed. A plot of force versus distance is constructed, and the elastic work is simply the area of the region between the force versus distance curve and the ordinate. The resistive or frictional work is shown in the middle panel. When resistive work is added to the curve, it becomes convex to the right, and the area between the line depicting elastic work and the new curve (shaded) is the additional work required to overcome friction. Both areas combined (bottom panel) represent all the work done on the rectilinear block system. Note that this excludes inertial work, which is generally considered negligible in the respiratory system and is not considered here. Inertial work may play a role in morbid obesity, however.[19]

The identical analysis can be applied to the respiratory system by substituting pressure for force and volume for displacement. A curve such as that shown in Figure 2-14 results. This particular curve represents a tidal breath from FRC (point A). Thus, area A-C-B represents the elastic work during inspiration, and A-I-C represents the flow-resistive work. The C-E-A area is the flow-resistive work during expiration, and

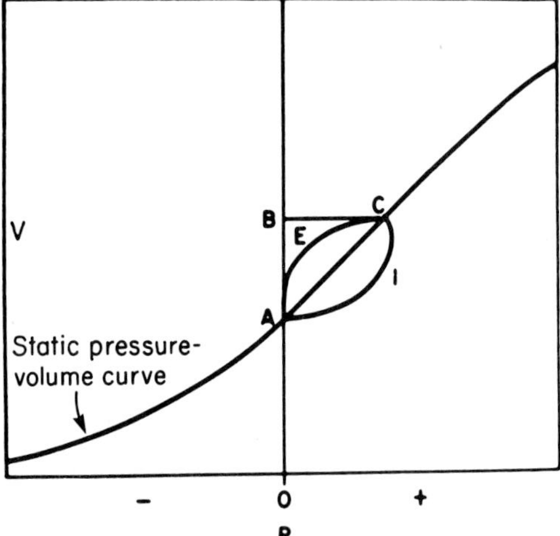

Figure 2-14. Pressure volume loop generated during a single tidal breath from FRC (point A). Work of breathing may be computed from various areas subtended by the curve (see text). (Modified, with permission, from Otis AB. The work of breathing. In: Fenn WO, Rahn H, eds. Handbook of physiology. Section 3: Respiration, Volume 1. Washington, DC: American Physiological Society, 1964: 467.)

area C-B-A is the work stored in the elastic properties of the respiratory system during inspiration and returned during expiration, just as a spring can give back its stored energy when it is allowed to relax. Some of this energy is used to perform the flow-resistive work during exhalation, and the rest (area A-B-C-E in Fig. 2-14) is dissipated in the respiratory system and lost. More complex respiratory cycles (such as forced exhalation) are analyzed in exactly the same way, using areas subtended by the pressure-volume curve. For the details of these analyses, the interested reader is referred elsewhere.[20]

In theory, calculation of respiratory muscle work by the method detailed above should be possible. Unfortunately, the pressure gradient produced by the respiratory muscles across the lungs and thorax cannot be readily measured because the respiratory muscles are actually a part of the thorax.[20] Ignoring the work done on the thorax and limiting the calculation to work done on the lungs is an easier approach. The transpulmonary pressure gradient is required for this calculation, measured with an esophageal balloon. In the recent literature on work of breathing during weaning from mechanical ventilation, such calculations are numerous. Unfortunately, it is not clear what may be lost when work done on the thorax is discarded.

Total work of breathing can be measured if the pressure used to drive the system is derived externally. This corresponds to an intubated subject on a positive-pressure ventilator, or a patient placed in a negative-pressure (Drinker) respirator. In such cases the integral of the pressure exerted by the ventilator and the volume change produced is easily calculated. The work thus computed may poorly correlate with the work of spontaneous breathing, however, if the subject does not relax completely. The correlation is probably highest for the paralyzed, ventilated patient in the operating room.

Lung Volumes and Pulmonary Function Tests

Spirometry (Dynamic Lung Volumes)

Figure 2-15 shows the graphic output obtained when a patient performs various breathing maneuvers into a simple spirometer. All of the listed volumes and capacities (sum of two or more volumes) may be measured by simple spirometry, except residual volume (RV) or any capacity containing residual volume as one of its constituents (also known as static lung volumes). This is obvious from the definition of residual volume, which is that volume of air contained in the lungs after maximal exhalation. Quite simply, spirometry measures exhaled gas volumes, and residual volume cannot

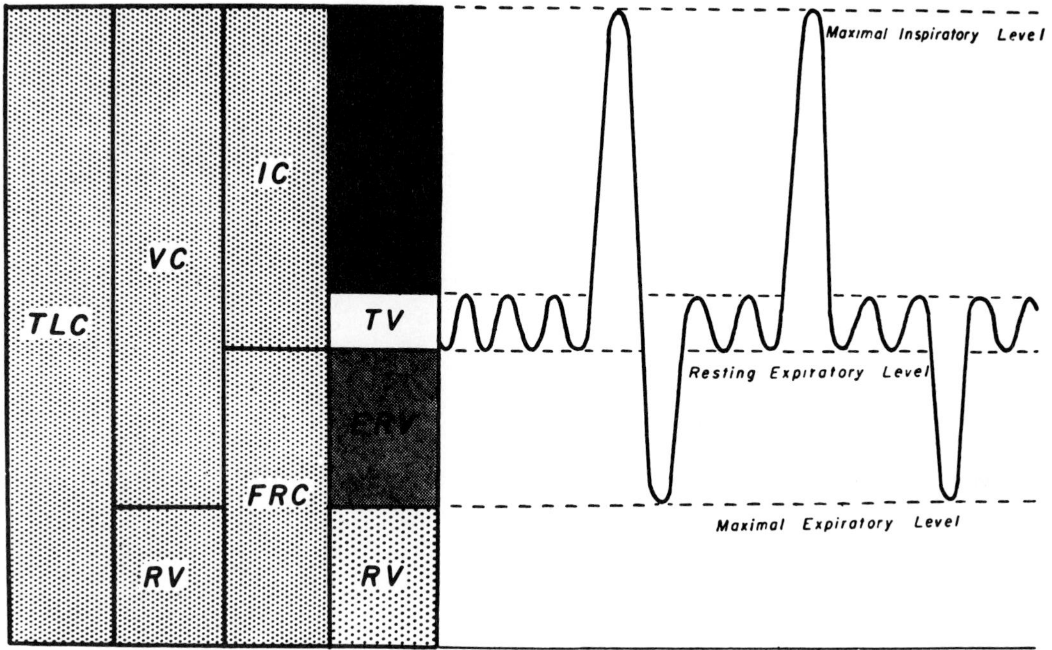

Figure 2-15. Spirometric tracing illustrating standard volumes and capacities. TLC = total lung capacity; VC = vital capacity; RV = residual volume; IC = inspiratory capacity; FRC = functional residual capacity; IRV = inspiratory reserve volume; TV = tidal volume; and ERV = expiratory reserve volume. (Used with permission from Comroe JH, Forster RE, DuBois AB, et al. The lung. Chicago:Year Book, 1962:8.)

be exhaled. Other methods are available for measuring static lung volumes (see below.)

The most important use of the spirometer, as originally perfected by John Hutchinson in 1846, was to measure vital capacity (VC). VC was usually measured during a slow maximal inspiration or expiration. Although this maneuver is still performed, commonly in conjunction with the measurement of static lung volumes, the spirometer is now most often used to measure exhaled volume during a forced, maximal expiration. The patient, usually seated and wearing noseclips, inhales to total lung capacity (TLC) and then exhales "as hard and fast as you can until no air is left" (RV). Such a spirometric maneuver (a spirogram) is depicted in Figure 2-16. VC, now termed forced vital capacity (FVC), is used to diagnose restrictive ventilatory impairment (Table 2-2). This condition may be the result of pulmonary parenchymal disorders (eg, interstitial lung disease, alveolar filling disease, lung resection) or restrictive chest wall disease. Such restrictive chest wall disease may be further classified into neuromuscular diseases that lead to respiratory muscle weakness (eg, myasthenia gravis) and deforming chest wall abnormalities that reduce the volume of the thorax or limit its expansion (eg, kyphoscoliosis).

The expiratory reserve volume (ERV) is defined as the volume difference between FRC (the end of a normal, tidal expiration) and RV

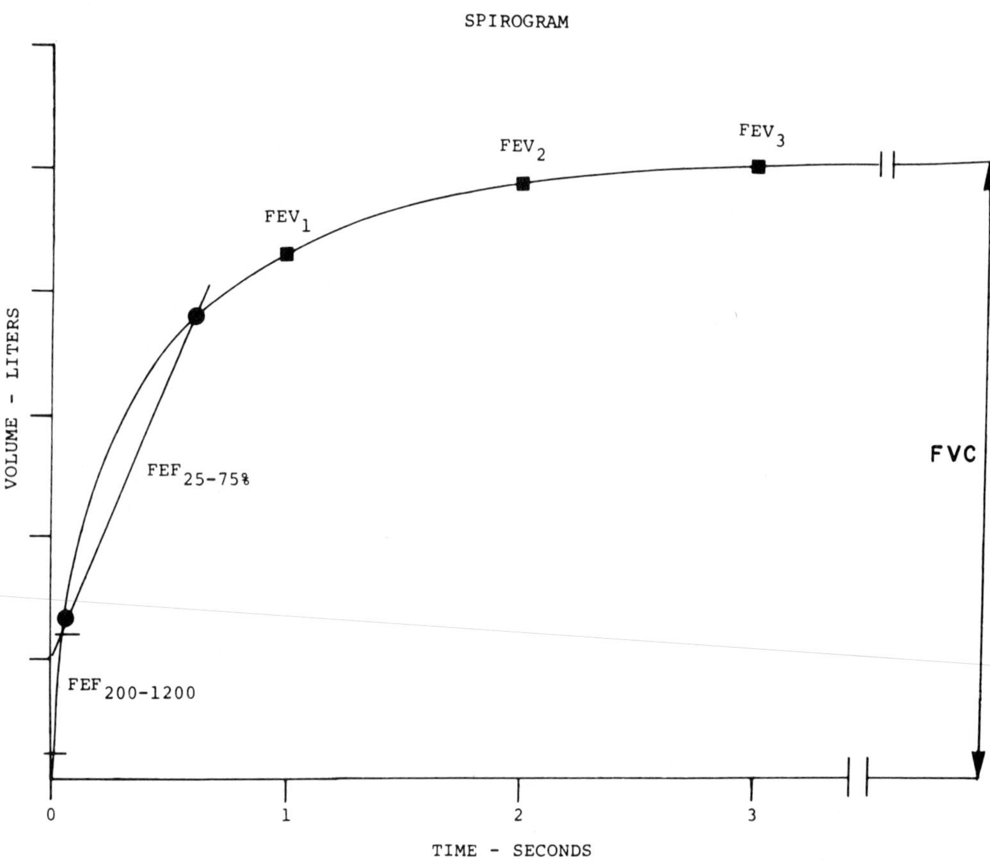

Figure 2-16. Spirogram depicting a forced expiration from TLC to RV. FVC (forced vital capacity) is generally an index of restrictive impairment; FEV_1, FEV_2, and FEV_3 are the forced expiratory volumes in 1, 2, and 3 seconds, respectively, and usually reflect obstructive impairment. $FEF_{25\%-75\%}$ is the average flow during the "middle half" of the maneuver and is also an index of obstruction. (Modified, with permission from Sobol BJ. Spirometry and forced flow studies. In: Chusid EL, ed. The selective and comprehensive testing of adult pulmonary function. Mt Kisco, NY: Futura, 1983:37.)

(the end of a maximal expiration) (Fig. 2-15). Like the FVC, this volume is reduced in certain restrictive disorders. Unlike the FVC, ERV is decreased primarily in diseases that affect diaphragmatic function (eg, neuromuscular disorders, obesity [abdominal obesity reduces the mobility of the diaphragm]) and immediately following abdominal surgery (the incision reduces diaphragmatic motion either directly due to pain or possibly through neural reflex pathways).

The diagnostic capabilities of forced expiratory spirometry were expanded to include obstructive ventilatory impairment in 1947 and 1951 in work by Tiffeneau and Gaensler.[21,22] These researchers noted that a parameter equivalent to flow (volume/time) could be obtained from the spirogram by measuring the volume

Table 2-2. Patterns of Abnormal Spirometry*

Impairment	Abnormal Parameter	Pathophysiology	Example
Restriction (chest wall)	Reduced FVC; reduced flows in proportion to FVC	Impaired thoracic expansion	Myasthenia gravis; kyphoscoliosis
Restriction (parenchymal)	Reduced FVC; reduced flows in proportion to FVC	Loss of lung parenchyma	Lung resection; interstitial lung diseases
Diaphragmatic dysfunction	Reduced ERV	Reduced diaphragmatic excursion	Myasthenia gravis; obesity
Obstruction (upper airway)	Depending on site and degree of variability: reduced FEV_1, FIV_1, FEF_{50}, FIF_{50}	Intrinsic obstruction or extrinsic compression of upper airway	Vocal cord paralysis; goiter; tracheal tumor
Obstruction (large airway)	Reduced timed volumes (eg, FEV_1) flows; FVC may be reduced due to air trapping and elevated RV	Obstruction of airways; loss of lung elastic recoil with expiratory airway collapse	Asthma; chronic bronchitis; pulmonary emphysema
Obstruction (small airway)	Normal timed volumes; reduced flows at low lung volumes; prolonged $FET_{25-75\%}$. FVC may be reduced due to air trapping.	Obstruction of small (less than 2mm) airways	Asthma in remission; cigarette smokers; early COPD
Obstruction and Restriction	Reduced FVC; reduced timed volumes and flows out of proportion to FVC; prolonged $FET_{25-75\%}$	See entries under "Restriction" and "Obstruction"	Bronchiectasis; sarcoidosis

* FVC = forced vital capacity; ERV = expiratory reserve volume.

exhaled in a given time interval (eg, forced expiratory volume at 1 second, or FEV_1). Timed volumes (actually average flows) were reduced when normal subjects exhaled through narrow tubes, thus simulating obstructive airways disease. The reduction correlated with the degree of obstruction imposed.[22] Although FEV_1 enjoys the greatest popularity for diagnostic purposes, several other timed volumes (FEV_2, FEV_3) are shown (Fig. 2-16). With one major exception, reduction in FEV_1 signals the presence of obstructive airways disease, such as bronchial asthma or chronic obstructive bronchitis. The exception occurs when FVC is decreased due to restrictive disease. When this occurs, FEV_1 may be reduced, roughly in proportion to FVC, simply because less volume for exhalation is available and not because of an obstructive limitation to airflow. The fact that FEV_1 falls in proportion to FVC in pure restrictive disease led to the use of the FEV_1/FVC ratio. If FEV_1 is reduced out of proportion to FVC, concurrent obstructive and restrictive impairment may be diagnosed.

FEV_1 and FEV_1/FVC are determinants of relatively high degrees of airway obstruction, which are often said to reside in the larger airways (conventionally, those >2 mm in diameter). Spirometric tests of small airways obstruction (also termed minimal airways dysfunction) are based on the concept of dynamic compression and the equal pressure point. During a forceful exhalation, alveolar ("upstream") pressure exceeds the positive pleural driving pressure by an amount equal to the elastic recoil pressure of the lung parenchyma. This continues to hold true for airways "downstream" from the alveoli until the pressure drop caused by airways resistance results in an airway pressure equal to pleural pressure. At this point (the "equal pressure point"), any increase in expiratory force (pleural pressure) causes the airway to compress and occlude. Should this happen, flow ceases, airway pressure rises, and the airway opens once again. In practice, the airway probably does not open and close, but reaches some equilibrium position such that increases in expiratory effort do not result in increased flow; this situation is termed "effort independence." Theory holds that, under conditions of effort independence, flow is inversely proportional to the upstream airways resistance representing airways less than 2 mm in diameter.

Effort independence does not occur throughout the forced expiratory effort.[23] At high lung volumes, an isovolume plot of expiratory flow versus pleural pressure shows that flow increases along with pleural pressure (Fig. 2-17). When lung volume declines to less than approximately 70% of TLC, effort independence may be demonstrated. Thus, the flows at these lower lung volumes may be used as indicators of minimal airways dysfunction. The maximal mid-expiratory flow, (or $FEF_{25\%-75\%}$), first defined by Leuallen and Fowler in 1955,[24] is an average flow at low lung volume which may be calculated from the spirogram by drawing a line between the curve at 25% and 75% of FVC. The slope of this line, which is $FEF_{25\%-75\%}$, correlates well with the presence of airways obstruction. In the same manner as FEV_1, $FEF_{25\%-75\%}$ is also reduced in restrictive lung disorders. The mid-expiratory time ($FET_{25-75\%}$),[24] or the time

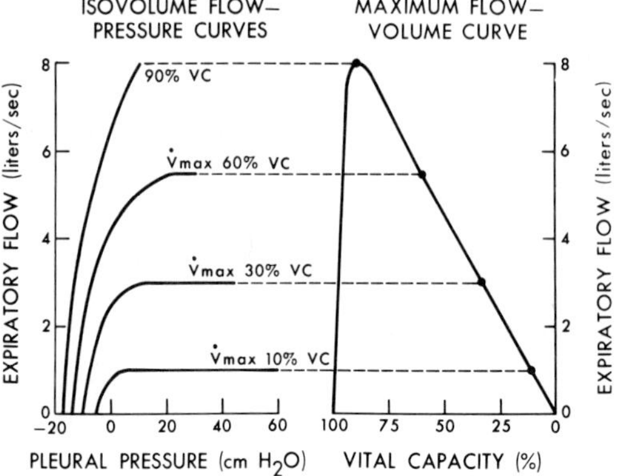

Figure 2-17. Demonstration of effort-independence of expiratory airflow at lower lung volumes. A family of isovolume pressure-flow curves (left) is related to the maximal expiratory flow-volume curve (right). Note that increased pleural pressure results in increased flow at 90% of VC. At 60% of VC and below, however, flow does not increase once a threshold of pleural pressure is exceeded. (Used with permission from Murray JF. The normal lung: the basis for diagnosis and treatment of pulmonary disease. Philadelphia: WB Saunders, 1976:102.)

required to exhale between 25% and 75% of FVC, has been developed to solve this problem. Mathematically, $FET_{25-75\%}$ is related to $FEF_{25-75\%}$

$$FET_{25-75\%} = FVC/2FEF_{25-75\%} \quad (2\text{-}10)$$

The presence of the FVC term in the equation normalizes this value for changes in FVC. Prolonged $FET_{25-75\%}$ is thus a useful indicator of obstructive impairment even in the presence of restrictive disease.

Because of the perceived usefulness of knowledge of the flows at various lung volumes during the forced expiratory maneuver, Bartlett and Phillips proposed that, rather than spirographic (volume versus time) displays, flow versus volume plots be used (Fig. 2-18).[25] Such a format has several useful properties.

1. All of the previous spirographic parameters are still obtainable providing a timing mark

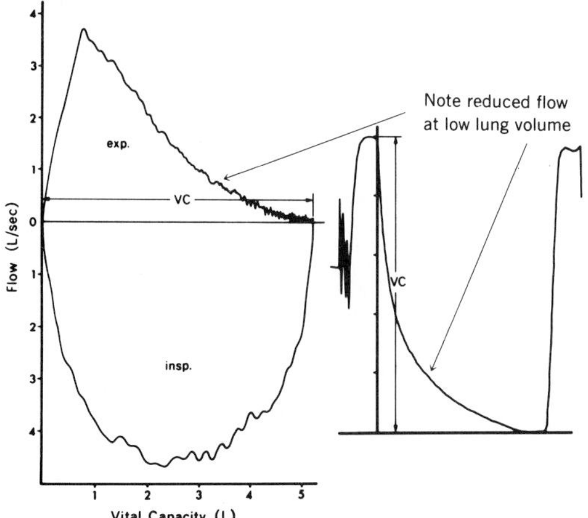

Figure 2-18. Maximal flow-volume loop (expiration and inspiration) and associated spirogram. Note that VC (actually, FVC) and all instantaneous flows are easily obtainable from the flow-volume loop. This loop exhibits the concave "tail" resulting from reduced flows at low lung volumes in small airways obstruction. (Used with permission from Petty TL, Lakshminarayan S. Practical pulmonary function tests. In: Petty TL, ed. Pulmonary diagnostic techniques. Philadelphia:Lea & Febiger, 1975:23.)

appears on the trace at the appropriate interval(s) to obtain timed volumes.

2. Instantaneous flows at various lung volumes are easily read. These include $FEF_{50\%}$ and $FEF_{75\%}$, used as parameters of small airways dysfunction, and peak flow, or FEF_{max}. This is the maximal flow, inscribed early in expiration, and is an effort-dependent indicator of large airways obstruction.
3. The shape of the expiratory flow volume loop can be used qualitatively to define the presence of impairment. For instance, a flow-volume loop with a long, concave "tail", which indicates that a large proportion of the terminal FVC is being exhaled at low flows (Fig. 2-18), heralds the presence of small airways obstruction.

Additional information may be obtained in certain disorders if the flow-volume loop is inscribed for forced expiration and inspiration. The inspiratory-expiratory flow-volume loop is useful for establishing the presence of upper airway obstruction (eg, bilateral mainstem bronchus, trachea, larynx, etc.) and can also give some indication of etiology (Fig. 2-19). In these disorders, peak flow is truncated, and a relatively flat plateau is inscribed during the midportion of the flow volume loop. In fixed upper airway obstruction at all sites, this truncation occurs during both inspiration and expiration (Fig. 2-19). Causes may include tracheal stenosis or sessile tumors. In other cases, obstruction may vary with the part of the respiratory cycle being inscribed.[26] For instance, the obstruction caused by bilateral vocal cord paralysis (an extrathoracic obstruction above the thoracic inlet) increases during inspiration when pressure gradients are such that they force the cords together. This obstruction decreases during expiration, when the pressure gradient pushes the cords apart. The flow-volume loop inscribed in variable, extrathoracic obstruction therefore exhibits a truncated inspiratory limb and a near-normal expiratory limb (Fig. 2-19). Conversely, variable intrathoracic obstruction eg, tracheomalacia below the thoracic inlet, or a polypoid mass in a similar location) may inscribe a flow volume loop with a flat expiratory limb and a near-normal inspiratory limb. Positive intrathoracic pressure reduces the caliber of the trachea at the site of the lesion, and negative intrathoracic pressure pulls the tracheal lumen outward and increases the cross-sectional area for air flow (Fig. 2-19).

In addition to performing spirometry or flow-volume loops for the baseline assessment of pulmonary function, parameters obtained from these tests may be used in tests for the presence of reversible airways obstruction (eg, bronchial asthma.) Most commonly, spirometry is performed before and after the administration of an aerosolized bronchodilator, and

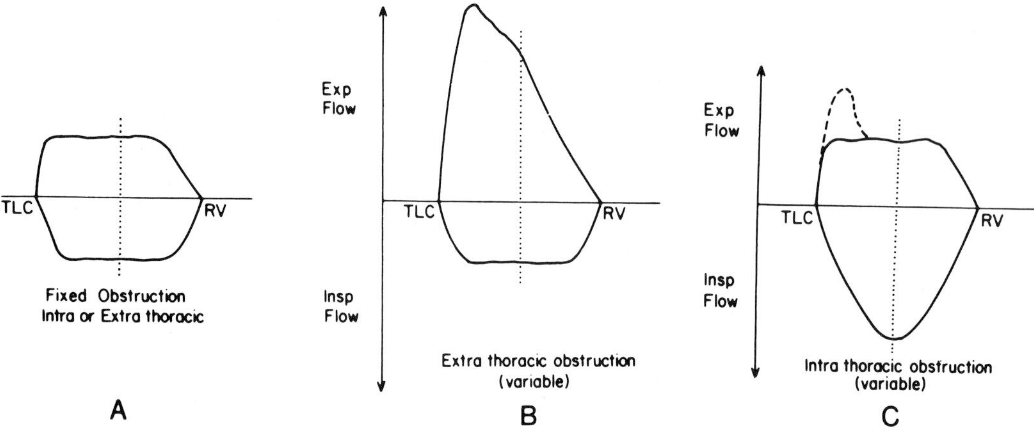

Figure 2-19. Maximal flow-volume loops in upper airways obstruction. A, fixed extra-or intrathoracic obstruction; B, variable extrathoracic obstruction; C, variable intrathoracic obstruction. A small peak flow (dashed line) is sometimes observed in variable intrathoracic obstruction. (Used with permission from Kryger M, Bode F, Antic R, et al. Diagnosis of obstruction of the upper and central airways. Am J Med 1976;61:87.)

changes in FEV_1 or FVC are assessed. Because of the inherent variability of these spirometric measurements, a positive response is recorded only if either parameter increases by 12% or more. Note that FVC may increase with decreasing airways obstruction because of the phenomenon of air-trapping (see below).

Spirometry may also be used in so-called provocational tests in which an aerosolized agent (eg, methacholine, histamine) known to provoke a bronchoconstrictor response in susceptible individuals is administered.[27] FEV_1 is measured before and after the agent is given; a decrease of greater than 20% is considered a positive response. Traditionally this test is used to diagnose atypical bronchial asthma that is manifested by symptoms of chronic cough with normal baseline pulmonary function. Similar tests may be useful in diagnosing the causes of occupationally related asthma in which the agent believed to be responsible for the symptom is administered in the laboratory.

Maximum Voluntary Ventilation

A properly equipped spirometer can be used to perform another useful test of ventilatory function, maximum voluntary ventilation (MVV). An archaic term for this test is the maximum breathing capacity (MBC). MVV is defined as the maximum minute ventilation that can be sustained over a 10–15-second period. This value is obtained by coaching the patient to breathe "in and out as hard and as fast as you can" on a spirometer for 10–15 seconds. The total volume either inhaled or exhaled is determined and expressed as the volume that would have been measured if the effort had continued for one minute.

MVV, which is actually a flow, is characteristically reduced in obstructive lung disease and is highly correlated with FEV_1:

$$\text{MVV} = 37.5 \times \text{FEV}_1 \quad \text{(2-11)}$$

In upper airway obstruction, however, MVV may be lower than the above equation would predict. This may be principally true in variable extrathoracic obstruction (eg, vocal cord paralysis) when expiratory flows such as FEV_1 are preserved and inspiratory flows (and thus MVV) are reduced.

MVV is also lowered in restrictive chest wall disease. MVV, which parallels the integrity of the chest bellows portion of the respiratory system, declines in such disorders as myasthenia gravis (respiratory muscle dysfunction) or kyphoscoliosis (reduced distensibility of the thorax). MVV generally falls below the value predicted by FEV_1 (Equation 2-11) in these disorders.

In restrictive parenchymal disease, MVV is generally quite well preserved, because what ventilatory volume is lost can simply be replaced by breathing more rapidly. MVV begins to decrease only when FVC is severely reduced and the compensatory mechanism of increasing respiratory rate no longer suffices. A reduction of MVV in mild-to-moderate obstructive parenchymal disease is a warning of possible additional disease, such as concomitant restrictive or neuromuscular disease. A convenient way of expressing this numerically is the air velocity index:

$$\text{(2-12)} \quad \text{Air velocity index} = \frac{\text{Percent predicted MVV}}{\text{Percent predicted VC}}$$

When this index falls below 0.8, concomitant disease should be suspected.

Static Lung Volumes

As noted above, the volume of air remaining at the end of a forced expiration (residual volume [RV]) cannot be measured directly. Therefore RV and any lung capacities containing RV (collectively termed static lung volumes) must be determined using specialized techniques. Most of these techniques measure FRC, considered the most easily reproducible static lung volume because no respiratory effort is necessary to maintain it (see above). RV and TLC may then be calculated using appropriate spirometrically measured volumes:

$$\text{(2-13)} \quad RV = FRC - ERV$$

$$\text{(2-14)} \quad TLC = FRC + IC$$

where IC is inspiratory capacity.

FRC is commonly measured either by a gas dilution technique or by body plethysmography. Gas dilution techniques depend on the law of conservation of mass, that is, in a closed system the mass of a given constituent remains constant. In the "wash-in" dilutional technique, a known concentration of an insoluble marker gas (usually helium) is contained within a reservoir of known volume (Fig. 2-20). The patient must rebreathe from this reservoir, starting at FRC, until the helium has equilibrated between the reservoir and the lungs. The final concentration of helium is then measured, and FRC is calculated using the conservation of mass equation:

$$\text{(2-15)} \quad \underset{\text{Initial quantity (mass) of marker gas}}{C_I \times V_I} = \underset{\text{Final quantity (mass) of marker gas}}{C_F \times V_F}$$

where C_I is the initial concentration of helium, V_I is the initial volume of the system, C_F is the final concentration of helium, and V_F is the final volume of the system

Using Vapp for the initial volume of the apparatus containing the helium mixture, FRC + Vapp for the final volume of the system, and V_{MP} for the dead space volume of the mouthpiece, equation 13 becomes (after rearranging terms):

$$\text{(2-16)} \quad FRC = Vapp\,(C_I - C_F)/C_F - V_{MP}$$

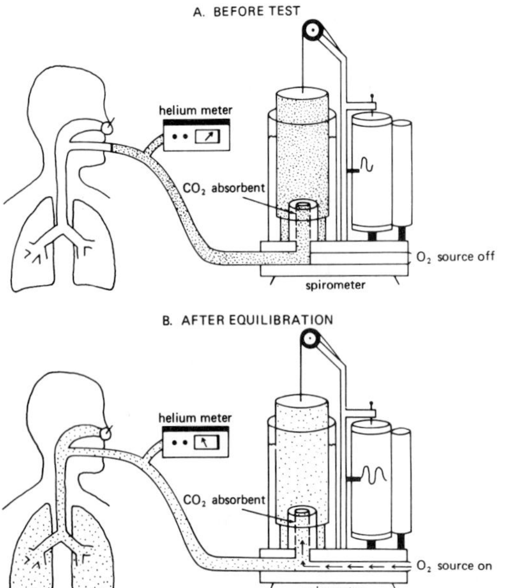

Figure 2-20. Schematic representation of the helium (He) wash-in determination of FRC. The dots represent He molecules contained in the spirometer and tubing before the test (upper panel). They are distributed throughout the apparatus and the lungs following equilibration (bottom panel). (Used with permission from Levitzky MG. Pulmonary physiology 3rd ed. New York: McGraw-Hill, 1991:60.)

FRC may also be measured by a "washout" method, utilizing nitrogen resident within the lungs as the marker gas. Using an apparatus such as that shown in Figure 2-21, the known concentration of nitrogen within the patient's lungs starting at FRC is washed out by 100% oxygen. The exhalate is collected in a large reservoir (eg, Tissot gasometer.) After equation 13 is again applied, FRC may be calculated:

(2-17) $$\text{FRC} = \frac{\text{V}_{\text{EXP}} \times \text{C}_{\text{EXP}}}{0.79 - \text{C}_{\text{ALV(final)}}}$$

where V_{EXP} is the volume of exhalate collected in the gasometer, C_{EXP} is the concentration of N_2 in the gasometer, 0.79 is the initial concentration of N_2 resident in the lungs (essentially the same as room air), and $\text{C}_{\text{ALV(final)}}$ is the concentration of N_2 left in the alveoli after the washout (approaches but does not reach zero).

Although these gas dilution methods are capable of determining FRC with good accuracy and speed in most patients, they necessitate reasonably complete equilibration by the end of the test period. Such equilibration depends on satisfactory distribution of ventilation within the lungs. Patients with impaired distribution of ventilation, such as those suffering from pulmonary emphysema or other severe obstructive lung disease, may require an inordinate amount of time before equilibration can occur. In addition, dilutional methods are not capable of measuring lung volumes that include bullae, because bullae do not participate in ventilation to the extent that equilibration can occur within them.

A technique using the body plethysmograph was developed (see previous description of the basic body plethysmograph) to bypass these deficiencies. This method applies Boyle's Law, which states that, in a closed system at constant temperature, the product of pressure and volume within the system remains constant:

(2-18) $$P_1V_1 = P_2V_2$$

In the plethysmographic determination of FRC, the patient's lungs are converted to a closed system by having the patient pant against a shutter. As inspiration is attempted against the occlusion, thoracic gas is rarified, and thoracic pressure decreases and volume increases. When applied to such an inspiratory effort, Equation 18 yields:

(2-19) $$\text{P}_{\text{FRC}}\text{V}_{\text{FRC}} = (\text{P}_{\text{FRC}} - \Delta\text{P})(\text{V}_{\text{FRC}} + \Delta\text{V})$$

where P_{FRC} equals alveolar pressure at FRC, or atmospheric pressure (remember, air flow is 0 because the airway is occluded), V_{FRC} equals

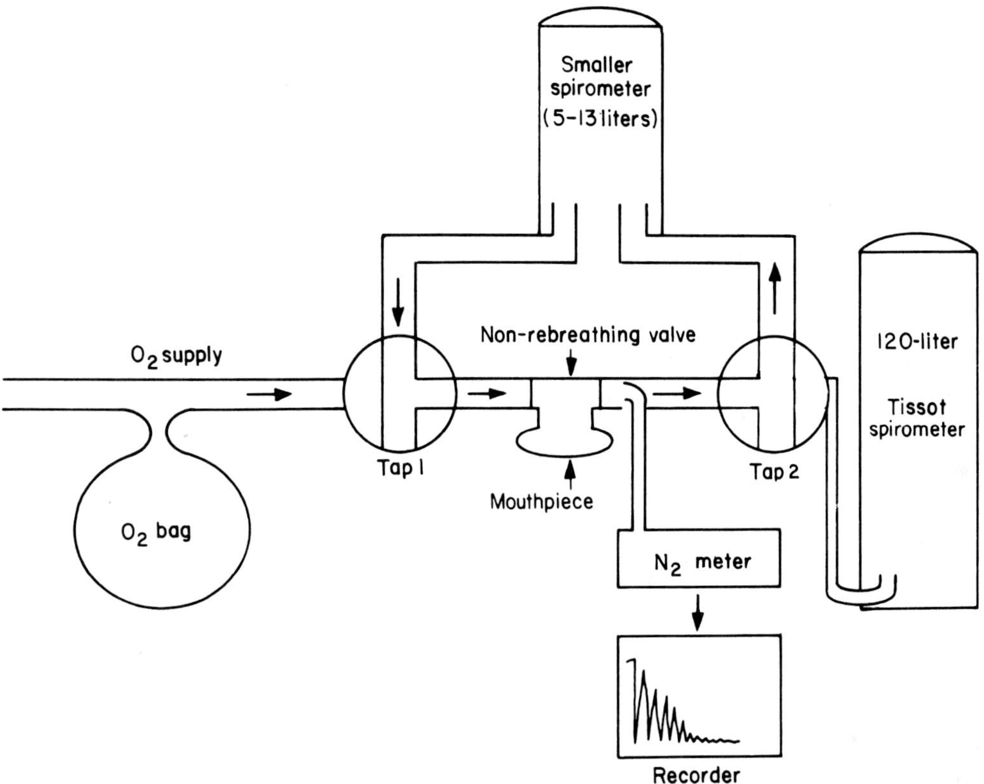

Figure 2-21. Apparatus for nitrogen washout determination of FRC. A separate spirometer circuit (top) is shown to allow observation of FRC during tidal breathing for correct timing of the transfer into the washout phase. (Used with permission from Jalowayski AA, Dawson A. Measurement of lung volume: the multiple breath nitrogen method. In: Clausen JL, ed. Pulmonary function testing. Guidelines and controversies. New York: Academic Press, 1982:117.)

lung volume at FRC, ΔP equals the small decrease in alveolar pressure that occurs with the inspiratory effort, and ΔV equals the small increase in lung volume that occurs with the inspiratory effort.

Solving for V_{FRC}:

$$V_{FRC} = \frac{\Delta V}{\Delta P}(P_{FRC} - \Delta P) \tag{2-20}$$

Because ΔP is so small, $P_{FRC} - \Delta P$ can be assumed to equal P_{FRC}. Thus:

$$V_{FRC} = \frac{\Delta V}{\Delta P}(P_{FRC}) \tag{2-21}$$

where P_{FRC}, as noted above, is simply atmospheric pressure (less the partial pressure of water vapor at saturation.)

A mouth pressure transducer in the body plethysmograph is used for measuring ΔP. ΔV is obtained by converting the change in box pressure into the volume change of the thorax within the sealed box (see above). In practice, the patient simply pants briefly against the shutter while ΔV/ΔP is measured.

In addition to greater speed in determining V_{FRC}, the body plethysmographic measurement also includes the volume of bullae or other poorly communicating air spaces. These structures expand during inhalation along with the better-communicating spaces. For this reason, plethysmographically-determined FRC is also referred to as thoracic gas volume (TGV).

Although static lung volumes are altered in a large variety of diseases, their role in pulmonary function evaluation is mainly adjunctive; they help clarify the findings of basic spirometry. Ries and Clausen summarized the physiologic mechanisms that affect these volumes.[29] TLC varies with lung size, chest wall and lung elastic recoil, structural changes in thoracic cage size, and strength of the inspiratory muscles. FRC is affected by lung size, the balance between chest wall and lung elastic recoil, structural changes in thoracic cage size, and air trapping (failure of lung units to empty due to closure of airways at low lung volumes in obstructive lung disease). RV changes with lung size, chest wall elastic recoil, size of the thoracic cage, air trapping, and expiratory muscle strength. Lung elastic recoil may also affect RV, although to a lesser extent than the other volumes. Knowledge of these mechanisms usually makes the effect of any disease process readily apparent.

Such knowledge about the alteration of static lung volumes is not necessarily clinically useful. These determinations are most helpful in cases where the forced expiratory spirogram indicates both obstruction and restriction (eg, reduced FVC and decreased FEV_1/FVC ratio). It is important to determine whether two types of impairment exist or whether the reduction in FVC is merely due to an elevated RV from air trapping. The difference between predicted RV and measured RV is added to measured FVC. If this results in a normal FVC value, then only obstructive impairment is present.

One other situation in which static lung volume determination is helpful concerns using the TLC as a "gold standard" test for restrictive impairment. Occasionally, both TLC and RV may be reduced by approximately the same amount so that FVC (TLC − RV) remains normal. In these cases, determination of TLC readily demonstrates the presence of the restrictive impairment.

Closing Volume/Closing Capacity

The concept of closing volume explains many of the abnormalities of gas exchange that are characteristic of anesthesia, which makes it important in the physiology of anesthesia practice. A simplified view of closing volume states that gravity-dependent forces may affect the dimensions of certain airways, principally the small airways (those <2 mm in diameter). This means that in the normal subject, small airways leading to alveolar units in dependent areas of lung (those being compressed by the weight of the lung above) become occluded at some volume below FRC. This effect may be demonstrated by a resident gas technique (single breath nitrogen washout) or a marker gas technique (single breath helium bolus), both of which are related to the methods for determining static lung volumes (see above). Although most frequently demonstrated by the nitrogen method, the helium method is more straightforward in its physiologic implications.

A characteristic helium concentration versus expired volume curve is shown in Figure 2-22. It is generated by inducing a patient to exhale all the way to RV. While the subject is breathing in slowly to TLC, a 300-mL bolus of helium gas is introduced at the beginning of the inhalation. Room air is supplied for the remainder of the inhalation. The patient then slowly exhales back to RV while the helium concentra-

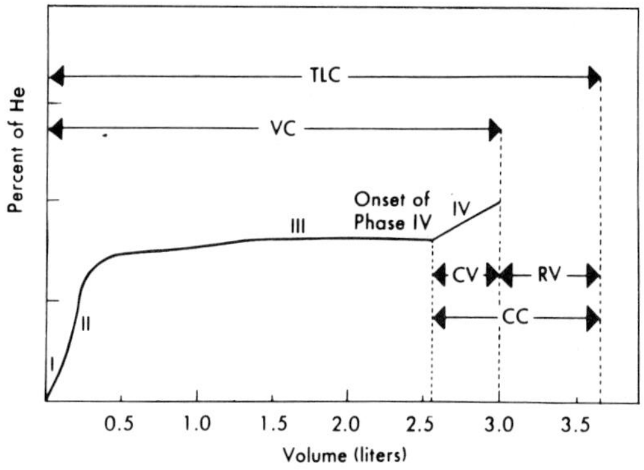

Figure 2-22. The single breath helium-bolus washout curve. Phases I–IV of the curve are defined in the text. (Modified, with permission, from Ruppel GL. Manual of pulmonary function testing. St Louis: Mosby-Year Book, 1991:74.

tion at the mouth versus exhaled volume is plotted. The gas delivered early in inspiration results in a higher concentration of He in nondependent lung zones whose small airways are open even near RV. This contrasts with lung units associated with small airways in dependent zones, which presumably are closed at the time the helium bolus is delivered; by the time they open, only room air is inhaled.

The resulting curve (Fig. 2-22) is partitioned for ease of analysis. Proceeding from the origin, phase I represents anatomic dead space that contains no helium. Phase II, the transition between anatomic dead space and alveolar air, is a gradual rather than abrupt transition because of the different lengths of conducting airways leading to alveolar units. Phase III, also known as the alveolar plateau, represents the gradual emptying of a mixture of nondependent lung units (containing helium) and dependent units (containing little or no helium.) The slope of this phase is affected by ventilatory inhomogeneity. In obstructive lung disease, with a mixture of well and poorly ventilated lung units, the slope of this phase becomes steeper. Finally, phase IV marks the closure of dependent lung units, which then stop contributing their low-helium contents to the total expirate.

The point at which phase IV begins is termed closing volume (CV)[30]; CV plus RV is termed closing capacity (CC). The physiologic importance of CC relates to the fact that under certain conditions, CC can exceed FRC, which means that part of each tidal breath occurs below the volume at which dependent lung zones close. These are lung units that are perfused but are now poorly ventilated; hence, a shunt is produced, and oxygenation can decline.

In practice, this situation can take place either if CC is increased or FRC declines. CC is known to be higher in obstructive diseases of small airways (eg, asthma, chronic bronchis) and in cigarette smokers.[30,31] In addition, CC increases with age and may rise during anesthesia due to changes in lung elastic recoil.[30,31,32]

FRC declines in many situations important to the conduct of anesthesia (eg, in the supine position, during general anesthesia, following abdominal or thoracic surgery.[33–36] FRC is also reduced in many pulmonary disorders (see above). All of these conditions, alone or in combination, may lead to a higher CC than FRC, increased shunting, and impaired oxygenation.

Diffusing Capacity

All of the tests previously discussed are measurements of the mechanical properties of the lungs and only indirectly concern gas exchange functions. Diffusing capacity is unique in that it allows direct assessment of gas exchange. Gas transport between the alveolus and the hemoglobin molecule occurs by the process of diffusion, that is, the movement of gas molecules from an area of high concentration to an area of low concentration. The path traversed is depicted schematically in Figure 2-23. Normally, this process of diffusion is sufficiently rapid such that pulmonary capillary Po_2 equals alveo-

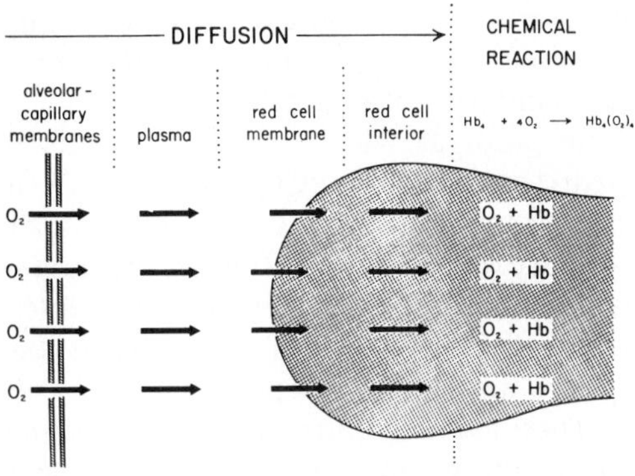

Figure 2-23. Schematic representation of the diffusion path for oxygen from alveolar space to hemoglobin molecule. (Used with permission from Comroe JH, Forster RE, DuBois AB, et al. The lung. Chicago:Year Book, 1962:113, with permission).

lar Po_2 by the time blood has traversed about one-third of the capillary length. In this normal situation, the amount of oxygen transported, which depends on blood flow through the capillary, is said to be perfusion limited.

When pulmonary disease lengthens the path that the oxygen molecule must traverse, reduces the surface area available for gas exchange, or attenuates the pulmonary vascular bed, capillary Po_2 may not equilibrate with alveolar Po_2 before the pulmonary capillary is traversed. Oxygen transport is then said to be diffusion limited. The ability of oxygen to diffuse from the alveolus to the hemoglobin molecule is described in terms of the diffusion capacity (DLO_2), which is defined as the rate of transfer (flow) of the gas divided by its partial pressure gradient. DLO_2 is thus equivalent to a conductance, defined as flow divided by pressure (see section on Mechanics of Breathing), as shown below

$$\text{(2-22)} \quad DLO_2 = \frac{O_2 \text{ flow}}{O_2 \text{ driving pressure}} = \frac{\text{Uptake of } O_2 \text{ (mL/min)}}{PAO_2 - PCO_2}$$

where PAO_2 and PCO_2 are partial pressures of O_2 in the alveoli and pulmonary capillaries, respectively.

There are two main components to DLO_2: DM, which is diffusion across the alveolar capillary membrane, and θV_c, which relates to gas transport within the erythrocyte and the chemical reaction of oxygen with hemoglobin. "θ" is the reaction rate of the gas with hemoglobin, and V_c is the pulmonary capillary blood volume. Each of these components also represent conductances, and therefore add as reciprocals:

$$\text{(2-23)} \quad \frac{1}{DL} = \frac{1}{DM} + \frac{1}{\theta V_c}$$

DM and θV_c are not generally measured independently. Other readily obtained parameters (eg, hemoglobin concentration) usually indicate which component is responsible for a reduction in diffusion capacity (DL). Clinical decision-making can then proceed.[37]

In practice, the direct measurement of DLO_2 is difficult because of problems in measuring the partial pressure of oxygen in the pulmonary capillary. An alternate method was developed by Krogh in which the diffusion of a small concentration of carbon monoxide (CO) is measured, and this has become the standard technique today.[38] CO is employed because it binds very avidly with hemoglobin, so that if small enough amounts are used, PCCO may be assumed to be zero. In addition, because the molecular size of CO is close to that of O_2, its diffusion characteristics are very similar.

The most widely used technique is the single breath method, and the parameter obtained is the single-breath lung-diffusing capacity for CO (DLCOSB). One possible apparatus that may be used is shown in Figure 2-24. In practice, the reservoir (B) is filled with 0.3% CO, 10% helium (He), 21% O_2, and 68.7% N_2. The patient exhales

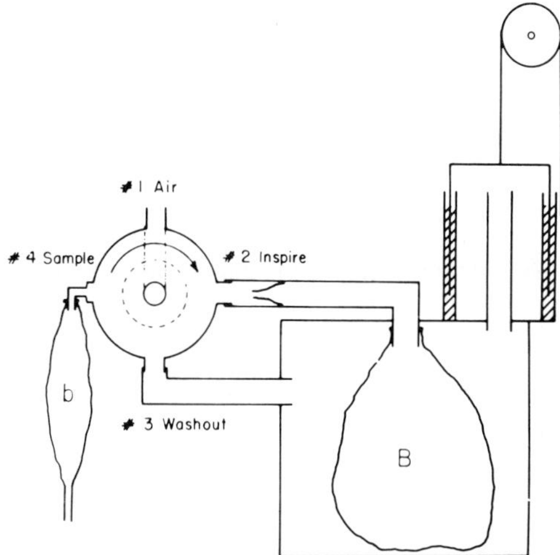

Figure 2-24. Bag-in box system for measurement of D_LCO_{SB}. A valve allows for switching the subject between the four phases of the measurement: 1, breathing room air, then expiration to RV; 2, inhalation of CO-He mixture from bag B to TLC; 3, breathhold for 10 seconds, then exhale deadspace; 4, continued exhalation while alveolar gas sample being collected. (Used with permission from Gaensler EA, Smith AA. Attachment for automated single breath diffusing capacity measurement. Chest 1973; 63:137.)

to RV, inhales rapidly to TLC from the reservoir, and holds his or her breath for 10 seconds. While the subject exhales rapidly to RV, a sample of alveolar gas is obtained (approximately 750 mL of dead space gas should be discarded) The fractional concentration of He and CO is measured in the initial reservoir gas (F_IHe and F_ICO, respectively) and in the expired alveolar sample (F_AHe and F_ACO, respectively).

The calculation of D_LCO_{SB} from these values starts with the computation of alveolar volume (V_A) from the initial and final helium concentrations. This technique is identical to that used in the determination of static lung volumes by gas dilution (see above).

$$\text{(2-24)} \quad V_A\,(\text{STPD}) = V_1\,(\text{ATPD})\,\frac{F_1He}{F_AHe} \times 1.05 \times (\text{ATPD} \rightarrow \text{STPD})$$

where V_I is the volume of test gas inhaled from the reservoir and (ATPD → STPD) is the factor for converting gas volumes between atmospheric temperature and pressure, dry (ATPD) and standard temperature and pressure, dry (STPD).

The concentration of CO in the alveoli at the start of the breathhold (F_ACO_0) is then calculated:

$$\text{(2-25)} \quad F_ACO_0 = F_ICO\,\frac{F_AHe}{F_IHe}$$

and D_LCO_{SB} computed:

$$\text{(2-26)} \quad D_LCO_{SB} = V_A\,(\text{STPD}) \times \frac{60}{t} \times \frac{1}{P_{BOX} - 47} \times \ln\frac{F_ACO_0}{F_ACO}$$

where t is breathhold time, and P_{BOX} is barometric pressure.

As noted previously, D_LCO_{SB} is reduced by diseases that attenuate the pulmonary vascular bed or decrease the surface area available for gas exchange. Processes that lengthen the path traversed by molecular oxygen in moving from the alveoli to the erythrocytes, such as interstitial fibrosis, also decrease D_LCO_{SB}. However, these disorders are invariably associated with an attenuated pulmonary vascular bed or a reduced surface area for gas exchange. It is believed that these mechanisms play a more important role than the so-called "alveolar capillary block" of increased path length.

Table 2-3 summarizes the pathophysiology involved in changes in D_LCO_{SB}. Note the utility of defining a measure of gas transfer per unit of alveolar volume (diffusing capacity divided by alveolar volume or D_L/V_A) as proposed by

Table 2-3. Causes of Abnormal DLCOSB*

Abnormality	Pathophysiology	Examples
Decreased	1. Loss of pulmonary capillary bed with normal lung volume (reduced DL/VA)	Multiple pulmonary emboli; early interstitial lung disease; primary pulmonary hypertension
	2. Loss of pulmonary capillary bed with increased lung volume (reduced DL/VA)	Pulmonary emphysema
	3. Loss of functioning alveolar-capillary bed due to decreased lung volume (normal DL/VA)	Pulmonary resection; pleural effusion
	4. Reduced red blood cell volume	Anemia
	5. CO back-pressure	Cigarette smokers; multiple repetition of DLCOSB test
Increased	1. Increase in pulmonary capillary blood volume	Early mitral stenosis, left-to-right shunts (eg, atrial septal defect); exercise (recruitment); supine position
	2. Increased red blood cell volume	Polycythemia
	3. Pulmonary hemorrhage	Goodpasture's Syndrome

* DL/VA = diffusing capacity divided by alveolar volume; DLCOSB = single breath diffusing capacity for carbon monoxide.

Krogh.[38] This definition may give further insight into the pathophysiology of the abnormality. For instance, pulmonary emboli or other pulmonary vascular disease (including the attenuated pulmonary vasculature of pulmonary emphysema) results in low values of DL/VA, indicating that the impairment in gas transfer is not simply caused by reduced alveolar volume. Conversely, the reduced DLCOSB associated with lung resection is accompanied by a normal or increased DL/VA; alveolar/capillary units are normal but their numbers are low.

DLCOSB is reduced by anemia, which is functionally an attenuation of the pulmonary vascular bed. Various equations are available for correcting DLCOSB in cases of decreased hemoglobin, such as that of Cotes[39].

$$\text{(2-27)} \quad \text{DLCOSB (corrected)} = \text{DLCOSB (observed)} \times \frac{10.2 + \text{Hgb}}{1.7 \times \text{Hgb}}$$

where Hgb is the patient's measured hemoglobin concentration in g/100 mL.

DLCOSB may also be reduced by CO back-pressure, since no measurement of pulmonary capillary CO is used in the calculation (the value is assumed to be zero). This assumption is usually true except in some patients who smoke cigarettes (such patients have elevated levels of carboxyhemoglobin) or after too many repetitions of the DLCOSB test. The former problem may be corrected by using smoking-specific predictive equations[40] or correcting for venous CO. The latter situation is easily controlled by allowing at least 4 minutes between determinations so that CO in the test gas may be excreted.

Table 2-4 lists specific situations in which determination of DLCOSB is useful. DLCOSB is the only easily measured laboratory parameter that reliably correlates with morphologic degree of pulmonary emphysema in patients with chronic obstructive pulmonary disease (COPD).[41] Tobacco abuse that leads to pulmonary disease may cause either chronic obstructive bronchitis or pulmonary emphysema, both of which result in spirometric evidence of ob-

Table 2-4. Conditions in Which DLCOSB Determinations Are Helpful

Condition	Use
Chronic obstructive pulmonary disease	Differentiate chronic bronchitis from pulmonary emphysema
Restrictive spirometric impairment	Distinguish parenchymal from chest wall disease
Sarcoidosis and interstitial lung diseases	Follow clinical course; determine need for treatment and assess results
Acquired immunodeficiency syndrome (AIDS)	Detect pulmonary sequelae
Pulmonary vascular diseases	Frequently the only abnormal pulmonary function test

structive impairment. Any given patient may exhibit predominantly one disease or the other, although both disorders commonly coexist. Both lung compliance (CL) and DLCOSB correlate with the degree of emphysema; although CL is difficult to obtain, DLCOSB is readily measured.

DLCOSB has several uses in evaluating patients with interstitial lung disease. DLCOSB measurement can help determine whether patients who present with a restrictive spirometric impairment have pulmonary parenchymal or chest wall disease. Generally, patients with reduced FVC and DLCOSB have pulmonary parenchymal disease, whereas patients with normal DLCOSB likely have restrictive chest wall disease. DLCOSB is useful in the early detection of interstitial lung diseases such as interstitial pulmonary fibrosis or sarcoidosis and may be used as a guide in treating an interstitial lung disease. A falling DLCOSB, for instance, indicates clinically active pulmonary sarcoidosis, while an increase in this value following therapy confirms the response to treatment.[42] The level of DLCOSB usually decreases long before FVC or TLC declines or chest radiographs become abnormal.[43] For that reason, DLCOSB is one of the best screening tests for the presence of opportunistic pulmonary infection in acquired immunodeficiency syndrome.[44]

DLCOSB is reduced in pulmonary vascular disease (eg, multiple pulmonary emboli, primary pulmonary hypertension, pulmonary vasculitis).[45,46] Spirometry and static lung volumes are generally normal, since these disorders are usually not associated with pulmonary fibrosis or airways disease. DLCOSB may thus provide an important clue to the diagnosis of these disorders.

Interpreting Pulmonary Function Studies

Knowing when to order specific pulmonary function tests and interpreting these studies can be complicated, as is evident from the detail involved in the brief survey of pulmonary function testing presented above. Tables 2-2 and 2-5 categorizes diseases by patterns of normal and abnormal tests and allow at least a "first approximation." Nuances and exceptions cannot be incorporated in such a schematic outline, however. Just as a physician would consult the radiologist for interpretation of a radiographic study or recommendations concerning appropriate follow-up studies there is no substitute for reviewing the results of pulmonary function studies with the laboratory professional staff.

Spirometry is universally required as the first step. Depending on the result, additional tests (DLCOSB, body plethysmography to measure static lung volumes, MVV) can further classify the disorder. Note that only a disease classification, not actual diagnosis, is usually possible, since many different diseases can commonly result in a single pattern of impairment.

Table 2-5. Simplified Interpretation of Pulmonary Function Tests*

Test	Restrictive Parenchymal Disease (pulmonary fibrosis)	Restrictive Chest Wall Disease (kyphoscoliosis or myasthenia gravis)	Upper Airway Obstruction	Bronchial Asthma	Pulmonary Emphysema	Chronic Obstructive Bronchitis	Small Airway Obstruction (asthma in remission)	Combined Obstruction and Restriction (bronchiectasis or sarcoidosis)	Pulmonary Vascular Disease (pulmonary emboli)
Spirometry	See Table 2-2	See Table 2-2	See Table 2-2	See Table 2-2 Must demonstrate reversibility of obstruction with bronchodilator or positive challenge test	See Table 2-2	See Table 2-2	See Table 2-2	See Table 2-2	N
D_LCO_{SB}	↓	N	N	N	↓	N	N	↓	↓
Static lung volumes	↓ TLC ↓ or N FRC, RV	↓ TLC	N	↑ FRC, RV	↑ TLC, FRC, RV	↑ FRC, RV	N or ↑ TRC, RV	↓ TLC ↓, N, or ↑ FRC, RV	N
MVV	N unless severe disease; % predicted MVV/% predicted VC > 0.8	↓	↓	↓	↓	↓	N	↓	N

* N = normal; ↓ = decreased; ↑ = increased; TLC = total lung capacity; FRC = functional residual capacity; RV = residual volume; MVV = maximum voluntary ventilation; VC = vital capacity

Suitable criteria for abnormality were developed by Miller and are presented in Table 2-6.[64] Almost universally, reports of pulmonary function tests give a predicted value for each test. These normal values are determined from statistically analyzed population studies, just as in chemistry reports. Unlike typical chemistry reports, however, pulmonary function reports rarely list a range of normal values. Instead, they give a single predicted value for each test, which is usually determined from appropriate regression equations. Typically, independent variables such as gender, age, and height are used in these equations. In the past, the use of criteria such as those outlined in Table 2-6 to determine whether a given value was normal compared to the predicted value was common. Increasingly, however, many laboratories include 95% confidence limits based on these predictive equations. When such limits are available, the guidelines of Table 2-6 should be discarded; any value beyond the 95% confidence limit should be considered abnormal.

Using Pulmonary Function Tests in Preoperative Evaluation

Preoperative pulmonary function testing is indicated under certain conditions, such as those associated with increased risk of surgery and general anesthesia. Such testing is also indicated before certain procedures that are associated with increased risk (Table 2-7).

Conditions that contribute to the risk of surgery include preexisting pulmonary disorders, which increase the probability of atelectasis, pneumonia, pulmonary embolus, respiratory failure, and bronchospasm in the postoperative period.[47–51] Tobacco abuse constitutes a separate indication for preoperative evaluation apart from its known association with cardiopulmonary disease, as this habit is strongly associated with postoperative morbidity.[52] Researchers have demonstrated that advanced age is a predictor of postoperative problems, including respiratory complications[53] and need for postoperative ventilatory support.[54] Obesity profoundly affects pulmonary and cardiovascular function and increases the risk of postoperative morbidity.[55,56]

Certain procedures significantly affect respiratory function, and when they are contemplated, preoperative evaluation is helpful. Procedures that require an incision closely adjacent to the diaphragm (upper abdominal or standard thoracotomy incisions) result in severely reduced VC, FEV_1, and presumably other

Table 2-6. Criteria for Abnormality (in the absence of actual 95% confidence limits)

1. Spirometry and flow-volume loops
   FVC, FEV_1, MVV: < 80% of predicted values
   $FEF_{25\%-75\%}$ (MMF): < 75% of predicted value
   FEV_1/FVC: < .75 (age < 40 years)
   < .70 (age between 40 and 59 years)
   < .65 (age > 59 years)
2. Body plethysmography (static lung volumes)
   RV: < 80% or > 135% of predicted value
   TLC: < 80% or > 120% of predicted value
3. DLCOSB: < 75% of predicted value

Table 2-7. Indications for Preoperative Pulmonary Function Testing*

Conditions likely to increase the risk of surgery
- Known cardiopulmonary disease
- Cigarette smoking
- Age > 70 years
- Obesity

Contemplated surgery profoundly affecting pulmonary function
- Lung resection
- Upper abdominal surgery
- Nonresectional thoracic surgery

* Used with permission from Brown LK. Surgical considerations: effects of surgery on lung function; preoperative evaluation. In: Miller A, ed. Pulmonary function tests in clinical and occupational lung disease. Philadelphia: WB Saunders 1986:345.

timed volumes and flows. These measurements may fall to as little as 35% of preoperative values[57,58]; analgesia leads to only incomplete reversal. This has suggested a reflex neurologic alteration in diaphragmatic function.[59] An important component of the morbidity caused by alteration in postoperative pulmonary function is the need for postoperative ventilatory support. The prediction of this need is the object of much work in the field of preoperative assessment.[49,60]

Theoretically, the changes in ventilatory function induced by a surgical incision are fully reversible given sufficient time after the procedure. Resectional lung surgery, however, results in irreversible alteration in ventilatory function, which must also be considered in computing surgical risk. The calculation of post-resection pulmonary function is discussed in Chapter 7. In addition, it should be stressed that preoperative testing be performed following suitable medical therapy (including smoking cessation) for preexisting pulmonary disorders. Such testing avoids counseling against surgery unnecessarily and improves surgical outcome in general.[61] This subject is discussed in more detail in Chapter 8.

Various schemes for quantitative assessment of operative risk based on pulmonary function studies have been published. One of the earliest is that of Miller et al.[47], who defined the "K" index, based on observed $FEV_{0.5}$ and FVC, and predicted FVC:

$$K = \frac{\text{observed } FEV_{0.5}/\text{observed FVC}}{\text{observed FVC/predicted FVC}} \qquad (2\text{-}28)$$

Note the inclusion of both an index of obstruction and an index of restriction, similar in principle to the air velocity index previously discussed. Miller used the value K to quantitate impairment; K of less than 0.15 constitutes severe surgical risk (see Table 2-8).[47,62]

Subsequently, numerous studies have advanced other combinations of parameters. Peters found that $FEF_{75\%-85\%}$ and maximal expiratory pressure ($P_E[max]$) could predict the need for ventilatory support in cardiac surgery patients (Table 2-8)[49]; FEV_1 alone was accurate in only two-thirds of cases. In an investigation

Table 2-8. Criteria for Assessing Postoperative Risk Based on Preoperative Pulmonary Function Testing

Source	Parameter	Limits	Risk
Miller[62]	K (see Equation 28)	> 0.5	Normal
		0.35–0.5	Mild
		0.25–0.35	Moderate
		0.15–0.25	Severe
		< 0.15	Extreme
Peters[49]	2.303 ($FEF_{75-85\%}$) +0.0271 ($P_E[max]$)	< 3.387	Ventilatory support needed
Gracey[63]	MVV	< 50% predicted	High probability of complications
	+		
	$FEF_{25\%-75\%}$	< 50% predicted	
	+		
	FVC	< 75% predicted	
Wanner[60]	Predicted $MSV_{post\ op}$	< 10 L/min	Ventilatory support needed

Used with permission from Brown LK. Surgical considerations: effects of surgery on lung function; preoperative evaluation. In: Miller A, ed. pulmonary function tests in clinical and occupational lung disease. Philadelphia: WB Saunders 1986:346.

of patients with chronic obstructive lung disease undergoing major surgery, Gracey et al. concluded that patients with MVV and $FEF_{25\%-75\%}$ less than 50% of predicted, in combination with FVC less than 75% of predicted had a high risk of pulmonary complications when there was no significant improvement following bronchodilator therapy.[63] This combination of parameters predicted the need for postoperative ventilatory support especially well.

More recently, Wanner described a method based on preoperative FEV_1 and the type of surgical incision contemplated that attempts to predict sustainable MVV in the immediate postoperative period.[60] This value would then predict the necessity for postoperative ventilatory assistance. First, MVV is calculated from FEV_1 based on a known regression:

(2-29) $$MVV = 37.5(FEV_1)$$

Only about 60% of MVV is sustainable indefinitely, so maximum sustained MVV (MSV) is calculated:

(2-30) $$MSV = 0.6(37.5)(FEV_1)$$

Next the effect of the planned surgical incision is calculated, based on data such as that of Latimer[57] or Howatt[58]:

(2-31) $$MSV_{postop} = (\text{Fraction of } FEV_1 \text{ remaining}) \times (0.6)(37.5)(FEV_1)$$

This value is then compared to 10 L/min, the minimum postoperative minute ventilation assumed to be necessary to avoid mechanical ventilation. For example, consider a patient with preoperative FEV_1 of 0.8 L who undergoes thoracotomy and will have a postoperative FEV_1 of 35% of the preoperative level:

(2-32) $$MSV_{postop} = (0.35)(0.6)(37.5)(0.8) = 6.3 \text{ L/min}$$

This indicates that postoperative ventilatory assistance will probably be necessary.

References

1. Mead J. Mechanical properties of lungs. Physiol 1961;41:281.
2. Mead J, Gaensler EA. Esophageal and pleural pressures in man, upright and supine. J Appl Physiol 1959;14:81.
3. Baydur A, Behrakis PK, Zin WA, et al. A simple method for assessing the validity of the esophageal balloon technique. Am Rev Respir Dis 1982; 126:788.
4. Fry DL, Ebert RV, Stead WW, et al. The mechanics of pulmonary ventilation in normal subjects and in patients with emphysema. Am J Med 1954;16:80.
5. Rahn H, Otis AB, Chadwick LE, et al. The pressure-volume diagram of the thorax and lung. Am J Physiol 1946;146:161.
6. Michaelson ED, Grassman ED, Peters WR. Pulmonary mechanics by spectral analysis of forced random noise. J Clin Invest 1975;56:1210.
7. Comroe JH, Forster RE, DuBois AB, et al. The lung—clinical physiology and pulmonary function tests. Chicago:Year Book, 1962:172.
8. Begin R, Renzetti AD Jr, Bigler AH, et al. Flow and age dependence of airway closure and dynamic compliance. J Appl Physiol 1975;38:199.
9. Stead WW, Fry DL, Ebert RV. The elastic properties of the lung in normal men and in patients with chronic pulmonary emphysema. J Lab Clin Med 1952;40:674.
10. Macklem PT, Becklake MR. The relationship between the mechanical and diffusing properties of the lung in health and disease. Am Rev Respir Dis 1962;87:47.
11. Gibson GJ, Pride NB. Lung distensibility. The static pressure-volume curve of the lungs and its use in clinical assessment. Br J Dis Chest 1976;70:143.
12. Finucane KE, Colebatch HJH. Elastic behavior of the lung in patients with airway obstruction. J Appl Physiol 1969;26:330.
13. DuBois AB, Botelho SY, Comroe JH Jr. A new method for measuring airway resistance in man using a body plethysmograph: values in normal subjects and in patients with respiratory disease. J Clin Invest 1956;35:327.

14. Mead J, Whittenberger J. Physical properties of human lungs measured during spontaneous respiration. J Appl Physiol 1953;5:779.
15. Briscoe WA, DuBois AB. The relationship between airway resistance, airway conductance, and lung volume in subjects of different age and body size. J Clin Invest 1958;37:1279.
16. McFadden ER Jr, Kiser R, deGroot WJ. Acute bronchial asthma. Relations between clinical and physiologic manifestations. N Engl J Med 1973;288:221.
17. Wanner A. Interpretation of pulmonary function tests. In: Sackner MA, ed. Diagnostic techniques in pulmonary disease. New York: Marcel Dekker, 1980:353.
18. Miller RD, Hyatt RE. Evaluation of obstructing lesions of the trachea and larynx by flow-volume loops. Am Rev Respir Dis 1973;108:475.
19. Brown LK, Schwartz J, Miller A, et al. Respiratory drive and pattern during inertially-loaded CO_2 rebreathing: implications for models of respiratory mechanics in obesity. Respir Physiol 1990;80:231.
20. Otis AB. The work of breathing. In: Fenn WO, Rahn H, eds. Handbook of Physiology. Section 3: Respiration. Volume 1. Washington, DC: American Physiological Society, 1964:463.
21. Tiffeneau R, Pinelli A. Air circulant et air captif dans l'exploration de la fonction ventilatrice pulmonaire. Paris Med 1947;37:624.
22. Gaensler EA. Analysis of the ventilatory defect by timed vital capacity measurements. Am Rev Tuberc 1951;64:256.
23. Fry DL, Hyatt, RE. Pulmonary mechanics. A unified analysis of the relationship between pressure, volume and gasflow in the lungs of normal and diseased human subjects. Am J Med 1960;29:672.
24. Leuallen EC, Fowler WS. Maximal midexpiratory flow. Am Rev Tuberc 1955;72:783.
25. Bartlett RG Jr, Phillips NE. The velocity volume loop: a composite pulmonary function test. Dis Chest 1962;42:482.
26. Kryger M, Bode F, Antic R, et al. Diagnosis of obstruction of the upper and central airways. Am J Med 1976;61:85.
27. Chai H, Farr RS, Froehlich LA, et al. Standardization of bronchial inhalation challenge procedures. J Allergy Clin Immunol 1975;56:323.
28. Pepys J, Hutchcroft BJ. Bronchial provocation tests in etiologic diagnosis and analysis of asthma. Am Rev Respir Dis 1975;112:829.
29. Ries AL, Clausen JL. Lung volumes. In: Pulmonary function testing: indications and interpretations. CA: Monterey California Thoracic Society, 1982: 6–1.
30. McCarthy DS, Spencer R, Greene R, et al. Measurement of "closing volume" as a simple and sensitive test for early detection of small airway disease. Am J Med 1972;52:747.
31. Knudson RJ, Lebowitz MD, Burton AP, et al. The closing volume test: evaluation of Nitrogen and bolus methods in a random population. Am Rev Respir Dis 1977;115:423.
32. Westbrook PR, Stubbs SE, Sessler AD, et al. Effects of anesthesia and muscle paralysis on respiratory mechanics in normal man. J Appl Physiol 1973;34:81.
33. Hewlett AM, Hulands GH, Nunn JF, et al. Functional residual capacity during anaesthesia. II. Spontaneous respiration. Br J Anaesth 1974;46:486.
34. Hewlett AM, Hulands GH, Nunn JF, et al. Functional residual capacity during anaesthesia. III. Artificial ventilation. Br J Anaesth 1974;46:495.
35. Anscombe AR, Buxton R St J. Effect of abdominal operations on total lung capacity and its subdivisions. BMJ 1958;2:84.
36. Boushy SF, Billig DM, North LB, et al. Clinical course related to preoperative and postoperative pulmonary function in patients with bronchogenic carcinoma. Chest 1971;59:383.
37. Quanjer PH. Standardized lung function testing. Report of working party on "Standardization of Lung Function Tests" of the European Community for Coal and Steel. Bull Eur Physiopathol Respir 1983;19(Suppl 5):39.
38. Krogh M. The diffusion of gases through the lungs of man. J Physiol (Lond) 1915;49:271.
39. Cotes JE, Dabbs JM, Elwood PC, et al. Iron deficiency anemia: its effect on transfer factor for the lung and ventilation and cardiac frequency during submaximal exercise. Clin Sci 1972;49:325.
40. Miller A, Thornton JC, Warshaw R, et al. Single breath diffusing capacity in a representative sample of the population of Michigan, a large industrial state: predicted values, lower limits of normal, and frequencies of abnormality by smoking history. Am Rev Respir Dis 1983;127:270.
41. Berend N, Woolcock AJ, Marlin GE. Correlation between the function and structure of the lung in smokers. Am Rev Respir Dis 1979;119:695.
42. Miller A, Teirstein AS, Chuang MT. The sequence of physiologic changes in pulmonary sarcoidosis: correlation with radiographic changes and response to therapy. Mt Sinai J Med 1977;44:852.

43. Epler GR, McCloud TC, Gaensler EA, et al. Normal chest roentgenograms in chronic diffuse infiltrative lung disease. N Engl J Med 1978;298:934.
44. Stover DE, White DA, Romano PA, et al. Spectrum of pulmonary diseases associated with the acquired immune deficiency syndrome. Am J Med 1985; 78:429.
45. Jones NL, Goodwin JF. Respiratory function in pulmonary thromboembolic disorders. BMJ 1965;1:14.
46. Fuster V, Steele PM, Edwards WD, et al. Primary pulmonary hypertension: natural history and the importance of thrombosis. Circulation 1984; 70:580.
47. Miller WF, Wu N, Johnson RL Jr. Convenient method of evaluating pulmonary ventilatory function with a single breath test. Anethesiology 1956; 17:480.
48. Hodgkin JE, Dines DE, Didier EP. Preoperative evaluation of the patient with pulmonary disease. Mayo Clin Proc 1973;48:114.
49. Peters RM, Brimm JE, Utley JR. Predicting the need for prolonged ventilatory support in adult cardiac patients. J Thoracic Cardiovasc Surg 1979;77:175.
50. Kafer ER. Respiratory and cardiovascular functions in scoliosis and the principles of anesthetic management. Anesthesiology 1980;52:339.
51. Mittman C. Assessment of operative risk in thoracic surgery. Am Rev Respir Dis 1961;84:197.
52. Morton HJV. Tobacco smoking and pulmonary complications after operation. Lancet 1944;1:368.
53. Burnett W, McCaffrey J. Surgical procedures in the elderly. Surg Gynecol Obst 1972;134:221.
54. Djokovic JL, Hedley-Whyte J. Prediction of outcome of surgery and anesthesia in patients over 80. JAMA 1979;242:2301.
55. Gould AB. Effect of obesity on respiratory complications following general anesthesia. Anesth Analg 1962;41:448.
56. Putnam L, Jenicek JA, Allen CR, et al. Anesthesia in the morbidity obese patient. South Med J 1974; 67:1411.
57. Latimer RG, Dickman M, Day WC, et al. Ventilatory patterns and pulmonary complications after upper abdominal surgery determined by preoperative and postoperative computerized spirometry and blood gas analysis. Am J Surg 1971;122:622.
58. Howatt WF, Talner NS, Sloan H, et al. Pulmonary function changes following repair of heart lesions with the aid of extracorporeal circulation. J Thoracic Cardiovasc Surg 1962;43:649.
59. Simonneau G, Vivien A, Sartene R, et al. Diaphragm dysfunction induced by upper abdominal surgery. Role of postoperative pain. Am Rev Respir Dis 1983;128:899.
60. Wanner A. Interpretation of pulmonary function tests. In: Sackner MA, ed. Diagnostic techniques in pulmonary disease. New York:Marcel Dekker, 1980:353.
61. Stein M, Cassara EL. Preoperative pulmonary evaluation and therapy for surgery patients. JAMA 1970;211:787.
62. Miller WF. Preoperative evaluation of pulmonary function in the surgical patient. In: Chusid EL, ed. The selective and comprehensive testing of adult pulmonary function. Mt Kisco NY: Futura, 1983:283.
63. Gracey DR, Divertie MB, Didier EP. Preoperative pulmonary preparation of patients with chronic obstructive pulmonary disease. Chest 1979;76:123.
64. Miller A. The role of the computer in pulmonary function testing. In: Miller A, ed. Pulmonary function tests in clinical and occupational lung disease. Orlando: Grune & Stratton, 1986:285.

CHAPTER

3

Ventilation-Perfusion Distribution and Pulmonary Gas Exchange

Andrew T. Costarino, Jr.
Bryan E. Marshall

The primary function of the lung is to exchange respiratory gases between the external environment and the arterial blood. The efficiency of this gas transfer is influenced by cardiopulmonary disease and by the effects of surgery and anesthetic medications or other drugs. The purpose of this chapter is to introduce the principles that govern respiratory gas transfer during thoracic anesthesia.

Figure 3-1 depicts an idealized respiratory system that illustrates some important features of external respiration but eliminates the complexity present in the mammalian lung. Convection carries both fresh gas and mixed venous blood to juxtapose at the alveolar epithelial/capillary endothelial membrane (approximately 0.1 μm thick in the human lung). At that juxtaposition of the gas space and blood space of the lung, O_2 enters and CO_2 exits the blood by diffusion. The driving force for the diffusion of O_2 and CO_2 is the partial pressure gradient for each gas between the alveoli (gas phase) and the pulmonary capillary (blood phase). Respiratory gas transfer is completed as convection returns both the arterialized pulmonary capillary blood to the systemic arterial circulation and the O_2-depleted alveolar gas laden with CO_2 back to the external environment. If a state of equilibrium is achieved, during each minute the quantities of the respiratory gases that are exchanged in the lung match exactly the volumes of O_2 consumed ($\dot{V}O_2$) and CO_2 produced ($\dot{V}CO_2$) by all of cellular metabolism.

Respiratory gas exchange in mammalian lungs is more complicated than the idealized model shown in Figure 3-1 for several reasons:[1]

1. Relatively dry environmental gas is warmed and diluted with water vapor as it passes through the mouth, nose, and proximal trachea before reaching the alveoli.
2. Convective flow within the gas space of the lung is tidal in nature so the alveoli and conducting passages are not completely emptied at the end of each exhalation (functional residual capacity [FRC]). As a result, fresh gas entering the lung is mixed with a gas volume that has already equilibrated with the blood. Although FRC provides a reservoir for exchange of gas during exhalation,[2] tidal flow reduces the efficiency of the lung by wasting some proportion of each tidal breath (respiratory dead space).

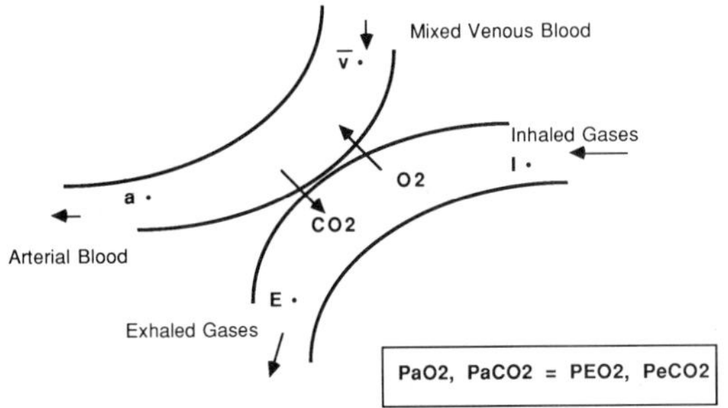

Figure 3-1. Simplified diagram of the respiratory system. Convective flow carries fresh inhaled gas and mixed venous blood to the O_2-CO_2 exchange area. Transfer of both O_2 and CO_2 is driven by the partial pressure gradient for each gas between the alveoli (gas phase) and the capillary (blood phase). Partial pressures for O_2 and CO_2 at point "a" are equal to their partial pressures at point "E" unless the epithelial/capillary endothelial membrane a barrier to diffusion. The amount of O_2 and CO_2 at point "a" compared to that at point "E" depend on the partial pressure-volume relationships of O_2 and CO_2 in the gas phase versus the blood (see text).

3. A proportion of the blood reaching the lung is never in juxtaposition with alveolar gas but instead returns to the systemic arterial circulation with O_2 and CO_2 concentrations unchanged from that of the mixed venous blood. This "shunted" blood represents wasted perfusion.
4. In the alveoli (gas phase), the relationship of gas pressure to gas volume is linear as described in the physical laws for ideal gases.[3] In the blood, the relationship of partial pressure to volume for O_2 and CO_2 is determined by the red blood cell, its hemoglobin, and other blood buffers. The partial pressure to volume relationships in blood for O_2 and CO_2 are nonlinear. The oxygen-hemoglobin and carbon dioxide-whole blood association curves interact with each other (Bohr and Haldane effects) to modify these relationships further.[4]
5. The human lung is made of some 300 million compartments.[5] Each unit exchanges gas in proportion to the balance of its fresh gas flow and blood flow (ventilation-perfusion ratio [$\dot{V}_A/\dot{Q}_{c'}$]). The total O_2 uptake or CO_2 excretion in the lung is equal to the sum of the exchange occurring in all compartments.[6] The O_2 and CO_2 concentrations in the mixed arterial blood are mean values for all the lung compartments, each of which contributes in proportion to its blood flow. Similarly, the O_2 and CO_2 concentrations in the mixed alveolar gas are ventilation weighted mean values for all lung units.[7]

These five factors are the sources of the nonlinearity and inefficiency that characterize mammalian lung function in both healthy and diseased states. To illustrate the role of each of the factors in governing the nature of external respiration in the following sections, three conceptual models of the lung are presented sequentially. Each model builds on the previous concepts and uses algebraic relationships and graphic representations to aid understanding.

Students of respiration have been aided greatly by the establishment, in 1950, of a set of universal terms and symbols (Table 3-1).[8] Familiarity with this system is necessary for any clinician or investigator who is interested in the literature on the normal and abnormal function of the lung.

How Oxygen and Carbon Dioxide Behave in the Gas Space of the Lung

The molecules of an ideal gas or a mixture of ideal gases behave as an enormous number of particles separated by distances large in comparison to their own dimensions and in continuous random motion. No energy is dissipated and no chemical reactions occur during the col-

Table 3-1. Useful Symbols and Abbreviations Used in the Description of Respiratory Gas Exchange*

General Symbols
- $\dot{V}$ = Gas volume (mL or L)
- $\dot{V}$ = Gas volume Per unit time (mL or L/min)
- P = Gas pressure (mmHg = torr)
- F = Fraction concentration of gas in the dry phase
- R = Respiratory exchange ratio ($\dot{V}CO_2/\dot{V}O_2$)
- $\dot{Q}$ = Volume of blood per unit time (L/min)
- C = Concentration in blood phase (mL of gas per 100 mL blood)
- f = Respiratory frequency (breaths/min)

Gas Phase Symbols
- I = Inspired gas
- E = Expired gas
- A = Alveolar gas
- B = Barometric
- D = Dead space

Blood Phase Symbols
- a = Arterial
- $\bar{v}$ = Mixed venous
- c′ = End pulmonary capillary

Abbreviations
- STPD = (Standard temperature, pressure and dry = 0.0°C, 760 mmHg PH_2O = 0)
- BTPS = (Body temperature, pressure, saturated with water = 37.0°C ambient pressure, Pressure, PH_2O = 47.0)

* From Pappenheimer.[8]

lisions that each gas particle has with its neighbors or the walls of the chamber. The frequency of collisions is proportional to the kinetic energy of the gas molecules (absolute temperature), and the total force of all the collisions is reflected in the pressure of the gas.[3] The relationship of ideal gas pressure, volume, and temperature is summarized in two laws derived in the 1700s.

Gas Laws

Boyle's Law

The product of the gas pressure (P) and the gas volume (V) is constant when the temperature is unchanging:[9]

$$P \cdot V = \text{Constant} \quad (3\text{-}1)$$

Charles's Law

The pressure of an ideal gas is proportional to its absolute temperature (T) when volume is constant[9]:

$$P = \text{Constant} \cdot T \quad (3\text{-}2)$$

Universal Gas Law

Combining Boyle's and Charles's laws gives the Universal Gas Law, which is written:[3]

$$P \cdot V = \text{Constant} \cdot T \quad (3\text{-}3)$$

The Universal Gas Law constant is equal to the number of molecules per unit volume of the gas multiplied by Boltzman's constant ($1.38 \cdot 10^{-23}$),[9] thus:

$$P \cdot V = [(\text{number of molecules per unit volume}) \cdot (1.38 \cdot 10^{-23})] \cdot T. \quad (3\text{-}4)$$

If the quantity of gas under consideration is one kilogram molecular weight (kilogram-mole), then the number of molecules is equal to Avogadro's number ($6.02 \cdot 10^{23}$).[9] Boltzman's constant multiplied by Avogadro's number, known as the "Molar Gas Constant" or the "Universal Gas Constant," is designated *R* (8314 Joules/[kg-mole] · [degrees Kelvin]). Thus the Universal Gas Law can be expressed as:[3]

$$P \cdot V = n \cdot R \cdot T \quad (3\text{-}5)$$

where n is equal to the number of moles of gas and P is expressed in atmospheres. Using this relationship, the volume of one mole of an ideal gas at standard temperature and pressure is derived.

$$V = \frac{n \cdot R \cdot T}{P} \quad (3\text{-}6)$$

Since n = number of moles (1), *R* = Molar Gas Constant, P = one atmosphere, and T = 273°K, then $(1) \cdot V = (1) \cdot (8314$ Joules/[kg-mole] $\cdot$ [degree Kelvin]) $\cdot$ (273), and

(3-7) $V = 22.4\ m^3$/kg-mole or 22.4 L/g-mole

Other Relationships of Ideal Gases

Two other principles of the behavior of ideal gases are also important.

Dalton's Law

In a mixture of ideal gases, the pressure exerted by each component gas is equal to the pressure it would exert if it occupied the entire volume. In this case its pressure is independent of the other gases. The total of a mixture of gases is then equal to the sum of the separate gas pressures.[10] For example, if the total pressure of gases in the alveoli is equal to the barometric pressure (P_B) and the gases present included O_2, CO_2, N_2, and water vapor (H_2O), then:

(3-8) $P_B = P_{O_2} + P_{CO_2} + P_{N_2} + P_{H_2O}$

and

(3-9) $P_{total} = 1 \cdot P_B = (F_{O_2} \cdot P_B) + (F_{CO_2} \cdot P_B) + (F_{N_2} \cdot P_B) + (F_{H_2O} \cdot P_B)$

where F_{O_2}, F_{CO_2}, F_{N_2} are equal to the fractional concentration of oxygen, carbon dioxide, and nitrogen, respectively.

Partial Pressure of Gas in a Liquid

When gas molecules are in a liquid solution they continually escape from the liquid surface into the gas and return from the gas into solution. When the partial pressure of a gas in solution is equal to its partial pressure in the gas space above the surface, the system is an equilibrium for the particular gas. The liquid is said to contain gas at that partial pressure.[10]

It is often necessary to apply the above ideal gas laws in calculations of respiratory gas exchange. For example, by convention, minute utilization of oxygen or production of carbon dioxide $\dot{V}_{O_2}$ and $\dot{V}_{CO_2}$) is expressed as volume at STPD, whereas minute ventilations (total minute ventilation = $\dot{V}_E$) are expressed at BTPS. When both minute volume of oxygen or carbon dioxide and minute ventilation of $\dot{V}_{O_2}$ or $\dot{V}_{CO_2}$ are present in the same equation, as is frequently be the case, the BTPS volume must be converted to the STPD volume.[8]

(3-10) STPD: $Pressure_1 = (P_1)$, $Volume_1 = (V_1)$, $Temperature_1 = (T_1)$

(3-11) BTPS: $Pressure_2 = (P_2)$, $Volume_2 = (V_2)$, $Temperature_2 = (T_2)$

In addition, $P_1 = P_B$ (usually 760 torr), $P_2 = P_B - P_{H_2O}$ (760 torr $-47 = 713$), V_1 (usually expressed in milliliters), V_2 (usually expressed in liters), and $T_1 = 273°$ K and $T_2 = 273 + 37°$K. Since $P_1 \cdot V_1 = n \cdot R \cdot T_1$ and $P_2 \cdot V_2 = n \cdot R \cdot T_2$ and because the quantity of gas is the same under both conditions:

(3-12) $P_1 \cdot V_1/T_1 = P_2 \cdot V_2/T_2 = n \cdot R$

By rearrangement:

(3-13) $V_1 = [(P_2 \cdot T_1)/(P_1 \cdot T_2)] \cdot V_2$, and

therefore

(3-14) V_1 (STPD) = V_2 (BTPS) $\cdot$ 0.826

How Oxygen and Carbon Dioxide Behave in Blood Space of the Lung

Some lower animals, insects, have air-filled tubes (tracheoles) that provide a path for atmospheric gas to flow sufficiently close to each body cell so that respiratory gases exchange directly by diffusion with mitochrondria.[11] In contrast, the bodies of mammals are too large for this arrangement, necessitating a medium (blood) to facilitate cellular respiration. The blood must carry the respiratory gases in sufficient quantity to satisfy tissue oxygen consumption and carbon dioxide production at physiologic blood flow rates and gas tension. The blood meets these requirements primarily through mechanisms contained the red blood cell.

Oxygen

Oxygen is relatively insoluble in plasma. Each 100 mL of plasma, if equilibrated with O_2 at a partial pressure of 100 mmHg, holds 0.3 mL.[12] More simply stated, the solubility of oxygen in plasma is 0.003 (mL O_2) per 100 mL plasma per mmHg. If blood could carry only that oxygen that is dissolved in plasma, then a 70-kg man with a $\dot{V}O_2$ of 250 mL would have to circulate about 83 liters of blood each minute to satisfy his body's needs. The erythrocytes and their hemoglobin augments the blood's capacity for carrying oxygen.[13]

Hemoglobin, a complex molecule composed of a globular protein and an iron pigment (heme), has a molecular weight of 64500.[12,14] The protein is composed of four polypeptide chains (two α and two β chains), and each chain is in conformation with one heme group. Heme is composed of four pyrrole components ($[CH]_4$ NH) arranged in a ring structure (porphyrin) with a ferrous ion (Fe^{++}) bound to the ring center (Fig. 3-2). One molecule of oxygen binds to each heme ferrous ion; each hemoglobin molecule can carry up to four molecules of oxygen, which translates, in theory, to 1.39 milliliters of oxygen per gram of fully saturated hemoglobin (Fig. 3-2). However, fully saturated human blood is often found to have only 1.34 milliliter per gram, so this volume is more commonly used.[14,15]

When hemoglobin is found to four molecules of oxygen it is called oxyhemoglobin (HbO_2), whereas oxygen-free hemoglobin is called deoxyhemoglobin (Hb). The presence or absence of oxygen binding to the heme pigment affects the absorption of both visible and infrared light by hemoglobin. Such absorption gives oxyhemoglobin its characteristic red appearance as compared to the violet color of deoxyhemoglobin and allows spectrophotometric methods to quantify the relative percentages of oxyhemoglobin and deoxyhemoglobin.[16,17]

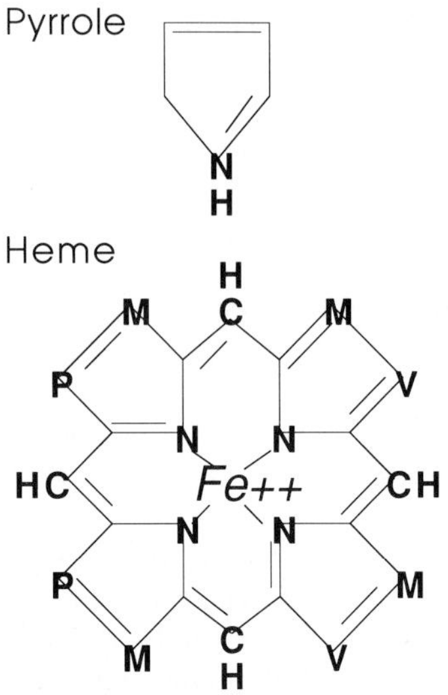

Figure 3-2. Schematic representation of the structure of hemoglobin. Hemoglobin is composed of a globular protein and an iron pigment. The iron pigment (heme) is made of four pyrrole groups linked in a ring structure by methylene bridges, with ferrous iron (Fe^{++}) bound in the ring center. M = methyl group; V = vinyl; P = propionic acid.

The globular protein is has four polypeptide chains (two α and two β chains); each chain contains one heme group and is capable of binding one molecule of oxygen. Four molecules of oxygen binding to each molecule of hemoglobin translates in the following way:

1 · g-mole O_2 = 22.4 liters (22,400 mL)

1 · g-mole hemoglobin = 64,500.0 g

Fully saturated HbO_2 = (4 · g-mole O_2) /(1 · g-mole Hb), or (89.6 L O_2)/(64,500 g Hb) = 1.39 mL O_2/g Hb

The structure of hemoglobin imparts characteristics that enhance the molecule's ability to take up oxygen from the lung and deliver it to the cell. One, interaction among the four iron-globin-porphyrin units during oxygen binding enhances the binding of each successive oxygen molecule. This cooperation causes the familiar s-shape in the hemoglobin saturation-oxygen partial pressure curve (Fig. 3-3).[7,17–21] Second, binding of oxygen to hemoglobin is altered by temperature, pH, and products of red cell metabolism (2,3-diphosphoglycerate).[19,20] At high pH the hemoglobin saturation-oxygen partial pressure curve is shifted to the left, whereas at low pH the curve is shifted to the right. Both the sigmoid hemoglobin saturation-oxygen partial pressure curve and its interaction with pH enhance the uptake of oxygen into the blood in the lung and the delivery of oxygen to body tissues. Adaptations to altitude, chronic hypoxemia, and carbon monoxide exposure (eg, cigarette smoking) alter the usual relationships.[22,23]

Figure 3-3. Plot of the hemoglobin saturation-O_2 partial pressure curve. The content of oxygen in the blood is the sum of the dissolved plus the hemoglobin bound portions. The figure represents the bound and dissolved oxygen in a patient with a blood hemoglobin concentration of 15 g/100 mL blood and normal lung function. The quantity of oxygen bound to the hemoglobin at the oxygen partial pressures represented on the x-axis is depicted by the line of solid circles. The total volume of oxygen per 100 mL of blood contains the additional oxygen dissolved in the plasma (0.003 mL/100 mL mmHg) and is represented by the line of open circles. Interestingly, the oxygen content of 100 mL of arterial blood (PaO_2 = 100 mmHg) is very similar to the oxygen content of 100 mL of the atmosphere at sea level. (Figure drawn using the equations developed by Kelman[18] and hemoglobin oxygen capacity of 1.39 mL O_2/g.)

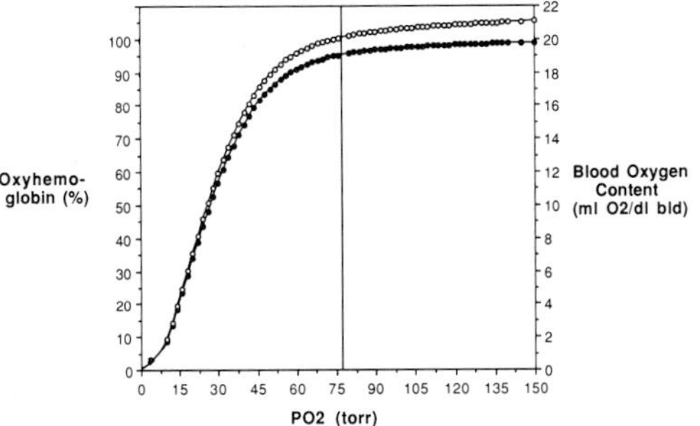

Carbon Dioxide

Carbon dioxide is ten times more soluble in plasma than oxygen. At a partial pressure of 47 mmHg, approximately 1.35 mL of CO_2 dissolves in 100 mL of venous blood.[24] Therefore, if blood carried CO_2 only in plasma, a 70-kg man with a $\dot{V}CO_2$ of 200 mL would have to circulate at least 14 liters of venous blood into his lungs in order to excrete this volume of CO_2![13] Thus despite its tenfold improvement in solubility in comparison to O_2, the exchange of CO_2 also demands mechanisms to enhance its transport in the blood. As with O_2, the necessary strategies are linked to the red blood cell and its hemoglobin, including:

1. Red cell carbonic anhydrase (CA). This enzyme catalyzes the combination of CO_2 with water to form carbonic acid (H_2CO_3). The H_2CO_3 molecule then rapidly dissociates into one hydrogen ion (H^+) and one bicarbonate ion (HCO_3^-).[25]

   $$CO_2 + H_2O \leftrightarrow (CA)\ H_2CO_3 \leftrightarrow H^+ + HCO_3^- \quad (3\text{-}15)$$

   Most of the hydrogen ions produced by this reaction attach to proton-accepting amino acid groups on the hemoglobin molecule, thus buffering the change in pH within the red blood cell. The bicarbonate ions diffuse into the plasma.
2. Carbamino compounds. CO_2 binds with terminal amino acid structures of the hemoglobin globin as well as other blood pro-

teins. These CO_2-amino acid structures are called carbamino compounds.[26]

Under usual physiologic conditions the mechanisms for CO_2 transport in the blood are partitioned in following way: 65% of the blood CO_2 is accounted for by the carbonic anhydrase bicarbonate mechanism, 30% by carbamino compounds (most of these are CO_2 hemoglobin structures), and 5% by direct solution of carbon dioxide in plasma.[22] Therefore, the 70-kg man with a $\dot{V}CO_2$ of approximately 200 mL/min who needs circulate only 4500 mL of venous blood to his lungs each minute liberates about 4.5 milliliters of CO_2 for each 100 milliliters of blood circulated:[13]

(3-16) $$4500\ \text{mL}/100 \cdot 4.5 = 202.5\ CO_2\ (\text{mL/min})$$

Three milliliters (65%) of the excreted CO_2 are due to a change in red cell $HCO_3^- = H_2CO_3$ mechanism, 1.30 milliliters (30%) to a change in carbamino compounds, and 0.2 milliliters (5%) to a change in the volume of dissolved CO_2.

Unlike the O_2 partial pressure-blood O_2 content curve (Fig. 3-3), the CO_2 partial pressure-blood CO_2 content curve is parabolic rather than sigmoid (Fig. 3-4).[26] In addition, within the range of the usual physiologic blood gas tensions, the curve is almost straight. The mechanisms that provide for carbon dioxide transport in the blood are augmented by the concurrent changes in the blood oxygen content and are analogous to the interactions of oxygen transport with blood pH. The CO_2-blood dissociation curve is shifted from the left to the right as the amount oxyhemoglobin increases from 70% to 100% (Fig. 3-4).[26,27] Without this interaction, mixed venous blood in the 70-kg man described above with a partial pressure of 47 mmHg would need a 10 mmHg

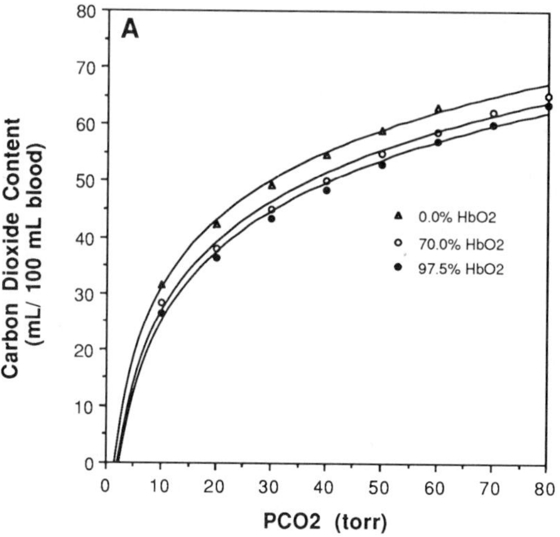

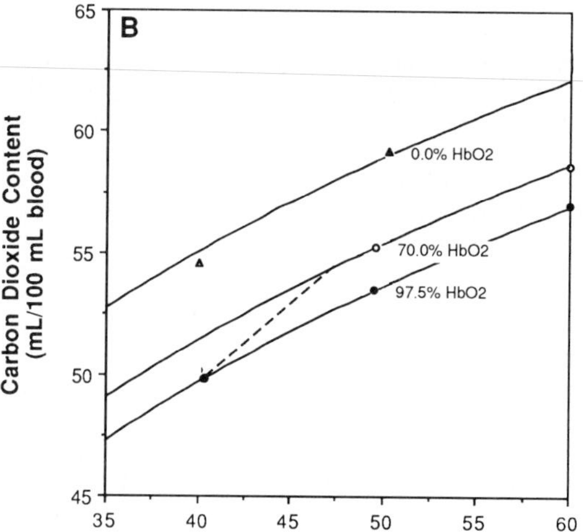

Figure 3-4. Plots of the carbon dioxide blood content-CO_2 partial pressure curves. The carbon dioxide blood content-CO_2 partial pressure curve is parabolic rather than sigmoid. Within the range of the usual physiologic blood gas tensions, the curve is almost straight. As the percentage of oxyhemoglobin increases from zero (triangles) to 97.5% (closed circles), the curve shifts from the left to the right. The mechanisms that provide for carbon dioxide transport in the blood are augmented by the concurrent changes in the blood oxygen content. Because of the right shift of the curve associated with the simultaneous uptake of oxygen in the lung, the unloading of carbon dioxide from the blood is enhanced. The necessary volume of CO_2 is excreted, and the P_{CO_2} only changes 5–7 mmHg. (Modified, with permission from Comroe.[38])

change in CO_2 partial pressure in order to liberate 4.5 mL CO_2 per 100 mL of blood as it is arterialized in its passage through the lung. However, because of the rightward shift of the CO_2 partial pressure-blood CO_2 content curve associated with the simultaneous uptake of O_2 in the lung, the unloading of CO_2 is enhanced. The necessary volume of CO_2 is excreted, and the P_{CO_2} falls only to 40 mmHg (only a 5–7 mmHg change) (Fig 3-4).[26–28]

The interaction of O_2 transport with CO_2 transport in the blood are summarized as two "effects," which are named for the respiratory physiologists who first noted them. The Bohr effect is the rightward movement of the partial pressure O_2 saturation curve due to increasing pH (or CO_2), and the Haldane effect is the leftward shift of the partial pressure-CO_2 content curve with decreasing oxygen saturation of hemoglobin.[21,29]

In summary, the behavior of O_2 and CO_2 in the blood is different from their behavior in the atmosphere, although both behaviors are predictable from the partial pressure. In gas, O_2 and CO_2 behave similarly to ideal gases. Their concentrations and volumes are linearly related to their partial pressures and the total pressure of the surrounding atmosphere. In blood, O_2 and CO_2 are carried in plasma in solution and by the mechanisms associated with the red cell and its hemoglobin molecules. The concentrations of the respiratory gases are dependent on the quantity of red cells and the concentration of hemoglobin, the partial pressure of each individual gas (O_2 or CO_2), and interaction of one with the other (Bohr and Haldane effects). Because most of the circulation equilibrates with the atmosphere during passage through the lung, the sum of partial pressures of all the gases in the arterial blood approximates that of the ambient atmosphere. In mixed venous blood, however, after uptake of O_2 and excretion of the sum of partial pressures of all gases no longer equals atmospheric pressure CO_2.[22]

The Oxygen-Carbon Dioxide Diagram

The O_2-CO_2 diagram, also known as the Rahn-Fenn diagram, was developed in the 1940s as a useful tool for representing the relationship of respiratory gas volume and pressure in both the gas phase and in the blood.[22] It is introduced here because of the simplicity with which the graphic analysis represents both the linear and nonlinear relationships that characterize the behavior of O_2 and CO_2 in the blood. This diagram later helps to illustrate the presentation of pulmonary gas exchange, which is often difficult to understand conceptually and algebraically. The graphic representation will be particularly useful in the later discussion of lung ventilation to perfusion balance in health and disease.

The two dimensional O_2-CO_2 diagram has the partial pressure of O_2 as its abscissa and the partial pressure of CO_2 on the ordinate (Fig. 3-5). This allows the composition of any atmospheric alveolar gas blood or blood gas to be represented by a single point. Comparison of the top with the bottom part of Figure 3-5 illustrates the difference between the partial pressure-content relationship of the O_2 and CO_2 in the gas phase compared to the blood.

Mammalian Respiratory System

One-Compartment Model

A one-compartment schematic model of the mammalian respiratory system the lung is depicted in Figure 3-6. Only the the gas space (alveoli) of the lung is considered in this model, which consists of a single chamber connected to the atmosphere by a single, tubelike conduct-

A.

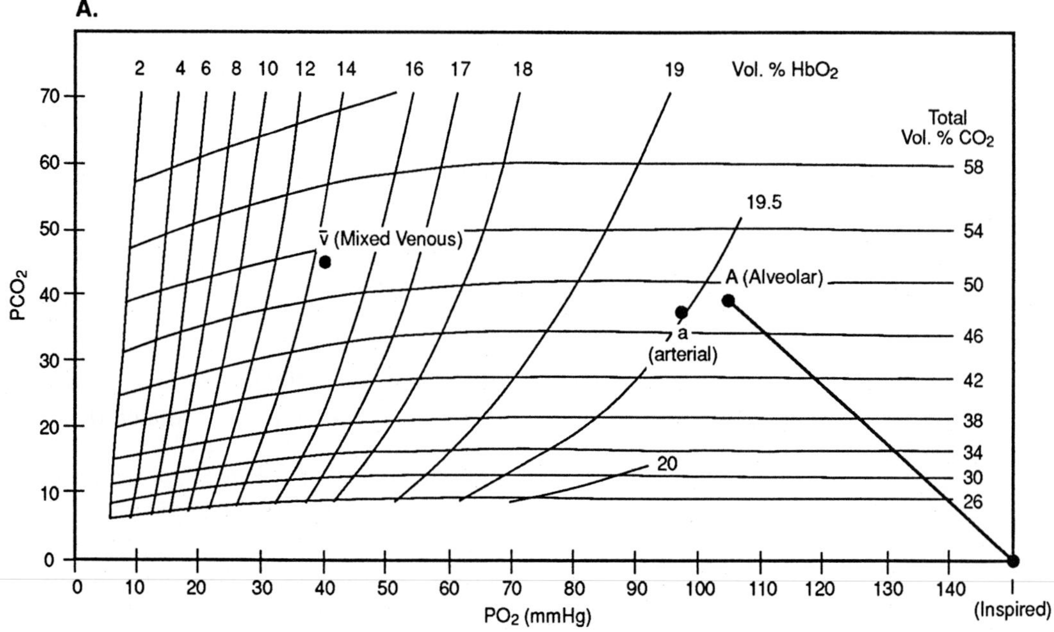

2 4 6 8 10 12 14 16 17 18 19 Vol. % HbO2
Total Vol. % CO2
58
54
50
46
42
38
34
30
26
19.5
20
v̄ (Mixed Venous)
A (Alveolar)
a (arterial)
PCO2
PO2 (mmHg)
(Inspired)

B.

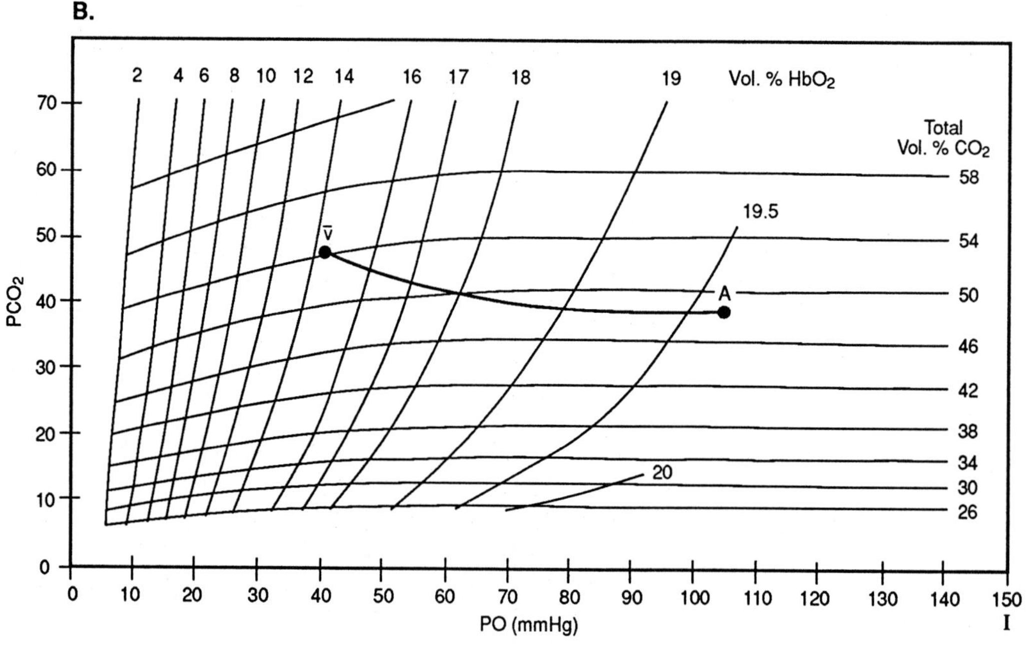

2 4 6 8 10 12 14 16 17 18 19 Vol. % HbO2
Total Vol. % CO2
58
54
50
46
42
38
34
30
26
19.5
20
v̄
A
PCO2
PO (mmHg)
I

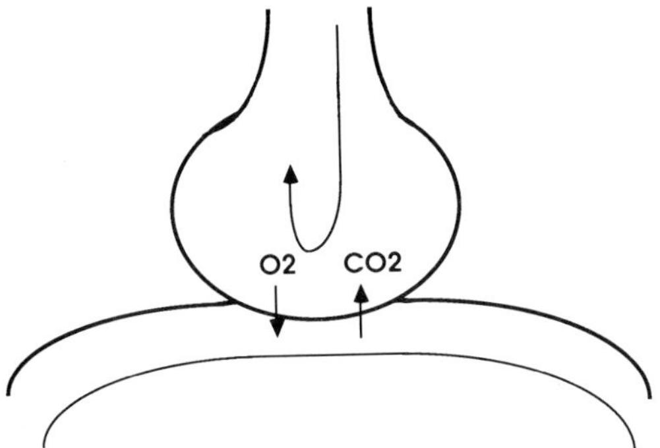

Figure 3-6. One-compartment model of the external respiratory system. In this model of the respiratory system, the lung is viewed as a simple expandable chamber (alveoli) connected to the atmosphere by a single tube-like conducting passage (nose, mouth, trachea, and intrathoracic airways to the 16th generation of branches). All respiratory gas exchange with the blood occurs in the alveolar portion of the model. At the end of exhalation some gas remains within the conducting tube. This gas mixes with the inspired volume of the subsequent breath.

ing passage. A volume of gas (tidal volume) enters the chamber through the tube during inhalation and then exits by the same route during exhalation. The total gas volume entering or exiting the chamber each minute is the summation of the periodic tidal breaths as expressed in Equations 3-17 and 3-18.[30]

$$\dot{V}_I = f \cdot V_{TI} \quad (3\text{-}17)$$

$$\dot{V}_E = f \cdot V_{TE} \quad (3\text{-}18)$$

where $\dot{V}_I$ and $\dot{V}_E$ are the total inspired and exhaled minute volumes, respectively; $\dot{V}_{TI}$ and $\dot{V}_{TE}$ are the average inspired and exhaled tidal volumes; and f is the respiratory frequency. When air is breathed the inhaled tidal gas is composed of O_2, N_2, and H_2O. In the exhaled volume some O_2 has been removed and CO_2 added. By convention, pulmonary ventilation is considered to be the exhaled volume, rather than the inhaled volume, unless otherwise specified.

Figure 3-5. Representation of the O_2-CO_2 Diagram. The two dimensional $O_2 - CO_2$ diagram has the partial pressure of oxygen as its abscissa and the partial pressure of carbon dioxide on the ordinate, which allows the composition of any atmospheric alveolar gas blood or blood gas to be represented by a single point. The composition of atmospheric air at sea level (after humidification at body temperature) is represented by the inspired point (I), alveolar gas by (A), arterial blood by (a), and mixed venous blood by ($\bar{v}$). The relationships of the respiratory gases in the blood is depicted in the figures by shaded isopleths. The more vertical lines are the isopleths of blood oxygen content. The diagonal direction and curve, which is a result of the Bohr effect, is more pronounced at higher oxygen partial pressures. The horizontal lines are isopleths that represent equal blood carbon dioxide volumes per unit volume of blood (milliliters CO_2 per 100 milliliters blood). The downward curve of each isopleth at its left side (low partial pressure of oxygen) is due to the Haldane effect; this is more pronounced as the blood carbon dioxide tension increases.

In A, the line *I-A* connecting points A and I represents the oxygen and carbon dioxide tensions that would exist in the lung gas spaces as carbon dioxide enters a given volume of humidified air and oxygen is taken up. The proportion of carbon dioxide increases linearly with the increase in its partial pressure. The volume and partial pressure of oxygen falls in a like manner. The I-A line represents the uptake of one molecule of oxygen for the excretion of each molecule of carbon dioxide (exchange ratio [R] of 1.0). The curved line $\bar{v}$-a in B represents all possible oxygen and carbon dioxide partial pressures in the blood as the volume of oxygen increases from the mixed venous point ($\bar{v}$), in a one:one ratio with decreasing carbon dioxide. As a result of the interaction of oxygen and carbon dioxide transport in the blood, the change in partial pressures on the O_2-O_2 diagram follows a curving path that is more pronounced on the left portion of the curve.

(Figure modified with permission from Rahn and Fenn.[22])

These volumes are expressed in BTPS after warming and humidification has occurred in the nose, mouth, and trachea.

Since only the gas space is considered here, the relationships of volume, concentration, and partial pressure are linear and the sum of the partial pressures of all component gases must equal the barometric pressure. From these basic principles a series of algebraic relationships can be presented. The following expressions are derived for air breathing at one atmosphere (760 mmHg) and when no CO_2 is present in the inspired gas. The negligible quantities of gases in air other than O_2, N_2, CO_2 and H_2O are ignored.[30]

(3-19) $$F_{I}O_2 + F_{I}N_2 + F_{I}H_2O = 1$$

(3-20) $$P_{I}O_2 + P_{I}N_2 + P_{I}H_2O = P_B$$

(3-21) At BTSP, $P_{I}H_2O = 47$, therefore $$P_{I}O_2 + P_{I}N_2 = P_B - 47$$

(3-22) Similarly, $$F_{E}O_2 + F_{E}N_2 + F_{E}CO_2 + F_{E}H_2O = 1$$

and

(3-23) $$P_{E}O_2 + P_{E}N_2 + P_{E}CO_2 = P_B - 47$$

The total volume of exhaled gas must be equal to the sum of the fractions of the component gases, therefore:

(3-24) $$(F_{E}O_2 \cdot \dot{V}_E) + (F_{E}N_2 \cdot \dot{V}_E) + (F_{E}CO_2 \cdot \dot{V}_E) + (F_{E}H_2O \cdot \dot{V}_E) = \dot{V}_E$$

The same would hold true for total volume and fractional components of the inhaled gases.

The principle of conservation of mass dictates that net respiratory exchange of any component gas is equal to the difference between its inhaled and exhaled volumes. Thus:

(3-25) $$\dot{V}O_2 = k \cdot (F_{I}O_2 \cdot \dot{V}_I) - (F_{E}O_2 \cdot \dot{V}_E)$$

(3-26) $$\dot{V}CO_2 = k \cdot (F_{E}CO_2 \cdot \dot{V}_E) - (F_{CO_2} \cdot \dot{V}_I)$$

Equation 3-26 can be simplified if no CO_2 is present in the inhaled mixture.

(3-27) $$\dot{V}CO_2 = F_{E}CO_2 \cdot \dot{V}_E$$

By convention, VO_2 and VCO_2 are expressed in milliliters at STPD, and $\dot{V}_E$ and $\dot{V}_I$ are expressed as liters in BTPS. Therefore, equations 3-25, 3-26, and 3-27 must include a constant ($k \sim 0.823$) to correct the respiratory volumes.

In a steady state, whole lung gas exchange is equal to the metabolic gas exchange for VO_2 and $\dot{V}CO_2$. The ratio of the volume of CO_2 excreted per minute to net volume of O_2 taken up by the lung (the respiratory exchange ratio [R]) is then equal to the tissue consumption of O_2 divided by the production of CO_2 (the respiration quotient [RQ]).[22]

(3-28) $$\frac{\dot{V}CO_2}{\dot{V}O_2} = R$$

Dead Space versus Alveolar Ventilation

Breathing is tidal, that is, the lung empties by reversing the direction of flow through the same passages used to inflate it. Since no exchange of oxygen and carbon dioxide between gas and blood occurs in the proximal portion of these conducting passages, a portion of the tidal volume, and total minute ventilation, is "wasted" in ventilating the conducting passage (Fig. 3-7).

This wasted ventilation, or dead space, can be described algebraically by considering minute ventilation as a combination of two separate components: the effective portion (alveolar ventilation, $\dot{V}_A$) and wasted ventilation (dead space, $\dot{V}_D$).[30]

(3-29) $$\dot{V}_E = \dot{V}_A + \dot{V}_D$$

Dead space ($\dot{V}_D$) does not participate in the exchange of respiratory gases, so the composition of the dead space gas is the same as that of the

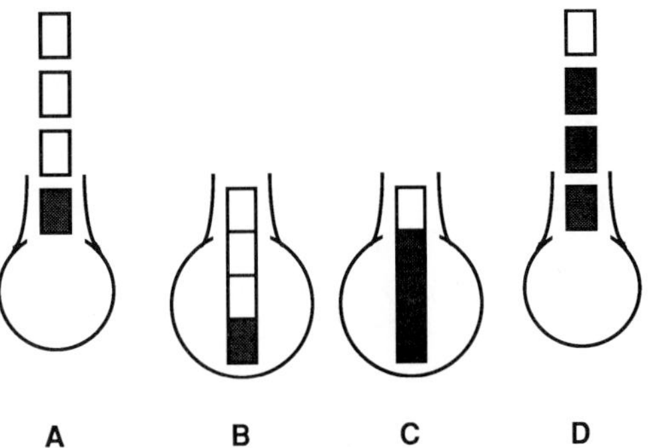

Figure 3-7. Simplied representation of dead space ventilation. In A, before the start of an inhalation the gas within the lung (functional residual capacity [FRC]) has previously equilibrated with the gas in the pulmonary capillary blood. In B, as the next tidal volume fills the lung, the fresh gas entering the alveoli is diluted with the gas remaining after the previous exhalation. The diagram in C shows the exchange of oxygen and carbon dioxide between the alveolar gas and the pulmonary blood. The last of the inspired gas does not past the 16th generation of airways, so this portion of inspired tidal volume remains unchanged. This keeps the concentrations of oxygen, nitrogen, and water vapor the same as those of the inspired air; no carbon dioxide is present. At the beginning of the next exhalation (D) the portion of inhaled gas that remains in the conducting passages in C leaves the lung unchanged. Again, at the end of this exhalation the alveolar gas, having already equilibrated with the blood, stays in the lung.

The combined affect of the dilution of the fresh gas and the failure of a portion of the inspired tidal volume to participate in oxygen and carbon dioxide exchange with the blood reduces the efficiency of ventilation. (Modified, with permission, from Comroe.[38(p 29)])

inspired gas. CO_2 production can therefore be expressed as:

$$\text{(3-30)} \quad \dot{V}_{CO_2} = \dot{V}_E \cdot F_{ECO_2} = (\dot{V}_A \cdot F_{ACO_2}) + (\dot{V}_D \cdot F_{ICO_2})$$

or:

$$\text{(3-31)} \quad \dot{V}_E \cdot F_{ECO_2} = (\dot{V}_A \cdot F_{ACO_2}) + (\dot{V}_D \cdot F_{ICO_2})$$

Rearrangement and solving for $\dot{V}_D$ gives:[31]

$$\text{(3-32)} \quad \dot{V}_D = \frac{(F_{ACO_2} - F_{ECO_2})}{(F_{ACO_2} - F_{ICO_2})} \cdot \dot{V}_E$$

If (1) no CO_2 is present in the inspired gas (eg, air breathing), (2) the fractional concentrations are replaced with partial pressure, and (3) the pressure of CO_2 in the arterial blood is assumed to be the same as (or very similar to) its pressure in the alveolar gas, then the equation 3-32 can be rearranged:[32]

$$\text{(3-33)} \quad \frac{\dot{V}_D}{\dot{V}_E} = \frac{P_{ACO_2} - P_{ECO_2}}{P_{ACO_2}}$$

The so-called "Bohr dead space" equation expresses dead space as a fraction of the total.

The Bohr dead space is sometimes measured clinically by collecting mixed exhaled gas and sampling arterial blood. Both samples are analyzed for partial pressure of CO_2. Normal values are 0.32 ± .07.[33] Values greater than 0.70 are associated with the need for mechanical assistance for breathing.[34, 35]

The Ideal Alveolar Gas

In the one compartment (Fig. 3-8) model, the whole lung is viewed as a single chamber (the ideal alveoli).[36] The composition of the gas in the ideal alveoli is the end product after the inspired gas is humidified, mixed with the dead space, and has exchanged both O_2 and CO_2 with the blood. In addition, because the exchange of O_2 and CO_2 between the chamber and the pulmonary capillary blood approach equilibrium, the composition of gases in the blood leaving the lungs is the same as that in the chamber.

The partial pressure of any gas in the ideal alveoli is determined by three factors:[7]

1. The partial pressure of that gas in the inhaled gas mixture.
2. The alveolar ventilation.

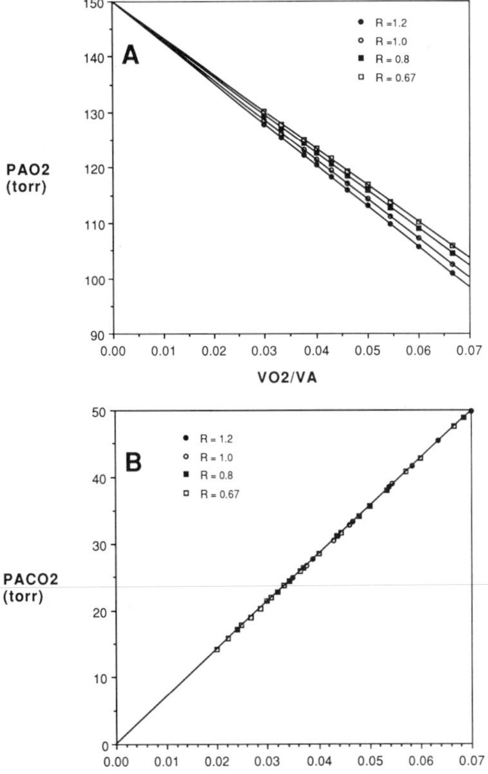

Figure 3-8. The three determinants of the ideal alveolar gas (see text) expressed in the familiar form of a linear equation y = mx + b. The independent variable (x) is the ratio of the respiratory exchange of the gas to the alveolar ventilation ($\dot{V}O_2/\dot{V}A$ [A] or $\dot{V}CO_2/\dot{V}A$ [B]), the dependent variable (y) is the alveolar partial pressure of the gas, and the y-axis intercept is the inhaled tension of the gas. The slope of the line (A) is proportional to R because in the ideal alveoli no exchange of nitrogen occurs, and the balance of oxygen to carbon dioxide exchange is expressed in the term R. The slope of the alveolar gas equation for carbon dioxide (B) remains one at any value for R only if there is no inspired carbon dioxide in the inspired gas (see equation below).

A: $$PAO_2 = PIO_2 - [(PB - 47) - PIO_2 \cdot (1 - R)] \cdot \frac{\dot{V}O_2}{\dot{V}A}$$

$$y \quad = \quad b \quad + \quad m \quad x$$

B: $$PACO_2 = PICO_2 + \left[(PB - 47) - PICO_2 \cdot \frac{(1 - R)}{R}\right] \cdot \frac{\dot{V}CO_2}{\dot{V}A}$$

3. The uptake of the gas from the alveoli (for O_2) or excretion of the gas into the alveoli CO_2).

The algebraic description of the interaction of these factors is known as the alveolar gas equation and its derivation is important to understanding lung gas exchange. This equation is based on principle that the lung exchange of respiratory gases is equal to the net difference between their inhaled and exhaled minute volumes. In order to develop these algebraic expressions, it is necessary to break with the convention mentioned above temporarily by distinguishing between inhaled ($\dot{V}AI$) and exhaled ($\dot{V}A$) minute alveolar ventilation.[30] The ideal alveolar gas equation is also considerably simplified if the discussion is limited to breathing mixtures that include only O_2, CO_2 and N_2 and a steady state is assumed. Under these conditions the exchange of nitrogen is zero, and the exchange of O_2 and CO_2 in the lung is equal to metabolic consumption of oxygen and production of carbon dioxide.[37]

(3-34) $$\dot{V}N_2 = 0$$

(3-35) $$\dot{V}CO_2/\dot{V}O_2 = R = RQ$$

Under these conditions, the difference between $\dot{V}AI$ and $\dot{V}A$ is due to the volume of O_2 that is removed from the alveoli ($\dot{V}O_2$). The volume of CO_2 added ($\dot{V}CO_2$) and the exchange of any individual gas is equal to the difference between its inhaled and exhaled concentrations.

(3-36) $$\dot{V}AI - \dot{V}A = \dot{V}CO_2 - \dot{V}O_2 \text{ or } \dot{V}AI = \dot{V}A + \dot{V}CO_2 - \dot{V}O_2$$

For carbon dioxide:

(3-37) $$\dot{V}CO_2 = (FACO_2 \cdot \dot{V}A) - (FICO_2 \cdot \dot{V}AI)$$

For oxygen:

(3-38) $$\dot{V}O_2 = (FIO_2 \cdot \dot{V}AI) - (FAO_2 \cdot \dot{V}A)$$

With these basic principles established, the derivation of ideal alveolar concentration for O_2 and CO_2 proceeds as follows. Substitution of equations 3-36 into 3-37 and 3-38 gives:

$$(3\text{-}39) \quad \dot{V}CO_2 = (FACO_2 \cdot \dot{V}A) - (FICO_2 \cdot [\dot{V}A - \dot{V}O_2 + \dot{V}CO_2])$$

and

$$(3\text{-}40) \quad \dot{V}O_2 = (FIO_2 \cdot [(\dot{V}A - \dot{V}O_2 + \dot{V}CO_2]) - (FAO_2 \cdot \dot{V}A)$$

since

$$R = \frac{\dot{V}CO_2}{\dot{V}O_2},\ \dot{V}CO_2 = \frac{R}{\dot{V}O_2},\ \text{and } \dot{V}O_2 = \frac{\dot{V}CO_2}{R}$$

Rearrangement and conversion of fractional concentrations to partial pressures gives the desired expressions[30]:

$$(3\text{-}41) \quad PACO_2 = PICO_2 + \left[(PB - 47) - PICO_2 \cdot \frac{(1 - R)}{R}\right] \cdot \frac{\dot{V}CO_2}{\dot{V}A}$$

$$(3\text{-}42) \quad PAO_2 = PIO_2 - [(PB - 47) - PIO_2 \cdot (1 - R)] \cdot \frac{\dot{V}O_2}{\dot{V}A}$$

y	=	b	+	m	x
dependent variable		Y-intercept		slope	independent variable

Equations 3-41 and 3-42 include the three determinants of the ideal alveolar gas listed above and can be arranged in the familiar form of a linear equation $y = mx + b$. Figure 3-8 gives graphic representations of these relationships. The independent variable (x) is the ratio of the respiratory exchange of the gas to the alveolar ventilation ($\dot{V}O_2/\dot{V}A$ or $\dot{V}CO_2/\dot{V}A$), the dependent variable (y) is the alveolar partial pressure of the gas, and the y-intercept is the inhaled tension of the gas.

The slope of the line is proportional to R because in the ideal alveoli there is no N_2 exchange and the balance of O_2 to CO_2 exchange is expressed in as R. The slope of the linear alveolar gas equation for each individual gas is proportional to the exchange of the other gas (ie, proportional to R).[22]

Two commonly employed simplifications of these derivations that are worth mentioning. One, under usual conditions, no CO_2 is present in the inspired gas (the y intercept is zero). Equation 3-41 simplifies to:

$$(3\text{-}43) \quad PACO_2 = \frac{\dot{V}CO_2}{\dot{V}A} \pm k$$

where VCO_2 is milliliters STPD, VA is expressed as liters BTPS, and $k = 0.863$).[37] Two, since $\dot{V}O_2 = \dot{V}CO_2/R$, when there is no CO_2 in the inspired gas, $\dot{V}A = \dot{V}CO_2/PACO_2$. Substitution into equation 3-42 gives:

$$(3\text{-}44) \quad PAO_2 = PIO_2 - \frac{PACO_2}{R} \cdot [(PB - 47) - PIO_2\,(1 - R)]$$

Algebraic rearrangement gives a more popular form of the equation[38]:

$$(3\text{-}45) \quad PAO_2 = PIO_2 - PACO_2 \cdot \left[FIO_2 + \frac{(1 - FIO_2)}{R}\right]$$

which is often radically simplified to the form.

$$(3\text{-}46) \quad PAO_2 = PIO_2 - \frac{PACO_2}{R}$$

These forms (Equations 3-44, 3-45, and 3-46) of the ideal alveolar gas equation for oxygen are consistent with the three determinants of alveolar gas, and they eliminate the awkward $\dot{V}O_2/\dot{V}A$ term: $PACO_2/R$ appears instead.

Although these substitutions emphasize the principles that determine alveolar gas tensions, they may introduce errors when assumptions are made about the value of R. This ratio normally varies between 0.7 and 1.2 in steady, stable conditions with a mean value of 0.8 within the limits of normal metabolism. The value 0.8 is often assumed when the alveolar gas equation for O_2 is used in the clinical setting. Similarly, the P_ACO_2 is assumed to be identical to the $PaCO_2$. These assumptions are reasonable when metabolism and lung function are normal, but they can generate significant errors when alveolar O_2 use is determined in critically ill patients with or under the influence of varied therapies or anesthetics to evaluate gas exchange.[39]

The composition of ideal alveolar gas and its three determinants as defined in the one-compartment model can be graphically represented on the O_2-CO_2 diagram.[22] In Figure 3-9, the point I_1 represents the inspired air at sea level (after humidification at normal body temperature), and the ideal alveolar point (A_1) is at the position equal to O_2 and CO_2 partial pressures of 110 and 40 mmHg, respectively. These values for alveolar O_2 and CO_2 result from their exchange and the minute ventilation as determined by the linear relationships expressed in Equations 3-41 and 3-42. In the diagram, alveolar ventilation is inversely proportional to the straight line distance between the inspired and ideal alveolar points, and the slope of the alveolar line is related to the ratio of CO_2 to O_2 exchange (R). Doubling the alveolar ventilation while breathing air and maintaining the same O_2 consumption and CO_2 production would move the alveolar point from A_1 to A_2. A similar

Figure 3-9. Determinants of ideal alveolar gas on the O_2-CO_2 diagram. Point I_1 represents inspired air (at sea level after humidification at 37°C normal body temperature, the oxygen tension is 150 mmHg and carbon dioxide is negligible). Point A_1 (oxygen tension of 110 mmHg and a carbon dioxide tension of 40 mmHg) represents the typical ideal alveolar gas in a healthy patient with normal alveolar ventilation, oxygen consumption, and an R of 1.0 (see text for further details).

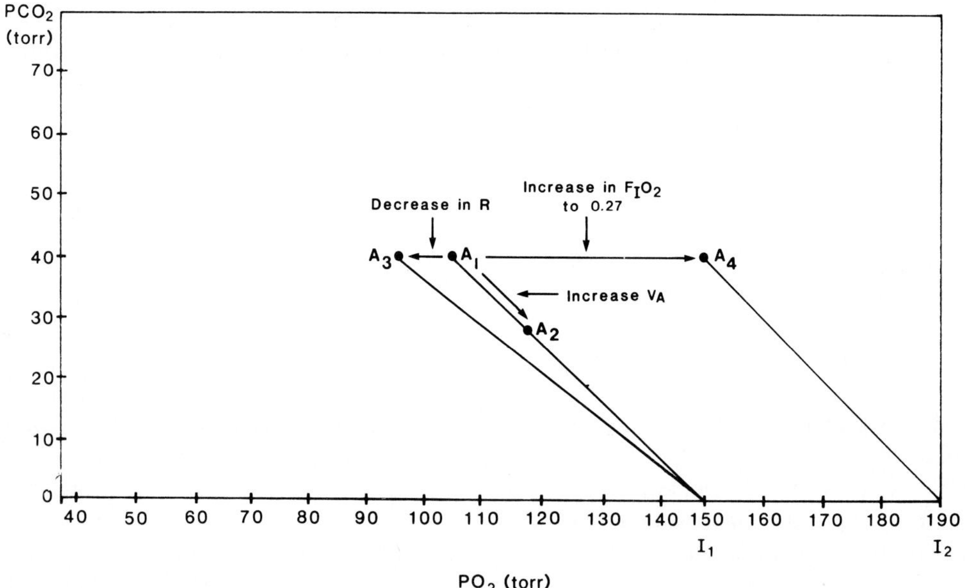

change would occur if the both O_2 consumption and CO_2 production were reduced by half while alveolar ventilation remained constant. Alterations to R change the slope of the line (A_3), and increasing the inspired concentration of oxygen moves the line to the right. The inspired point is repositioned at I_2 and the alveolar gas is thus represented by A_4.

Three-Compartment Model

Although the one-compartment lung described above is a useful simplification, it does not explain many of the abnormalities in gas exchange present in diseased lungs. These sources of inefficiency can be conceptualized by expansion to a three-compartment lung model.[7,40]

The three-compartment model (Fig. 3-10) is composed of three similar lung units that differ only by the presence or absence of (1) fresh gas flow (ventilation) or (2) venous blood flow (perfusion). The first compartment or shunt (compartment A in Fig. 3-10) receives perfusion but no ventilation. The ideal alveoli (compartment B in Figure 3-10) have both ventilation and perfusion, and the third compartment, the alveolar dead space (compartment C in Figure 3-10), receives ventilation but no perfusion.

Figure 3-10. Diagram of the three-compartment model. Compartment A (shunt) receives no fresh gas but is perfused by venous blood, compartment B (ideal alveoli) has equal ventilation and blood flow, and compartment C (alveolar dead space) is the converse of compartment A (ventilated but not perfused). All perfused compartments (A and B) receive the same mixed venous blood, whereas the compartments B and C receive the same fresh inspired gas. The respiratory gas tensions in compartment A are identical to the mixed venous blood, reflecting the lack of contribution from fresh inhaled gas. Without interaction with the blood, compartment C has the respiratory gas tensions present in humidified inspired air. Compartment B, with matched ventilation and perfusion, behaves according to the rules derived for the ideal alveolar gas in the one-compartment model described in the text. (Modified, with permission, from West.[40])

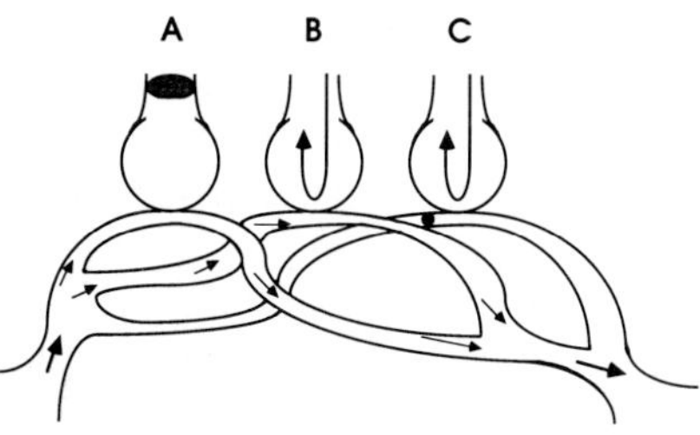

Each of the ventilated compartments receive the same inspired gas, and all perfusion involves the same mixed venous blood.[7] The tensions of respiratory gases that exist in each of the three lung units are the product of the total quantity of oxygen and carbon dioxide brought to that unit by inhaled gas and venous blood. Thus compartment A (no ventilation) has partial pressures of O_2 and CO_2 identical to those of mixed venous blood. At the other extreme, compartment C, which has no interaction with the blood, has the same respiratory gas tensions as in humidified, inspired air. Compartment B, with matched ventilation and perfusion, is the only part of the model that participates in the exchange of gases between the environment and the circulation. Compartment B behaves according to the rules derived for the ideal alveolar gas in the one-compartment model. Therefore the composition of its alveolar gas depends on (1) the inspired tensions of that gas, (2) the fresh gas flow (alveolar ventilation), and 3) the uptake of O_2 and the excretion of CO_2 ($\dot{V}O_2$ or $\dot{V}CO_2$).

The efficiency of whole lung function in the three-compartment model depends on the proportions of the total ventilation and total perfusion that are distributed to each of the three compartments.[7,36,41] If, for example, none of an individual's pulmonary blood flow is distributed to lung units that behave as shunt (compartment A) and none of the ventilation is distributed to alveolar dead space lung units (compartment B), then whole lung gas exchange is identical to the one-compartment model. Many diseases of the heart and lung cause the lung to behave as if it has regions that are not ventilated and regions that are not perfused, however. Arterial hypoxemia is caused by inefficient gas exchange associated with shunt compartments, whereas the presence of alveolar dead space is reflected in high minute ventilations necessary to achieve normal arterial CO_2 tensions or hypercardia.

The value of a three-compartment model in conceptualizing inefficient gas exchange is best demonstrated using an example. Consider a hypothetical patient: a 60-year-old, 70-kg man with mild emphysema and pneumonia causing consolidation of the right middle lobe. He is breathing air, with a minute ventilation ($\dot{V}_E$) of 8.5 liters at a respiratory frequency (f) of 15 (tidal volume [$\dot{V}_T$] = 8.5/15 or 0.567 liters). His cardiac output ($\dot{Q}_T$) is 5.5 liters and the conducting passage volume of his lung is 0.150 liters. On a regular diet, his oxygen consumption and CO_2 production are 0.300 liters and 0.250 liters per minute, respectively (R = 0.83). The mixed venous blood has a $P\bar{v}O_2$ of 40 mmHg and a $P\bar{v}CO_2$ of 47 mmHg. His hemoglobin is 15 g/dL. For the purpose of this example, it is assumed that the right middle lobe has no ventilation (shunt) and receives 15% of this cardiac output. Much of the ventilated portions of the lungs are emphysematous with disrupted airways and blood vessels; these regions behave like compartment C of the model.[41,42] In this hypothetical example such alveolar dead space regions receive 20% of the total minute ventilation. The remaining 85% percent of the cardiac output and 80% of the ventilation are distributed to the regions the lung that receive both ventilation and perfusion (ideal alveolar compartment).

Ideal Alveolar Compartment

Compartment B, the ideal alveoli, is the only compartment with effective ventilation. Therefore all alveolar ventilation is associated with this compartment. Eighty percent of the total ventilation is delivered to this compartment ($8.5 \cdot 0.8 = 6.8$ L). Similarly, 80% of the volume of the 0.150-liter conducting passage (anatomic dead space) is associated with the ideal alveolar compartment ($0.150 \cdot 0.8 = 0.120$ L). At 15 breaths/min, ventilation of these passages consumes 1.8 L/min ($0.120 \cdot 15 = 1.8$ L). Since: $\dot{V}_A = \dot{V}_{total} - \dot{V}_D$, then for compartment B of this example, $\dot{V}_A = 6.8 - 1.8$ liters $= 5.0$ liters.

Because the ideal alveolar compartment the only compartment of this model that participates in respiratory gas exchange, the algebraic expressions developed for the one-compartment model apply. Using Equation 3-43 when $\dot{V}CO_2 = 250$ mL, STPD applies, body temp is assumed to be 37°, V_A is liters BTPS, and k = 0.863:

$$(3\text{-}47) \quad P_ACO_2 = \frac{0.250 \text{ L/min}}{5.0 \text{ L/min}} \cdot 0.863 = 43.1 \text{ mmHg}$$

From equation 3-45

$$(3\text{-}48) \quad P_AO_2 = P_IO_2 - \frac{P_ACO_2}{R} - F_IO_2 \cdot \frac{(1-R)}{R}$$

Since R = 0.83 and P_IO_2 = 150 mmHg:

$$(3\text{-}49) \quad P_AO_2 = 150 - \frac{43.1}{0.83} + 0.21 \cdot \frac{(1-0.83)}{0.83} \cdot 43.1 = 108.75 \text{ mmHg}$$

Both the exhaled alveolar gas and effluent blood have the P_AO_2 and P_ACO_2 tensions calculated above because the pulmonary capillary blood and alveolar gas in each compartment are assumed to reach equilibrium.

The blood content of O_2 ($Cc'O_2$) is calculated and the CO_2 ($Cc'CO_2$) content is obtained from the nomogram.

(3-50) $Cc'O_2 = [(15.0 \cdot 1.34) \cdot .99(\% \text{ sat})] + (108.75 \cdot .003) = 20.23$ mL O_2/100 mL blood

(3-51) $Cc'CO_2$ (at a $PaCO_2$ of 43.1 mmHg and HbO_2 of 99%) = 47.0 mL CO_2/100 mL blood

Eighty-five percent of the cardiac output (5.5 L · 0.85 = 4.675 L [4675 mL]) is distributed to this compartment. Therefore:

(3-52) 4675 mL · 20.22/100 mL = 945.3 mL/min of O_2, and

(3-53) 4675 mL · 47.0/100 mL = 2197.3 mL/min of CO_2

These enter the arterial circulation from this compartment.

Alveolar Dead Space Compartment

In the one-compartment model, dead space ventilation was associated with the conducting passages. This ventilation was defined as the ineffective portion of the total ventilation. Considering first the conducting passage ventilation, their volume in the hypothetical patient is 0.150 L. At a respiratory frequency of 15 L they consume 2.25 L of the total minute ventilation (0.150 B/min · 15 = 2.25 L), and 20% of it (2.25 · 0.2 = 0.450 L) is associated with compartment C.

Using the more general definition of dead space ventilation as ineffective ventilation, its volume can be calculated by determining the difference between total ventilation and alveolar ventilation ($\dot{V}_D = \dot{V}_E - \dot{V}_A$ from Equation 3-29).[30] The total ventilation for this patient was given as 8.50 L and alveolar ventilation was determined above to be 5.00 L. Therefore:

(3-54) $\dot{V}_D = 8.5 - 5.0 = 3.5$ L

The discrepancy between the volume of dead space ventilation as calculated in Equation 3-29 and the volume of conducting passage ventilation (3.5 − 2.25 = 1.25 L) is due to the ventilation of nonperfused alveoli (compartment C). The conducting passage dead space is sometimes called "anatomic dead space," and the dead space associated with nonperfused alveoli is referred to as "alveolar dead space." The total dead space associated with compartment C is equal to its alveolar dead space and its portion of the conducting passage dead space (1.25 + 0.45 = 1.70 L). This total $\dot{V}_D$ equals compartment C's portion of the total ventilation (20%) as given above:

(3-55) $\dot{V}_D$ (compartment C) = 8.5 · 0.2 = 1.7 L

Shunt Compartment

No gas exchange occurs in the shunt compartment. The 15% of cardiac output distributed to these consolidated lung regions enters and leaves with the same partial pressures and contents of O_2 and CO_2 in mixed venous blood. In the hypothetical patient, this results in entering the arterial circulation from the shunt compartment of 122.3 mL of O_2 and 441.4 mL of CO_2 each minute.

$Cc'O_2 = (15 \cdot 1.34) \cdot (0.7) + (40 \cdot 003) = 14.82$ mL/100 mL blood

$Cc'CO_2$ (at a PCO_2 of 47 mmHg and HbO_2 of 70%) = 53.5 mL/100 mL blood

The blood flow to the compartment is 5.5 LP · 0.85 = 825.0 mL, therefore:

(825.0/100) · 14.82 = 122.3 mL/min of O_2, and (825.0/100) · 53.5 = 441.4 mL CO_2/min

These enter the arterial circulation from this compartment.

Impact of the Three-Compartment Model on PO_2 and PCO_2 in Mixed Arterial Blood and Exhaled Gas

Variations in the quantity of ventilation and blood flow to each of the three compartments in this lung model affect the efficiency of respiratory gas transfer in the lung. The partial pressure of gases in the arterial blood and mixed exhaled gas reflect these variations.

EXHALED GASES

Volume and Pressures in the Mixed Exhaled Gas ($\dot{V}E$ and PE). The mixed exhaled carbon dioxide in the hypothetical patient is calculated from equation 3-30:

$$\text{(3-56)} \quad PECO_2 = \frac{(\dot{V}D \cdot PICO_2 + \dot{V}A \cdot PACO_2)}{\dot{V}E}$$

The total dead space associated with this patient is 3.25 L, the alveolar ventilation is 5.0 L, and the partial pressure of inspired carbon dioxide is 0.0 mmHg.

$$\text{(3-57)} \quad PECO_2 = \frac{(3.25 \text{ L} \cdot [0]) + (5.0 \text{ L} \cdot [43.1])}{8.5} = 25.3 \text{ mmHg}$$

A similar-sized patient with the same alveolar ventilation and little or no alveolar dead space (compartment C) would have a total dead space of only 2.25 L. Minute ventilation would also be smaller.

$$\text{(3-58)} \quad \dot{V}D_{total} = \dot{V}D_{anatomic} + \dot{V}D_{alveolar} = 2.25 \text{ L} + 0.0 \text{ L} = 2.25 \text{ L}$$

$$\text{(3-59)} \quad \dot{V}E = \dot{V}D + \dot{V}A = 2.25 \text{ L} + 5.0 \text{ L} = 7.25 \text{ L}$$

The partial pressure of the mixed expired carbon dioxide is:

$$\text{(3-60)} \quad PECO_2 = \frac{(2.25 \text{ L} \cdot [0]) + (5.00 \text{ L} \cdot [43.1])}{7.50 \text{ L}} = 28.7 \text{ mmHg}$$

Volume and Pressures in the End Tidal Gas ($\dot{V}ET$ and PET). The end tidal gas ($\dot{V}ET$) is the last gas to be exhaled. In the three-compartment model, the composition of $\dot{V}ET$ is a mixture of the alveolar gases from compartment B and compartment C.[7] The contribution from compartment B is equal to its portion of the entire tidal volume minus its proportion of the conducting passage tidal ventilation. Similarly, the contribution of compartment C is proportional to its fraction of the total ventilation less the proportion of the conducting passage ventilation associated with C. The total end tidal volume is equal to the sum of $\dot{V}ET$ compartment B and $\dot{V}ET$ compartment C.

Thus:

$$\text{(3-61)} \quad \dot{V}ET \text{ (compartment B)} = (80\% \ \dot{V}T) - (80\% \text{ of the conducting passage volume}), \text{ so}$$

$$\dot{V}ET \text{ (compartment B)} = \frac{(0.8 \cdot 8.5)}{15} - (0.8 \cdot 0.150) = 0.333 \text{ L.}$$

$$\text{(3-62)} \quad \dot{V}ET \text{ (compartment C)} = (20\% \ VT) - (20\% \text{ of the conducting passage volume})$$

$$\dot{V}ET \text{ (compartment C)} = \frac{(0.2 \cdot 8.5)}{15} - (0.2 \cdot 0.120) = 0.089 \text{ L}$$

$$\text{(3-63)} \quad \text{Total end tidal volume } (\dot{V}ET \text{ total}) = \dot{V}ET \text{ compartment B} + \dot{V}ET \text{ compartment C}$$

$$\dot{V}ET_{total} = 0.333 + 0.089 = 0.422 \text{ L}$$

The partial pressure of CO_2 in the end tidal gas is a result of the mixture of compartment B and compartment C gases. Compartment B contributes gas with a partial pressure equal to the ideal alveolar CO_2, whereas compartment C contains CO_2 at a partial pressure equal to that of the inspired gas.

$$\text{(3-64)} \quad PETCO_2 = \frac{(\dot{V}ET \text{ (compartment B)} \cdot PACO_2) + (\dot{V}ET \text{ (compartment C)} \cdot PICO_2)}{\dot{V}ET \text{ total}}$$

$$PETCO_2 = \frac{(0.333 \text{ L} \cdot 43.1 \text{ mmHg} + (0.089 \text{ L} \cdot 0 \text{ mmHg})}{0.422 \text{ L}} = 34.0 \text{ mm}$$

In a similar-sized patient with the same alveolar ventilation and little or no alveolar dead space (compartment C), the end tidal CO_2 tension would equal the ideal alveolar CO_2 of 43.1 mmHg. Thus alveolar dead space (compartment C) is reflected in lower than expected values for both end tidal CO_2 ($P_{ET}CO_2$) and mixed expired CO_2 ($P_{ET}CO_2$) tensions.

ARTERIAL BLOOD. The partial pressures of gases in the arterial blood are also of interest. Contribution to the arterial blood comes only from compartments A (shunt) and B (ideal alveoli). Compartment B receives 85% of the cardiac output ($5.5 \cdot 0.85 = 4.68$ L/min), and the blood leaving this compartment contains the O_2 and CO_2 at the same partial pressure as that present in the alveoli. In compartment A, however, no gas exchange with the alveoli occurs. The 15% of the cardiac output ($5.5 \cdot 0.15 = 0.825$ L/min) distributed to compartment A enters the arterial circulation with respiratory gas composition identical to that of mixed venous blood. The mixed arterial blood contains O_2 and CO_2 in concentrations equal to the sum of the contents of each gas (O_2 and CO_2), leaving the two perfused compartments divided by the total blood flow leaving the two compartments.

Table 3-2 demonstrates that the resulting arterial blood has an O_2 content of 18.9 mL/dL and CO_2 content of 47.0 mL/100 mL blood; therefore has an O_2 partial pressure is 80.2 mmHg and the CO_2 partial pressure is 40 mmHg. However, the cardiac output is entirely distributed to the ideal alveoli (compartment B), then the arterial blood would have the same respiratory gas partial pressures as in the ideal alveolar gas (P_AO_2 of 108 mmHg, P_ACO_2 of 43.1 mmHg. However, in the example, 20% of the total cardiac output is distributed to regions of the lung that behave as shunt (compartment A). The effect of shunt compartments is to reduce the arterial O_2 tension to values lower than the ideal alveoli with minimal increase in arterial carbon dioxide tensions.

The Shunt Equation

The Bohr expression (equation 3-33) provides a useful algebraic expression to calculate wasted ventilation. An analogous expression can be derived to quantitate the shunt (compartment A). Underlying this derivation is the principle that the size of the difference in the O_2 tension between the ideal alveoli and the arterial blood is proportional to the percentage of total circulation directed to the shunt compartment.[7] Thus the shunt compartment perfusion can be quantified through comparison of the ideal alveoli to the mixed arterial blood.

O_2 consumption can be calculated by examining the difference between the mixed arterial and the mixed venous blood.[43]

$$\dot{V}O_2 = (\text{volume } O_2 \text{ arterial blood per minute}) - (\text{volume } O_2 \text{ venous blood per minute}) \qquad (3\text{-}65)$$

By rearrangement and dividing both sides by the total cardiac output (Q_T):

Table 3-2. Arterial Blood Gas Contents and Pressures (Three-Compartment Model)

Compartment	O_2 Content/ (Partial Pressure)	CO_2 Content/ (Partial Pressure)	Flow	Total O_2	Total CO_2
A	14.5 mL/dL (40 mmHg)	52 mL/dL (47 mmHg)	5.25 dL	130.5 mL	468 mL
B	20 mL/dL (108.8 mmHg)	47 mL/dL (43.1 mmHg)	46.8 dL	1020 mL	2397 mL
C	0.0 mL/dL	0.0 mL/dL	0 dL	0 mL	0 mL
Total	18.9 mL/dL (80 mmHg)	47 mL/dL (40 mmHg)	55 dL	1150.5 mL	2865.0 mL

$$\text{(3-66)} \quad \frac{\text{Volume } \dot{O}_2 \text{ arterial blood per minute}}{\dot{Q}T} = \frac{\text{(Volume } \dot{O}_2 \text{ venous blood per minute)}}{\dot{Q}T} + \frac{\dot{V}O_2}{\dot{Q}T}$$

Since total volume of O_2 per minute divided by cardiac output (volume of blood per minute) is equal to the O_2 concentration, equation 3-66 can be written:

$$\text{(3-67)} \quad CaO_2 = C\bar{v}O_2 + \frac{\dot{V}O_2}{\dot{Q}T}$$

Rearrangement gives:

$$\text{(3-68)} \quad (CaO_2 - C\bar{v}O_2) = \frac{\dot{V}O_2}{\dot{Q}T}$$

Since gas exchange with the environment occurs only in the lungs, O_2 consumption is also determined by examining the volume of O_2 entering via the lungs each minute. In the three compartment model, only the ideal alveoli participates in the exchange.

$$\text{(3-69)} \quad \dot{V}O_2 = [O_2 \text{ (mL) exiting the ideal alveolar compartment}] - [O_2 \text{ (mL) carried to the ideal alveolar compartment}]$$

The minute volumes of O_2 are the products of blood concentration and flow, thus:

$$\text{(3-70)} \quad \dot{V}O_2 = (\text{ideal compartment blood flow} \cdot Cc'O_2) - (\text{ideal compartment blood flow} \cdot C\bar{v}O_2)$$

where $Cc'O_2$ is the concentration of oxygen in the pulmonary capillary of the ideal compartment.

If the blood flow to the shunt compartment is $\dot{Q}s$, then blood flow to the ideal alveoli must be equal to the total cardiac output minus the shunt flow ($\dot{Q}T - \dot{Q}s$). Equation 3-70 can then be written:

$$\text{(3-71)} \quad \dot{V}O_2 = ([\dot{Q}T - \dot{Q}s] \cdot Cc'O_2) - ([\dot{Q}T - \dot{Q}s)] \cdot C\bar{v}O_2)$$

By rearrangement:

$$\text{(3-72)} \quad \dot{V}O_2 = (\dot{Q}T - \dot{Q}s) \cdot (Cc'O_2 - C\bar{v}O_2)$$

Combining the two expressions for oxygen consumption (equations 3-68 and 3-72) gives:

$$\text{(3-73)} \quad \dot{Q}T\,(CaO_2 - C\bar{v}O_2) = (\dot{Q}T - Qs) \cdot (Cc'O_2 - C\bar{v}O_2)$$

Rearrangement to solve for the fraction of total cardiac output distributed to the shunt compartment[44]:

$$\text{(3-74)} \quad \frac{\dot{Q}s}{\dot{Q}T} = \frac{CaO_2 - Cc'O_2}{Cc'O_2 - C\bar{v}O_2}$$

In order to determine the content of oxygen in the ideal compartment pulmonary capillary blood ($Cc'O_2$), the partial pressure of O_2 in the pulmonary capillary blood is assumed to be the same as that in the ideal alveolar gas (3-15). The concentration of hemoglobin in the capillary is assumed to be the same as in both the mixed venous and arterial blood. The O_2 content in the pulmonary capillary is calculated from these variables.[39]

$$\text{(3-75)} \quad PAO_2 \text{ (ideal alveolar compartment)} = 107.0 \text{ mmHg (saturation 99\%)}$$

$$Cc'O_2 = (1.34 \cdot 15.0 \text{ g/100 mL}) \cdot (0.99) + 107 \cdot (0.003 \text{ mL/100 mL/mmHg}) = 20 \text{ mL/100 mL blood}$$

Using the values from the hypothetical patient above where: CaO_2 = 18.9 mL/100 mL blood, $C\bar{v}O_2$ = 14.5 mL/100 mL blood, Hgb = 15.0 g/100 mL blood, and $\dot{Q}T$ = 5.5 L/min, and substituting all variables into Equation 3-73:

$$\text{(3-76)} \quad \frac{\dot{Q}s}{QT} = \frac{(18.9 - 20.0) \text{ mL/100 mL blood}}{(20.0 - 14.5) \text{ mL/100 mL blood}} = \frac{1.1 \text{ mL/100 mL blood}}{5.5 \text{ mL/100 mL blood}} = 0.2, \text{ or } 20\%$$

The respiratory gas tensions associated with the three compartments of the model for the hypothetical patient can be depicted on the O_2-CO_2 diagram in Figure 3-11. The points v, A_i, and I are the mixed venous, ideal alveolar, and inspired gas tensions, respectively. These points also correspond, to the compartments A, B, and C, respectively in Figure 3-10. The patient's whole O_2 consumption and CO_2 production result in an R value of 0.8 which define the blood gas R lines. The straight line extending from the inspired point I is the gas R line. The distance between any two points on that line represents a ratio of change in content of O_2 to CO_2 of 0.8. Similarly, the blood R line is the curve extending from point $\bar{v}$; this blood line follows a course such that the distance between any two points represents a ratio of change in O_2 and CO_2 contents of 0.8. The intersection of blood and gas R lines occurs at point A_i. At A_i, the respiratory gas tensions are equal to the ideal alveolar gas tensions and can be calculated using the algebraic relationships developed for the one-compartment model.

The values derived for the sample patient, for the mixed expired (E), mixed alveolar (A) and arterial (a) tensions are plotted in the figure. The mixed expired and mixed alveolar points fall on the gas R line at higher O_2 and lower CO_2 tensions than the ideal alveolar point. Similarly, the arterial blood point is on the blood R line at lower O_2 and higher CO_2 partial pressures than the ideal alveolar gas. The distance that the arterial point is displaced from A_i along the blood R line is proportional to the percentage of cardiac output that perfuses

Figure 3-11. The respiratory gas tensions associated with the three-compartment model. For the hypothetical patient, these tensions can be depicted on the $O_2 - CO_2$ diagram. The points $\bar{v}$, A_i, and I show the mixed venous, ideal alveolar, and inspired gas tensions, respectively. These points also correspond to the compartments A, B, and C of Figure 3-10. For this hypothetical patient.

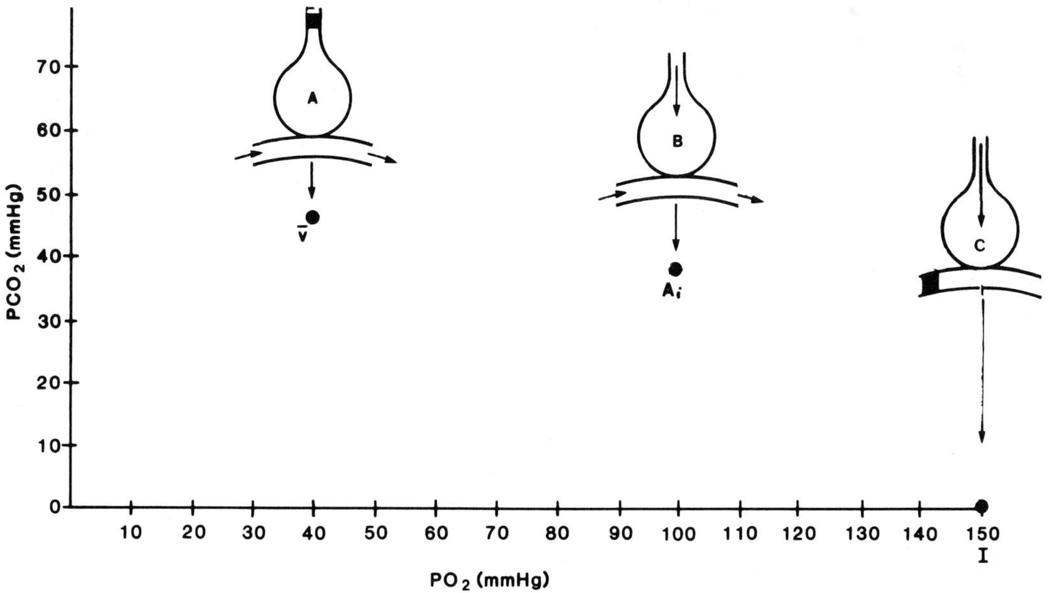

shunt regions (compartment A) of the lung.[20] Note that even a small amount of shunt (compartment A) has a great impact on the difference between the alveolar and arterial O_2 tension but minimal a effect on the CO_2 tension (see below).

Multicompartment Model

Two lungs of a human adult together have approximately 300 million alveoli. Therefore it is unlikely that each of these many units behaves identically or even that just three variations account for all the possible functional differences of such a large number of gas exchanging units. Despite the very useful concepts derived with the one- and three-compartment schemes, these model are incomplete. The three-compartment model does, however, provide a clue to the variable missing from these more simple schemes. The ideal alveolar compartment behaves just like the one-compartment model and is joined by two compartments that are the most extreme cases of ventilation perfusion imbalance. Thus the three-compartment model introduces ventilation-perfusion ratio ($\dot{V}A/\dot{Q}c'$) as a factor in the efficiency of respiratory gas exchange. The infinite number of other possible combinations of ventilation and perfusion that fall in between shunt, ideal alveoli, and alveolar dead space are not included in the three-compartment model. A multicompartment model is necessary to include the impact of ventilation to perfusion balance on pulmonary gas exchange.

Source of Variation in Ventilation and Perfusion

A complete discussion of the many influences on the distribution of gas flow and blood flow the lung is beyond the scope of this chapter. Brief mention of some of these factors is necessary, however, to demonstrate the importance of $\dot{V}A/\dot{Q}c'$ as a cause of inefficient gas exchange in respiratory or circulatory disease.

DISTRIBUTION OF VENTILATION. Variation in the fresh gas flow to different regions in the lung is produced by several mechanisms, including (1) uneven distribution of the forces that pull the lung open on inspiration[45,46]; (2) regional differences in airways resistance (pressure to flow relationships)[47]; (3) regional differences in lung compliance (pressure-volume relationship[48]; (4) regional differences in the interaction of resistance and compliance (the time constant for lung filling and emptying); and (5) regional differences in the gas volume present at end exhalation (FRC).[49]

In healthy lungs, these factors interact in many ways. The net result is an increased distribution of ventilation to the dependent portions of the lung.[50] In diseased states, much more variation in these factors occurs, and the distribution of gas flow within the lung cannot easily be predicted. Chest wall deformity, trauma, pain, pleural fluid, and air collections and encroachment by intra-abdominal structures alter the regional distribution of the forces of inspiration during spontaneous breathing.[39] Positive-pressure mechanical ventilation redistributes fresh gas flow to the nondependent lung fields.[45] Bronchospasm, mucosal swelling, increased quantity of airway secretions, and airway compression from adjacent structures (interstitial water, enlarged pulmonary or bronchial blood vessels, or inflammatory cellular infiltrate) increase airway resistance. Increased volume of water, inflammatory infiltrate, or fibrosis in the interstitium and reduced production of alveolar surfactants alter lung compliance.[51] Extreme heterogenicity of the regional time constants for gas flow into and out of the lung occur in patients with chronic lung disorders who may also have coexisting acute disease. Regional differences in end-expiratory volume and alveolar dead space are present in many lung diseases, notably emphysema and asthma.[52,53]

REGIONAL BLOOD FLOW. The distribution of blood flow within the lung depends on the interaction of the hydrostatic pressure change from pulmonary artery to veins and the pulmonary vascular resistance. Several factors influence this balance, including (1) the hydrostatic pressure within the pulmonary blood vessels, which in turn, is related to the force generated by the heart and the effect of gravity; (2) the smooth muscle tone of the pulmonary blood vessels, which in turn is related to the lung volume, perivascular oxygen tension, and acid-base balance, age, and other factors; and (3) the pressure outside the vessels, which is the net result of alveolar, interstitial and pleural pressures.[54,55]

Perfusion distribution within a healthy lung demonstrates a pattern depicted in Figure 3-12. Diseases greatly influence this pattern, however.[55] Heart disease and anesthetic agents affect the hydrostatic forces with the pulmonary vasculature profoundly by altering the force generated by the heart. Positional changes alone have only a small influence on pulmonary hydrostatics by altering the influence of gravity. In combination with variations in cardiac function, however, such changes may greatly affect blood flow distribution.[56] Chronic lung and heart disease and anesthetic medications dramatically affect pulmonary vascular tone. Positive-pressure ventilation influences pleural and alveolar pressures.[56–58]

SOURCE OF VARIATION IN $\dot{V}A/\dot{Q}c'$. The interaction of all the above mentioned factors on ventilation and perfusion distribution results in marked variation of $\dot{V}A/\dot{Q}c'$ in disease.[59] A model of pulmonary gas exchange that includes $\dot{V}A/\dot{Q}c'$ as a variable is required for multiple compartments in order to explain the inefficiency in lung function that results from disease or medications.[59,60]

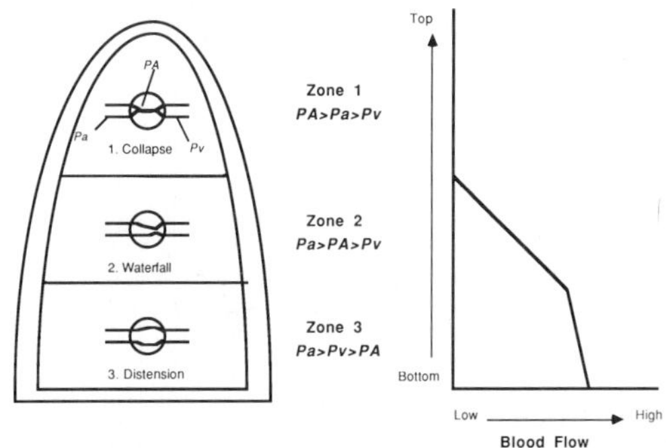

Figure 3-12. Schematic presentation of the distribution of blood flow within the lung, which depends on the balance between the hydrostatic pressure change from pulmonary artery to veins and the pulmonary vascular resistance. In the healthy lung of an upright human this balance is most dramatically influenced by the interaction between the hydrostatic effects of gravity and the distribution of alveolar and pleural pressure. In the upper portion of the lung (zone 1), alveolar pressure (*PA*) is greater than both the pulmonary arterial pressure (P_a) and pulmonary venous pressure (P_v). In the middle portion of the lung (zone 2), P_a is greater than *PA*. This in turn is greater than venous pressure; therefore, the vessels tend to constrict towards the outlet end. Flow in zone 2 is proportional to the difference between the arterial and alveolar pressures.[54] In the lower lung (zone 3), both the arterial and venous pressures exceed PA so the capillaries are distended, and blood flow is maximized. (Modified, with permission, from West.[37])

Algebraic Derivation of $\dot{V}A/\dot{Q}c'$

In order to place the concept of $\dot{V}A/\dot{Q}c'$ within the principles introduced with the one- and three-compartment lung models, a visual analogy (Fig. 3-13) and demonstration of the algebraic relationships between $\dot{V}A/\dot{Q}c'$, respiratory gas exchange, and the alveolar gas tensions is useful.[61] As with the derivations of the alveolar

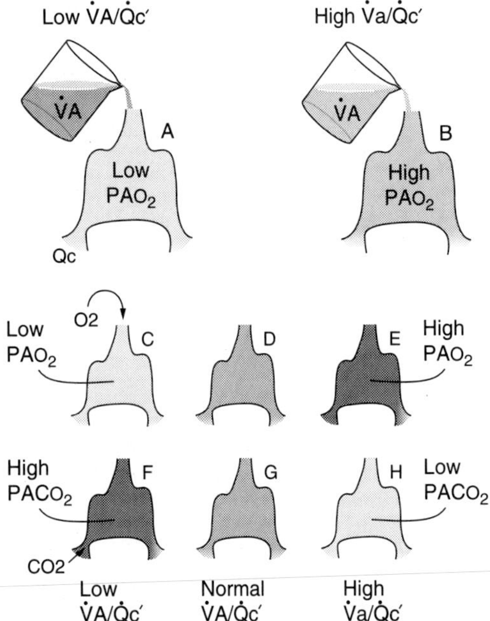

Figure 3-13. Schematic presentations of the impact of $\dot{V}_A/\dot{Q}c'$ ratio on the partial pressures and content of oxygen and carbon dioxide of a given lung unit. This effect is often represented by the analogy of dye being added to a chamber with continuously flowing water.[38] The concentration of the dye within the chamber depends on the balance between the mass of dye poured in per unit time ($\dot{V}_A$) and the volume of water flowing through the chamber per unit time ($\dot{Q}c'$). Thus in A, $\dot{V}_A/\dot{Q}c'$ is equal to dye concentration in grams per liter. At higher $\dot{V}_A/\dot{Q}c'$ ratios, increased dye entry ($\dot{V}_A$) or decreased rate of water flowing through the chamber results in a higher concentration of dye in the chamber until at infinitely high $\dot{V}_A/\dot{Q}c'$ the concentration of dye in the chamber is equal to its concentration as it is poured (B).

Similarly, the effect of $\dot{V}_A/\dot{Q}c'$ on alveolar concentration of oxygen in the alveoli of lung units with varying $\dot{V}_A/\dot{Q}c'$ ratios is shown in C and D. At high $\dot{V}_A/\dot{Q}c'$ ratios alveolar oxygen tension approaches that of the inspired gas; conversely, at low $\dot{V}_A/\dot{Q}c'$ ratios, the alveolar oxygen concentration is much lower (E). The effect of $\dot{V}_A/\dot{Q}c'$ on alveolar concentration of carbon dioxide is represented by simply reversing the analogy so that the dye enters from the venous circulation ($\dot{Q}c'$) and ventilation ($\dot{V}_A$) is the diluting water. The diagrams in F, G, and H demonstrate that high $\dot{V}_A/\dot{Q}c'$ results in a lower concentration of carbon dioxide, whereas a low $\dot{V}_A/\dot{Q}c'$ increases its concentration toward that in the mixed venous blood.

Viewed together, the diagrams in C through H show the impact of $\dot{V}_A/\dot{Q}c'$ on both oxygen and carbon dioxide. In lung units with low $\dot{V}_A/\dot{Q}c'$ the oxygen concentration is low, whereas the carbon dioxide concentration is high (the respiratory gas tensions approach that of the mixed venous blood). As $\dot{V}_A/\dot{Q}c'$ increases, oxygen tension rises while the carbon dioxide tension falls; the lung unit gas concentrations approach that of the inspired gas. (Modified, with permission, from West.[37])

gas equations, these relationships are based on the principle that at equilibrium the lung exchange of respiratory gases equals the metabolic consumption of O_2 and production of CO_2. The exchange of N_2 is zero. To reduce complexity, these interactions are described under the simple conditions of air breathing and in the absence of inspired CO_2.

Either O_2 or CO_2 can be used to illustrate the relationship. Carbon dioxide can be expressed using its gas phase equation:

$$\text{(3-77)} \quad \dot{V}CO_2 = (P_ACO_2 \cdot \dot{V}_A) \cdot (P_B - 47) \cdot k$$

For the blood phase:

$$\text{(3-78)} \quad \dot{V}CO_2 = \dot{Q} \cdot (C\bar{v}CO_2 - CaCO_2)$$

At equilibrium the CO_2 exchange in the gas phase must equal its exchange in the blood. Thus:

$$\text{(3-79)} \quad P_ACO_2 \cdot \dot{V}_A \cdot (P_B - 47) \cdot K = \dot{Q}c' \cdot (C\bar{v}CO_2 - CaCO_2)$$

By rearrangement:

$$\text{(3-80)} \quad \frac{\dot{V}_A}{\dot{Q}c'} = K \cdot \frac{(C\bar{v}CO_2 - CaCO_2)}{P_ACO_2}$$

The constant K equals 8.63 and is necessary to reconcile CO_2 blood content expressed in mL at STPD. VA is expressed in L at BTPS).

This derivation demonstrates the relationship central to understanding the importance of $\dot{V}A/\dot{Q}c'$ in lung function. The $\dot{V}A/\dot{Q}c'$ ratio links total respiratory gas exchange ($\dot{V}CO_2$ in the example above) to the gas content changes in the alveoli ($PACO_2 - 0$ in the example) and the blood ($C\bar{v}CO_2 - CaCO_2$). Substitution into 3-41 and 3-45 gives:

$$PACO_2 = PICO_2 + \frac{(C\bar{v}CO_2 - CaCO_2)}{\dot{V}A/\dot{Q}c'} \cdot \left([PB - 47) - PICO_2 \cdot \frac{[1 - R]}{R}\right) \quad (3\text{-}81)$$

and

$$PAO_2 = PIO_2 - \frac{(CaO_2 - C\bar{v}O_2)}{\dot{V}A/\dot{Q}c'} \cdot [(PB - 47) - PIO_2 (1 - R)] \quad (3\text{-}82)$$

The above expressions demonstrate that the $PACO_2$ increases from the inspired value to a level inversely proportional to the $\dot{V}A/\dot{Q}c'$ ratio, whereas the PAO_2 is lowered from the inhaled value to a value inversely proportional to the $\dot{V}A/\dot{Q}c'$. In other words, PAO_2 is directly related to $\dot{V}A/\dot{Q}c'$, and $PACO_2$ is related inversely to $\dot{V}A/\dot{Q}c'$. In the one-compartment model, alveolar gas tensions were determined by examining the following factors: (1) the inspired partial pressure of the gas, (2) the alveolar ventilation, and (3) the uptake of the gas. The above relationships for ventilation and perfusion allow the list of influences of alveolar gas tension to be condensed to (1) the inspired partial pressure of the gas, (2) the alveolar uptake or excretion of the gas, and (3) the $\dot{V}A/\dot{Q}c'$ ratio.[61]

The $\dot{V}A/\dot{Q}c'$ Distribution, the O_2-CO_2 Diagram, and the $\dot{V}A/\dot{Q}c'$ Line

The relationship of the $\dot{V}A/\dot{Q}c'$ distribution to the more simple one- and three-compartment models can be illustrated with the O_2-CO_2 diagram.[22] Figure 3-14 shows the now familiar two-axis diagram with partial pressure of O_2 on the abscissa and the partial pressure of CO_2 on the ordinate. The inspired composition of gas and mixed venous blood points are indicated by points at I and v, respectively. The straight lines radiating from point I are the gas R lines. For each line the change in gas tensions between any two points represents the partial pressures of O_2 and CO_2 that result if the ratio of change in CO_2 to O_2 is equal to the R value depicted above the line. The gas R lines are straight because the relationship between partial pressure and volume for O_2 and CO_2 in the gas phase is linear. The curved lines radiating from the mixed venous point ($\bar{v}$) are the blood R lines are the exchange ratio isopleths for O_2 and CO_2 in the pulmonary capillary blood. The blood R lines are curved because of the nonlinear partial pressure-volume relationships for O_2 and CO_2 in the blood.

Assuming that the consumption of O_2 and production of CO_2 by the alveolar tissue is trivial in comparison to exchanged volumes, then for each lung unit the volume of O_2 leaving the gas phase must be equal to the volume entering the blood. Similarly, the volume of CO_2 exiting the blood must be equal to that entering the gas phase. More simply stated, in each lung compartment at steady state, the gas R must equal the blood R. Assuming that there is little limitation to diffusion of gases as well, the values of PO_2 and PCO_2 in the alveolar gas of the compartment are identical to that in the compartment pulmonary capillary blood. Thus, the point of intersection of the blood and gas R lines of equal value identifies the O_2 and CO_2 partial pressures that must exist in the lung compartment that is exchanging gas at the defined R value.[22,61] Furthermore, the line that connects the blood-gas R intersection points defines a curve that represents the only possible values for oxygen and carbon dioxide tensions in the multiple compartments of a lung receiving in-

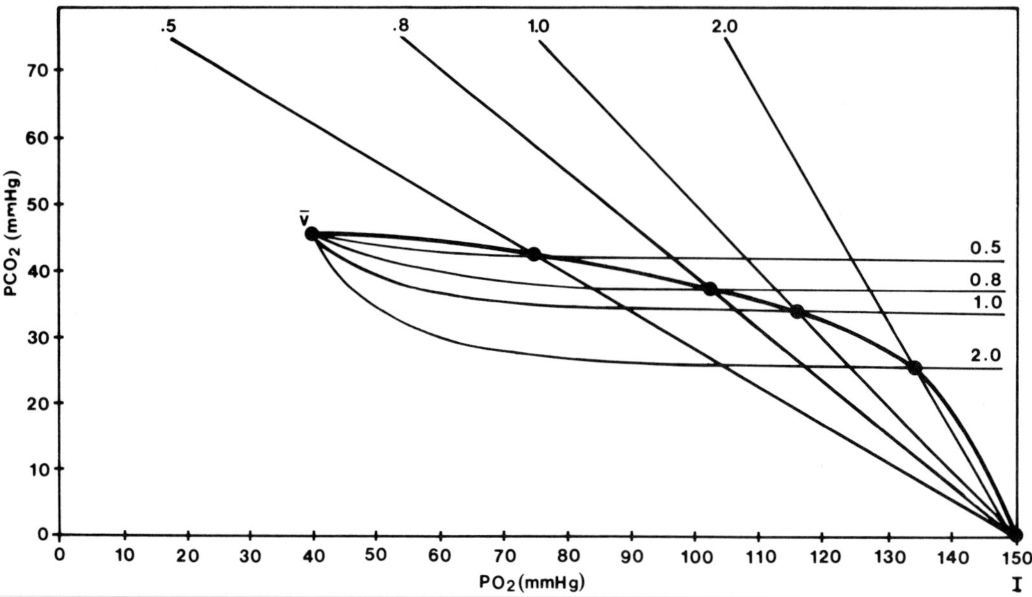

Figure 3-14. The $\dot{V}A/\dot{Q}c'$ distribution, the $O_2 - CO_2$ diagram, and the $\dot{V}A/\dot{Q}c'$ line. The figure shows the now familiar two-axis diagram with partial pressure of O_2 on the abscissa and the partial pressure of CO_2 on the ordinate. The inspired composition of gas and mixed venous blood points are indicated by the inspired point (I) and the mixed venous point ($\bar{v}$), respectively. The straight lines radiating from point I are the gas R lines. For each line, the change in gas tensions between any two points represents the partial pressures of oxygen and carbon dioxide that result if the ratio of change in carbon dioxide to oxygen is equal to R value above the line. The curved lines that radiate from $\bar{v}$ are the blood R lines depict the exchange ratio isopleths for oxygen and carbon dioxide in the pulmonary capillary blood.

In each lung compartment at steady state, the gas R must equal the blood R. The point of intersection of the blood and gas R lines of equal value identifies the oxygen and carbon dioxide partial pressures that must exist in the lung compartment that is exchanging gas at the defined R value (see text). The line connecting the blood-gas R intersection points (the $\dot{V}A/\dot{Q}c'$ line) defines a curve that represents the only possible values for oxygen and carbon dioxide tensions in the multiple compartments of a lung receiving inspired gas defined by I and mixed venous blood defined by $\bar{v}$. (Modified with permission from Rahn and Fenn.[22])

spired gas defined by point I and mixed venous blood defined by point $\bar{v}$.[22,61]

If a lung compartment has a very low ventilation in proportion to its perfusion (low $\dot{V}A/\dot{Q}c'$), then the gas tensions in the compartment approach the values of the mixed venous blood (similar to compartment A of the three-compartment model). Alternatively, if a compartment has excess ventilation compared to its perfusion (high $\dot{V}A/\dot{Q}c'$), then its gas tensions approach that of the inspired gas (similar to compartment C). In the O_2-CO_2 diagram of the multiple compartment model, as the compartment's $\dot{V}A/\dot{Q}c'$ ratio increases from zero to infinity, the gas tensions move from left ($\bar{v}$) to right (I) along the line. The relationship of the three-compartment model to the continuous distribution of $\dot{V}A/\dot{Q}c'$ ratios depicted with the O_2-CO_2 diagram is illustrated in Figure 3-15.

The $\dot{V}A/\dot{Q}c'$ for any compartment is quan-

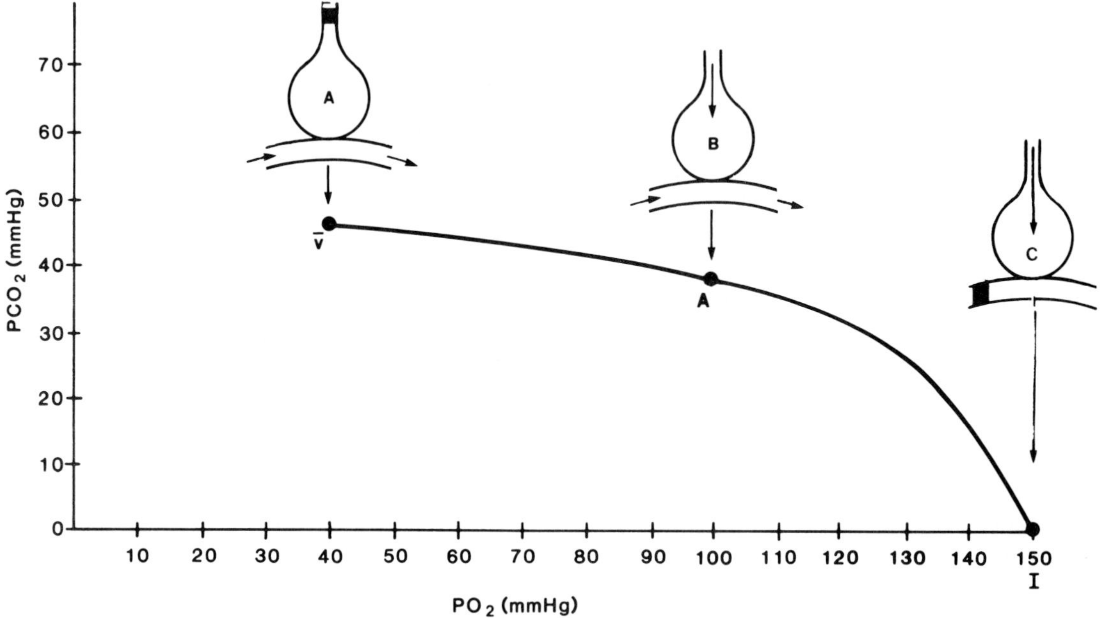

Figure 3-15. Relationship of the three-compartment model to the continuous distribution of $\dot{V}A/\dot{Q}c'$ ratios depicted with the O_2-CO_2 diagram. If a lung compartment has a low $\dot{V}A/\dot{Q}c'$, then the gas tensions in the compartment approach the values of the mixed venous blood (similar to compartment A). Alternatively, if a compartment has excess ventilation compared to its perfusion (high $\dot{V}A/\dot{Q}c'$) then its gas tensions approach that of the inspired gas (similar to compartment C). In the O_2-CO_2 diagram of the multiple compartment model, as the compartment's $\dot{V}A/\dot{Q}c'$ ratio increases from zero to infinity, the gas tensions are identified by moving from left ($\bar{v}$) to right (I) along the line. (Modified, with permission, from West.[37])

tified by solving equation 3-79 using the values for PO_2, and PCO_2 identified by the $\dot{V}A/\dot{Q}c'$ line or R lines. For example, at the intersection of the blood and gas R lines with a value of 0.8, the PO_2, and PCO_2 are 105 mmHg and 40 mmHg, respectively. The mixed venous to pulmonary capillary content difference for CO_2 is 4.3 mL CO_2/liter blood (determined from the CO_2 partial pressures identified from the diagram and from a blood nomogram or reference to Fig. 3-4). Substitution of these values into the equation allows precise determination of the $\dot{V}A/\dot{Q}c'$ ratio for that compartment:

$$\text{(3-83)} \quad \frac{\dot{V}A}{Qc'} = K \cdot \frac{(C\bar{v}CO_2 - CaCO_2)}{PACO_2} = \frac{(8.63) \cdot (4.3)}{40} = 0.93$$

The points of the line represent not only PO_2, PCO_2, and R, but also the $\dot{V}A/\dot{Q}c'$ for each compartment of a lung with the given values for inspired gas and mixed venous blood. Thus the curve connecting the intersecting blood and gas R lines in Figure 3-14 is often called the $\dot{V}A/\dot{Q}c'$ line.[22,61] Since the shape and course of the line is established by position of the mixed venous and inspired points, the location of any given gas exchanging compartment on the line is determined if any one of the variables P_{O_2}, P_{CO_2}, R, or $\dot{V}_A/\dot{Q}c'$ is also known.

The relationship of the three-compartment model to the continuous distribution of $\dot{V}_A/\dot{Q}c'$ ratios depicted with the O_2-CO_2 diagram is again illustrated in Figure 3-15. The basic determinants of partial pressures of the respiratory gases in any lung compartment can be simplified to (1) the composition of the inspired gas, (2) the composition of the mixed venous blood, and (3) the ventilation-perfusion ratio of the compartment. Each compartment in the multiple compartment model exchanges respiratory gases at different rates and with different values for P_{O_2}, P_{CO_2}, R, and $\dot{V}_A/\dot{Q}c'$. In addition, each compartment contributes to whole lung gas exchange in proportion to its percent of the total cardiac output and total ventilation.

Impact of $\dot{V}_A/\dot{Q}c'$ Heterogeneity on Pulmonary Gas Exchange

The impact of the $\dot{V}_A/\dot{Q}c'$ heterogeneity on the efficiency of lung function is illustrated in Figure 3-16 and Table 3-3.[62] Differences in pulmonary blood flow and alveolar ventilation in the normal, upright lung result in regional differences in the $\dot{V}_A/\dot{Q}c'$ ratio and therefore regional differences in the respiratory gas tensions.[62, 63] The regions of differing $\dot{V}_A/\dot{Q}c'$ ratio are represented by the 11 points on the $\dot{V}_A/\dot{Q}c'$ line. The hypothetical values for ventilation and perfusion to each of the 11 compartments and the composition of the mixed venous blood, the inhaled gas, are given in table 3-3. These values determine the $\dot{V}_A/\dot{Q}c'$ ratio of each compartment and P_{O_2}, P_{CO_2}, and R for each compartment. The $\dot{V}_{O_2}$ and $\dot{V}_{CO_2}$ for each compartment can be calculated from either the gas or blood phase. Using the gas phase, the product of the inhaled to compartment partial pressure differences for each gas is multiplied by the ventilation to each compartment. Alternatively, using the blood phase, the capillary to mixed venous blood content difference for each gas multiplied by the compartmental blood flow gives the same values. The sum CO_2 excretion divided by the sum of O_2 uptake for all compartments gives the whole lung R (equal to the metabolic RQ). Similarly, the sum of all compartment ventilations divided by the sum of all blood flows gives the mean lung $\dot{V}_A/\dot{Q}c'$.

The point of intersection of the blood and gas R lines of equal value to the whole body respiratory quotient (RQ) identifies point A_i on Figure 3-16. This point is called the ideal point because it represents the respiratory gas tensions of a single compartment lung or a multiple compartment lung in which there is no heterogeneity of $\dot{V}_A/\dot{Q}c'$.[36, 62, 63] The partial pressures for O_2 and CO_2 in the mixed alveolar gas (point A) may be obtained by multiplying the partial pressure of respiratory gases in each compartment by the compartment ventilation and dividing the sum of these values by the total alveolar ventilation. The partial pressure of the respiratory gases in the arterial blood (point a) is obtained in a similar manner by summing the products of compartment blood flow and respiratory blood gas content and dividing by the total flow. The mean gas content must then be converted to gas tension.

In Figure 3-16 the points representing the different regions within the normal lung are scattered to either side of the ideal point; they illustrate the variation around a central value for $\dot{V}_A/\dot{Q}c'$ for different segments of a normal lung. This heterogeneity of $\dot{V}_A/\dot{Q}c'$ in the normal lung leads to slightly different values for O_2 and CO_2 partial pressures at the mixed alveolar, ideal, and arterial points, but each value is related to the whole lung R lines. The ideal point (A_i) sits on the $\dot{V}_A/\dot{Q}c'$ line at the intersection of blood and gas R lines, the mixed alveolar point (A) occupies a place on the gas R line slightly closer to the inspired gas point (I) and the arte-

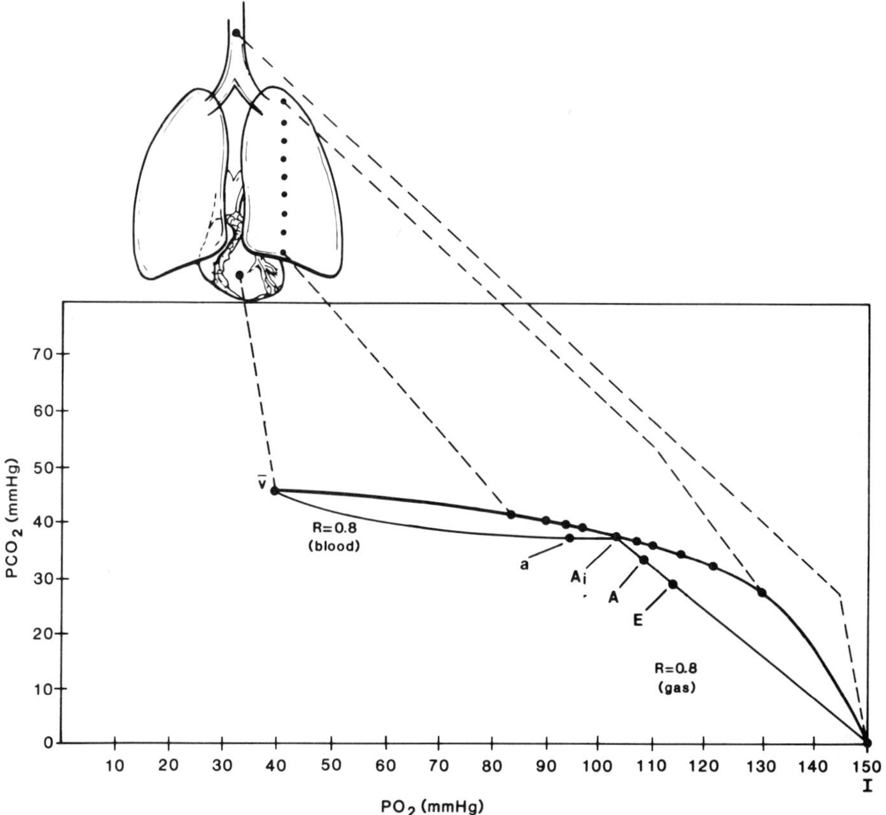

Figure 3-16. Multiple compartment model and the $O_2 - CO_2$ diagram illustrating the impact of the $\dot{V}A/\dot{Q}c'$ heterogeneity on the efficiency of lung function (also shown in Table 3-3). Differences in pulmonary blood flow and alveolar ventilation within the normal, upright lung result in regional differences in the $\dot{V}A/\dot{Q}c'$ ratio and therefore, differences in the respiratory gas tensions. The regions of varying $\dot{V}A/\dot{Q}c'$ ratio are represented by the 11 points on the $\dot{V}A/\dot{Q}c'$ line and the hypothetical values for ventilation and perfusion to each of the nine compartments. The composition of the mixed venous blood and the inhaled gas are listed in Table 3-3. (See text for further details.) (Modified, with permission, from West.[38 (p37)].

rial point (a) lies on the blood R line closer to the mixed venous blood ($\bar{v}$).

Figure 3-17 provides a magnified view of the three points in the normal lung described above. The distance along the gas R line that the mixed alveolar point (A) is displaced from the ideal point (A_i) is proportional to the fraction of total ventilation delivered to compartments; $\dot{V}A/\dot{Q}c'$ is higher than the mean $\dot{V}A/\dot{Q}c'$ of the entire lung.[22, 62, 63] Similarly, the distance on the blood R line that the arterial point (a) ranges from the ideal point is proportional to the amount of blood flow delivered to lung units; $\dot{V}A/\dot{Q}c'$ is lower than the mean $\dot{V}A/\dot{Q}c'$ for the entire lung.[22, 62, 63] In the three-compartment model the combined effect of all $\dot{V}A/\dot{Q}c'$ com-

Table 3-3. Impact of $\dot{V}A/\dot{Q}c'$ Heterogenicity of Pulmonary Gas Exchange

Gas Tension Entering Lung	Po_2	O_2 content	Pco_2	CO_2 content
Inhaled Gas	149.0	21.6	0	0
Mixed Venous Blood	40.0	14.6	45.0	53.0

Compartment	Ventilation (L/min)	Blood Flow (L/min)	$\dot{V}A/\dot{Q}c'$	Po_2 (mmHg)	O_2 Content (mL/100 mL)	Pco_2 (mmHg)	CO_2 Content (mL/100 mL)	R	$\dot{V}o_2$ (mL/min)	$\dot{V}co_2$ (mL/min)
1	2.55	0	∞	—	—	—	—	∞	0	0
2	0.24	0.07	3.43	132.0	21.50	28.0	42.50	2.00	4.83	7.35
3	0.33	0.19	1.74	121.0	20.24	34.0	45.90	1.30	10.72	13.49
4	0.42	0.33	1.27	114.0	19.76	37.0	47.44	1.10	17.03	18.35
5	0.52	0.50	1.04	108.0	19.54	39.0	48.10	0.92	24.70	24.50
6	0.59	0.66	0.89	102.0	19.47	40.0	48.70	0.85	32.14	28.38
7	0.67	0.83	0.81	98.0	19.35	41.0	49.30	0.78	39.43	30.71
8	0.72	0.98	0.73	95.0	19.20	41.0	49.60	0.73	45.08	33.32
9	0.78	1.15	0.68	92.0	19.08	42.0	49.90	0.68	51.52	35.65
10	0.82	1.29	0.64	89.0	19.02	43.0	50.10	0.65	57.02	37.41
11	0	0.32	0	40.0	14.60	45.0	53.00	0	0	0
									Total	Total
$\dot{V}E$ =	7.71	6.32							282.46	229.16
$\dot{V}A$ =	5.09	6.00	0.85							

Resultant mean values exiting the lung

	R	Po2	PCo2	$\dot{V}A/\dot{Q}c'$
Ideal Point	0.81	102.00	40.00	0.93
Mixed Alveolar	—	106.00	39.00	
Mixed Arterial	—	97.00	41.00	

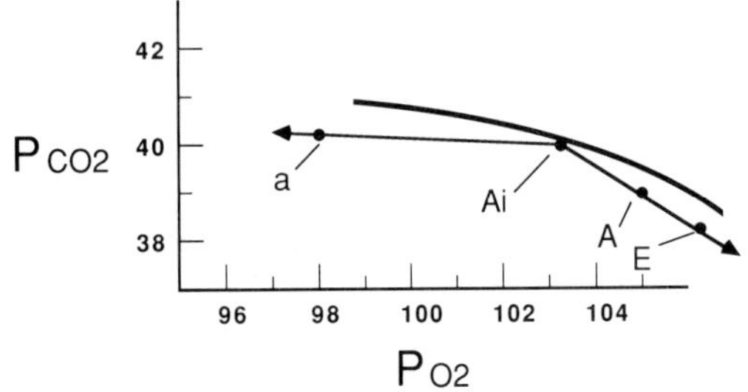

Figure 3-17. A magnified view of the three points in the normal lung described above. The distance along the gas R line that the mixed alveolar point (A) is displaced from the ideal point (A_i) is proportional to the fraction of total ventilation delivered to the compartments; $\dot{V}_A/\dot{Q}c'$ is higher than the mean $\dot{V}_A/\dot{Q}c'$ of the whole lung. The mixed exhaled gas point (E) is displaced further to the right due to the combined effect of dead space in the conducting passages and high $\dot{V}_A/\dot{Q}c'$ compartments. The distance on the blood R line that the arterial point (a) is from the ideal point is proportional to the amount of blood flow delivered to lung units. $\dot{V}_A/\dot{Q}c'$ is lower than the whole lung mean $\dot{V}_A/\dot{Q}c'$ and the shunt.

partments to the right of the ideal point is called the physiologic dead space, and the combined effect of the compartments to the left of the ideal point constitutes the physiologic shunt.

In disease, the heterogeneity of $\dot{V}_A/\dot{Q}c'$ in the lung is increased.[41, 42] The mixed alveolar (A) and mixed arterial (a) points are displaced further from the ideal point (A_i) (the mean $\dot{V}_A/\dot{Q}c'$ point) as a result. Large differences in partial pressure of O_2 between the arterial and ideal points but little difference in the partial pressure of CO_2. Alternatively, the difference in partial pressure of CO_2 in the mixed alveolar versus ideal points is a sensitive measure of region of high $\dot{V}_A/\dot{Q}c'$. The underlying premise reflect the increased number of lung units with low $\dot{V}_A/\dot{Q}c'$. All clinical assessments of gas exchange lies in quantifying the relationship in respiratory gas tensions between (1) the ideal point and the arterial blood or (2) between the ideal point and the exhaled gas (see section on Clinical Evaluation of Respiratory Gas Exchange).[62]

The efficiency of the whole lung function is determined by the relationship of whole body O_2 consumption and CO_2 production to the average $\dot{V}_A/\dot{Q}c'$ ratio of all lung units, including the degree of variation around that average value. The ideal point (A_i), the point of intersection of the $\dot{V}_A/\dot{Q}c'$ line and the blood and gas R lines, represents the gas tensions of a completely efficient lung. If all lung compartments have the same ventilation and perfusion and there is no dead space ventilation or shunt (Fig. 3-18A), then the arterial blood (a), the mixed alveolar gas (A), and the mixed exhaled gas (E) would all have the same gas tensions as those identified by the ideal alveolar point (A_i). In such a "superefficient" lung, the $\dot{V}_A/\dot{Q}c'$ ratio identified by the ideal alveolar point would also equal the ratio of total ventilation to total cardiac output ($\dot{V}_A/\dot{Q}c' = \dot{V}_E/\dot{Q}_T$).

If conducting airways that do not participate in the exchange of respiratory gases with the blood are introduced into the hypothetical model (Fig. 3-18B), then the mixed exhaled gas is diluted. The partial pressure of O_2 in the exhaled gas is increased and the partial pressure of CO_2 tension is lowered; this shifts the mixed exhaled point (E) down the gas R line, as shown. The $\dot{V}_A/\dot{Q}c'$ ratio is no longer equal to the ratio of total minute ventilation to cardiac output ($\dot{V}_A/\dot{Q}c' \neq [\dot{V}_A + \dot{V}_D]/[\dot{Q}_T]$).

Figure 3-18C illustrates "shunt" added to the model. Shunt occurs when a portion of the cardiac output does not exchange with the inspired gases (eg, bronchial and thebesian (coronary) circulations. Shunt dilutes the mixed arterial blood with mixed venous blood, therefore reducing the arterial O_2 tension and raising the arterial CO_2 tension. The arterial point (a) is displaced leftward on the blood R line ($\dot{V}_A/\dot{Q}c' \neq \dot{V}_E/\dot{Q}_T = \dot{V}_A/[\dot{Q}c' + \dot{Q}_s]$).

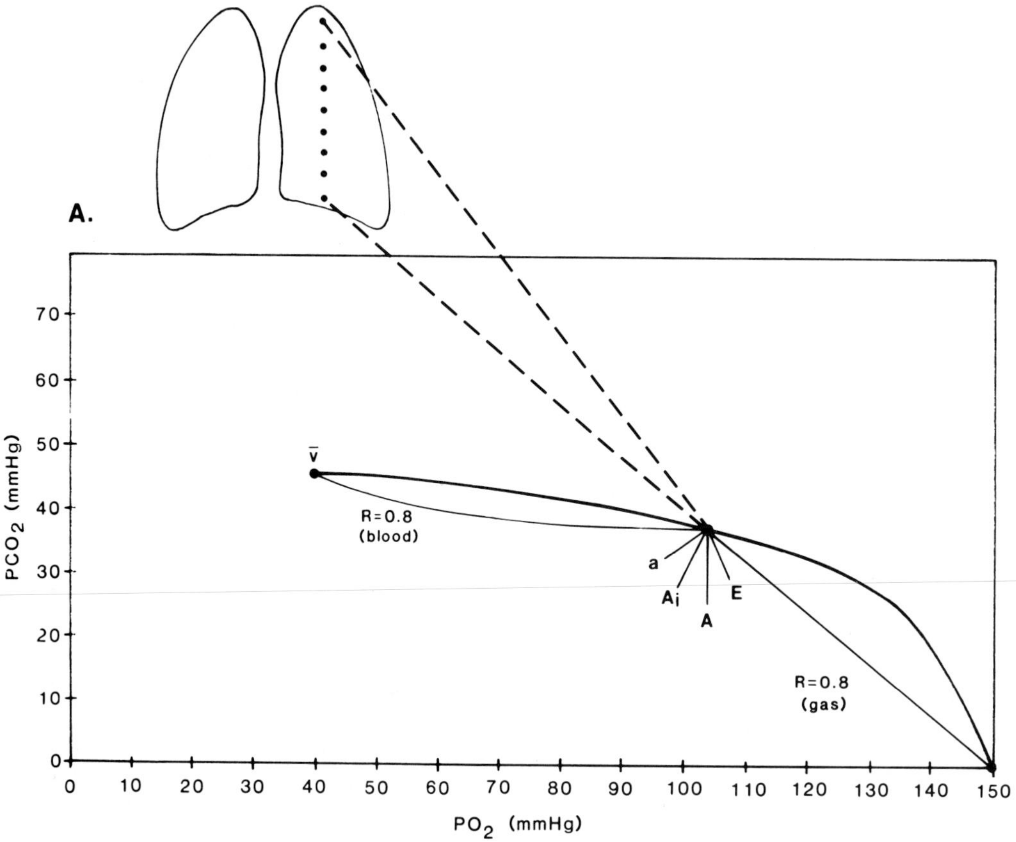

Figure 3-18. A: All lung compartments have the same ventilation and perfusion; no dead space ventilation or shunt exists. In such a superefficient lung, the $\dot{V}A/\dot{Q}c'$ ratio identified by the ideal alveolar point also equals the ratio of total ventilation to total cardiac output ($\dot{V}A/\dot{Q}c' = \dot{V}E/\dot{Q}T$). The arterial blood (a), the mixed alveolar gas (A), and the mixed exhaled gas (E) all have the same gas tensions as those identified by the ideal alveolar point (A_i).

Figure 3-18D, similar to the three-compartment shunt presented above, represents the lung with both dead space and shunt. An ideal compartment has the gas tensions and a $\dot{V}A/\dot{Q}c'$ ratio of the ideal point (A_i), and shunt and dead space compartments dilute the exhaled gas and arterial blood displacing points (eg, E, a) along the blood and gas R lines ($\dot{V}A/\dot{Q}c' \neq \dot{V}E/\dot{Q}T = [\dot{V}A + \dot{V}D]/[\dot{Q}c' + \dot{Q}s]$).

The effect of broadening the distribution of $\dot{V}A/\dot{Q}c'$ ratios around the ideal point is illustrated with an O_2-CO_2 diagram of a hypothetical lung without shunt or conducting passage dead space (Fig. 3-18E). In the lung compartments with low $\dot{V}A/\dot{Q}c'$, the O_2 tension is lower and the CO_2 tension is higher relative to the average of all alveolar gases. By definition these compartments have more blood flow then ventilation;

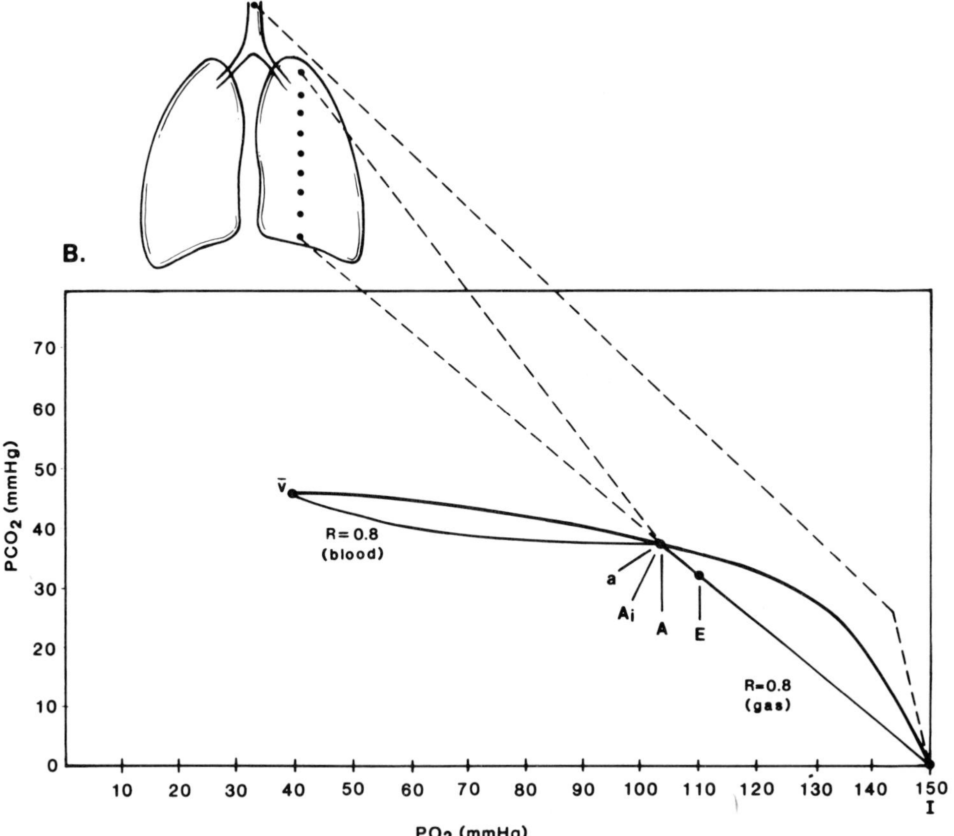

Figure 3-18 (Continued). B: Conducting airways that do not participate in the exchange of respiratory gases with the blood are introduced into the hypothetical model. The mixed exhaled gas is diluted so the partial pressure of oxygen in the exhaled gas is increased and the partial pressure of carbon dioxide tension is lowered. The mixed exhaled point (E) is moved down the gas R line as depicted. The $\dot{V}_A/\dot{Q}_C'$ ratio is no longer equal to the ratio of total minute ventilation to cardiac output [$\dot{V}_A/\dot{Q}_C' \neq (\dot{V}_A + \dot{V}_D)/(\dot{Q}_T)$].

therefore the composition of the mixed arterial blood is weighted toward these lung compartments. Conversely, in the regions of higher $\dot{V}_A/\dot{Q}_C'$, the partial pressures of O_2 and CO_2 are closer to the gas tensions in the inspired gas as compared to the average. Thus the composition of the mixed alveolar gas (A) is weighted toward the compartments to the right of the ideal point. In other words, as the distribution of $\dot{V}_A/\dot{Q}_C'$ compartments around the mean value is increased, the arterial point (a) moves leftward on the blood R line and the mixed alveolar gas point (A) moves away from the ideal point on the gas R line.[62, 63]

The complete multiple compartment model combining conducting passage dead space, shunt, and a wide distribution of $\dot{V}_A/\dot{Q}_C'$ compartments is shown in Figure 3-16. These

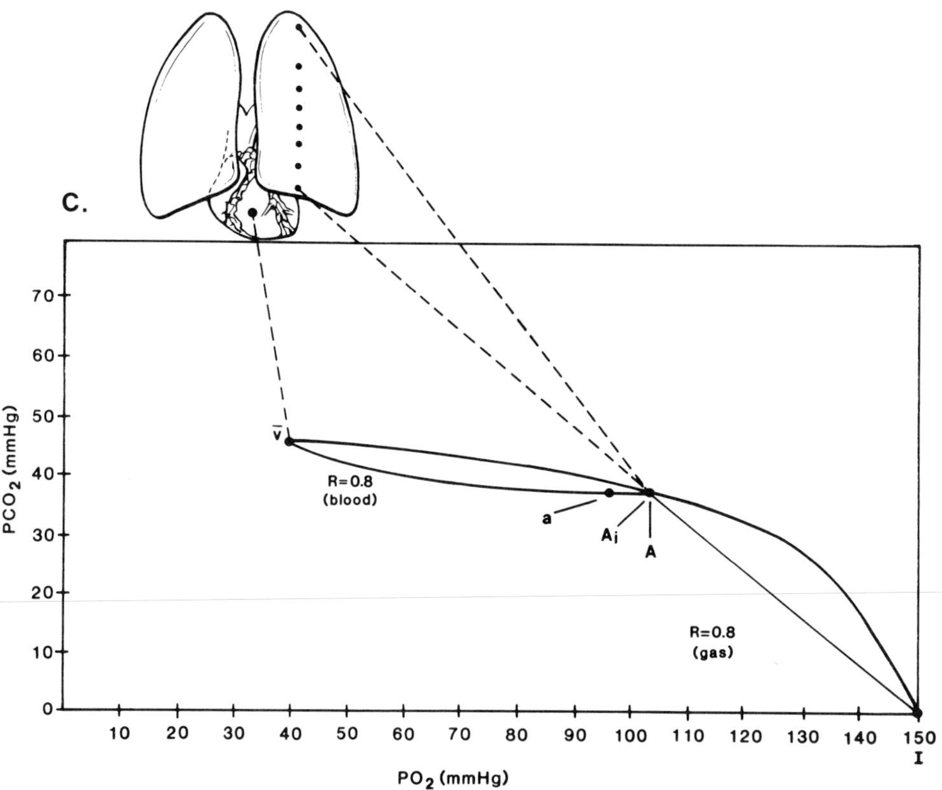

Figure 3-18 (Continued). C: "Shunt" is added to the model (eg, bronchial and thebesian [coronary] circulations), which dilute the mixed arterial blood with mixed venous blood. The arterial oxygen tension is reduced, and the arterial carbon dioxide tension is increased. The arterial point (a) is displaced to the left on the blood R line [$\dot{V}A/\dot{Q}c' \neq \dot{V}E/\dot{Q}T = \dot{V}A/(\dot{Q}c' + \dot{Q}s)$].

causes of inefficient gas exchange result in (1) displacement of the arterial point leftward along the blood R line due to the combined effect of shunt and low $\dot{V}A/\dot{Q}c'$ compartments, (2) displacement of the mixed exhaled gas point (E) rightward on the gas R line due to the combined effect of conducting passage dead space and high $\dot{V}A/\dot{Q}c'$ compartments, and (3) displacement of the mixed alveolar gas point (A) a lesser distance along the gas R line due to the effect of only the high $\dot{V}A/\dot{Q}c'$ lung compartments (alveolar dead space) (Fig. 3-17).

Figure 3-19 illustrates three hypothetical examples of how lung pathology and respiratory treatments affect the distribution of $\dot{V}A/\dot{Q}c'$ among lung compartments. In Figure 3-19A, a portion of the left lower lobe is atelectatic but retains a significant proportion of the pulmonary blood flow, which results in compartments with $\dot{V}A/\dot{Q}c'$ ratios of zero. The ventilation that would have gone to the atelectatic regions is distributed to the remaining compartments of the lung so that they have $\dot{V}A/\dot{Q}c'$ ratios that are slightly higher than in the normal state. The entire lung continues to have an exchange ratio (R) of 0.8 and its mean $\dot{V}A/\dot{Q}c'$

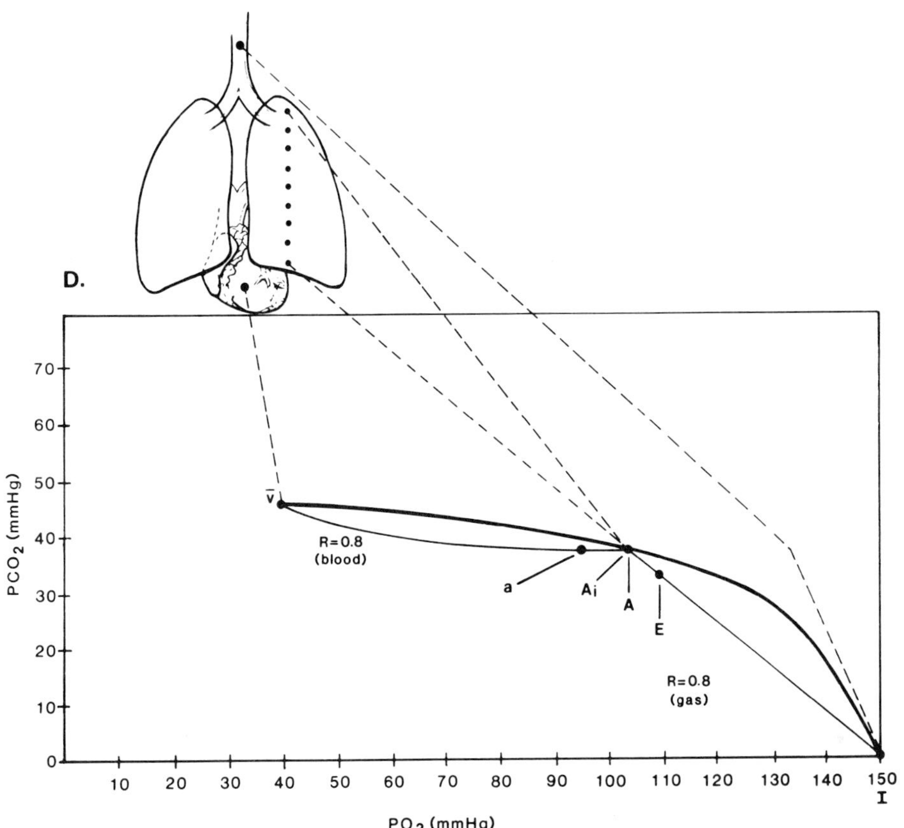

Figure 3-18 (Continued). D: The lung with both dead space and shunt (similar to the three-compartment shunt presented earlier) has an ideal compartment with gas tensions and VA/Qc′ ratio of the ideal point (A_i). The shunt and dead space compartments dilute the exhaled gas (E) and arterial blood (a) and displace them along the blood and gas R lines [$\dot{V}A/\dot{Q}c' \neq \dot{V}E/\dot{Q}T = (\dot{V}A+\dot{V}_d)/(\dot{Q}c' + \dot{Q}s)$].

remains at approximately 0.9. Therefore the ideal point (A_i) is placed at a PO_2 of 100 mmHg and a PCO_2 of 41 mmHg. As a result of the increase in regions of zero $\dot{V}A/\dot{Q}c'$, however, the arterial point is moved back along the blood R line, where PaO_2 is 70 mmHg and $PaCO_2$ of 42 mmHg. The mixed alveolar gas point (A) and mixed exhaled gas points are closer to the inhaled point along the gas R line because of the lung units with slightly high $\dot{V}A/\dot{Q}c'$ (alveolar dead space).

Figure 3-19B shows the results of hypothetical conditions in which there is (1) reduced pulmonary arterial hydrostatic pressure and (2) overinflation of the lungs. These conditions exaggerate the normal top-to-bottom distribution of pulmonary blood flow. An example of a clinical situation where this may occur is during the initiation of positive-pressure mechanical ventilation (PEEP) in a critically ill or anesthetized patient. Under such conditions, a large increase in the number of lung compartments with high

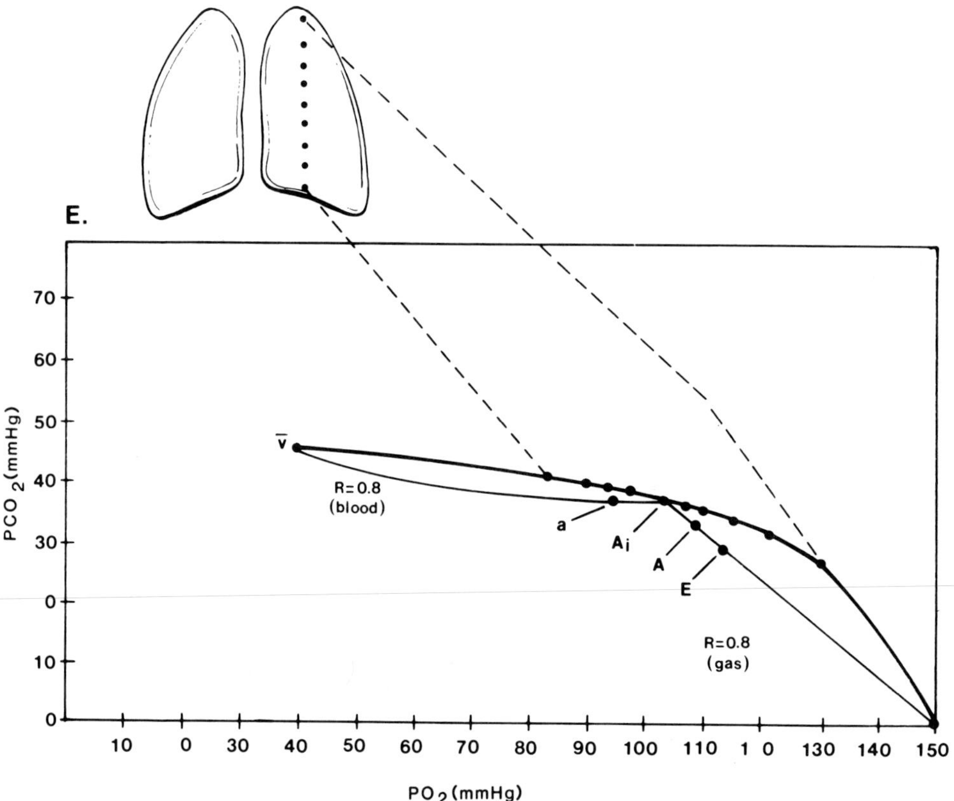

Figure 3-18 (Continued). E: This graph broadens the distribution of V̇A/Q̇c′ ratios around the ideal point without shunt or conducting passage dead space. Lung compartments with low V̇A/Q̇c′ have lower oxygen tensions and higher carbon dioxide tensions relative to the average. By definition, these compartments have more blood flow then ventilation, weighting the the mixed arterial blood toward these lung compartments. The regions of higher V̇A/Q̇c′, with respiratory gas tensions closer to inspired gas, as compared to the whole lung average, weight the composition of the mixed alveolar gas (A) values to the right of the ideal point. (Figure modified, with permission from West.[37])

V̇A/Q̇c′ occurs, and the number of regions with low V̇A/Q̇c′ shows only a small increase.[41] The whole lung R and mean V̇A/Q̇c′ remain 0.8 and 0.9, respectively, so the ideal point is unchanged as compared to Figure 3-19A. The mixed alveolar (A) and mixed exhaled (E) points, however, are displaced on the gas R line and are positioned much closer to the inspired point (I); ideal point (A_{i-1}), the arterial point (a) is shifted a bit closer to the mixed venous point (v) along the blood R line.

The effect of a decreased cardiac output on a normal lung is illustrated in Figure 3-19C. Again, the whole lung R and V̇A/Q̇c′ are approximately 0.8 and 0.9, respectively, and the distribution of V̇A/Q̇c′ within the lung is normal. The inspired point (I), mixed venous point $\bar{v}_1$, and arterial points a_1 are the same as in the other

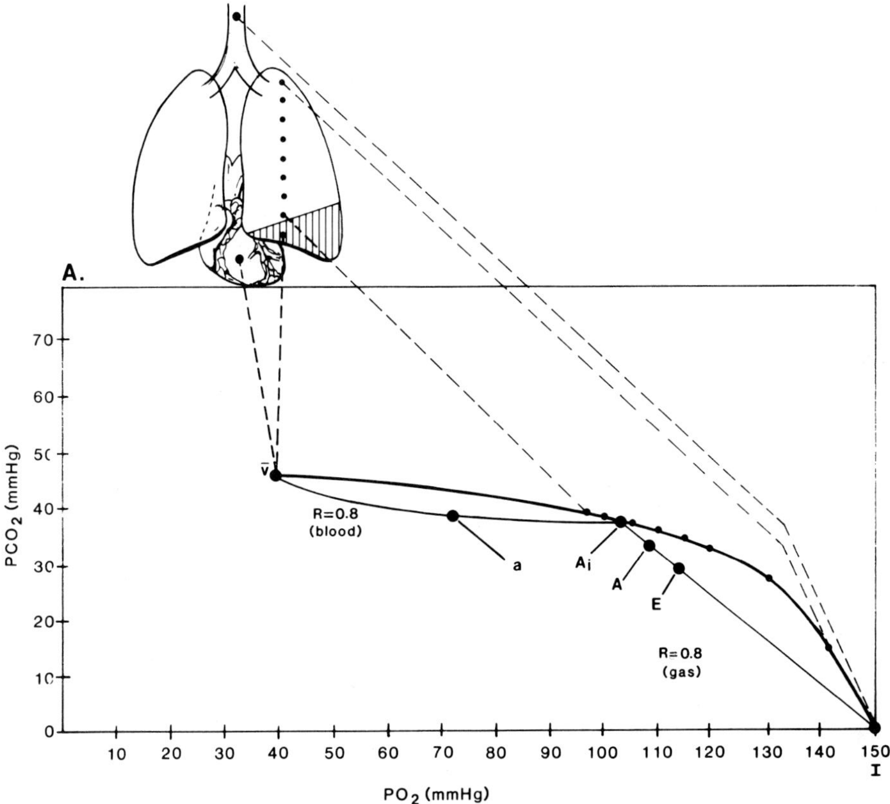

Figure 3-19. The effect of three hypothetical examples of relatively uncomplicated lung pathology on the distribution of $\dot{V}_A/\dot{Q}c'$ among lung compartments are illustrated. A: A portion of the left lower lobe is atelectatic but retains a significant proportion of the pulmonary blood flow resulting in compartments with $\dot{V}_A/\dot{Q}c'$ ratios of zero. B: Hypothetical conditions caused by (1) reduction in the pulmonary arterial hydrostatic pressure and (2) overinflation of the lungs that exaggerate the normal top-to-bottom distribution of pulmonary blood flow. Under such conditions, a large increase in the number of lung compartments with high $\dot{V}_A/\dot{Q}c'$, and only a small increase in the number of regions with low $\dot{V}_A/\dot{Q}c'$ occurs. C: The effect of a decreased cardiac output on a normal lung is illustrated. The distribution of $\dot{V}_A/\dot{Q}c'$ within the lung is normal and the inspired point I, mixed venous point $\bar{v}_1$, ideal $A_{i\text{-}1}$, and arterial point a_1, are the same as previous figures. A new $\dot{V}_A/\dot{Q}c'$ line results that displaces the ideal point, the arterial point, and the mixed alveolar point to $A_{i\text{-}2}$, a_2, and A_2 as illustrated. (Figure modified, with permission, from West.[37])

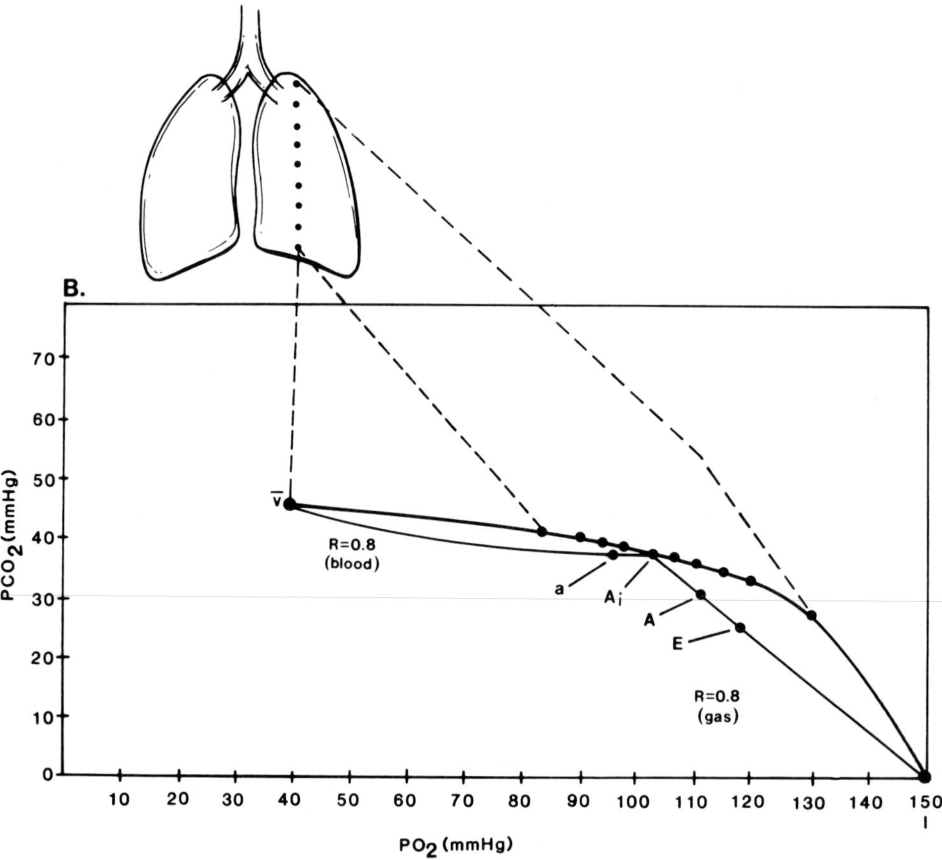

Figure 3-19 (Continued).

graphs in Figure 3-19. When the cardiac output is decreased, the body's extraction of O_2 and production of CO_2 unit volume of systemic blood flow increases, thus raising the mixed venous point to $\bar{v}_2$. Whole lung O_2-CO_2 exchange (R) and $\dot{V}A/\dot{Q}c'$ distribution do not change. As a result, this alteration in the mixed venous point sets a new $\dot{V}A/\dot{Q}c'$ line displacing the ideal point, the arterial point, and the mixed alveolar point to A_{i-2}, A_2, and A_2 as shown.

It must be emphasized that the graphs in Figure 3-19 illustrate the result of relatively uncomplicated variations from the normal state. In the clinical setting numerous compensatory adjustments may occur in response to pathologic conditions which change lung gas exchange efficiency. For example, a shift to lower $\dot{V}A/\dot{Q}c'$ distribution when whole lung and whole body R do not change will likely cause an increase in cardiac output, thus moving the mixed venous point and resetting the $\dot{V}A/\dot{Q}c'$ line. Finally, the arterial point returns close to the original, normal.arterial point.

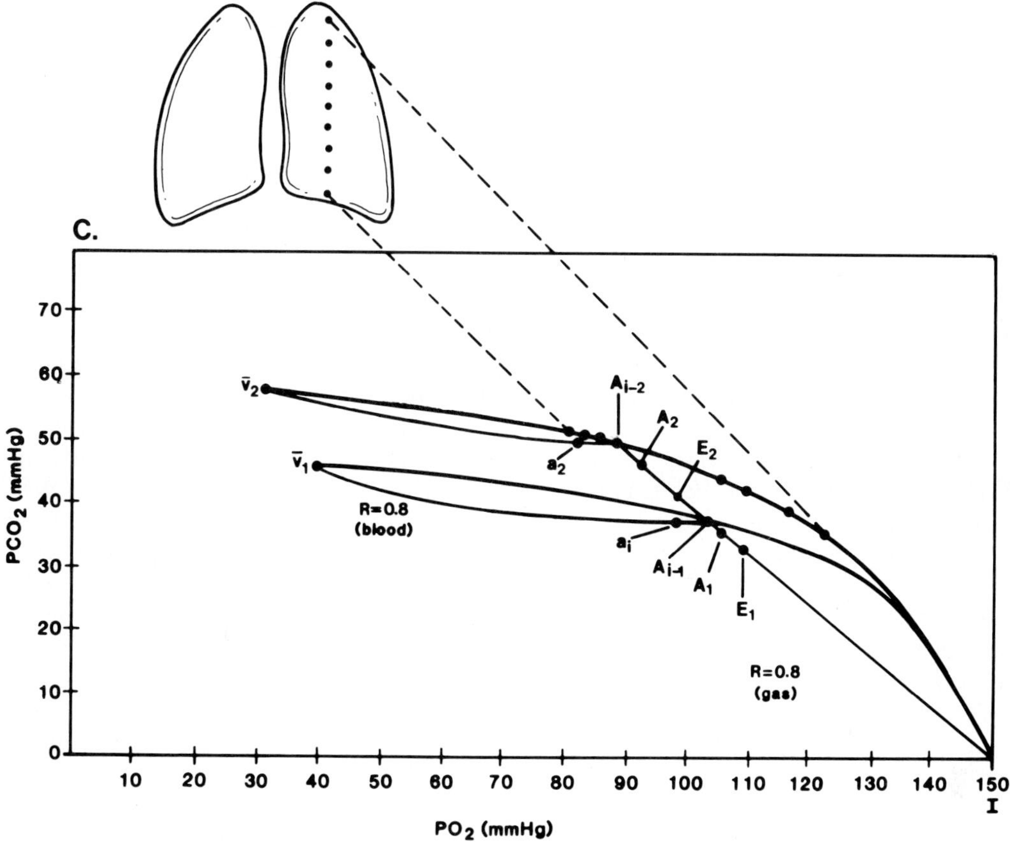

Figure 3-19 (Continued).

Clinical Evaluation of Respiratory Gas Exchange

The introduction to this chapter states that (1) the primary function of the respiratory system is to exchange respiratory gases between the external environment and the arterial blood and (2) the efficiency of this gas transfer reflects the state of health or magnitude of disease of the lung. In addition, the effect of therapies directed at the lung or indirect effects associated with surgery and anesthesia also affect the efficiency of this transfer. Measurements of gas exchange allow comparisons of the same patient at different times during the disease and its treatment as well as comparisons among those with similar diseases and among those that receive the same therapy.[64,65] Accurate measurement of gas exchange also allows precise titrations in treatment of individual patients.

Clinical assessment of respiratory gas exchange has been greatly improved by technical advances over the last 30 years. Proper use of these methods requires an understanding of the physiologic principles presented earlier. Before the approach of the clinical assessment of pulmonary gas exchange is discussed, the important points presented previously are summarized[64,65]:

1. Respiratory gas exchange occurs when convection carries atmospheric gas and blood to juxtaposition at that point, equilibration of gas tensions occur across a thin barrier by passive diffusion.
2. In the steady state the composition of respiratory gases in the alveoli and pulmonary capillary blood (gas-exchanging compartment) can be predicted based on the nature of ideal gases and the way in which respiratory gases are carried in the blood.
3. The composition of respiratory gas composition in any lung unit is determined by three factors: (1) the composition of respiratory gases in the inhaled mixture, (2) the composition of respiratory gases in the mixed venous blood, and (3) the balance of ventilation and perfusion to that gas exchange compartment.
4. The lung is composed of millions of gas-exchanging compartments that all behave according to the principles listed in 1–3 above. Each compartment potentially receives the same inhaled gas and the same mixed venous blood but has its own individual ventilation-perfusion ratio ($V_A/Q_{c'}$). Therefore each has its own composition of respiratory gases.
5. Gas transfer to the entire lung is the sum of the transfer occurring in each of the many compartments. If all lung units had the same $\dot{V}_A/\dot{Q}_{c'}$ ratio, then the mixed arterial blood and the mixed alveolar gas would have the gas tensions predicted from the inhaled mixture, the mixed venous blood, and the whole lung $\dot{V}_A/\dot{Q}_{c'}$. If many compartments have $\dot{V}_A/\dot{Q}_{c'}$ ratios that vary widely from the mean value, the mixed arterial blood and mixed alveolar gas will have gas tensions that differ from those predicted by the whole lung $\dot{V}_A/\dot{Q}_{c'}$ ratio.

The mean value for gas tensions in the multitude of lung compartments is reflected in mixed arterial blood and the mixed alveolar gas. The arterial blood gas tensions is biased to those compartments with a higher percentage of the total blood flow (a lower $\dot{V}_A/\dot{Q}_{c'}$). The mixed alveolar gas tensions is biased toward compartments with a higher $\dot{V}_A/\dot{Q}_{c'}$.

When lung pathology results in increased variation in $\dot{V}_A/\dot{Q}_{c'}$ ratios among lung units, the efficiency of pulmonary gas exchange is then decreased. Furthermore, this inefficiency is reflected in the size of the difference between the mixed arterial blood and the mixed alveolar gas or the difference between the ideal compartment gas tensions and the mixed blood or mixed alveolar gas.[62,64]

What variable is most useful in quantifying the efficiency of the gas exchange in the lung is controversial. The literature on this subject is further complicated because authors disagree on terminology.[66] However, interest is limited to the respiratory exchange for O_2 and CO_2 under usual clinical circumstances; either or both gases may be examined. The characteristics of the hemoglobin-oxygen association and carbon dioxide-whole blood association relationships as well as the opposite direction of exchange for the two gases (O_2 enters the blood, whereas CO_2 exits) results in quantitative differences in how each gas is affected by various abnormalities in lung function.[67] We believe that both O_2 and CO_2 exchange should be examined to assess the efficiency of lung function most accurately.

Examination of the O_2-CO_2 diagram and the algebraic relationships presented in previous sections suggest several methods in such studies. Figure 3-20 represents a lung with both dead space and shunt that is similar to the-three compartment model presented earlier in the chapter. It has an ideal compartment with gas tensions and V̇A/Q̇c′ ratio of the ideal point (A_i) and shunt and dead space compartments that dilute the exhaled gas and arterial blood, displacing the mixed inhaled gas point (E) and the arterial point (a) along the blood and gas R lines. The displacement of the arterial point from the ideal point due to shunt has a much greater impact on O_2 tensions than it does on the CO_2 tensions. The length of line $X_{Ai}X_a$, (alveolar-arterial O_2 difference) along the ordinate in Figure 3-20A is much greater than the length of $Y_{Ai}Y_a$ (arterial-ideal alveolar CO_2 difference). In fact, unless the shunt is extremely large, the difference in CO_2 tensions between the ideal compartment and the arterial blood are so close that they are assumed to be equal. In contrast to the effect of the shunt, the displacement of the mixed exhaled gas point (E) from the ideal point (A_i) due to dead space has a large effect on the difference in CO_2 tensions Figure 3-20B. The length of line $Y_{Ai}Y_E$, which equals the CO_2 difference, is longer than line $X_{Ai}X_E$, the difference

Figure 3-20. Graphical representation of a lung with both dead space and shunt similar to the three-compartment model presented earlier. Shunt has a much greater impact on oxygen tensions that it does on the carbon dioxide tensions. In A the length of line $X_{a\text{-}Ai}$, the alveolar-arterial oxygen difference, along the ordinate is much greater in length than the line Y_{Ai}-Y_a, the arterial-ideal alveolar difference for carbon dioxide, along the abscissa (B).

The effect of dead space has a large impact on carbon dioxide tension differences. The length of line YAI-YE (B), the difference in carbon dioxide between the ideal alveolar and mixed exhaled gas (similar to the arterial to alveolar difference), is proportional to the total or physiologic dead space. The line YA-YA(ET), the arterial to end tidal (mixed alveolar) difference for carbon dioxide, is proportional to the dead space due to lung units with V̇A/Q̇c′ higher than the mean. (Modified, with permission, from West.[37])

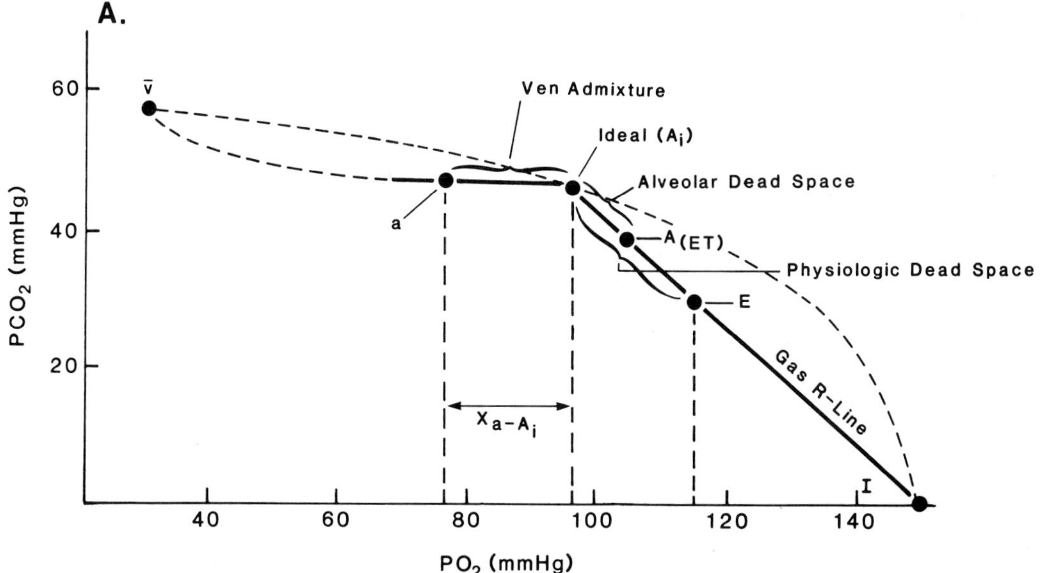

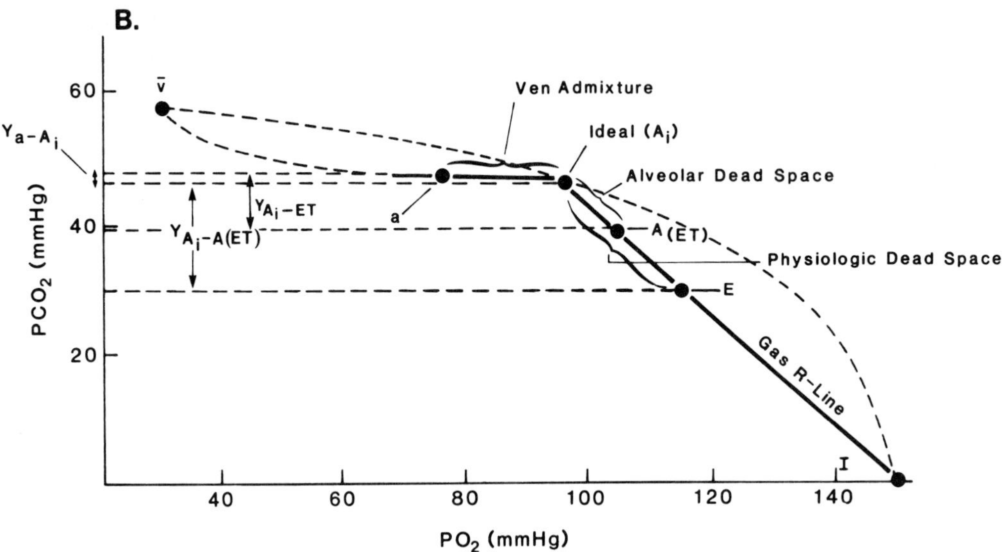

Figure 3-20 (Continued).

in partial pressure of oxygen. Thus Figure 3-20 illustrates how the arterial to ideal alveolar difference for O_2, $P(A_i - a)O_2$, is valuable in the quantification of the magnitude of the shunt. In contrast, the ideal to mixed exhaled difference in CO_2 $P(A_i - E)CO_2$, (or more commonly the respiratory dead space equation) is a more sensitive measure of respiratory dead space. Because of the similarity of the arterial and ideal compartment CO_2 tensions, the measured $PaCO_2$ is used in determination of the respiratory dead space and in place of P_ACO_2 when the ideal alveolar O_2 tension is calculated using the alveolar gas equation.

Gas Exchange for Oxygen

Figure 3-21 illustrates the many factors that cause a low O_2 partial pressure in the arterial blood.[66] Proper patient management requires examination of the contribution of each of the causes of hypoxemia. Measurement of the arterial O_2 tension alone is insufficient to evaluate the gas exchange abnormality. The arterial blood gases must be examined in relation to the inspired gases and the mixed venous gases. The dashed boxes in the figure represent groupings of factors that can be evaluated by commonly used calculations.

The causes for lower than normal arterial O_2 tension (hypoxemia) include (1) low inspired O_2 tension, (2) hypoventilation (in relation to O_2 consumption [ie, high $\dot{V}O_2/\dot{V}_A$ ratio], (3) diffusion abnormality, (4) venous to arterial shunt (as in congenital heart disease or with completely nonventilated perfused regions of the lung), (5) increased proportion of lung compartments with low $\dot{V}_A/\dot{Q}c'$ ratio, and (6) low mixed venous O_2 tension.[39] Distinguishing among these causes is often a considerable challenge. (Low inspired O_2 tension, the first possibility, is an uncommon etiology, but anesthesiologists are among the few clinicians who must carefully consider this. The operating room is one of the few hospital settings where a patient's inspired O_2 tension may well be lower

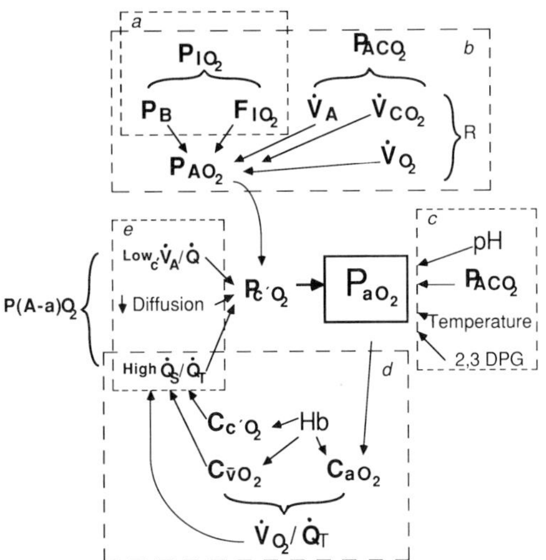

Figure 3-21. The multiple factors of a low partial pressure of oxygen in the arterial blood. Measurement of the arterial oxygen tension is insufficient alone to evaluate the gas exchange abnormality. The arterial blood gases must be examined in relation to the inspired gases and the mixed venous gases. The dashed boxes represent groupings of factors that can be evaluated through commonly used tools, including *a*, the PaO_2/FIO_2 ratio; *b*, the alveolar gas equation; *c*, the oxygen hemoglobin saturation curve; *d*, the shunt equation; and *e*, the $P(A - a)O_2$. See text for further details. (Used with permission from Cruz JC, and Metting PJ.[66])

than 150 mmHg (21% of humidified atmospheric gas at sea level). Low inspired O_2 tension is a cause of hypoxemia that is not due to inefficiency of lung function.

Low alveolar ventilation in proportion to O_2 consumption, the second cause of hypoxemia, is a relatively common phenomenon in patients recovering from the effects of surgery and anesthesia.[39,68] Often it is not a result of inefficient lung function; for example, it may occur when alveolar ventilation is low in relation to O_2 consumption because of a massive increase in O_2 consumption, such as malignant hypothermia or shivering. In these situations the lungs may be relatively healthy, but the capacity for ventilation of the respiratory system is overwhelmed. Similarly, in patients with residual neuromuscular blockade, low alveolar ventilation indicates absence of function rather than inefficient function. Alternatively, a large number of the compartments in a diseased lung may have high ventilation-perfusion ratios, which waste a significant volume of the total ventilation and thus reduce the alveolar ventilation.[33] In such instances the hypoxemia due to hypoventilation is associated with inefficient lung function. In any case, when alveolar hypoventilation is the cause of hypoxemia, the arterial O_2 tension is decreased in proportion to the rise in the arterial CO_2 tension.

When hypoxemia is caused by the two causes described above or when it results from low mixed venous O_2 (associated with high mixed venous CO_2), little if any discrepancy between the O_2 tension predicted by the ideal alveolar gas equation and that measured in the arterial blood exists.[33] The other three causes of hypoxemia, diffusion abnormality, shunt, and low $\dot{V}A/\dot{Q}c'$ always indicate inefficient respiratory function; all of these factors result in a difference between the gas tensions predicted by the ideal alveolar gas equation and those measured in the arterial blood.[62] For the clinician, quantifying the magnitude of shunt and low $\dot{V}A/\dot{Q}c'$ and distinguishing between these two contributions to hypoxemia, are the most difficult tasks.

The PaO_2/FIO_2 Ratio

The simplest calculation of all simply accounts for variation in the arterial O_2 tension associated with variation of the fraction of inspired O_2. This calculation does not allow differentiation of the cause of PaO_2 abnormalities resulting from variation in barometric pressure, hypoventilation, intrapulmonary shunt, $\dot{V}A/\dot{Q}c'$ abnormalities, or variations in the relationship of O_2 consumption to CO_2 production or their relationship to cardiac output. In addition, as demonstrated in Figure 3-22, the relationship between the PaO_2/FIO_2 ratio and FIO_2 is nonlinear. It is exaggerated when the $PaCO_2$-barometric pressure respiratory exchange ratio varies from the assumed values. However, because the PaO_2/FIO_2 ratio is simple, can be accurately measured, and takes into account the most important variable that is altered therapeutically (the FIO_2), it has become popular.[69,70]

The P(A − a)O₂ and (a/A)Po₂

In the 1940s and 1950s technological advances that allowed convenient measure of arterial blood gas tensions contributed to the recognition of the factors that determined steady state gas exchange (the ideal alveoli of the one-compartment model). Calculation of the ideal alveolar O_2 partial pressure (Equation 3-45) and direct measure of the mixed arterial tension accounted for the factors contained in boxes *b* and *e* in Figure 3-21. The differences between the ideal alveolar and measured arterial gas tensions ($P(A - a)O_2$) became a widely used tool in the study the inefficiency of pulmonary gas exchange.[69] The three most important causes of the $P(A - a)O_2$ including alveolar-capillary diffusion abnormalities, direct contribution of venous blood (true shunt), and low $\dot{V}A/\dot{Q}c'$ (distribution factor, are contained in box *e* of the figure

$$(3\text{-}84)\quad PAO_2 = PIO_2 - PACO_2 \cdot \left[FIO_2 + \frac{(1 - FIO_2)}{R}\right]$$

$$(3\text{-}85)\quad PaO_2 = \text{Measured value}$$

$$(3\text{-}86)\quad P(A - a)O_2 = PAO_2 - PaO_2$$

Farhi and Rahn presented a theoretical analysis of the $P(A - a)O_2$ that suggested that the relative contribution of the three major factors may be distinguished by varying the in-

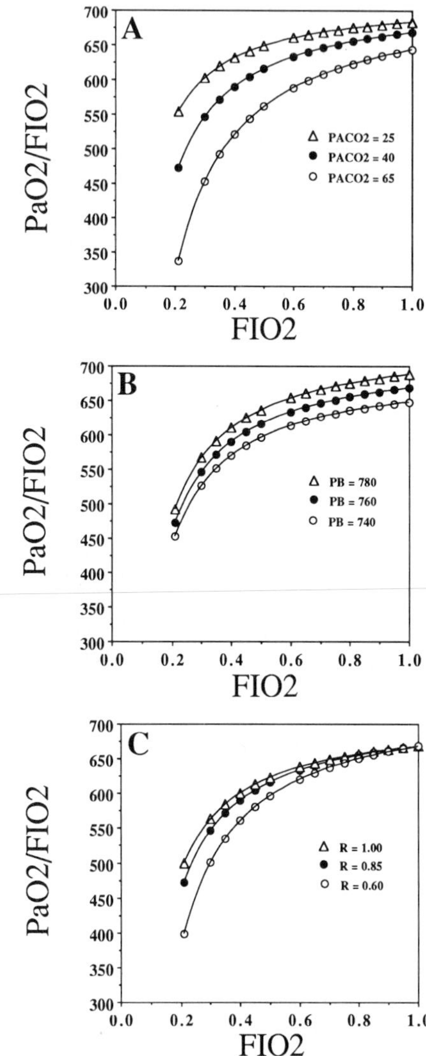

Figure 3-22. The PaO_2/FIO_2 Ratio. The simplest calculation for judging the efficiency of gas exchange for oxygen is the PaO_2/FIO_2 ratio. This calculation does not allow differentiation of the cause of PaO_2 abnormalities resulting from variation in barometric pressure, hypoventilation, intrapulmonary shunt, $\dot{V}A/\dot{Q}c'$ abnormalities, or variations in the relationship of oxygen consumption to carbon dioxide production or their relationship to cardiac output. Another disadvantage to this calculation is nonlinearity of the relationship of the PaO_2/FIO_2 ratio to FIO_2. When the $PaCO_2$, (A) barometric pressure (B), respiratory exchange ratio (C) vary from the assumed values, the nonlinear relationship is exaggerated.

spired O_2 tension.[62] Normal diffusing capacity of O_2 is approximately 35 mL · min · mmHg and results is less than a 1 mmHg difference between the ideal alveoli and arterial O_2 tension. When diffusing capacity falls to less than half its normal value, only then does a significant discrepancy develop between the ideal alveolar and arterial O_2 tensions. At low inhaled O_2 tensions, such as at high altitude or in lung compartments with poor ventilation, diffusion limitation becomes more important.[62,71,72] This effect is exaggerated if, for example, a patient with fibrotic lung disease who is exercising at high altitude becomes significantly hypoxemic due to diffusion limitation. Even a small increase of the partial pressure of O_2 in the alveoli will overcome large abnormalities in alveolar-pulmonary capillary diffusion.[67] Although many patients may have diffusion abnormalities, they are rarely the principal cause of arterial hypoxemia in hospitalized patients breathing oxygen-enriched mixtures. Determination of the $P(A - a)O_2$ while the patient is breathing more than 30%–40% O_2 helps eliminate this possibility from consideration.

Farhi and Rahn also suggested the differentiation of shunt from lung regions of low $\dot{V}A/\dot{Q}c'$ is accomplished through breathing 100% O_2.[62,63] Greatly raising the inspired O_2 tension means that even poorly ventilated lung units contain an O_2 volume sufficient to saturate all the pulmonary capillary blood delivered to that compartment fully. In contrast, completely unventilated lung units do not receive the enriched mixture and continue to contribute desaturated blood to the systemic arterial circulation. Low $\dot{V}A/\dot{Q}c'$ is "responsive," and shunt is "unresponsive" to O_2.

The theoretical analysis of the $P(A - a)O_2$ presented by Farhi and Rahn can be summarized as follows. The contribution of alveolar to capillary diffusion abnormality is maximized at low inspired O_2 levels and minimized when the ideal alveolar O_2 tension is greater than 200 mmHg. The effect of shunt on the $P(A - a)O_2$ in the normal lung increases to a maximum of 30–50 mmHg at ideal alveolar O_2 tensions up to 200 mmHg, whereas the contribution of low $\dot{V}A/\dot{Q}c'$ is greatest at ideal alveolar O_2 tensions between 70–90 mmHg and small at higher PAO_2. By examining the $P(A - a)O_2$ during 100% oxygen breathing, diffusion and distribution (low $\dot{V}A/\dot{Q}c'$) factors are eliminated. This gives an estimate of the contribution of shunt regions to the observed hypoxemia. A comparison to $P(A - a)O_2$ determined at lower FIO_2 would provide an estimate of the contribution of low $\dot{V}A/\dot{Q}c'$. For example, if at an FIO_2 of 0.3–0.4, the $P(A - a)O_2$ is greater than 10–15 mmHg but less than 50 mmHg when FIO_2 is 1.0, then a significant $\dot{V}A/\dot{Q}c'$ abnormality is present.

Experimental results, especially for normal lungs, have generally supported the theoretical treatment of Farhi and Rahn. However, when the percentage of cardiac output distributed to shunt or the amount of lung with low $\dot{V}A/\dot{Q}c'$ varies as a result of lung disease, the predictions have several pitfalls. One, the calculation of the ideal alveolar O_2 tension contains two variables (the barometric pressure [PB] and the respiratory exchange ratio [R]) that are usually assumed rather than measured. Figure 3-23 illustrates how variation in PB from the usually assumed value of 760 mmHg and, changes in R from the usually assumed value of 0.8 affect $P(A - a)O_2$. The combined effects may add as much as 25 mmHg in calculated versus arterial PAO_2. The contribution of these assumptions is often ignored when examining the value of the $P(A - a)O_2$ as a measure of pulmonary gas exchange efficiency.

In addition, O_2 breathing may result in the collapse of lung compartments with a very low ventilation-perfusion ratio. And increase the amount of intrapulmonary shunt may occur as an artifact.[73] Because regions of low $\dot{V}A/\dot{Q}c'$ have

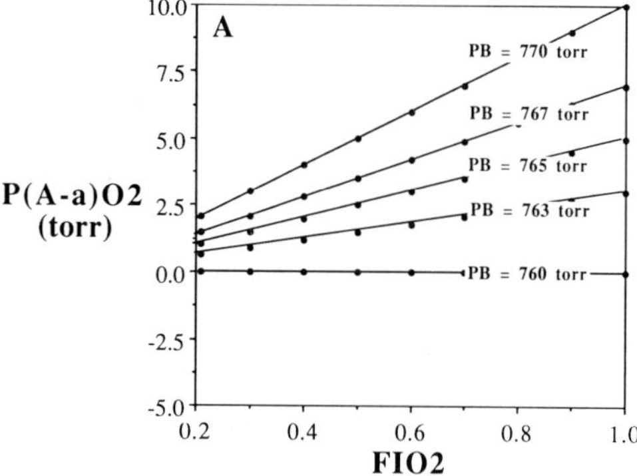

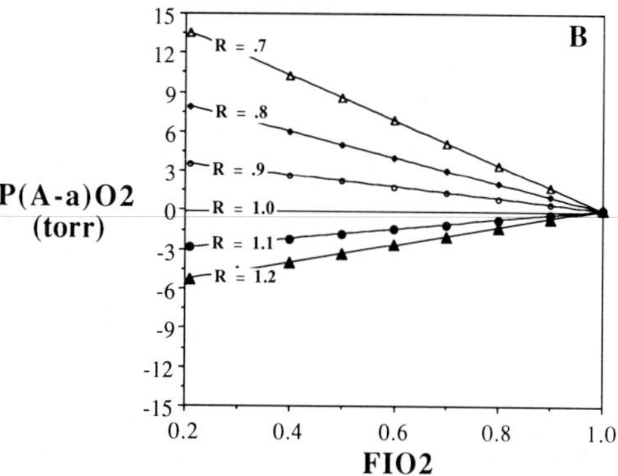

Figure 3-23. The P(A − a)O_2. The calculation of the ideal alveolar oxygen tension contains two variables (the barometric pressure (PB) and the respiratory exchange ratio [R]) that are usually assumed rather than measured. A illustrates the effect on P(A − a)O_2 of variation in PB from the usually assumed value of 760 mmHg. B illustrates the effect on P(A − a)O_2 due to variation in R from the usually assumed value of 0.80. The combined effect of the variation may be as much as 25 mmHg) in calculated versus arterial PAO_2. The contribution of these assumptions is often ignored when examining the value of the P(A − a)O_2 as a measure of pulmonary gas exchange efficiency.

a low R, when the inhaled mixtures contain only O_2 (FiO_2 = 1.0), alveolar gas is removed without replacement by either CO_2 from the blood or fresh gas from ventilation; atelectasis occurs as a result.[73] At high inspired O_2 tensions, the size of the shunt may actually increase due to the collapse of poorly ventilated areas. Alternately, when oxygen-enriched mixtures are inhaled, inhibition of hypoxic pulmonary vasoconstriction may occur in the regions of low $\dot{V}A/\dot{Q}c'$; this causes a redistribution perfusion to these areas, thus decreasing the proportion of the cardiac output distributed to shunt.[74,75]

The arterial-alveolar partial pressure ratio ([a/A]Po_2) is a more recently advocated calculation that involves the same considerations as the P(A − a)O_2, but may be algebraically more resilient to variation associated with shunt and low $\dot{V}A/\dot{Q}c'$.[76–78] Figures 3-24 and 3-25 compare changes in the P(A − a)O_2 and (a/A)Po_2 as FiO_2, size of shunt, and severity of low $\dot{V}A/\dot{Q}c'$ areas change.[77] These figures illustrate that when a shunt predominates over lung disease, P(A − a)O_2 rises with increasing FiO_2, whereas if the percentage of pulmonary shunt is low, the P(A − a)O_2 plateaus. Alternatively, the (a/A)Po_2 demonstrates a flatter curve at high FiO_2. In lungs with a high degree of shunt, the biggest changes in (a/A)Po_2 occur at low FiO_2, and the curve is flat at the clinically useful FiO_2. This is true even in patients with a high percentage of shunt. The comparison of P(A − -a)O_2 and (a/A)Po_2 in a lung with shunt fixed at 2% but regions of low $\dot{V}A/\dot{Q}c'$ have variable severity of abnormality (Fig. 3-25) illustrates abnormalities in pulmonary gas exchange that predominantly result from low $\dot{V}A/\dot{Q}c'$ (eg, bronchitis, asthma). The abnormalities vary in severity. At low FiO_2 and P(A − a)O_2 the curves rise steeply, and (a/A)Po_2 lines fall. For some FiO_2 the curves suddenly change slope; P(A − a)O_2 falls and (a/A)Po_2 rises. The dramatic change in the curves occurs at the point where the Pco_2 of the

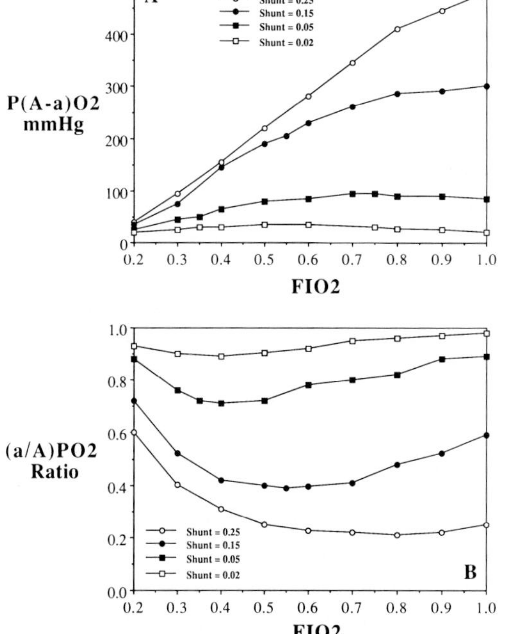

Figure 3-24. Comparison of $P(A - a)O_2$ and a/A Po_2 ratio with varying FiO_2 in patients with shunt. The arterial-alveolar partial pressure ratio ($[a/A]Po_2$) includes the same considerations as the $P(A - a)O_2$, but may be algebraically more resilient to variation associated with shunt and low $\dot{V}A/\dot{Q}c'$. The figure utilizes a theoretic lung model that contains high and low $\dot{V}A/\dot{Q}c'$ compartments plus anatomic shunt (Qs). In the model, oxygen consumption is assumed to be 300 mL/min, total alveolar ventilation is 5 L/min, and cardiac output ($\dot{Q}T$) is 6 L/min. The blood flow to areas of low $\dot{V}A/\dot{Q}c'$ is always 50% of the $\dot{Q}T - \dot{Q}s$. A and B compare changes in the $P(A - a)O_2$ and $(a/A)Po_2$ as FiO_2 and the size of shunt is altered as shown. In contrast, the low $\dot{V}A/\dot{Q}c'$ region is held constant at a ratio of 0.7 (see text for further details). (Modified, with permission, from Gilbert R et al.[77])

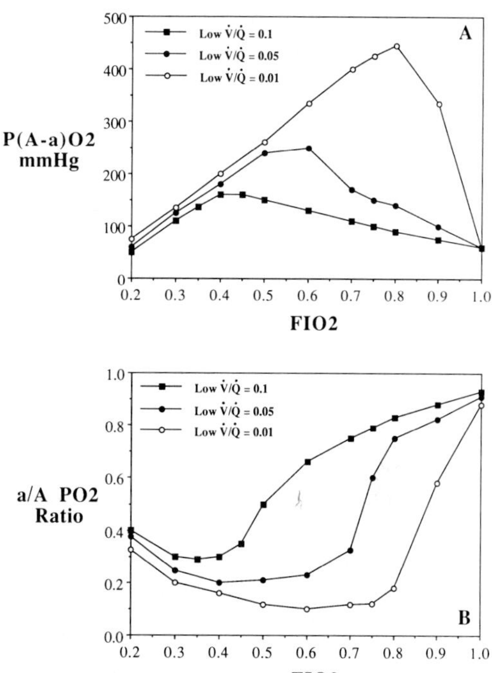

Figure 3-25. Comparison of $P(A - a)O_2$ and a/APo_2 ratio with varying FiO_2 in patients with $\dot{V}A/\dot{Q}c'$ mismatch. Like Figure 3-24, Figure 3-25 uses a theoretic lung model that contains high and low $\dot{V}A/\dot{Q}c'$ compartments plus anatomic shunt ($\dot{Q}s$). In the model, oxygen consumption is assumed to be 300 mL/min, total alveolar ventilation is 5 L/min, and cardiac output ($\dot{Q}T$) is 6 L/min. In addition, the blood flow to the low $\dot{V}A/\dot{Q}c'$ regions is always 50% of the $\dot{Q}T - \dot{Q}s$. A and B compare changes in the $P(A - a)O_2$ and $(a/A)Po_2$ as FiO_2. the low $\dot{V}A/\dot{Q}c'$ region is altered as shown, and the size of shunt is held constant at 2%.

Figures 3-24 and 3-25 illustrate that when lung disease is predominated by shunt, $P(A - a)O_2$ rises with increasing FiO_2, whereas if the percentage of pulmonary shunt is low, the $P(A - a)O_2$ plateaus. Alternatively, the $(a/A)Po_2$ demonstrates a flatter curve at high FiO_2. In lungs with a high degree of shunt, the largest changes in $(a/A)Po_2$ occur at low FiO_2 and the curve is flat at the clinically useful FiO_2. (Modified, with permission, from Gilbert R et al.[77])

low $\dot{V}A/\dot{Q}c'$ reaches the flat portion of the hemoglobin-oxygen saturation curve at a higher FIO_2 in the lungs with a larger degree of low $\dot{V}A/\dot{Q}c'$ abnormality.[77]

These differences suggest to some investigators that the $(a/A)PO_2$ is a more useful measure of gas exchange efficiency in the clinical setting because it allows the clinician to predict more accurately the resultant change in PaO_2 when FIO_2 is altered.[78] In addition, in lungs with a combination of shunt and low $\dot{V}A/\dot{Q}c'$ resulting in arterial hypoxemia, the $(a/A)PO_2$ does not vary as much with changing FIO_2, especially in the probable therapeutic range (≥ 0.4) Fig. 3-26).[77]

In summary, due to the multiple influences on the size of the $P(A - a)O_2$, this value may increase, decrease, or remain constant as the FIO_2 is altered. When the shunt fraction is about 5% and $\dot{V}A/\dot{Q}c'$ variability is minimal, the $P(A_i - a)O_2$ plateaus at 35 to 50 mmHg as the FIO_2 is increased above 0.4. At high shunt fractions, however, a higher FIO_2 is necessary to reach the $P(A - a)O_2$ plateau. When the shunt fraction exceeds 20% the $P(A - a)O_2$ continues to increase as FIO_2 rises to 1.0. The ratio of the arterial to the ideal alveolar oxygen tension, $a/A)PO_2$, is more resistant to change from strictly mathematical considerations as compared to the $P(A_i - a)O_2$. This is particularly true in patients where the major abnormality is shunt rather than regions of low $\dot{V}A/\dot{Q}c'$. For this reason a/APO_2 may be a more useful tool for adjusting oxygen therapy in critically ill patients.[78]

Figure 3-26. Comparison of $P(a\text{-}A)O_2$ and a/APO_2 ratios with varying FIO_2 in patients with a combination of shunt and $\dot{V}A/\dot{Q}c'$ mismatch. The figure compares changes in the $P(A - a)O_2$ and $(a/APO_2$ as FIO_2 varies in a lung with a combination of shunt and low $\dot{V}A/\dot{Q}c'$; these factors cause arterial hypoxemia. The $(a/A)PO_2$ does not vary as much with changing FIO_2, especially in the probable therapeutic range (≥ 0.4). This figure uses the same lung model as in Figures 3-24 and 3-25 (high and low $\dot{V}A/\dot{Q}c'$ regions plus shunt, oxygen consumption = 300 mL/min, total alveolar ventilation = 5 L/min, $\dot{Q}T$ = 6 L/min, blood flow to the low $\dot{V}A/\dot{Q}c'$ = 50% of the $\dot{Q}T - \dot{Q}S$), but the shunt is 15% and the region of low $\dot{V}A/\dot{Q}c'$ is 0.2. (Modified, with permission, from Gilbert R.[77])

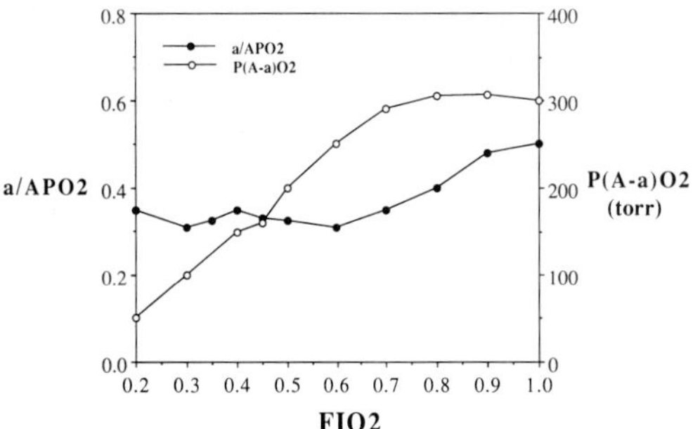

The Shunt Equation ($\dot{Q}S/\dot{Q}T$)

The shunt or venous admixture equation (Equation 3-74) developed by Berggren[44] is an expression of arterial hypoxemia in terms of the percentage of the total cardiac output that would have to pass through totally unventilated areas to produce such a degree of desaturation. Most commonly, the O_2 content in the arterial mixed venous blood is calculated from the measurement of the O_2 saturation of hemoglobin, O_2 partial pressure, and the hemoglobin concentration (Equation 3-75). In addition, the O_2 content in the mean pulmonary capillary blood is calculated; it is assumed that the hemoglobin concentration is the same as in arterial blood and that the O_2 partial pressure and O_2 saturation of hemoglobin is the same as would be obtained if the pulmonary capillary equilibrated with the mean alveolar gas as defined by the alveolar gas equation (Equation 3-45).

Normally, desaturated blood from venous circulation may enter the arterial blood from two sources: (1) the bronchial and thebesian (coronary) circulations (desaturated venous blood will also mix into the arterial circulation in disease states including structural heart disease when blood can flow from the right to the left chambers of the heart) and (2) lung disease where perfusion of completely unventilated regions within the lung may occur. These are often called "true" shunt. The contribution of bronchial and thebesian circulation to time shunt is relatively constant. In contrast, acquired or congenital structural heart disease exists in a limited number of patients who usually have coexisting physical findings or laboratory abnormalities that allow differentiation of these lesions from pulmonary causes of hypoxemia. Most commonly, venoarterial shunts are due to the presence within the lung of compartments that are completely airless or receive no ventilation. Thus the cause of the true shunt that is of most interest when diagnosing or treating patients with hypoxemia is unventilated portions of the lung.

If the Berggren equation is calculated at low inspired O_2 tensions ($F_{IO_2} < 1.0$), then many of the pulmonary mechanisms that contribute to hypoxemia, including diffusion abnormalities, regions of low $\dot{V}_A/\dot{Q}c'$ (distribution effect), and shunt (true venous admixture), contribute to the calculated shunt.[66] In other words, the calculated shunt fraction is "as if" all of the hypoxemia is due to true shunt. As discussed for $P(A - a)O_2$ and $(a/A)PO_2$ inhalation, O_2 FiO_2 of 1.0 has been advocated as a strategy to eliminate hypoxemia caused by low $\dot{V}_A/\dot{Q}c'$ and diffusion abnormality. At FiO_2 of 1.0 the $\dot{Q}_S/\dot{Q}_T$ will be smaller than when calculated at $FiO_2 < 1.0$ (as with a large $\dot{V}_A/\dot{Q}c'$ abnormality). It will be unchanged (no significant $\dot{V}_A/\dot{Q}c'$ abnormality) as compared to the $\dot{Q}_S/\dot{Q}_T$ obtained at low fractions of inspired O_2 if no $\dot{V}_A/\dot{Q}c$ abnormality is present.

Just as with the $P(A - a)O_2$ calculation, this practice has been criticized because several investigators have noted that after breathing 100% O_2, the shunt calculation appears to increase rather than decrease as would be expected if two of three potential causes of hypoxemia were eliminated.[79–81] However, other investigators have not noted a paradox,[66,82,83] and there are a number of explanations for the apparent difference in the calculated sums.[73] Alveoli with low output of ventilation may collapse during the breathing of 100% O_2 because once the N_2 is washed out, absorption of O_2 into the pulmonary blood removes more gas than enters from ventilation. Ultimately the gas volume is inadequate to distend to the alveoli. Inhibition of hypoxic pulmonary vasoconstriction that leads to dilation of vessels and perfusion of unventilated lung units is an often suggested but unproven cause of paradoxical change in shunt size.[66]

In addition to absorption atelectasis or release of hypoxic vasoconstriction, calculated Q_S/Q_T is influenced by changes in O_2 consumption, cardiac output, and the content of O_2 in the mixed venous blood.[84,85] Cruz and Metting[66] have algebraically modified the Berggren expression in order to call attention to the implicit variables in the traditional expression. In their derivation, O_2 consumption and its relationship to total cardiac output are included as explicit rather than implicit variables:

$$\dot{Q}_S/\dot{Q}_T = 1 - [(\dot{V}O_2/\dot{Q}_T)/(Cc'O_2 - C\bar{v}O_2)] \tag{3-87}$$

This expression of the shunt equation suggests an explanation for the unexpected change in the size of calculated shunt. The five variables ($Cc'O_2$, $CaCO_2$, $C\bar{v}O_2$, $\dot{V}O_2$, and $\dot{Q}_T$) in the the shunt fraction calculation that are assumed to remain the same when the $\dot{Q}_S/\dot{Q}_T$ is recalculated at varied F_{IO_2} may in fact change between calculations. Concomitant changes in these variables may result in variations in the $\dot{Q}_S/\dot{Q}_T$ on subsequent determinations without necessarily indicating a change in the amount of true shunt.

Gas Exchange for Carbon Dioxide

Examination of the gas exchange for CO_2 provides different information about the efficiency of lung function than O_2 measurements, although the same principles apply to the exchange of both gases. The reasons for this difference relate to the opposite direction of CO_2 exchange and three other factors: (1) there is usually no carbon dioxide in the inhaled gas, (2) there is a more linear relationship between partial pressure and volume for blood CO_2, and (3) the diffusion from capillary to alveoli is 10 times greater for CO_2 than for O_2. For these reasons, the CO_2 tension in the mixed arterial blood is depends only on the CO_2 production and the total alveolar ventilation. Gas diffusion abnormalities across the alveolar capillary membrane are rarely, if ever, important. The distribution factor, $\dot{V}A/\dot{Q}c'$ mismatch, is critical only if it results in a low total alveolar ventilation in proportion to the CO_2 production.

Arterial P_{CO_2}

Equation 3-41, the alveolar gas equation for CO_2, illustrates all the factors that determine the mean partial pressure of CO_2 in the alveolar gas. When no CO_2 is present in the inhaled gas, this equation can be considerably simplified to equation 3-43. Under usual circumstances then, the mean alveolar P_{CO_2} depends on the alveolar ventilation and the CO_2 production.[30]

The partial pressure-volume relationship for CO_2 in the blood, in contrast to O_2, and the

Figure 3-27. Alveolar ventilation, carbon dioxide production, and $PaCO_2$. The $PaCO_2$ (mixed arterial CO_2), which is a good estimate of the alveolar carbon dioxide, can be predicted from the simplified (no inspired carbon dioxide) alveolar gas equation for carbon dioxide (Equation 3-43 displayed in the figure). The two clusters of points show the relationship at two different ranges of carbon dioxide production. Curve A represents $\dot{V}CO_2$ between 120 and 170 mL/min and the curve B represents higher $\dot{V}CO_2$ (950 to 1200 mL/min). It is apparent that measurement of $PaCO_2$ alone is insufficient to predict the $\dot{V}A$. However, if it is assumed that the $\dot{V}CO_2$ in a resting or anesthetized patients is likely to be in the normal range (curve A) (150–250 mL/min or 3.5 ± 0.5 mL/kg/min [mean ± SD]), then a high $PaCO_2$ indicates a low $\dot{V}A$. In addition, manipulation to affect alveolar ventilation has direct and predictable influence on the $PaCO_2$ (as indicated in the figure).

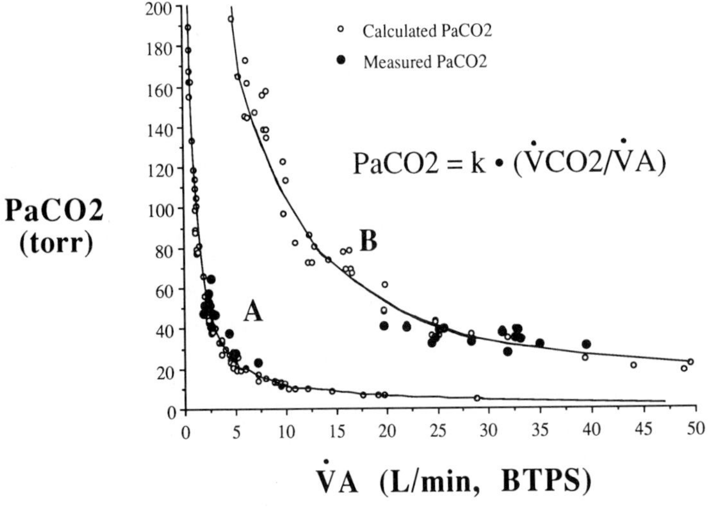

blood's capacity for CO_2 result in the P_{CO_2} a small effect by lung units with a low $\dot{V}A/\dot{Q}c'$ on the mixed arterial blood. The $PaCO_2$ (mixed arterial CO_2) is a good estimate of the alveolar CO_2 and is, therefore, affected by the same variables as in Equation 3-43.[30]

The interaction of alveolar ventilation, CO_2 production, and $PaCO_2$ is illustrated in Figure 3-27. The two clusters of points represent the $\dot{V}A$ to $PaCO_2$ relationship at two different ranges of CO_2 production. The left cluster (curve A) includes measured values and values predicted from equation 3-43 for V_{CO_2} (between 120 and 170 mL/min, (which were obtained from a series of 24 anesthetized patients),[33] and the right set (curve B) were obtained from exercising young male adults with high V_{CO_2}, (between 950 and 1200 mL/min).[86] An elevated Pa_{CO_2} indicates low alveolar ventilation in proportion to the $\dot{V}_{CO_2}$. Although it is apparent that measurement of $PaCO_2$ alone is insufficient to predict the absolute value of $\dot{V}A$, $\dot{V}_{CO_2}$ is likely to be in the range of the first curve (150 to 250 mL/min or 3.5 ± 0.5 mL/kg/min [mean ± SD]). If it is assumes that the $\dot{V}_{CO_2}$ is in the normal range of curve A, then a high $PaCO_2$ indicates a low $\dot{V}A$. In such a case, therapeutic manipulation to effect alveolar ventilation has direct and predictable influence on the $PaCO_2$ as indicated by Figure 3-27 and the relationship in Equation 3-43.

P(a − ET) CO_2

Infrared CO_2 monitors or mass spectrometers are now regularly available for routine measurement of exhaled CO_2 tensions in anesthetized and critically ill patients. These tools are most easily used in patients breathing through artificial tracheal airways.[87] Exhaled CO_2 measurements are useful for confirmation of placement of the artificial airway in the trachea and as less invasive measurements of P_{CO_2}, which ensure adequate ventilation during manipulation of mechanical respiratory support. Determination of the difference between simultaneously obtained end tidal (ET) and mixed arterial (a) P_{CO_2}, the P(a-ET) CO_2 has also been advocated as a useful measure of respiratory dead space and $\dot{V}A/\dot{Q}c'$ in homogeneity in the lung (increased distribution to high $\dot{V}A/\dot{Q}c'$ regions).[87,88]

Except for simple confirmation of airway placement in the trachea or airway patency, the clinical application of end tidal gas monitoring assumes that the end tidal measurement, which is usually displayed over time, reflects the mean alveolar CO_2 tension in some regular way.[90] However, since lung ventilation is tidal in nature, the P_ACO_2 fluctuates during the breathing cycle; therefore, whereas the arterial P_{CO_2} tends to reflect the mean alveolar CO_2, the end tidal P_{CO_2} approaches the peak alveolar CO_2. Increasing tidal volume, increasing CO_2 production, and decreasing respiration rate exaggerate this effect. Alternatively, when the contribution to the end tidal gas from regions of high $\dot{V}A/\dot{Q}c'$ is increased (high $\dot{V}A/\dot{Q}c'$ in homogeneity), then the $P_{ET}CO_2$ is most likely lower than the mean P_ACO_2 of the alveoli with matched ventilation and perfusion. Under such circumstances, the $P_{ET}CO_2$ is lower than the $PaCO_2$.[85,88]

Another complicating influence comes from the devices used to measure end tidal P_{CO_2} and the breathing circuit to which the patient is attached. A small (± 5%) error in CO_2 measurement using infrared flow through analyzers may occur, which is attributable to the electrical response time of the instrument and the rate at which the gas in the censoring chamber is changed (This in turn depends on expiration flow rate and respiratory frequency.)[90] This type of error is less of a problem with most spectroscopy. Water vapor and anesthetics gases (N_2O) affect the accuracy of end tidal CO_2 monitors, but most commercially available instruments have internal calibrations and heaters to prevent condensation of water to account for these effects.[91,92] The clinician, however, must be aware of these factors; the appropriate instrument for the patient should be used.

The breathing circuit to which the patient is attached may affect end tidal measurement. Whenever continuous fresh gas flow is near the patient airway, exhaled gas may be diluted by the fresh gas flow. These conditions are present when using modifications of the T-piece and partial rebreathing circuits (Mapleson D or Bain) or in many mechanical ventilators set in the IMV (intermittent mandatory ventilation) mode.[93–95] Low expiration flow rates and high fresh gas flow rates (Fig. 13-28) increase dilution of the end tidal gas by fresh gas flow.[94] These conditions are most likely to be present in infants and small children, the patient groups in whom these techniques are most frequently used.[93,94] Error due to these factors may be reduced by sampling the respiratory gas at a site as close to the patient as possible and using lower sampling flow rates (< 500 mL/min) for sidestream type devices.[93]

For to the reasons stated above, the partial pressure of CO_2 in the end tidal gas can be higher, the same, or lower than that in the arterial blood. Because of the varied number of factors that influence the measurement, caution must be exercised when estimating $PaCO_2$ and when making judgements about the efficiency of lung function from the P(a-ET) CO_2. Table 3-4 summarizes some findings of past investigations of P(a-ET)CO_2 and various influences in the magnitude of this variable.

In summary, the assessment of pulmonary gas exchange efficiency is necessary and useful for the diagnosis and management of patients. The O_2-CO_2 diagram, which illustrates the various factors that influence such gas exchange, suggests clinical methods to describe and quantify pulmonary gas transfer. Inspired, arterial, mixed venous, and exhaled gas tensions can be

Figure 3-28. Graph showing error in ET CO_2 due to fresh gas flow in the breathing circuit. Dilution of the end tidal gas by fresh gas flow results in widening of the P(a-ET)CO_2, which rises as the ratio of fresh gas flow to expiratory flow rates increases. (Figure drawn from the data of Gravenstein et al[96].)

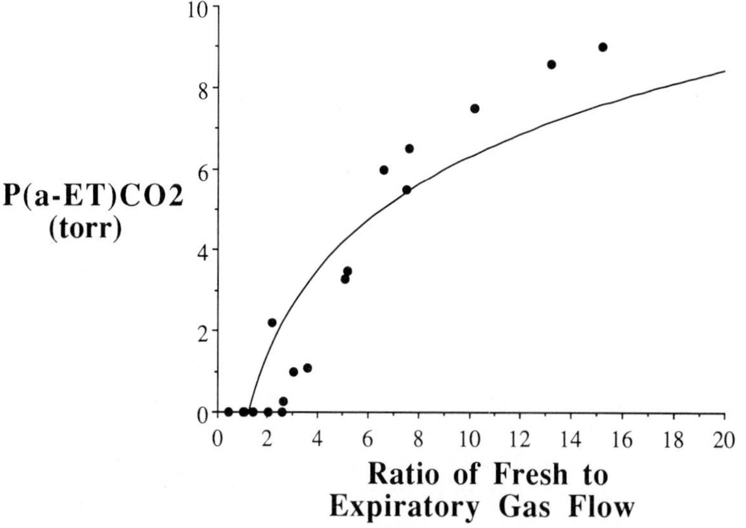

Table 3-4. Studies of Clinical Value of the Alveolar to End-tidal Difference for Carbon Dioxide

$P(a - ET) CO_2$				
Mean	±SD	Range	Setting	Reference
4.46	2.50	−0.40–+7.70	Healthy anesthetized adults; rebreathing circuit; spontaneous respiration	Nunn & Hill[33]
4.72	2.47	−1.70–+9.10	Healthy anesthetized adults; mechanical respiration	Nunn & Hill[33]
5.50	5.20	−8.00–+2.10	Adults, postop (cardiac surgery (mean age 63 ± 9 years)	Russell & Graybeal[87]
0.70	0.04	+0.46–+0.95	Healthy women (mean age: 26 years) after general anesthesia for lower abdominal surgery	Shankar, et al[96]
0.10	0.09	−0.53–+0.90	Pregnant women (mean age: 23 years) after general anesthesia for caesarean section	Shankar, et al[96]
4.60	2.90		Anesthetized adults before cardiopulmonary bypass surgery	Bermudez & Lichtiger[97]
11.60	3.50		Anesthetized adults after cardiopulmonary bypass surgery	Bermudez & Lichtiger[97]
4.10	2.44	−12.00–+12.30	Anesthetized adults (mean age: 57 years)	Raemer et al[88]
−1.76	2.20	−3.30–+1.00	Healthy adults who exercise at maximum of 25–50% $\dot{V}O_2$	Jones[85]
8.40	5.60		Anesthetized healthy infants < 8.0 kg; rebreathing circuit; I/E ratio < 1/3.5	Bagwell et al[94]
4.30	4.80		Anesthetized infants < 8.0 kg; partial rebreathing circuit; I/E ratio > 1/3.5	Bagwell et al[94]
2.20	2.00		Anesthetized infants < 8.0 kg; partial rebreathing circuit; I/E ratio > 1/3.5	Bagwell et al[94]

accurately measured with commonly available clinical tools. Examination of the arterial blood and consideration of the inhaled gas mixture, the exhaled gas tension and the mixed venous blood gases provide clinicians with an estimate of the efficiency of the pulmonary gas exchange. Several shortcomings are inherent in each of these techniques, however. Respiration gas measurements in arterial blood samples are accurate and simple to obtain, and it is reasonable to expect that such a sample represents completely mixed return from pulmonary circulation, but distinguishing the various influences on the partial pressure of respiratory gases in the blood is difficult. To partition the contribution of each of these influences, it is useful to perform certain calculations and consider both the exchange of O_2 and CO_2.

References

1. Weibel E R. The pathway for oxygen. Cambridge, MA: Harvard University Press, 1984:337.
2. Farhi L E, Rahn H. Gas stores of the body and the unsteady state. J Appl Physiol 1955;7:472.
3. Newbower R S. The physics of ideal gases. J Clin Anesth 1989;1:232.
4. Olszowka A J, Farhi L E. A system of digital computer subroutines for blood gas calculation. Resp Physiol 1968;4:270.
5. Dunnill M S. Postnatal growth of the lung. Thorax 1962;17:329.
6. Rahn H. A concept of mean alveolar air and the

ventilation-bloodflow relationship during pulmonary gas exchange. Am J Physiol 1949;153:21.
7. Riley R L, Courand A, Donald K W. Analysis of factors affecting partial pressure of oxygen and carbon dioxide in gas and blood of lungs: method. J Appl Physiol 1951;4:77.
8. Pappenheimer J. Standardization of definitions and symbols in respiratory physiology. Fed Proc 1950; 9:602.
9. Strickland D. Physical principles: Part I: Mechanical quantities in physical basis of the science of anaesthesia. In: Scurr C and Feldman S, eds. London: In William Heinemann, 1982:1.
10. Duffin J. Physics for anesthetists. Springfield IL: Charles C. Thomas, 1976:92.
11. Weibel E R. The pathway for Oxygen. Cambridge MA: Harvard University Press, 1984:10.
12. Perutz M F. The hemoglobin molecule. Sci Am 1964;64:211.
13. Farhi L E, Rahn H. Total flow requirements for gas transport. In: Studies in pulmonary physiology. Rahn H ed. Wright Air Development Center Technical Report 1960;60–1:147.
14. International Committee for Standardization in Hematology (ICSN) recommendations and requirements for haemoglobinometry in human blood. Nature 1965;206:491.
15. Gregory I C. The oxygen and carbon monoxide capacities of foetal and adult blood. J Physiol (Lond) 1974;236:625.
16. Comroe J H, Botelho S. The unreliability of cyanosis in the recognition of arterial anoxemia. Am J Med Sci 1947;214:1.
17. New W. Pulse oximetry. J Clin Monit 1985;1:126.
18. Kelman GR. Digital computer subroutine for the conversion of oxygen tension into saturation. J Appl Physiol 1966;21:1375.
19. Benesch R, Benesch RE. The effects of organic phosphates from the human erythrocyte on the allosteric properties of hemoglobin. Biochem Biophys Res Commun 1967;26:162.
20. Severinghaus JW. Blood gas calculator. J Appl Physiol 1966;21:1108.
21. Perutz MF. Stereochemistry of cooperative effects of haemoglobin. Nature 1970;228:726.
22. Rahn H, Fenn WO. A graphic analysis of respiratory gas exchange the O_2-CO_2 diagram. Washington DC: American Physiological Society, 1955: .
23. Oski FA, et al. The effects of deoxygenation of adult and fetal hemoglobin on the synthesis of red cell 2,3 diphosphoglycerate and its in vivo consequences. J Clin Invest 1970;49:400–407.
24. Austin WH, Lacombe E, Rand PW, et al. Solubility of carbon dioxide in serum from 15 to 38°C. J Appl Physiol 1963;18:301.
25. Maren TH. Carbonic anhydrase: chemistry, physiology and inhibition. Physiol Rev 1967;47:595.
26. Perutz MF. Hemoglobin structure and respiratory transport. Sci Am 1978;239:92.
27. Kelman GR. Digital computer procedure for conversion of P_{CO_2} blood CO_2 content. Respir Physiol 1967;4:270.
28. Grodins FS, Yamashiro SM. Optimization of the mammalian respiratory gas transport system. Annu Rev Biophys Bioeng 1973;4:115.
29. Klocke RA. Mechanism and kinetics of the Haldane effect in human erythrocytes. J Appl Physiol 1973; 35:673.
30. Otis AB. Quantitative relationship in steady-state gas exchange. In: Handbook of Physiology Sections, Volume 1. Respiration. Fern Wo, Rahn H, eds. Washington DC: American Physiological Society, 1964:681.
31. Bohr C. Ueber die Lungenathmung. Skand Arch Physiol 1891;2:236.
32. Enghoff H. Volumen inefficax. Benerkungen zur Frage des schädlichen raumes. Uppsala Läkaref Förh 1938;44:191.
33. Nunn JF, Hill DW. Respiratory dead space and arterial to end-tidal CO_2 tension difference in anesthetized man. J Appl Physiol 1960;15:383.
34. Sahn SA, Lakshminarayan S, Petty TL. Weaning from mechanical ventilation. JAMA 1976;235:2208.
35. Pontoppidan H, Laver MB, Geffin B. Acute respiratory failure in the surgical patient. Adv Surg 1970; 4:163.
36. Riley RL, Courand A. "Ideal" alveolar air and the analysis of ventilation-perfusion relationships in the lungs. J Appl Physiol 1949;1:825.
37. West JB. Ventilation blood flow and gas exchange. Oxford: Blackwell Scientific Publications, 1977: 103.
38. Comroe JH, Forester RE, Dubois AB, et al. The lung clinical physiology and pulmonary function tests. Chicago: Year Book, 1962:339.
39. Marshall BE Whyche MQ. Hypoxemia during and after anesthesia. Anesthesiology 1972;37:178–209.
40. West JB. Ventilation blood flow and gas exchange. Oxford: Blackwell Scientific Publications, 1977:59.
41. West JB. New advances in pulmonary gas exchange. Anesth Anal 1975;54:409.
42. Wagner PD, Dantzker DR, Dueck R, et al. Ventilation-perfusion in equality in chronic obstructive pulmonary disease. J Clin Invest 1977;59:203.

43. Weissman C. Measuring oxygen uptake in the clinical setting. In: Oxygen transport and utilization. Bryan-Brown C, Ayres SM, eds. Fullerton CA: Society of Critical Care Medicine, 1987:25.
44. Berggren SM. The oxygen deficit of arterial blood caused by nonventilation to parts of the lung. Acta Physiol Scand (Suppl 11) 1942;4:1.
45. Rehder K, Sessler AD, Rodarle JR. Regional intrapulmonary gas distribution in awake and anesthetized-paralysed man. J Appl Physiol 1977;42:391.
46. Machlem PT, Murphy B. The forces applied to the lung in health and disease. Am J Med 1974;57:371.
47. Bake B, Wood L, Murphy B, et al. Effect of inspiratory flow rate on regional distribution of inspired gas. J Appl Physiol 1974;37:8.
48. Hoppin PG, Hildebrandt J. Mechanical properties of the lung. In: Bioengineering aspects of the lung. West JB, ed.) New York: Marcel Dekker, 1977:83.
49. Milic-Emili J. Pulmonary statics. In: Widdecombe JG, ed. MTP international review of sciences: respiratory physiology. Physiology series. Volume 2. Baltimore: University Park Press, 1974:127.
50. Milic-Emili J. Regional distribution of inspired gas in the lung. J Appl Physiol 1966;21:749.
51. Ralph DD, Robetson T, Wenoli J, et al. Distribution of ventilation and perfusion during positive end expiratory pressure in adult respiratory distress syndrome. Am Rev Respir Dis 1985;131:54.
52. Campbell EJM. Mechanisms of airway obstruction in emphysema and asthma. Proc R Soc Med 1958; 51:108.
53. Mayfield JD, Paez PN, Nicholson DP. Static and dynamic lung volume and ventilation perfusion abnormalities in adult asthma. Thorax 1971;26:591.
54. West JB, Dollery CT, Naimark A. Distribution of blood flow in isolation lung: relation to vascular and alveolar pressures. J Appl Physiol 1964;19:713.
55. Hughes JMB, Glazier JB, Maloney JE, et al. Effect of lung volume on the distribution of pulmonary blood flow in man. Respir Physiol 1968;4:58.
56. Marshall BE. Hypoxic pulmonary vasoconstriction. Acta Anaesthesiol Scand 1990;34 (Supplement 94):37.
57. Benumof JL, Wahrenbrock EA. Local effects of anesthetics on regional hypoxic pulmonary vasoconstriction. Anesthesiology 1975;43:525.
58. Zapol WM, Rie MA, Frikker M. Pulmonary circulation during adult respiratory distress syndrome. In: Zapol WM and Falke KJ, eds. Acute respiratory failure. New York: Marcel Pekker, 1985:241.
59. Grant BJB, Davies EE, Jones HA, et al. Local regulation of pulmonary blood flow and ventilation-perfusion ratios in the coati mundi. J Appl Physiol 1976;40:216.
60. Grant BJB. Vasomotor tone and the optimization of gas exchange. In: Will JA, Dawson CA, Weir EK, et al, eds. The pulmonary circulation in health and disease. Boston: Academic Press, 1987:335.
61. West JB, Wagner PD. Pulmonary gas exchange. In: West JB, ed. Bioengineering aspects of the lung. New York: Marcel Dekker, 1977:361.
62. Farhi LE, Rahn H. A theoretical analysis of the alveolar difference with special reference to the distribution effect. J Appl Physiol 1955;7:699.
63. Rahn H, Farhi LE. Ventilation, perfusion and gas exchange the $\dot{V}_A/\dot{Q}$ concept. In: Fenn WO, Rahn H, eds. Handbook of Physiology. Section 3: Respiration. Volume 1. Washington DC, American Physiological Society, 1964.
64. Gilbert R, Auchimcloss JH, Kuppinger M, et al. Stability of the arterial/alveolar oxygen partial pressure ratio. Crit Care Med 1979;7:267.
65. Benatar SR, Hewlett AM, Nunn JF. The use of isoshunt lives for control of oxygen therapy. Brit J Anaesth 1973;45:711.
66. Cruz JC, Metting PJ. Understanding the meaning of the shunt fraction calculation. J Clin Monit 1987; 3:124.
67. Dantzker DR, Gutierz G. Effects of circulatory failure on pulmonary and tissue gas exchange. In: Schay SM, Cassidy SS, eds. Heart-lung interactions in health and disease. New York: Marcel Dekker, 1989:983.
68. Nunn JF, Payne JP. Hypoxemia after general anesthesia. Lancet 1962;1:631.
69. Covelli HD, Nessan VJ, Tuttle WK. Oxygen-derived variables in acute respiratory failure. Crit Care Med 1983;11:646.
70. Lawrence M. Abbreviating the alveolar gas equation: an argument for simplicity. Respir Care 1985; 30:964.
71. Wagner PD, Gale GE, Moon RE, et al. Pulmonary gas exchange in humans exercising at sea level and simulated altitude. J Appl Physiol 1986;60:260.
72. Wagner PD, West JB. Effects of O_2 and CO_2 time courses in pulmonary capillaries. J Appl Physiol 1972;33:62.
73. Dantzker DR, Wagner PD, West JB. Instability of lung units with low $\dot{V}_A/\dot{Q}$ ratios during O_2 breathing. J Appl Physiol 1975;38:886.
74. Benumof JL, Pirlo Af, Johanson I, et al. Interaction

of $P\bar{v}O_2$ with PAO_2 on hypoxic, pulmonary vasoconstriction. J Appl Physiol 1981;51:871.
75. Miller FL, Chen L, Malmkvist CT, et al. Mechanical factors do not influence blood flow distribution in atelectasis. Anesthesiology 1989;70:481.
76. Gilbert R, Keighley JF. The arterial/alveolar oxygen tension ratio. An index of gas exchange applicable to varying inspired oxygen concentrations. Am Rev Respir Dis 1974;109:142.
77. Gilbert R, Auchincloss JH, Kuppinger M, et al. Stability of the arterial/alveolar oxygen partial pressure ratio. Crit Care Med 1979;7:267.
78. Gross R, Israel RH. A graphic approach for prediction of arterial oxygen tension at different concentrations of inspired oxygen. Chest 1998;79:311.
79. Douglas ME, Downes JB, Dommemiller FJ, et al. Change in pulmonary venous admixture with varying inspired oxygen. Anesth Anal 1976;55:688.
80. Suter PM, Fairley HB, Scholbohn RM. Shunt, lung volume and perfusion during short periods of ventilation with oxygen. Anesthesiology 1975;43:617.
81. Oliven A, Abinader E, Bursztein S. Influence of varying inspired oxygen tensions on the pulmonary venous admixture (shunt) of mechanically ventilated patients. Crit Care Med 1980;8:99.
82. McAslan TC, Matjasko-Chin J, Turney SZ, et al. Influence of inhalation of 100% oxygen on intrapulmonary shunt in severely traumatized patients. J Trauma 1973;13:811.
83. Quan SF, Kronberg GM, Schlobohm RM, et al. Changes in venous admixture with alterations of inspired oxygen concentration. Anesthesiology 1980;52:477.
84. Dantzler DR, Lynch JP, Weg JG. Depression of cardiac output is a mechanism of shunt reduction in the therapy of acute respiratory failure. Chest 1980; 77:636.
85. Jones NL, Robertson DG, Kane JW. Difference between end-tidal and arterial PCO_2 in exercise. J Appl Physiol 1979;47:954.
86. Lillie PE, Roberts JG. Caron dioxide monitoring. Anaesth Intensive Care 1988;16:41.
87. Russell GB, Garybeal JM. Stability of arterial to end-tidal carbon dioxide gradients during postoperative cardiorespiratory support. Can J Anesth 1990;37: 560.
88. Raemer DB, Francis D, Philip JH, et al. Variation in PCO_2 between arterial blood and peak expired gas during anaesthesia. Anesth Anal 1983;62:1065.
89. Shapiro BA, Cove RD. Blood gas monitoring: yesterday, today and tomorrow. Crit Care Med 1989; 17:573.
90. Stock MC. Noninvasive carbon dioxide monitoring. Crit Care Clin 1988;4:511.
91. Severinghaus JW. Water vapor calibration errors in some capnometers: respiratory conventions misunderstood by manufactures? Anesthesiology 1989; 70:996.
92. Severinghaus JW, Larson CP, Eger EI. Correction factors for infrared carbon dioxide pressure broadening by nitrogen, nitrous oxide and cyclpropane. Anesthesiology 1961;22:429–432.
93. Pascucci RC, Schena JA, Thompson JE. Comparison of a sidestream and mainstream capnometer in infants. Crit Care Med 1989;17:560.
94. Bagwell JM, Heavner JE, May WS, et al. End-tidal PCO_2 monitoring with either a partial rebreathing or nonrebreathing circuit. Anesthesiology 1987; 66:405.
95. Gravenstein N, Lanpotong S, Beneken JEW. Factors influencing capnography in the brain circuit. J Clin Monit 1985;1:6.
96. Shankar KB, Moseley H, Kumar Y, et al. Arterial to end tidal carbon dioxide tension difference during caesarean section anaesthesia. Anaesthesia 1986; 41:698.
97. Bermudez J, Lichtiger M. Increases in arterial to end-tidal CO_2 tension differences after cardiopulmonary bypass. Anesth Analg 1987;66:690.

CHAPTER

4

Hypoxic Pulmonary Vasoconstriction and Choice of Anesthesia

Linda Chen
Bryan E. Marshall

In this chapter, the role of hypoxic pulmonary vasoconstriction (HPV) in oxygenation will be described and the considerations necessary to guide a choice of anesthetic for thoracic surgery will be discussed. HPV is viewed in terms of its two responses: a change in pulmonary artery pressure and a change in blood flow to hypoxic lung regions. In caring for patients, clinicians should consider not only the primary hypoxic stimulus but also the secondary variables that affect the HPV response such as disease, cardiac output, and drugs used during anesthesia.

In the past several years, a great deal of material concerning the pulmonary circulation has accumulated. Information about the hemodynamic, metabolic, humoral, mechanical, and gas exchanging function of the pulmonary circulation now provides a detailed understanding of many physiologic and pathophysiologic states.

Physiology

In 1946 Von Euler and Liljestrand[1] suggested that a local pulmonary vasoconstriction in response to hypoxia acts to redistribute pulmonary blood flow from poorly ventilated to more adequately ventilated regions. This observation received little attention until the work of Bjertnaes in Scandinavia[2], Sykes in the United Kingdom[3], and Benumof in the United States[4]. This research demonstrated the effects of anesthetics on HPV and suggested inhibition of HPV responses as a possible explanation for hypoxemia observed during anesthesia and surgery.

HPV is now recognized as a critical factor in the pathophysiology of several medical conditions. It is an important mechanism that reduces the severity of hypoxia by diverting blood flow away from hypoxic lung regions to oxygenated areas of the lung, thus diminishing systemic arterial hypoxemia. HPV is one cause of persistent pulmonary hypertension of the newborn,[5] adult respiratory distress syndrome,[6] chronic lung disease,[7] and high altitude sickness.[8] Although many factors influence the generally very low background pulmonary vascular tone, HPV is the only consistent and continuous active local mechanism that regulates the distribution of blood flow in the lung.

Blood Flow in the Lungs

The blood flow through the lungs is essentially equal to the cardiac output. The flow is able to accommodate at least a fivefold increase in cardiac output without developing so great a pulmonary hydrostatic pressure as to result in pulmonary edema. As the total flow increases, the pulmonary vascular resistance decreases for two reasons: one, because of the recruitment or opening of previously closed vessels, thus increasing the numbers of open vessels, and two, because of the distension of already open vessels, thus enlarging these opened vessels. But for adequate gas exchange it is important that blood be distributed to those lung segments where the alveoli are best oxygenated.

In the upright human lung, blood flow decreases from the bottom to the top, reaching very low values at the apex as compared to the base (see Chapter 2) (Fig. 4-1).[9,10] Posture and exercise affect this distribution. In the supine position, the distribution is similar; blood flow in the posterior regions of the lung (analogous to the bottom) exceeds flow in the anterior regions (analogous to the top). On mild exercise, blood flow through all areas of the lung increases so that regional differences become less.

Within the human lung inequality of blood flow is considerable.[11] The uneven distribution can be explained only partly by the vertical hydrostatic pressure gradient between the blood vessels at the bottom and top of the lung. For every centimeter of vertical distance up the lung, the decrease in pulmonary artery pressure is approximately 1 cm H_2O.

End expiration alveolar pressure is normally close to atmospheric pressure. At least in the upright posture, a region may exist at the top of the lung (zone 1) where the pulmonary arterial pressure is less than alveolar pressure ($P_A > Ppa$). If this is so, then all pulmonary arterial vessels are collapsed and no blood flow occurs. Under normal conditions such conditions do not occur when the pulmonary artery pressure is high enough to maintain perfusion to the top of the lung. Zone 1 may occur, however, if arterial pressure is reduced by severe hemorrhage or if alveolar pressure is raised by positive pressure ventilation. This ventilated but nonperfused lung does not participate in gas exchange and contributes to alveolar dead space.

Further down the lung (zone 2) the hydrostatic pressure is greater than at the top of the lung. Pulmonary arterial pressure now exceeds alveolar pressure ($Ppa > P_A$), which in turn exceeds venous pressure. Under these conditions, blood flow is determined by the difference between arterial and alveolar pressures and not by the usual arterial and venous difference. This has been called the Starling resistor or waterfall effect.

Since pulmonary artery pressure is greater towards the base of the lung than toward the apex and venous pressure now exceeds alveolar pressure ($Ppv > P_A$), which is the same throughout the lung, the blood flow in zone 3 is determined by the usual arterial venous pressure difference ($Ppa > Ppv$). The pressure immediately outside the vessels (ie, the pleural pressure) becomes only slightly less negative in more dependent lung regions, but the arterial-venous pressure within the vessels is increasing steadily down the zone. Thus the pressure across the walls of the vessels (ie, the transmural distending pressure or the intraluminal pressure relative to pleural pressure) is also rising, so that the mean width of the vessels is greater. Any further increase in blood flow to this lung region is accomplished primarily by distension of these vessels. As Ppa increases from moderate to high levels of vascular pressure, distension causes zone 2 vessels to become new zone 3 vessels.

In the most dependent regions of the lung, fluid may transudate out of the pulmonary capillaries and veins into the pulmonary interstitial

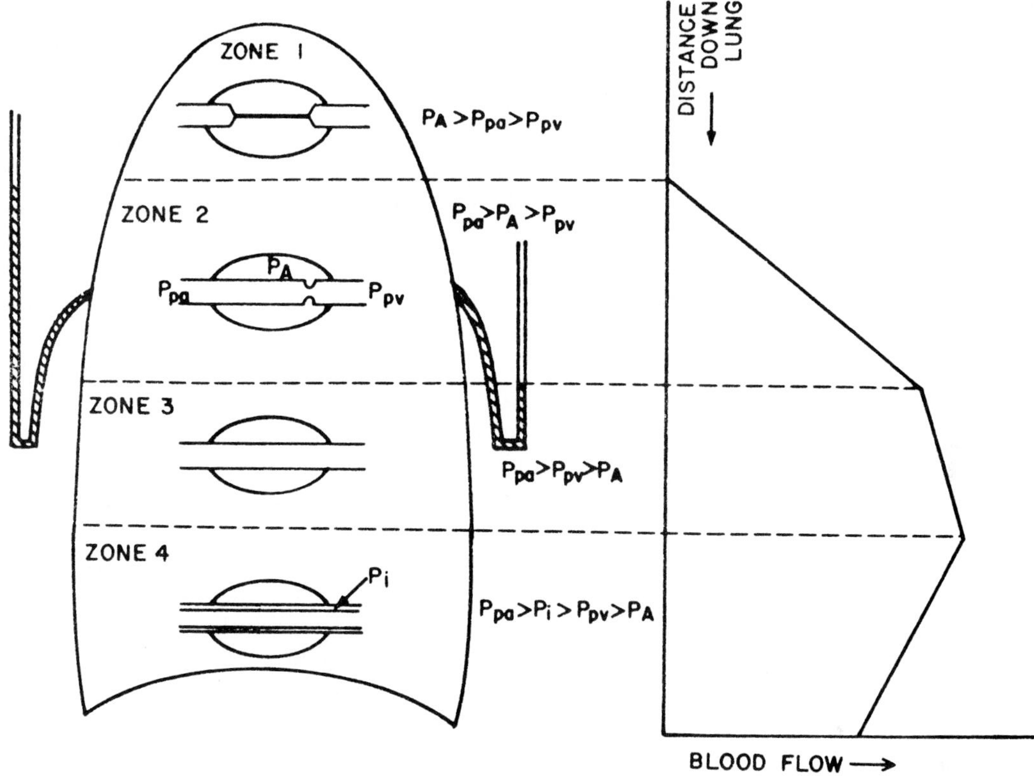

Figure 4-1. Distribution of pulmonary blood flow in the upright lung showing the gravity effect. In zone 1, the pulmonary artery pressure (Ppa) is less than alveolar pressure (PA), and no flow occurs as alveolar pressure compresses and collapses the vessels (PA > Ppa > Ppv). In zone 2, pulmonary blood flow is determined by the arterial-alveolar pressure difference. Since Ppa increases progressively down the lung and PA remains constant, the pulmonary blood flow increases down the zone (Ppa > PA > Pp v). In zone 3, pulmonary blood flow is determined by the arterial venous pressure difference (Ppa > Ppv > PA). The increase in blood flow is caused chiefly by distension of the capillaries, although recruitment of previously closed vessels is also a contributor to the increase in blood flow. In zone 4, the flow rate decrease is attributed to compression of vessels by increasing interstitial tissue pressure (PI). (Redrawn, with permission, from West.[10])

compartment, with conversion of the normally present negative pressure to a positive interstitial pressure. The interstitial pressure (PI) increases to compress and reduce the diameter of the vessels (zone 4), and thus may lead to decreased regional blood flow.

These concepts provide an explanation of the distribution of normal pulmonary blood flow, which may be considered to result from mechanical properties of the lung vasculature under the influence of gravity. With each unit increase in pulmonary artery pressure, however, the flow increase becomes larger. This pressure-flow relationship is due to both recruitment and distension of vessels and allows accommodation of a wide range of flows without the generation of excessive pulmonary vascular pressures.

Mechanism of Hypoxic Pulmonary Vasoconstriction

The HPV response may be viewed as a local mechanism for regulation of pulmonary blood flow by which the mismatching of ventilation-perfusion is reduced and oxygen exchange maintained. Although the two HPV responses are increases in pulmonary artery pressure and flow diversion, the relative contribution of each depends on how much of the lung is stimulated by HPV. At a certain point the gain in P_AO_2 stops because as more and more lung becomes hypoxic, the vascular resistance increases throughout the lung, and the capacity for flow diversion from hypoxic areas decreases (Fig. 4-2).[12] The greater the size of the hypoxic lung segment, the less effective is blood flow diversion and the greater the increase in pulmonary perfusion pressure. If the entire lung is maximally hypoxic, then blood flow diversion does not occur from one lung region to the other and the only observed response is an increase in perfusion pressure. The corollary to this statement is that if the hypoxic lung segment is very small, then the blood flow changes in that portion are large, whereas the perfusion pressure changes are very small.

Pressure-Flow Curves

Measurable HPV responses are one, a reduction of blood flow to hypoxic regions, with a concomitant increase of blood flow to the normoxic regions, and two an overall rise in pulmonary vascular resistance so that pulmonary arterial pressure and pulmonary perfusion pressure increase. These two major responses of the HPV phenomenon can be conveniently displayed simultaneously as a pressure-flow (P-Q) curve of the pulmonary circulation. Data pooled from several studies were used to generate the P-Q curves for normoxic and hypoxic lung;[12–17] some of these curves appear quite similar (Fig. 4-3).[18]

P-Q curves for normoxic and hypoxic states imply that pulmonary vascular resistance changes when cardiac output changes independently of HPV or any other stimulus to vascular contraction. Thus, to characterize a particular "state" of the pulmonary artery, operating information that describes the flow at each pressure when the relationship is no longer linear is needed. The calculation of resistance by dividing the perfusion pressure difference by the total flow is a useful convenience but may be misleading if these nonlinear characteristics are ignored. Calculation of resistance based on assumptions about an apparently linear portion of a pressure-flow relationship has been common, however. The concept of a critical opening pressure for pulmonary vessels arose from the extrapolation of such a curve through to the pressure axis that corresponds to zero flow. This concept appears to have little justification and permits no insight to physiologic or pathophysiologic mechanisms.

The fundamental importance of HPV for patients is primarily during pathological states. Although HPV plays only a minor role in the matching of ventilation and perfusion under normal circumstances, HPV has been found to play a critical role in diseased states, however. The fact that lung vessels in the body are unique in that they react to hypoxia with constriction rather than dilation has prompted many investigators to search for the site and mechanism of oxygen sensing for the pulmonary vessels. The stimulus for HPV is determined by both the alveolar oxygen tension (P_AO_2) and mixed venous oxygen tension ($P\bar{v}O_2$)[19] using the following equation:

$$(4\text{-}1) \qquad P_SO_2 = P_AO_2^{\,0.6} \times P\bar{v}O_2^{\,0.4}$$

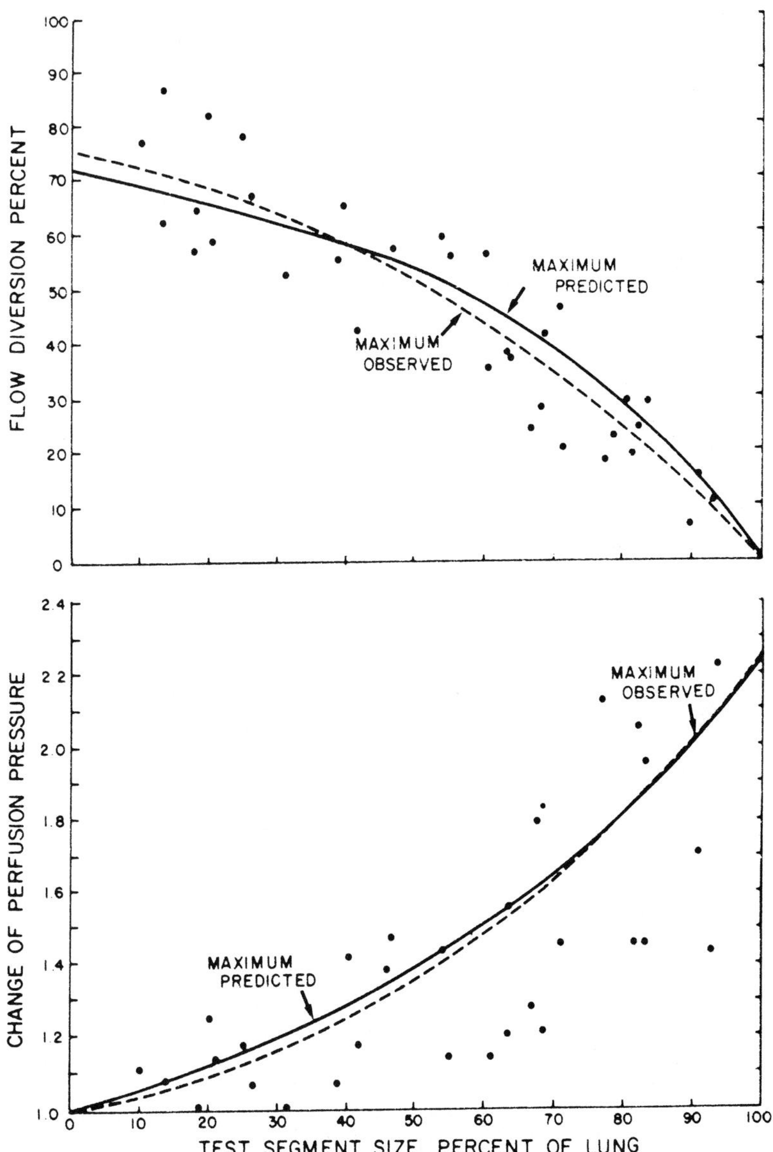

Figure 4-2. Relationship between hypoxic lung test segment size and the HPV responses of blood flow diversion percent and change in pulmonary perfusion pressure. As the test segment becomes larger, the only observed response is an increase in perfusion pressure, which are maximized when the entire lung is hypoxic. As the test segment becomes smaller, the only observed response is an increase in blood flow diversion (filled circles), which is minimized when the entire lung is hypoxic. (Reprinted, with permission, from Marshall et al.[12])

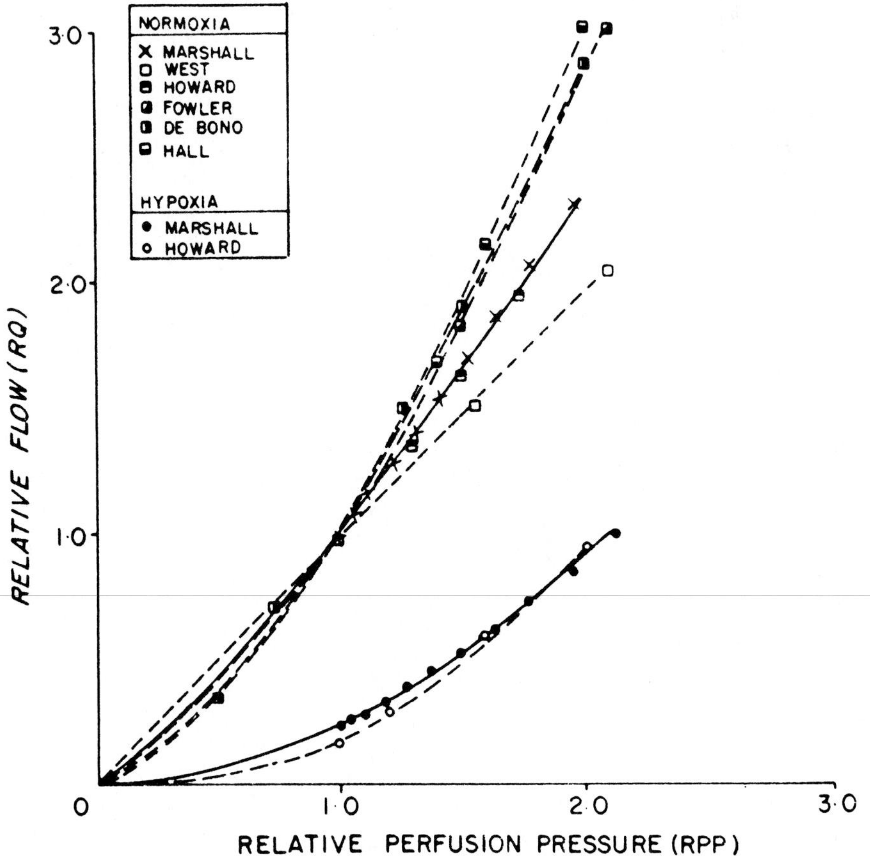

Figure 4-3. The two major HPV responses of changes in blood flow and changes in pulmonary perfusion pressure expressed in the form of pressure-flow curves. Pressure-flow curves are calculated for both the normoxic and the hypoxic lung. All data were calculated relative to the baseline control conditions defined by the point (1,1). (Data from references 12–17. Reprinted, with permission, from Marshall.[18])

The stimulus oxygen tension (PsO_2) may be defined as if the sensor were at a discrete site within the precapillary arterial smooth muscle wall (Fig. 4-4).[20–22] The quantitative contribution by intravascular blood gas tension is defined only when an in vitro isolated rat heart-lung model allowed perfusate and ventilating gas concentrations to be adjusted independently. Increasing perfusate oxygen tension reduces the pressor response to graded alveolar hypoxia (Fig. 4-5).[19]

Interestingly, the arterial oxygen tension also influences pulmonary vascular tone in other ways, that is, via the bronchial arteries that supply the vasavasorum to the pulmonary artery walls[23] as well as via stimulation of carotid chemoreceptors.[24] Although the stimulus for HPV (PsO_2) is determined predominately by

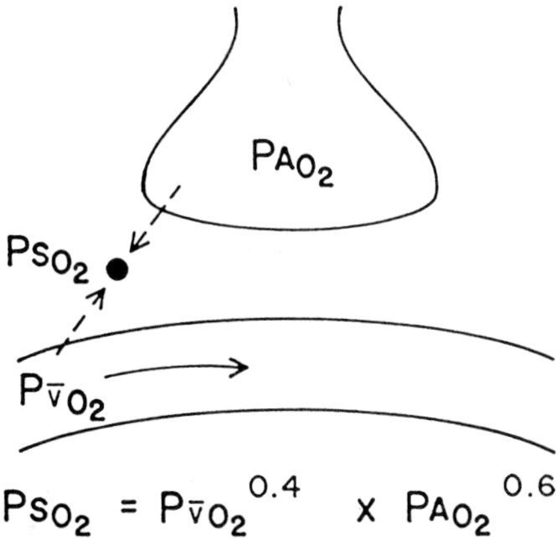

Figure 4-4. Illustration of the stimulus oxygen tension (PsO_2), which is shown as a discrete site in the wall of the precapillary arteriole influenced by both the alveolar (PAO_2) and mixed venous ($P\bar{v}O_2$) oxygen tensions. (Reprinted, with permission, from Marshall.[19])

the alveolar gas, the role of mixed venous oxygen tension on the pressor response increases if PAO_2 and $P\bar{v}O_2$ are reduced, so that with large regions of lung atelectasis, the main stimulus for HPV is $P\bar{v}O_2$.

Atelectasis and Blood Flow

The HPV response to either hypoxia or atelectasis in one lung is an active response that results in a rapid, large and persistent reduction of blood flow to that lung.[25,26] Burton and Patel[27] observed that the larger pulmonary arteries in atelectatic lung were "kinked and gnarly," and therefore they concluded that blood flow reduction through atelectatic lung was caused by mechanical obstruction. However, Barer et al[28] found that administration of vasodilating drugs prevented the usual decrease in blood flow to atelectatic lung, and thus they concluded that active vasoconstriction was responsible for the blood flow reduction observed in atelectatic lung. Benumof confirmed the presence of an active HPV response[29]; when a canine left lower lobe was exposed both to selective atelectasis or to ventilation with 95% N_2–5% CO_2, the lobar blood flow decreased by the same amount. In open-chest dogs, Domino et al[30] found that approximately 50% of blood flow was directed away from atelectatic lung when $P\bar{v}O_2$ was low (24 mmHg) or normal (46 mmHg), but that blood flow was normal when $P\bar{v}O_2$ was increased to greater than 100 mmHg. Miller et al[31] showed that passive mechanical factors did not measurably affect blood flow distribution during open-chest atelectasis; the decrease in blood flow during atelectasis was almost completely reversed with addition of a vasodilator (eg, sodium nitroprusside) infusion. Together these observations demonstrate that the mechanism of blood flow diversion accompanying atelectasis is entirely the result of hypoxic pulmonary vasoconstriction. Surprisingly, mechanical factors appear to have no significant influence.

Pressure-Flow Model

These concepts of segment size, the influence of the stimulus oxygen tension, and the active, rather than passive, nature of the HPV response have been incorporated into a model of the pulmonary circulation reproducing the pressure-flow (P-Q) relationship of the pulmonary circuit. The model was developed from data for cats that measured the branching pattern, number, diameter, length, compliance, apparent viscosity, and flow properties of all lung vessels.[32] When blood flow is converted to relative units for a variety of different animal models, the P-Q curves become essentially the same. Thus the general model based on the cat lung unit allows comparison between many species, including humans.[18,33–35] The model enables prediction of P-Q curves under a variety of circumstances based entirely on anatomic data and known physics of fluid flow. In addition, it also allows for active constriction by pulmonary artery segments so that the effects

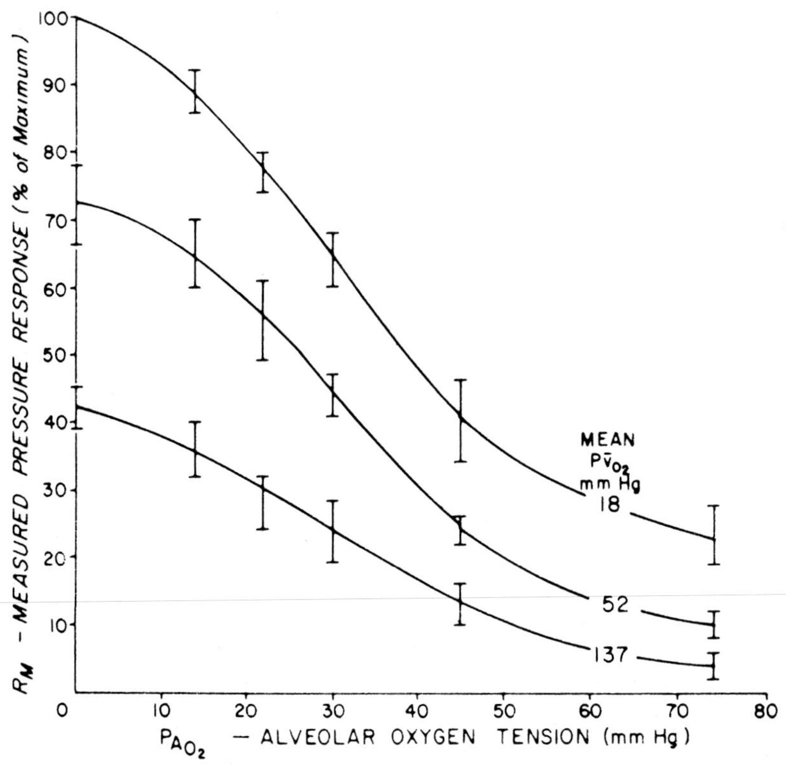

Figure 4-5. Mean rise in pulmonary artery pressure in response to varying concentrations of alveolar (PAO_2) and perfusate ($P\bar{V}O_2$) oxygen tension in isolated perfused rat lungs. The perfusion circuit is capable of degassing blood to deliver a $P\bar{V}O_2$ as low as 7 mmHg. The isolated lung is ventilated with 10 times the volume (plus 5.5% $FiCO_2$) with which it was perfused. In this way PAO_2 are completely divorced from $P\bar{V}O_2$. To enable comparison between individual animals, the rise in mean Ppa is expressed as a percentage of the maximum pressure rise during hypoxia. Increasing perfusate oxygen tension ($P\bar{V}O_a$) reduces the pressor response to graded alveolar hypoxia; as the mixed venous oxygen increases clinically, the stimulus for HPV decreases. As PAO_2 decrease, $P\bar{V}O_2$ assume greater importance. In an atelectatic lung, $P\bar{V}O_2$ is the sole deterrent of the stimulus for HPV. (Reprinted, with permission, from Marshall.[19])

of vasoconstrictors and vasodilators can be predicted.

Thus the model can be useful in assessing the influence of drugs with multiple effects (Fig. 4-6).[36] The action of dopamine, for example, is complicated because it not only causes vasoconstriction but also changes cardiac output and mixed venous oxygen tension. P-Q curves are shown for 100% oxygen (constriction ratio = 1.0), for maximum HPV (constriction ratio = 0.6), and for intermediate states of vasoconstriction (dashed lines). The amount of constriction, which is referred to as the constriction ratio, is the ratio of the diameter of the constricted vessel to the diameter of the relaxed vessel when the transmural pressure is zero. When both lungs are ventilated with a 100% oxygen (asterisk) and no constriction is present,

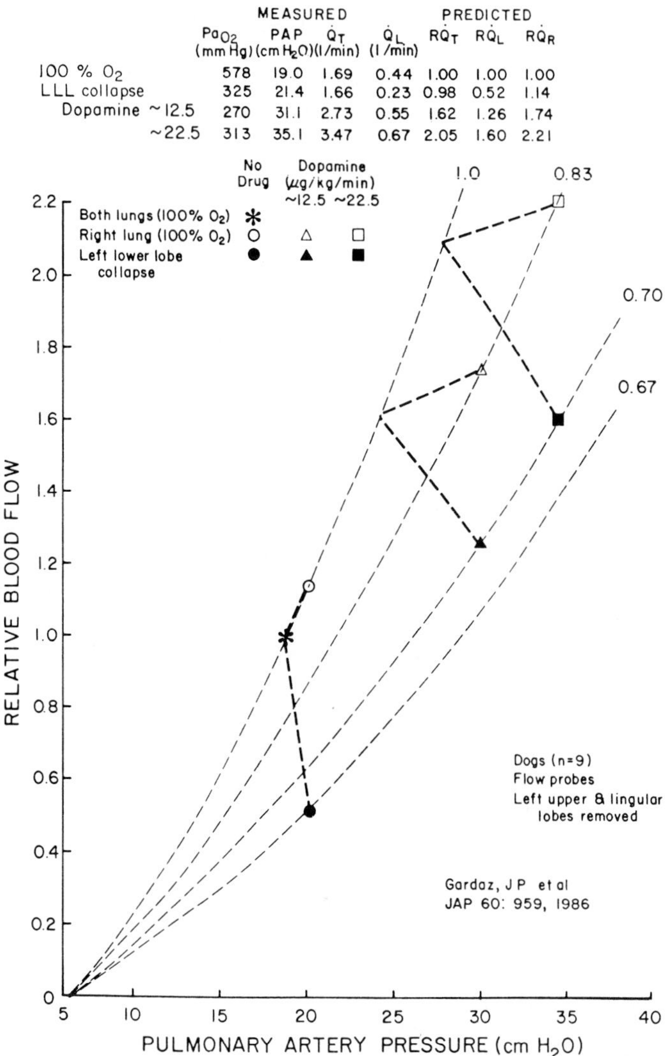

Figure 4-6. Influence of dopamine on HPV. Pressure-flow curves are shown for 100% oxygen (constriction ratio = 1.0), for maximum HPV (constriction ratio = 0.6), and for intermediate states of vasoconstriction (dashed lines). After the left lower lobe was collapsed, HPV was stimulated with constriction to 0.67 (solid circle) in the left lower lobe (LLL). Flow diversion caused flow to increase to the rest of the lung (open circle), which remained unconstricted. When dopamine (approximately 12.5 μg/kg/min or 22.5 μg/kg/min) was infused in the presence of left lower lobe atelectasis, the relative cardiac output was increased to 1.6 or 2.1, respectively, but the pulmonary artery pressure and left lung flow increased disproportionately. The model confirms the experimental observations that the predominant action of dopamine is to induce constriction of the normoxic lung (open triangle) and thereby decrease overall conductance and reduce flow diversion resulting from HPV. The model assigned predicted relative total cardiac output (RQT), relative left lung blood flow (RQL), and relative right lung blood flow (RQR). Arterial oxygen tension (PAO_2), pulmonary artery pressure (PAP), total cardiac output (QT) and left lung blood flow (QL) were measured variables given in the data from Gardaz JP et al.[36] (Reprinted, with permission, from Marshall.[34])

the pulmonary artery pressure is approximately 19 cm H_2O.

The left lower lobe is then collapsed. With the occurrence of the HPV response occurred and the vasoconstriction in the left lower lobe, the pulmonary artery pressure increases. This is represented by the rise in the pulmonary artery pressure from 19.0 to 21.4 cm H_2O and by the change in the constriction ratio from 1.0 to 0.67 (solid circle) for the left lower lobe. At the same time, flow diversion causes blood flow to increase to the rest of the lung (open circle) from a relative blood flow of 1.0 to 1.14.

When dopamine (12.5 μg/kg/min) is infused in the presence of left lower lobe atelectasis, the pulmonary artery pressure increases to 31.1 cm H_2O, and the relative cardiac output rises to 1.62 as would be expected from an inotropic drug. However, the left lower lobe is less constricted; the constriction ratio goes from 0.67 to 0.70. In addition, the blood flow to the hypoxic lung is increased from 0.52 to 1.26. Therefore, dopamine causes vasoconstriction in the entire pulmonary vascular bed and also increases blood flow through the hypoxic lung. This rise in blood flow contributes to a decrease in arterial PaO_2 and a reduction in the effectiveness of the HPV phenomenon.

The increase in cardiac output may have been expected to affect the stimulus oxygen tension, thus yielding a decreased HPV response due to the increase in the mixed venous $P\bar{v}O_2$. Alternatively, it may have been thought that the increase in pulmonary vasoconstriction would decrease the amount of blood flow through the hypoxic lung. However, the model confirms the experimental observations. The predominant action of this particular dopamine dose was to induce constriction in the 100%-O_2 ventilated lung (open triangle), thus decreasing the amount of blood flow diverted from the hypoxic lung region. The model allows (1) a quantitative evaluation of the active regulation of pulmonary blood flow distribution by the HPV phenomenon and (2) analysis, reinterpretation, and comparison of blood flow changes in studies performed by various investigators.

Influences on Hypoxic Pulmonary Vasoconstriction

The characteristically large variation in magnitude of HPV responses is attributable to the influence of several variables (Table 4-1).[37] Although the primary determinants are the vascular smooth muscle tone and responsivity, secondary variables act to change pressure or flow responses or the mechanical parameters that set the position of the P-Q curve.

The pulmonary artery pressure, or the intraluminal vascular pressure against which the pulmonary vessels must constrict, is a major determinant of the magnitude of HPV because even vessels constricted by hypoxia dilate when exposed to pressures exceeding 16–18 mmHg.[38,39] Clinical conditions that increase pulmonary vascular pressure and therefore inhibit clinically significant blood flow redis-

Table 4-1. Pulmonary Circulation with Hypoxia or Atelectasis

Stimulus	
PaO_2 and $P\bar{v}O_2$	
Response	
Increased pulmonary vascular resistance	
Results	
Flow diversion and pulmonary artery pressure	
Primary determinants	
Smooth muscle tone and responsivity	
Secondary variables	
Age	Trauma
Sex	Segment size
Temperature	P_AO_2
Species	Cardiac output
pH	Left atrial pressure
P_{CO_2}	Pleural pressure
Individual	Airway pressure
Drugs	Posture
Anesthetics	PaO_2
Disease	Pulmonary artery pressure

tribution away from hypoxic lung are mitral stenosis, left heart failure, volume overload, gross edema, administration of vasopressor drugs, ligation of pulmonary vessels, thromboembolism, and large hypoxic segments.[12]

When the left atrial pressure is raised, the HPV response is blunted.[38] Increasing the left atrial pressure distends the vein, venules, and capillaries in addition to the arteries. As the vessel diameter becomes greater, a further pressure increase has relatively less effect on the flow than when the vessel diameter is narrower. As left atrial pressure increases, recruitment and distension of all vessels occurs, so that blood flow diversion from hypoxic regions is less.

Positive end-expiratory pressure (PEEP) applied to a hypoxic lung tends to decrease conductance through that segment and hence enhances flow diversion away from that segment. The vessel size is determined by the transmural pressure at each end; blood flows only when the transmural pressure at the inflow to each vessel is greater than the transmural pressure at the outflow. However, the transmural pressure is the difference between the hydrostatic pressure inside the vessel and that on the outside. In the alveoli and in the small intra-alveolar arterioles and vessels, the outside pressure is the same as the alveolar pressure; thus PEEP narrows these vessels and enhances HPV. In all other vessels, the outside pressure is related to the pleural pressure.

Studies of the effects of lateral decubitus position on the distribution of pulmonary blood flow have demonstrated a 5–15% shift of flow from the nondependent to the dependent lung.[40] In the lateral decubitus position, the ventilated (down) lung usually has a reduced lung volume (functional residual capacity [FRC] as a result of the combined actions of induction of general anesthesia and paralysis and compression by the full weight of the abdominal contents, the upper lung, and the mediastinum.[41] To prevent dependent lung atelectasis from this cause as well as denitrogenation, the 2.5 cm of PEEP should be applied to the lower lung, particularly in obese patients, to preserve adequate level of oxygenation.[42] After the start of surgery, when the chest wall and pleura are opened, the negative intrapleural pressure is lost and becomes ambient. In open-chest animals, HPV causes blood flow diversion from lung regions exposed to either atelectasis or hypoxic ventilation. However, in closed chest animals the ineffectiveness of the HPV mechanism in studies of collapsed lungs[43] inflated lungs,[44–46] and isolated dog lung lobes,[47] has been attributed to changes in pleural pressure or lung volume on blood vessels. As a result of the negative intrapleural pressure generated during left lung resorption atelectasis when the animal's chest is closed, however, diversion of perfusion away from the collapsed lung may be reduced.[48] For this reason, HPV is less effective during closed-chest atelectasis.

Other factors affect HPV. HPV is maximal at normal pH. Decreases in $PaCO_2$ and P_ACO_2 below 30 mmHg were found to inhibit HPV.[49] Although the HPV response is attenuated more by alkalosis than acidosis, both metabolic and respiratory change in pH inhibit HPV.[38, 50, 51] In addition, the HPV response is greater in males than in females, probably because of hormonal differences.[52] The response is reduced by pregnancy in rats[53] and in dogs[54] where it appeared that the depressed hypoxic pressor response was due to some blood-borne substance other than estrogen and progesterone. Marked species differences are apparent in both the level of PO_2 required to elicit pulmonary vascular responses and the amplitude of these responses.[55]

There is some evidence that infection (eg, granulomatous pulmonary disease[56] and pneumococcal pneumonia)[57] may inhibit HPV. Some authors suggest that local hypoxic vasoconstriction is ineffective in directing blood flow away from diseased regions of the lung in which gas exchange is impaired or absent, whereas others dispute this.[58] Perhaps mediators of septic shock such as endotoxin, tumor necrosis factor, interleukins, prostaglandins, and leukotrienes play a role that is yet to be defined.

The ever-accumulating evidence suggests that in patients with severe lung disease, inhibition of HPV may produce marked increases of venous admixture that may prove to be hazardous to anesthetized patients. Bacterial endotoxins lead to both pulmonary vascular damage and enhanced prostaglandin $F_{2\alpha}$, prostacyclin, and thromboxane production by the lung.[59,60] In addition, pulmonary embolism and nonhemodynamic lung injury following acute myocardial infarction are associated with enhanced pulmonary prostanoid biosynthesis.[61]

In the surgical setting, physical trauma to pulmonary tissue may be of special concern. Moderate degrees of surgical manipulation of the nonventilated lung have been shown to significantly increase the shunt fraction as compared with two-lung ventilation with the chest open and one-lung ventilation with the chest closed.[62] When no chest wall surgery is performed, HPV responses are maximal from the outset, whereas after surgical manipulation, the HPV response is markedly reduced (Fig. 4-7).[63]

Figure 4-7. Data from dogs in which the flow diversion from the left lung was measured with an hypoxic shunt. In one group of animals, no surgery on the chest wall was undertaken, and the HPV responses are maximal from the beginning and throughout the approximately 90 min required for the four trials.[63] In the second group of animals, the chest wall was opened and the lung manipulated to attach electromagnetic flow probes.[26] Subsequently, the hypoxic response was found to be markedly reduced and was restored only after some 60–90 minutes without further manipulation. (Reprinted, with permission, from Chen.[63])

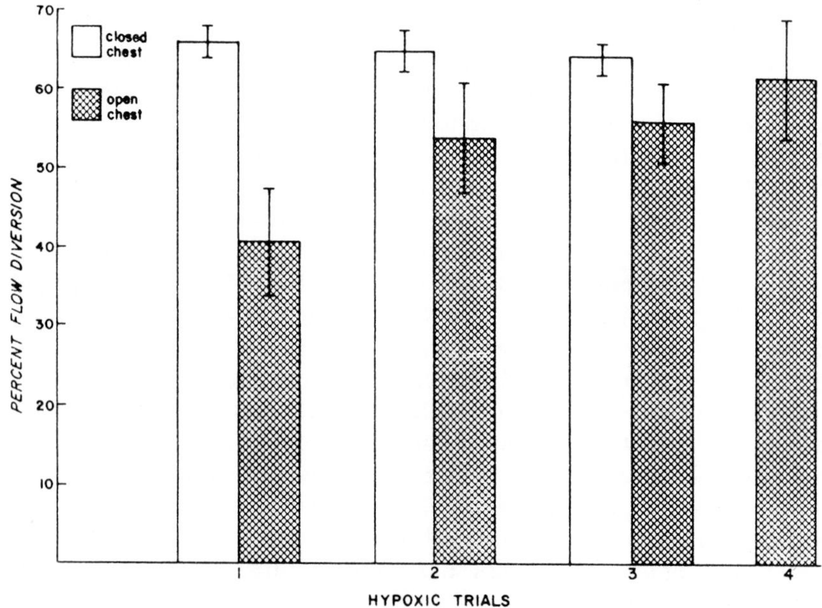

Trauma may also cause local release of vasodilator prostaglandins that may affect the HPV response.[64]

Body temperature has also been shown to have an effect on the HPV response. Hypothermia itself has been associated with a significant decrease in HPV.[65] Hypothermia is also associated with a significant increase in pulmonary vascular resistance in normoxic lung regions, however; therefore this may also contribute to the impaired effectiveness of HPV to divert blood flow. Similarly, hyperthermia to 42°C enhanced HPV.[66]

One of the major secondary variables that may obscure the interpretation of the effects of inhalational anesthetics on HPV is cardiac output, which is altered to a markedly different extent by the various inhaled agents. The dashed line in Figure 4-8 shows that when cardiac output is decreased, HPV is improved, but when cardiac output is increased, HPV is reduced without inhalational anesthetic.[35] However, with the administration of anesthesia is administered, however, and if the cardiac output remains the same as under control conditions, blood flow to the hypoxic lung would increase. Thus inhalational anesthetics actually reduce the HPV response.

On the other hand, if cardiac output is decreased with the administration of an anesthetic, the $P\bar{v}O_2$ decreases and the PsO_2 falls. Both of these reactions would tend to enhance the HPV response, but the overall effect may appear as an unchanged blood flow response. This results from the fact that as the cardiac output decreases, the true inhibition of HPV by the inhalational anesthetics becomes increasingly more obscured by a greater stimulus for HPV.

Drugs

Anesthetic Agent

The effect of inhalational anesthetic agents on HPV has been debated by various investigators. Particular concerns have arisen concerning species differences and the applicability of in vitro data to in vivo or clinical situations. Additional information on the clinical use of anesthetic agents can be found in Chapter 13.

In an isolated rat lung model, halothane, enflurane, and isoflurane were found to depress HPV in a dose-related manner.[2,67] The concentrations in minimum alveolar concentration (MAC) units for the rat at which 50% depression of HPV (ED_{50}) occurred were 0.47, 0.60, and 0.56 for halothane, isoflurane, and enflurane, respectively (Fig. 4-9). Among these agents, neither the ED_{50} values nor the slopes of the dose-response curves were significantly different. Thus the halogenated, inhalational anesthetics inhibit HPV in a dose-related manner with essentially the same potency (ie, ED_{50} = 0.5 MAC).

Bjertnaes in 1978[68,69] was one of the first to suggest that inhalational anesthetics inhibit HPV in humans (Fig. 4-10). The distribution of blood flow to the test lung was determined by pulmonary perfusion scanning or lung scintigraphy using human serum albumin macroaggregates labeled with either ^{99m}Tc or ^{131}I. After spontaneous breathing of room air occurred, anesthesia induction proceeded with thiopental, fentanyl, and pancuronium. Unilateral hypoxia was achieved by ventilating the test lung with 100% N_2 and the other lung with 100% O_2. After ipsilateral administration of either diethyl ether or halothane, blood flow to the test lung increased significantly. The researchers concluded that diethyl either and halothane inhibit HPV and that this contributes to the development of arterial hypoxemia during anesthesia in humans.

If inhalational anesthetics are administered to only a hypoxic segment of lung, then low systemic concentrations can be maintained such that the effects of these anesthetics on HPV can be studied without the occurrence of

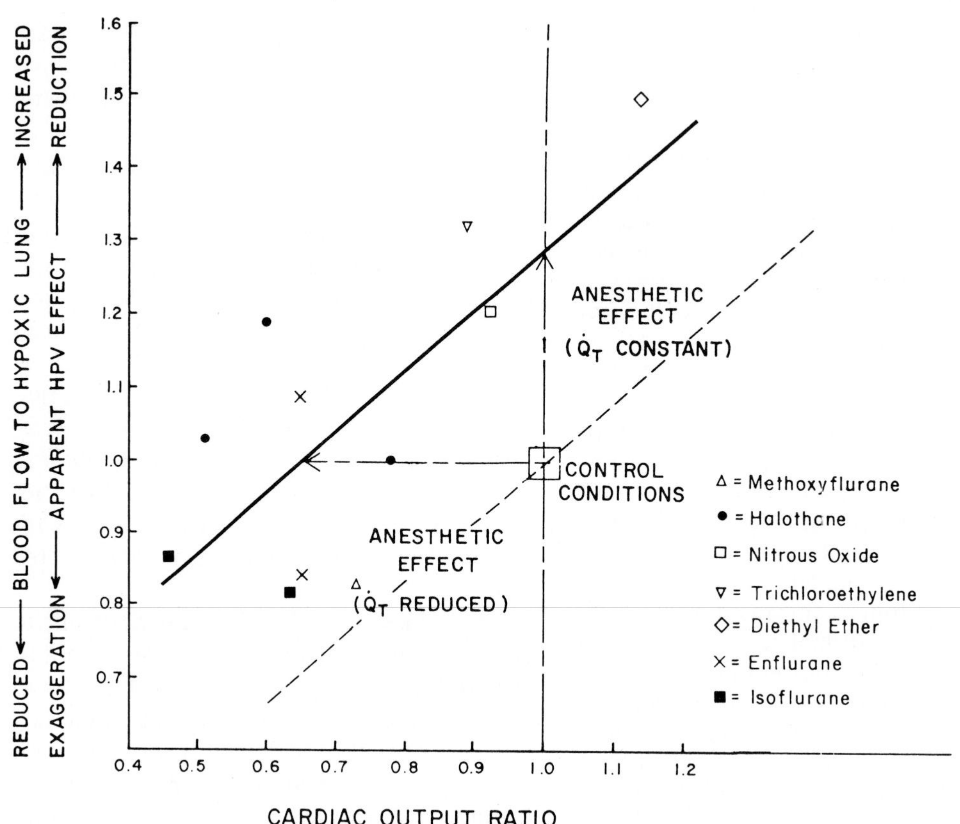

Figure 4-8. Influence of Q_T on inhalational anesthetics on observed HPV responses. Observed HPV response with inhalational anesthetics are compared with simultaneous changes in cardiac output. Data have been standardized to allow comparison between studies. The cardiac output ratio is:

$$\frac{\text{Cardiac output with anesthetic}}{\text{Cardiac output without anesthetic}}$$

where control cardiac output without anesthetic = 1.0. The HPV ratio is:

$$\frac{\text{Hypoxic segment blood flow with anesthetic}}{\text{Hypoxic segment blood flow without anesthetic}}$$

where the control hypoxic segment blood flow without anesthetic = 1.0. The regression line for the relationship is effect of anesthetic on the HPV ratio = 0.46 + 0.83 (cardiac output ratio), and r = 0.74. These results suggest that changes in cardiac output in the presence of inhalation agents are an important influence on whether the HPV response appears increased or decreased. Q = Halothane[74,81,84]; R = isoflurane[77,81]; Δ = methoxyflurane[88]; □ = nitrous oxide[75]; ∇ = trichloroethylene[85]; ◇ = diethylether[84]; and x = enflurane.[74] (Modified, with permission, from Marshall.[35])

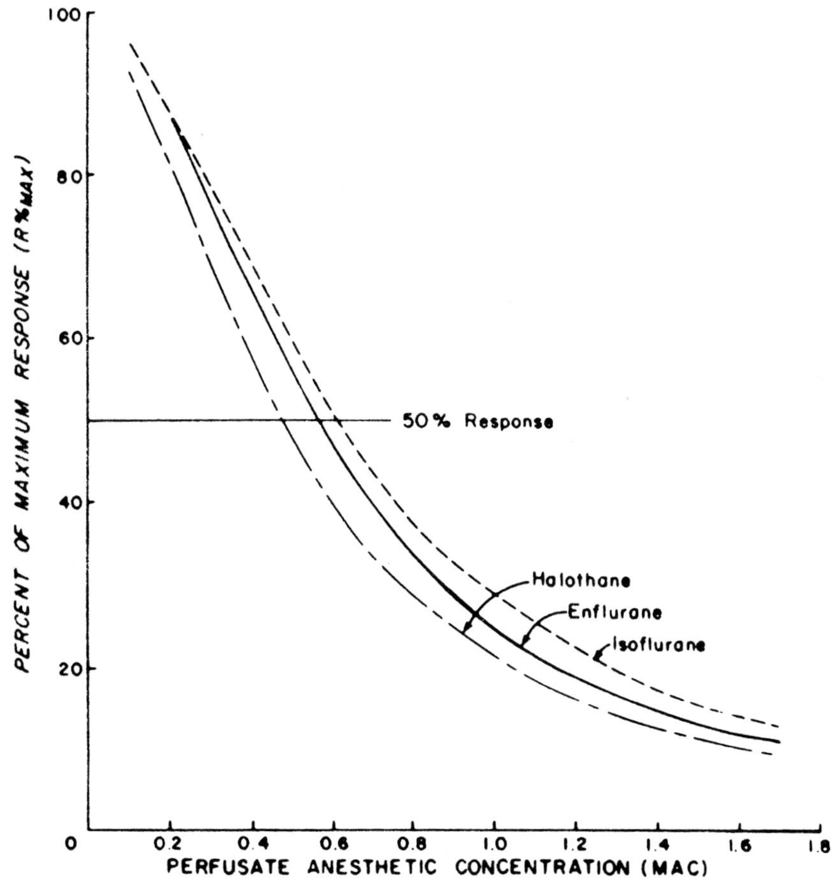

Figure 4-9. Dose-response curves for inhibition of HPV by halothane, isoflurane, and enflurane. In an isolated perfused rat lung model, the curves for the three anesthetic agents do not differ significantly in slope or in ED_{50} MAC units, and $r > 0.82$. (Reprinted, with permission, from Marshall.[67])

large hemodynamic alterations. When variables such as cardiac output and $P\bar{v}O_2$ are maintained constant, a dose-response curve can be derived for the influence of inhalational anes thetics for both humans and other animals thus demonstrating the inhibition of HPV by inhalational anesthetics (Fig. 4-11).[37,70–72]

The extent of the variability of the inhibition of HPV is not the same for different inhalational agents (Fig. 4-12).[37,73] Apparently, the mean PAO_2 in patients anesthetized with halothane is lower than in those patients receiving isoflurane. In addition, much more individual variability is evident with halothane as compared with isoflurane. This explains in part the clinical observation that although some patients do very well with an inhalational agent, others appear to be susceptible to hypoxemia. This latter group may actually benefit from a change to an injectable agent.

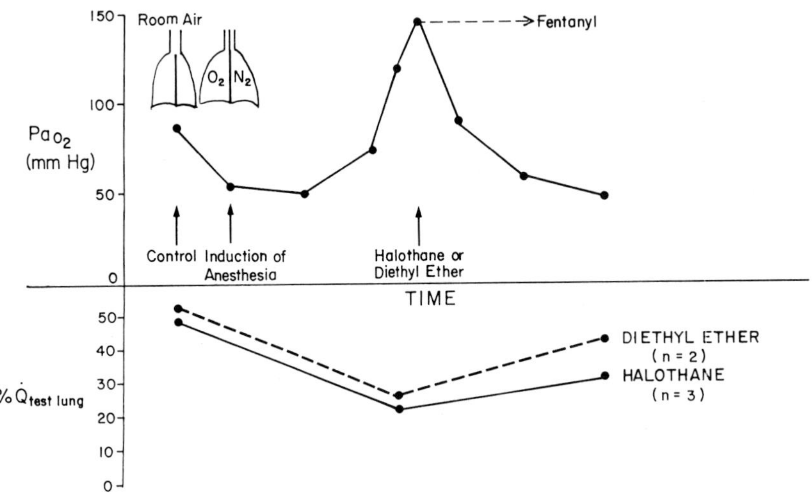

Figure 4-10. Effect of halothane and diethyl ether on HPV in humans. At baseline both lungs are ventilated with room air. After induction of anesthesia with thiopental, fentanyl and pancuronium, the test lung is ventilated with 100% N_2 and the other lung with 100% O_2. With development of a HPV response, the arterial oxygen tension (PAO_2) rises and the blood flow in the test lung (% $Q_{test\ lung}$) falls. With the presence of either halothane or diethyl ether, the PAO_2 falls and the % $Q_{test\ lung}$ rises, suggesting inhibition of the HPV response by the inhalational anesthetic agents (Courtesy of Bryan E. Marshall. Data from Bjertnaes[68] and Bjertnaes.[69])

Buckley and colleagues[74] studied N_2O using a dog model of global hypoxia and suggested HPV was enhanced by N_2O. Animal models using global hypoxia result in systemic hypoxemia, which has profound hemodynamic effects on the whole animal, however, and therefore must be interpreted cautiously. Most subsequent studies have found a small but consistent inhibition of HPV by N_2O.[4,75,76] In summary, the inhalational anesthetics that inhibit HPV are N_2O,[2,4,74–77] isoflurane,[4,67,73,75,78] enflurane,[67,75,79] halothane,[2,4,67,69,74,75,80–84] ether,[2,69,83–85] trichloroethylene,[83,86] fluroxene,[4,75] and methoxyflurane (Table 4-2).[2,87–89] Cyclopropane[90] does not appear to affect the HPV response, but no recent studies are available and this inconsistency may be spurious.

Intravenous anesthetics agents, on the other hand, have no detectable effect on the HPV response, for the most part. (Table 4-3). Bjertnaes[2,91] reported that pentobarbital sodium had no influence on HPV in an isolated rat lung preparation in marked contrast to ether or halothane. There has been some controversy concerning this issue, however. In 1972, Susmano et al[92] reported that in intact dogs anesthetized with pentobarbital, HPV was dampened compared with those that received fentanyl-droperidol anesthesia. Wetzel et al[93] found that in isolated sheep lungs, pentobarbital inhibited HPV in a concentration-dependent fashion. In both these studies, however, high doses of anesthetics were used. Intravenous drugs in clinical use, such as barbiturates, narcotics, benzodiazepines, local anesthetics,[94] droperidol, chlorpromazine, pentazocine, appear to have no significant effect on the HPV response. For emergency thoracic pro-

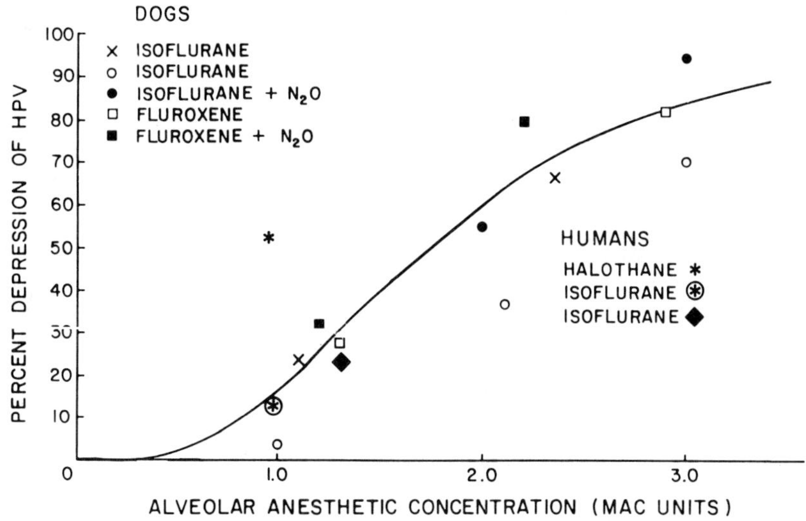

Figure 4-11. Depression of HPV by inhalational anesthetics in vivo. For the studies in dogs the anesthetic was administered only to hypoxic lung segments. All agents were associated with dose-related depression of HPV summarized as a sigmoid in the equation. The crosses are for isoflurane, while the open circles and squares refer to isoflurane and fluroxene, respectively, and the closed circles and squares are the same agents in the presence of nitrous oxide. (Data for isoflurane alone from Domino et al[70]; other dog data from Benumof[4]; and the human studies from Bjertnaes,[2] Zapol,[6] Foex,[71] and Carlsson.[72] Reprinted, with permission from Marshall.[37])

cedures the advantages of ketamine include sympathomimetic properties, rapid onset of anesthesia, induction, and ability to reduce bronchospasm. Ketamine, which appears to have no effect on hypoxic pulmonary vasoconstriction,[95] does not impair arterial oxygenation. Recently, claims have been made that propofol also has no effect on the HPV response.[96, 97]

Other Drugs

Many other drugs may eventually be necessary for patient care in the course of a surgical procedure. These drugs fall in a variety of classes, and each agent may be evaluated separately in terms of its effects on HPV (Table 4-4). Two generalizations should be considered concerning the action of vasoactive drugs on the pulmonary circulation. One, a number of drugs have dose-related, bimodal action, which means that they may inhibit or enhance HPV or have no effect depending on the dose administered. Two, the response of the pulmonary vasculature is often tone-dependent. In patients with regions of diseased lung and the presence of high pulmonary vascular tone, further vasoconstriction may lead to right heart failure; in regions constricted by HPV, drug induced vasodilation unfortunately may allow blood flow into these regions of lung that do not oxygenate well.

When the desired drug actions cannot be separated from effects on vascular tone, effects such as these make the selection of a particular drug and its dose difficult. One or both generalizations appear to account for the wide range of responses reported. Dopamine is a good example; which at a dose of 2.5 $\mu g \cdot kg^{-1} \cdot min^{-1}$ this

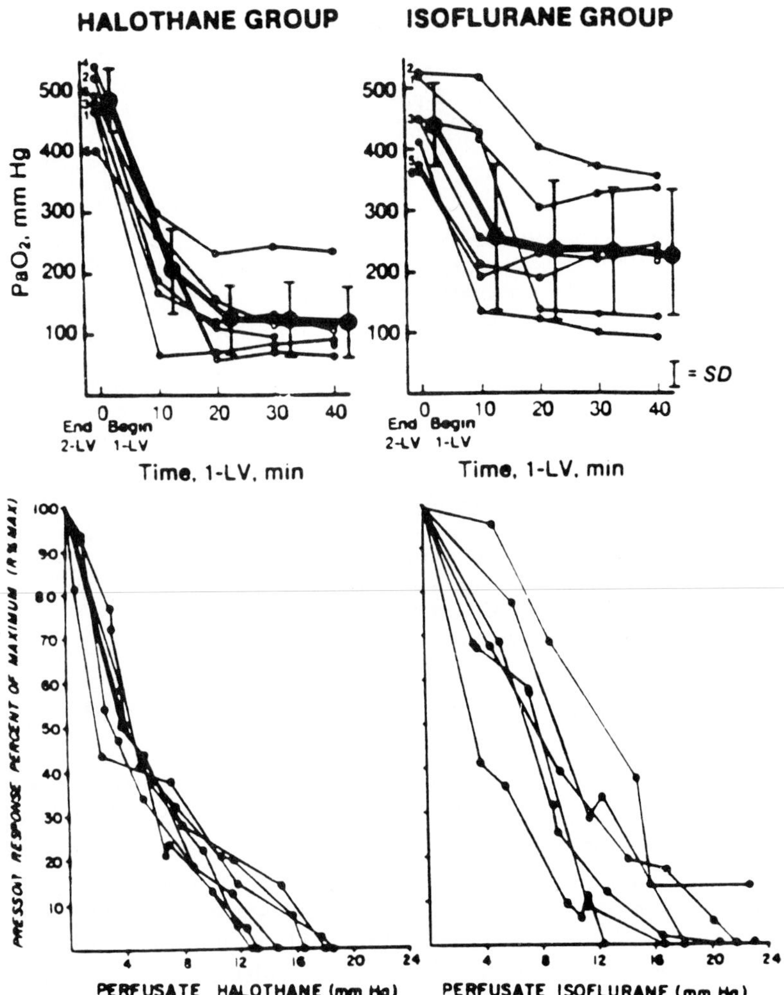

Figure 4-12. Comparison of effects of halothane and isoflurane on P_{AO_2} and hypoxic pressor response during one-lung anesthesia.[67,73] The upper panels show that following the introduction of one-lung anesthesia (1-LV) in human subjects, the mean P_{AO_2} is lower in the presence of halothane compared to isoflurane, but the variability among the individual subjects is less. The lower panels show that this conclusion is consistent with data obtained from rat lung-ventilated and perfused in vitro where the variability among the subjects for the two agents is striking. (Reprinted, with permission, from Marshall.[37])

Table 4-2. Effects of Inhalational Anesthetics on Hypoxic Pulmonary Vasoconstriction (HPV)*

Anesthetic Agent	Reference	Animal	Model	Effect
Nitrous oxide	Buckley[74]	Dog	5% O_2 whole lung	Enhance
	Hurtig[77]	Cat	3% O_2 isolated lung	Inhibit
	Bjertnaes[2]	Rat	2% O_2 isolated lung	None
	Sykes[76]	Dog	N_2 one lung	Inhibit
	Mathers[75]	Dog	N_2 LL lobe	Inhibit
	Benumof[4]	Dog	N_2 LL lobe	None
Isoflurane	Marshall[67]	Rat	3% O_2 isolated lung	Inhibit
	Benumof[73]	Human	N_2 one lung	None
	Benumof[4]	Dog	N_2 LL lobe	Inhibit
	Mathers[75]	Dog	N_2 LL lobe	Inhibit
	Saidman[78]	Dog	N_2 LL lobe	None
Enflurane	Marshall[67]	Rat	3% O_2 isolated lung	Inhibit
	Mathers[75]	Dog	N_2 LL lobe	None
	Carlsson[79]	Human	6% O_2 one lung	None
Halothane	Buckley[74]	Dog	5% O_2 whole lung	Inhibit
	Kaur[80]	Dog	10% O_2 whole lung	None
	Fargas-Babjak[81]	Dog	8% O_2 whole lung	None
	Sykes[83]	Dog	95% N_2 one lung	None
	Marshall[67]	Rat	3% O_2 isolated lung	Inhibit
	Sykes[82]	Cat	3% O_2 isolated lung	Inhibit
	Bjertnaes[2]	Rat	2% O_2 isolated lung	Inhibit
	Loh[84]	Cat	3% O_2 innervated lung	Inhibit
	Bjertnaes[69]	Human	N_2 one lung	Inhibit
	Benumof[4]	Dog	N_2 LL lobe	None
	Mathers[75]	Dog	N_2 LL lobe	None
Ether	Sykes[83]	Cat	3% O_2 isolated lung	Inhibit
	Bjertnaes[2]	Rat	2% O_2 isolated lung	Inhibit
	Loh[84]	Cat	3% O_2 innervated lung	Inhibit
	Bjertnaes[69]	Human	N_2 one lung	Inhibit
	Sykes[85]	Dog	N_2 left lung	Inhibit
Trichlorethylene	Sykes[83]	Cat	3% O_2 isolated lung	Inhibit
	Sykes[86]	Dog	N_2 one lung	Inhibit
Fluroxene	Benumof[4]	Dog	N_2 LL lobe	Inhibit
	Mathers[75]	Dog	N_2 LL lobe	Inhibit
Methoxyflurane	Sykes[87]	Cat	3% O_2 isolated lung	Inhibit
	Bjertnaes[2]	Rat	2% O_2 isolated lung	Inhibit
	Marin[88]	Dog	7% O_2 isolated lung	None
Cyclopropane	Tait[90]	Cat	3% O_2 isolated lung	None

* Modified, with permission, from Pavlin EG.[89]

agent had no effect on HPV, and yet at a clinically high dose 25 $\mu g \cdot kg^{-1} \cdot min^{-1}$ it inhibited HPV in dogs.[98] This suggests that predicting the dose at which the occurrence of HPV inhibition suddenly manifests itself as a decline in PaO_2. may be difficult for any given individual. At high doses, dopamine HCl is a pulmonary vasoconstrictor that appears to cause an increase in vasoconstriction of the normoxic lung as well as the hypoxic lung. This constriction of the normoxic lung shifts blood flow diverted from the hypoxic lung back into the hypoxic lung, with a resulting inhibition of HPV.[36, 98–100]

Epinephrine vasoconstricts both the hyperoxic and hypoxic lungs.[101] Of the inotropic drugs, isoproterenol is a pulmonary vasodilator

Table 4-3. Effects of Injectable Anesthetic Agents on Hypoxic Pulmonary Vasoconstriction (HPV)

Injectable Agent	Reference	Animal	Model	Effect
Barbiturates				
Pentobarbital	Bjertnaes[92]	Rat	2% O_2 isolated lung	None
	Wetzel[93]	Sheep	−4% O_2 isolated lung	Inhibit
	Susmano[92]	Dog	8% O_2 whole lung	Inhibit
Thiopental	Bjertnaes[2]	Rat	2% O_2 isolated lung	None
Hexobarbital	Bjertnaes[2]	Rat	2% O_2 isolated lung	None
Narcotics				
Fentanyl	Bjertnaes[2]	Rat	2% O_2 isolated lung	None
	Susmano[92]	Dog	8% O_2 whole lung	None
Morphine	Bjertnaes[2]	Rat	2% O_2 isolated lung	None
Demerol	Bjertnaes[2]	Rat	2% O_2 isolated lung	None
Benzodiazepines				
Diazepam	Bjertnaes[2]	Rat	2% O_2 isolated lung	None
Local Anesthetics				
Lidocaine	Bindslev[94]	Dog	7% O_2, LL lobe	None
Droperidol	Bjertnaes[2]	Rat	2% O_2 isolated lung	None
	Susmano[92]	Dog	8% O_2 whole lung	None
Chlorpromazine				
Pentazocine	Bjertnaes[2]	Rat	2% O_2 isolated lung	None
Ketamine	Bjertnaes[2]	Rat	2% O_2 isolated lung	None
	Rees[95]	Human	One-lung anesthesia	None
Propofol	Naeije[96]	Dog	10% O_2 whole lung	None
	VanKeer[97]	Human	One-lung atelectasis	None

Table 4-4. Effects of Inotropic Drugs on Hypoxic Pulmonary Vasoconstriction (HPV)

Injectable Agent	Reference	Animal	Model	Effect
Inotropes				
Dopamine				
12.5 μg/kg/min	Gardaz[36]	Dog	Lobar atelectasis	Inhibit
2.5 μg/kg/min	Marin[98]	Dog	7% O_2 one lung	None
25 μg/kg/min	Marin[98]	Dog	7% O_2 one lung	Inhibit
5 μg/kg/min	McFarlane[100]	Dog	7% O_2 LL lobe	None
20 μg/kg/min	McFarlane[100]	Dog	7% O_2 LL lobe	Inhibit
2,4,10,20 μg/kg/min	Furman[99]	Dog	6% O_2 isolated lung	None
Epinephrine	Hales[101]	Dog	100% N_2 one lung	Inhibit
Isoproterenol				
0.25 μg/kg/min	Marin[98]	Dog	7% O_2 one lung	Inhibit
0.25, 0.5, 1.25, 2.5 μg/kg/min	Furman[99]	Pig	6% isolated lung	Inhibit
Dobutamine				
5 μg/kg/min	McFarlane[100]	Dog	7% O_2 LL lobe	None
20 μg/kg/min	McFarlane[100]	Dog	7% O_2 LL lobe	Inhibit
2,4,10,20 μg/kg/min	Furman[99]	Pig	6% O_2 isolated lung	Inhibit
Ouabain	Haas[102]	Dog	10% O_2 whole lung	Enhance

and decreases pulmonary vascular resistance, thus inhibiting HPV.[98,99] Dobutamine also has a negative effect on HPV at higher doses, causing vasodilation in both the hypoxic/atelectatic lung as well as in the 100% O_2-ventilated other lung.[99,100]

Ouabain, a Na^+/K^+ pump inhibitor, may enhance HPV.[102] Clinically a patient may receive digoxin, a clinically useful drug of this class for cor pulmonale, left-sided congestive heart failure, or a supraventricular dysrhythmia with a rapid ventricular response. Digoxin may also benefit the thoracic surgical patient who is at risk for atrial dysrhythmia due to manipulation of the atrium during left pneumonectomy. (This is more important during a left than during a right pneumonectomy.)

Although no drugs are known to improve HPV unequivocally, various drugs in clinical use have been investigated for their effects on the HPV response (Table 4-5). Drugs whose primary action on pulmonary vasculature is vasodilation are inhibitors of HPV. These include sodium nitroprusside,[103–105] nitroglycerin,[105,106] hydralazine,[104] and alpha-blockers such as dibenzyline HCl.[28,107] The beta-blocker propranolol,[103,107] a vasoconstrictor, is reported to enhance HPV. Bretylium[28] reportedly has no effect on HPV. The bronchodilators aminophylline,[101,108] orciprenaline,[109] and salbutamol[110] inhibit HPV. The effect of almitrine bimesylate on HPV is biphasic and dose-dependent; a very low dose enhances HPV,[111,112] a moderate dose has no effect,[113] and a high dose inhibits HPV[114]

Table 4-5. Effects of Vasoactive Drugs on Hypoxic Pulmonary Vasoconstriction (HPV)

Injectable Agent	Reference	Animal	Model	Effect
Vasodilators				
Sodium Nitroprusside	Miller[103]	Dog	95% N_2 LL lobe	Inhibit
	Bishop[104]	Dog	10% O_2 whole lung	Inhibit
	D'Oliveira[105]	Dog	7% O_2 one lung	Inhibit
Nitroglycerine	D'Oliveira[105]	Dog	7% O_2 one lung	Inhibit
	Hales[106]	Dog	100% N_2 one lung	Inhibit
Hydralazine	Bishop[104]	Dog	10% O_2 whole lung	None
Alpha-Blockers				
Dibenzyline Hcl (dilator)	Porcelli[107]	Cat	8–10% O_2 isolated LL lobe	Inhibit
Phentolamine	Barer[28]	Cat	12.6% O_2 one lung	Inhibit
Beta-Blocker				
Propranolol (constrictor)	Porcelli[107]	Cat	8–10% O_2 isolated LL lobe	Enhance
	Miller[103]	Dog	95% N_2 LL lobe	None
Bretylium	Barer[28]	Cat	12.6% O_2 one lung	None
Bronchodilators				
Aminophylline	Hales[101]	Dog	100% N_2 one lung	Inhibit
	Benumof[108]	Dog	95% N_2 LL lobe	None
Orciprenaline				
0.1 μg/kg/min	Reyes[109]	Dog	9% O_2 LL lobe	None
1.0 μg/kg/min	Reyes[109]	Dog	9% O_2 LL lobe	Inhibit
0.5 mg IV bolus	Reyes[109]	Dog	9% O_2 LL lobe	Inhibit
Salbutamol	Reyes[110]	Dog	9% O_2 one lung	Inhibit
Almitrine				
3.3 μg/kg/min	Romaldini[115]	Dog	12% whole lung	Enhance
3.3 μg/kg/min	Chen[113]	Dog		None
14.3 μg/kg/min	Chen[114]	Dog	13% O_2 one lung	Inhibit
0.003,0.03,0.3,3.0 μg/kg/min	Chen[111]	Dog	8% O_2 one lung	Enhance
0.3,1,3,5 μg/kg/min	Nakanishi[112]	Dog	95% N_2 LL lobe	Enhance

resulting from nonspecific pulmonary vasoconstriction. In a dog model using global hypoxia, almitrine bimesylate enhanced HPV.[115] Clinicians continue to be concerned whether a particular drug will eliminate HPV in a patient who relies on HPV to improve ventilation-perfusion matching and oxygenation.

The search for a mediator of the HPV response has led investigators to study many of agents that affect pulmonary vascular tone (Table 4-6). The humoral factors, the products of arachidonic acid metabolism, and the endothelium-derived relaxing factor are all substances that can enter the circulation and potentially have affect pulmonary vascular tone. Histamine release with morphine sulfate and D-tubocurarine are well established. Although the ability of such vasoactive substances to affect HPV is known, the clinical relevance of this fact is still undetermined. In the bulk of reports, histamine emerges as a pulmonary vasoconstrictor with effects on the three major divisions of the pulmonary vascular bed (ie, venous more than capillary or arterial); yet in the systemic circulation, it is a vasodilator. Although histamine has been reported either to enhance, inhibit, or have no effect on HPV, it does not appear to mediate HPV as much as modulate the pulmonary vascular responses to hypoxia by opposing hypoxia-induced vasoconstriction.[116–123] Bradykinin is usually is considered to be a pulmonary vasodilator. Some investigators have suggested, that however, that it was a pulmonary vasoconstrictor in a rat model.[124, 125] Serotonin (5-hydroxytryptamine) is a pulmonary vasoconstrictor.[126]

Table 4-6. Humoral Modulators of Hypoxic Pulmonary Vasoconstriction (HPV)

Humoral Factors	Reference	Animal	Model	Effect
Histamine				
Vasoconstriction	Tucker[116]	Dog	3% O_2 isolated lung	Inhibit
Vasodilation	Silove[117]	Neonatal calf	10% O_2 isolated LL lobe	Inhibit
Mast cell histamine release	Storstein[118]	Dog	(None)	
Polymxin B	Dawson[119]	Cat	3% O_2 isolated lung	None
BW 48/80	Dawson[119]	Cat	3% O_2 isolated lung	Inhibit
BW 48/80	Hauge[120]	Cat	14–4% LL lobe	Inhibit
H_1-blockade				
Chlorpheniramine	Hoffman[121]	Cat	10% O_2 whole lung	Inhibit
	Tucker[116]	Dog	10% O_2 whole lung	None
	Hales[122]	Dog	N_2 one lung	None
H_2-blockade				
Metiamide	Hoffman[121]	Cat	10% O_2 wholelung	Enhance
	Tucker[116]	Dog	10% O_2 wholelung	Enhance
H_1-H_2 blockade				
Chlorphenamine	Hoffman[121]	Cat	10% O_2 wholelung	None
Metiamide	Tucker[116]	Dog	10% O_2 wholelung	None
″-block				
Dibenzyline Hcl	Porcelli[107]	Cat	8–10% O_2 LL lobe	Inhibit
Mast cell membrane-stabilizing agent				
Cromolyn sodium	Ahmed[123]	Sheep	13% O_2 wholelung	Inhibit
Bradykinin				
Vasodilator 2 μg/kg/min	Nyhan[124]	Dog	(None)	
Vasoconstrictor	Hauge[120]	Rat	2% O_2 isolated lung	None
Serotonin				
Vasoconstriction	Levy[126]	Dog	(None)	

The two major products of arachidonic acid metabolism, leukotrienes and prostacyclins, have opposite effects on HPV (Table 4-7). Leukotrienes appear to promote HPV, whereas prostacyclins are potent inhibitors. The observed HPV response depends on which of these two products predominates.[127–133] When prostaglandin $F_{2\alpha}$, a potent pulmonary vasoconstrictor,[134, 135] is infused directly into the pulmonary artery of an atelectatic lung, HPV is enhanced.[136] On the other hand, when $PGF_{2''}$ was administered via a continuous peripheral intravenous infusion, pulmonary vasoconstriction occurs without significantly changing blood flow to either lung.[137] Prostaglandin D_2 (PGD_2) dilates the fetal pulmonary circulation,[138] produces a dose-dependent biphasic response in the newborn lambs,[139] and causes pulmonary vasoconstriction in adults. Research has shown that reported to PGD_2 inhibits HPV in neonatal lambs.[140] Prostaglandin I_2 (PGI_2; prostacyclin) reportedly limits HPV[141] and may cause PaO_2 degradation during trauma. Prostaglandin E_1 (6-keto-PGE_1) is a potent direct vasodilator of the pulmonary systemic circulation.[142]

In addition, the cyclo-oxygenase inhibitors meclofenamate and indomethacin are pulmonary vasoconstrictors that may enhance the pulmonary pressor response to hypoxia; ibuprofen and aspirin also have the same result (Table 4-8).[143–149] Other factors include acetylcholine, which seems to be a pulmonary vasodilator and inhibitor of HPV[150, 151] and angiotensin II, which appears to be pulmonary vasoconstrictor.[152]

Endothelium-derived relaxing factor (EDRF) activates the soluble form of the enzyme guanylate cyclase, which converts guanosine triphosphate to cyclic guanosine monophosphate (cGMP). The concentration of cGMP correlates with vascular smooth muscle contraction. When guanylate cyclase activity is inhibited by methylene blue, the inhibition of HPV by halothane, isoflurane, and enflurane is not altered. This suggests that although EDRF may modulate HPV it does not mediate HPV.[153]

One-Lung Ventilation for Thoracic Procedures

If arterial hypoxemia is a constant concern during general anesthesia, it is even a more important consideration when one-lung ventilation is used for thoracic operations. In most cases, the patient is placed in the lateral decubitus position, and a double-lumen endobronchial tube is used to secure separate ventilation to the two lungs. The upper, or nondependent, lung is allowed to collapse to total atelectasis after the pleura has been opened. Gas exchange and administration of inhalational anesthetic is maintained by ventilation of the lower, or dependent, lung only.

The potential significance and importance of HPV as a homeostatic mechanism may be appreciated during anesthesia for thoracic surgery. For many thoracic procedures, it is advantageous to allow collapse of one lung and to maintain gas exchange by ventilation of the remaining lung. If the HPV response does not occur, the expected venous admixture is large, reflecting the fraction of blood flow to the unventilated lung. Clinical experience has demonstrated that the values of P_{AO_2} are not severely depressed and that measurements of venous admixture are reasonably low. These measurements correlate well with venous admixtures found in the presence of an active HPV response, which diverts blood flow away from the collapsed lung (Fig. 4-13).[154]

The contribution of HPV to patient oxygenation is important (Fig. 4-14).[155] For hypoxic or atelectatic lung regions (about 20% to 50%), HPV provides protection against arterial hypoxemia. In the absence of HPV, the expected P_{AO_2}

Table 4-7. Humoral Modulators of Hypoxic Pulmonary Vasoconstriction (HPV)

Humoral Factors	Reference	Animal	Model	Effect
Lipoxygenase pathway				
Leukotrienes (SRS-A)				
LTC4 (vasoconstrictor)	Morganroth[128]	Rat	3% O_2 isolated lung	Enhance
LTB4	McDonnell[129]	Rat	3% O_2 isolated lung	None
LTD4	Schnader[130]	Sheep	4.2% O_2 isolated lung	None
Leukotrienes synthesis inhibitors				
DEC	Morganroth[128]	Rat	3% O_2 isolated lung	Inhibit
	Schuster[131]	Dog	N_2 LL lobe	None
U-60257	Morganroth[128]	Rat	3% O_2 isolated lung	Inhibit
End organ antagonist of Leukotrienes Effects				
FPL55712	Morganroth[128]	Rat	3% O_2 isolated lung	Inhibit
	Ahmed[123]	Sheep		Inhibit
	Leffler[132]	Neonatal piglets	3% O_2 whole lung	None
Nordihydroguaiaretic acid (NDG)	Gottlieb[133]	Ferret		Inhibit
Cyclooxygenase pathway				
Prostaglandins				
$PGF_{2''}$				
Vasoconstrictor				
2 μg/kg IV bolus	Weir[135]	Dog	9% whole lung	Enhance
0.4–1.2 μg/kg/min intra PA	Scherer[136]	Dog	Atelectasis one lung	Enhance
1.0 μg/kg/min IV	Chen[137]	Dog	13% O_2 one lung	None
PGD_2				
Vasodilator	Gause[138]	Fetal lamb	Isolated LL lobe	—
	Cassin[139]	Fetal goat	Isolated LL lobe	—
	Philips[140]	Neonatal lamb	5% O_2 whole lung	Inhibit
Dose-dependent (biphasic)	Cassin[139]	Newborn lamb	Isolated LL lobe	—
Vasoconstrictor	Cassin[139]	Goat	Isolated LL lobe	—
PGI_2 (prostacyclin)	Sprague[141]	Dog	100% N_2 one lung	Inhibit
PGE_1 (vasodilator)	Tyler[142]	Newborn goat	5% O_2 whole lung	Inhibit
Lipoxygenase and cycloxygenase blocker				
BW755C	Garrett[143]	Dog	Atelectasis LL lobe	Enhance
	Marshall[144]	Rat	3% O_2 isolated lung	Inhibit
Thromboxane (vasoconstrictor)				
Thromboxane inhibitor				
Dazamgrel	Voelkel[145]	Rat	(None)	
Cycloxygenase inhibitors				
Meclofenamate	Weir[135]	Dog	9% O_2 whole lung	Enhance
	Rubin[146]	Dog	10% O_2 whole lung	None
Indomethacin (vasoconstrictor)	Weir[135]	Dog	9% O_2 whole lung	Enhance
	Lock[147]	Newborn lamb	12% O_2 whole lung	—
	Hales[148]	Dog	100% N_2 one lung	Enhance
	Ali[149]	Dog	LL Oleic Acid—pulmonary edema	Enhance
	Rubin[146]	Dog	10% O_2 whole lung	None
Ibruprofen	Marshall[144]	Rat	3% O_2 isolated lung	Enhance
	Rubin[146]	Dog	10% O_2 whole lung	None
Aspirin	Hales[148]	Dog	100% N_2 one lung	Enhance

Table 4-8. Humoral Modulators of Hypoxic Pulmonary Vasoconstriction (HPV)

Humoral Factors	Reference	Animal	Model	Effect
Acetylcholine				
Vasodilator	Fritts[150]	Human	12% whole lung	Inhibit
Vasoconstrictor	Catravas[151]	Dog	(None)	
Angiotensin II				
Vasoconstrictor	McMurtry[152]	Cat	95% air isolated lung	Enhance
Inhibition of EDRF*				
Methylene Blue	Marshall[153]	Rat	3% O_2 isolated lung	None

* EDRF = endothelium-derived relaxing factor.

Figure 4-13. Pulmonary physiological shunt measured in humans undergoing anesthesia for thoracic surgery.[154] At 1, the normal pulmonary shunt is less than 5% with the patient in the lateral position. At 2, when the chest is opened, this percentage increases only slightly. At 3, the upper lung is collapsed, which represents atelectasis in approximately 50% of the lung; ventilatory exchange is maintained only in the lower dependent lung. Although pulmonary shunt may be expected to increase along the dotted line to meet the line of identity, the percentage shunt increases along the line describing a maximal HPV response instead, causing blood flow to be diverted away from atelectatic areas. Most of this response appears to be due to HPV, although this distribution of blood flow to the dependent lung is assisted by gravity and offset by the increased airway pressure required to ventilate the lung in this position. At 4, the upper lung hilum is ligated and the shunt returned to the value expected for a normal dependent lower lung (Reprinted, with permission, from Marshall.[155])

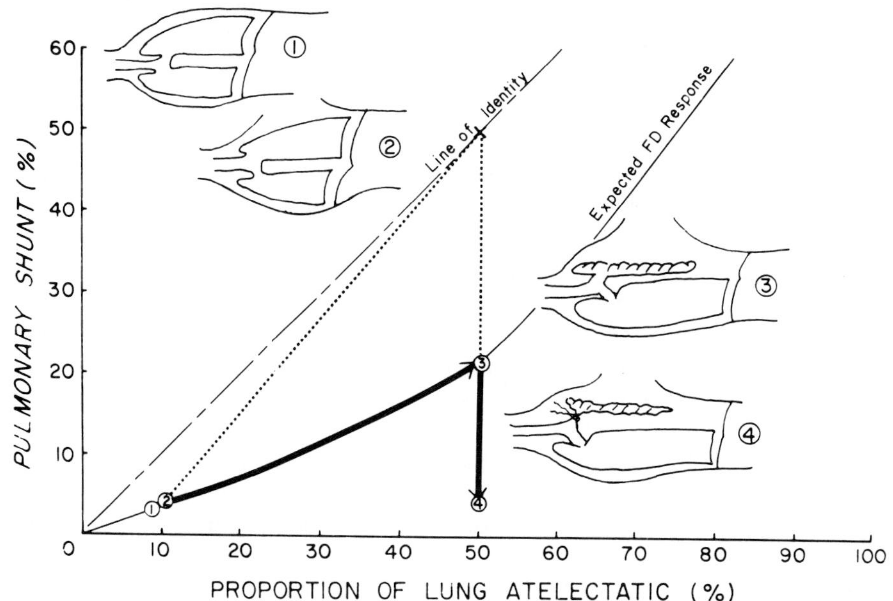

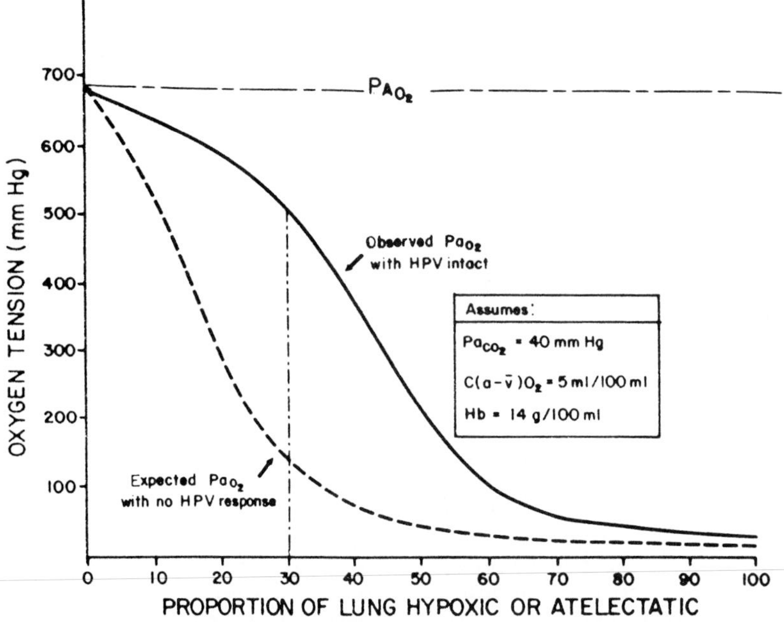

Figure 4-14. Role of HPV in preserving arterial oxygen tension in dogs. Assumptions are that $PACO_2$ = 40 mmHg, (CaO_2 − $C\bar{v}O_2$) = 5 mL · dL^{-1}, and hemoglobin = 14 g · dL^{-1}. The lung FIO_2 of 1.0, is ventilated with and increasing proportions of the lung are subjected to hypoxia or atelectasis. In the absence of HPV, the expected PAO_2 would follow the dashed line, whereas in the presence of an active HPV response, the observed PAO_2 is maintained closer to the solid line. For example, when 30% of the lung is atelectatic and the rest of the lung is ventilated with oxygen, the PAO_2 might be 130 mmHg in the absence of HPV, whereas the PAO_2 might be 500 mmHg with a maximal HPV response.[12,34] (Adapted, with permission, from McMurtry.[152])

may be unacceptably low, whereas in the presence of an active HPV response, the observed PAO_2 is clinically higher and acceptable.

The role of HPV in maintaining systemic oxygenation is a critical one for clinical practice. When the results from general studies in which the mean and standard deviation of arterial oxygen tension for patients during one-lung anesthesia are compared, the mean PAO_2 during one-lung ventilation with a fraction of inspired oxygen (FIO_2) of 1.0 is generally acceptable (ie, FIO_2 > 100 mmHg in patients with localized lung lesions but otherwise normal lung tissue) (Table 4-9).[37,156–159] It should be noted that the values differ considerably, however, so that the range of PAO_2 may be large and the actual PAO_2 can be quite low. Moreover, the fact that the standard deviations are so wide suggests that several patients will always have some degree of arterial hypoxemia. In some such patients, preoperative impairment of oxygen exchange as a result of chronic lung disease will alert the anesthesiologist to potential intraoperative problems, whereas in other patients arterial hypoxemia will occur suddenly and unexpectedly so that management of anesthetic care may be particularly demanding.

The anesthesiologist may wish to consider

Table 4-9. Intraoperative Arterial Oxygen Tension*

Study	Year	No. of Subjects	Anesthetic	Ventilation (mean mmHg plus SD range)	
				Two-Lung	One-Lung
Torda[156]	1974	10	Halothane/methoxyflurane	377 (472–282)	111 (165–57)
Kerr[154]	1974	9	Halothane	452 (562–342)	248 (449–47)
Capan[157]	1980	11	Halothane	376 (469–283)	155 (238–72)
Katz[158]	1982	17	Halothane	421 (471–372)	210 (334–86)
		10	Halothane	437 (524–350)	234 (336–132)
Rogers[159]	1985	10	Isoflurane	445 (520–370)	278 (400–156)
Benumof[73]	1987	6	Isoflurane	442 (500–384)	232 (329–135)
		6	Halothane	484 (533–432)	116 (177–55)

* Adapted, with permission, from Benumof.[4]

various strategies to preserve gas exchange. Simple measures include increasing the F_{IO_2} and avoiding atelectasis by maximizing tidal volume/respiratory rate during mechanical ventilation. Intermittent reinflation of the intentionally collapsed lung[160] to minimize the risk of hypoxemia during one-lung ventilation during thoracotomy has also been suggested.[161] Research has shown that when the collapsed lung is manually inflated on an intermittent basis, P_{AO_2} is increased and remains higher than in the control group, which does not receive intermittent reinflation.[162] Adequate hemoglobin (Hb) and cardiac output must be ensured. The anesthesiologist must consider the advantages of intravenous anesthetic agents versus inhalational anesthetics and the other drugs being taken by the patient must be considered. The use of drugs with vasodilating and vasoconstricting properties must be weighed carefully, and SaO_2 or P_{AO_2} should be closely monitored whenever any of these agents are given.

Summary

HPV is an important, sensitive control in the adjustment of ventilation-perfusion ratios in the lung. As one of the primary active regulators of pulmonary blood flow during atelectasis, HPV reduces the expected pulmonary shunt. It is the principal mechanism that causes reduction of blood flow to the atelectatic lung. Therefore the relative safety of one-lung anesthesia for thoracic surgery relies on HPV. The variability of individual HPV responses, inhibition by inhalation anesthetic agents and the effects of surgical manipulation and trauma explain the magnitude and range of arterial oxygen tensions seen in patients during anesthesia for thoracic surgery.

References

1. Euler US, von, Liljestrand G. Observation on the pulmonary arterial blood pressure in the cat. Acta Physiol Scand 1946;12:301.
2. Bjertnaes LJ. Hypoxia-induced vasoconstriction in isolated perfused lungs exposed to injectable or inhalation anesthetics. Acta Anaesthiol Scand 1977; 21:133.
3. Sykes MK, Loh L, Seed RF, et al. The effect of inhalational anaesthetics on hypoxic pulmonary vasoconstriction and pulmonary vascular resistance in the perfused lungs of the dog and cat. Br J Anaesth 1972;44:776.
4. Benumof JL, Wahrenbrock EA. Local effects of an-

esthetics on regional hypoxic pulmonary vasoconstriction. Anesthesiology 1975;43:525.
5. Rabinovitch M, Keane JF, Fellows KE. Quantitative analysis of the pulmonary wedge angiogram in congenital heart defects. Circulation 1981;63:152.
6. Zapol WM, Snider MT. Pulmonary hypertension in severe acute respiratory failure. N Engl J Med 1976; 296:476.
7. Harris P, Segal N, Bishop JM. The relationship between pressure and flow in the pulmonary circulation in normal subjects and in patients with chronic bronchitis and mitral stenosis. Cardiovasc Res 1968;2:73.
8. Wagner PD, Gale GE, Moon RE, et al. Pulmonary gas exchange in humans exercising at sea level and simulated altitude. J Appl Physiol 1986;60:260.
9. West JB. Regional differences in gas exchange in the lung of erect man. J Appl Physiol 1962;17:893.
10. West JB. Ventilation/blood flow and gas exchange. 4th ed. Boston: Blackwell Scientific Publications, 1985:12.
11. West JB. Respiratory physiology, the essentials. Baltimore: Williams & Wilkins, 1974:33.
12. Marshall BE, Marshall C, Benumof J, et al: Hypoxic pulmonary vasoconstriction in dogs: effects of lung segment size and oxygen tension. J Appl Physiol 1981;51:1543.
13. De Bono EF, Caro CG. Effect of lung-inflating pressure on pulmonary blood pressure and flow. Am J Physiol 1963;205:1178.
14. Fowler NO. The normal pulmonary arterial pressure-flow relationships during exercise. Am J Med 1969;47:1.
15. Hall PW III. Effects of anoxia on postarteriolar pulmonary vascular resistance. Circ Res 1953;1:238.
16. Howard P, Barer GR, Thompson B, et al. Factors causing and reversing vasoconstriction in unventilated lung. Respir Physiol 1975;24:325.
17. West JB, Dollery CT. Distribution of blood flow and the pressure-flow relations of the whole lung. J Appl Physiol 1965;20:175.
18. Marshall BE, Marshall C. Active regulation of the pulmonary circulation: a model for hypoxic pulmonary vasoconstriction, In: Will J, Weir K, Cassin S, et al, eds. Pulmonary circulation in health and disease. New York: Academic Press, 1986:249.
19. Marshall C, Marshall BE. Site and sensitivity for stimulation of hypoxic pulmonary vasoconstriction. J Appl Physiol 1983;55:711.
20. Hauge A. Hypoxia and pulmonary vascular resistance. The relative effects of pulmonary arterial and alveolar PO_2. Acta Physiol Scand 1969;76:121.
21. Fishman AP. Hypoxia on the pulmonary circulation: how and where it acts. Circ Res 1976;38:221.
22. Brower RG, Gottlieb J, Wise RA, et al. Locus of hypoxic vasoconstriction in isolated ferret lungs. J Appl Physiol 1987;63:58.
23. Marshall BE, Marshall C, Magno M, et al. Influence of bronchial arterial PO_2 on pulmonary vascular resistance. J Appl Physiol 1991;70:405.
24. Levitzky MG, Newell JC: Dutton RE. Effect of chemoreceptor denervation on the pulmonary vascular response to atelectasis. Respir Physiol 1978;35:43.
25. Glasser SA, Domino KB, Lindgren L, et al. Pulmonary blood pressure and flow during atelectasis in the dog. Anesthesiology 1983;58:225.
26. Domino KB, Chen L, Alexander CM, et al. Time course and responses of sustained hypoxic pulmonary vasoconstriction in the dog. Anesthesiology 1984;60:562.
27. Burton AC, Patel DJ. Effect on pulmonary vascular resistance of inflation of the rabbit lungs. J Appl Physiol 1958;12:239.
28. Barer AC, Howard P, McCurrie JR. Changes in the pulmonary circulation after bronchial occlusion in anesthetized dogs and cats. Circ Res 1969;25:747.
29. Benumof JL. Mechanism of decreased blood flow to atelectatic lung. J Appl Physiol 1979;46:1047.
30. Domino KB, Wetstein L, Glasser SA, et al. Influence of mixed venous oxygen tension ($P\bar{V}O_2$) on blood flow to atelectatic lung. Anesthesiology 1983; 59:428.
31. Miller FL, Chen L, Malmkvist G, et al. Mechanical factors do not influence blood flow distribution in atelectasis. Anesthesiology 1989;70:481.
32. Zhuang FY, Fung YC, Yen RT. Analysis of blood flow in cats lungs with detailed anatomical and elasticity data. J Appl Physiol 1983;55:1341.
33. Marshall BE, Marshall C. A model for hypoxic constriction of the pulmonary circulation. J Appl Physiol 1988;64:68.
34. Marshall BE. Pulmonary blood flow and oxygenation. In: Marshall BE, Longnecker DE, Fairley HB, eds. Anesthesia for thoracic procedures. Boston: Blackwell Scientific Publications, 1987:73.
35. Marshall BE, Marshall C. Anesthesia and the pulmonary circulation. In: Covino BG, Fozzard HA, Rehder K, et al, eds. Effects of anesthesia. Bethesda MD: American Physiological Society, 1985:121.
36. Gardaz JP, McFarlane PA, Sykes MK. Mechanisms by which dopamine alters blood flow distribution during lobar collapse in dogs. J Appl Physiol 1986; 60:959.

37. Marshall BE. Hypoxic pulmonary vasoconstriction. Acta Anaesthesiol Scand Suppl 1990;94:37.
38. Benumof JL, Wahrenbrock EA. Blunted hypoxic pulmonary vasoconstriction by increased lung vascular pressures. J Appl Physiol 1975;38:846.
39. Borst HG, McGregor M, Whittenberger JL, et al. Influence of pulmonary arterial and left atrial pressures on pulmonary vascular resistance. Circ Res 1956;4:393.
40. Kaneko K, Milic-Emili J, Dolvich MB, et al. Regional distribution of ventilation and perfusion as a function of body position. J Appl Physiol 1966;21:767.
41. Craig JOC, Bromley LL, Williams R. Thoracotomy and contralateral lung. A study of the changes occurring in the dependent and contralateral lung during and after thoracotomy in lateral decubitus. Thorax 1962;17:9.
42. Nunn JF, Williams IP, Jones JG, et al. Detection and reversal of pulmonary absorption collapse. Br J Anaesth 1978;50:91.
43. Elebute EA, Masood A, Fraulkner CS, et al. The effects of acute and chronic atelectasis on pulmonary hemodynamics. J Thorac Cardiovas Surg 1966; 52:292.
44. Finley TN, Hill TR, Bonica JJ. Effect of intrapleural pressure on pulmonary shunt through atelectatic dog lung. Am J Physiol 1963;205:1187.
45. Niden AH. The acute effects of atelectasis on the pulmonary circulation. J Clin Invest 1964;43:810.
46. Morgan BC, Guntheroth WG. Pulmonary blood flow and resistance during acute atelectasis in intact dogs. J Appl Physiol 1970;28:609.
47. Quebbeman EJ, Dawson CA. Influence of inflation and atelectasis on the hypoxic pressure response in isolated dog lung lobes. Cardiovasc Res 1976;10:672.
48. Chen L, Williams JJ, Alexander CM, et al. The effect of pleural pressure on the hypoxic pulmonary vasoconstrictor response in closed chest dogs. Anesth Analg 1988;67:763.
49. Benumof TL, Mathers TM, Wahrenbrock EA. Cyclic hypoxic pulmonary vasoconstriction induced by concomitant carbon dioxide changes. J Appl Physiol 1976;41:466.
50. Malik AB, Kidd BSL. Independent effects of changes in H^+ and CO_2 concentrations on hypoxic pulmonary vasoconstriction. J Appl Physiol 1973;34:318.
51. Marshall C, Lindgren L, Marshall BE. Metabolic and respiratory hydrogen ion effects on hypoxic pulmonary vasoconstriction. J Appl Physiol 1984;57:545.
52. Wetzel RC, Sylvester JT. Gender differences in hypoxic vascular response of isolated sheep lungs. J Appl Physiol 1983;55:100.
53. Fuchs KI, Moore LG, Rounds S. Pulmonary vascular reactivity is blunted in pregnant rats. J Appl Physiol 1982;53:703.
54. Moore LG, Reeves JT. Pregnancy blunts pulmonary vascular reactivity in dogs. Am J Physiol 1980; 239:H297.
55. Peake MD, Harabin AL, Brennan NJ, et al. Steady-state vascular responses to graded hypoxia in isolated lungs of five species. J Appl Physiol 1981; 51:1214.
56. Irwin RS, Martinez-Gonzalez-Rio H, Thomas HM III, et al.: The effect of granulomatous pulmonary disease in dogs on the response of the pulmonary circulation to hypoxia. J Clin Invest 1977;60:1258.
57. Light RB, Mink SN, Wood LDH. Pathophysiology of gas exchange and pulmonary perfusion in pneumococcal lobar pneumonia in dogs. J Appl Physiol 1981:50:524.
58. Hiser W, Penman RW, Reeves JT. Preservation of hypoxic pulmonary pressor response in canine pneumococcal pneumonia. Am Rev Respir Dis 1975;112:817.
59. Demling RH, Smith M, Gunther R, et al. Pulmonary injury and prostaglandin production during endotoxemia in conscious sheep. Am J Physiol 1981; 240:H348.
60. Hirose T, Ikeda T, Aoki E, et al. The protective effect of PGI_2 on increased lung vascular permeability caused by endotoxin in dogs. Nippon Kyobu Shikkan Gakkai Zasshi 1978;16:410.
61. Gee MH, Havill AM, Washburne JD, et al. Prostanoids and acute lung vascular injury. Microcirculation 1981;1:125.
62. Alfery DD, Benumof JL, Trousdale FR. Improving oxygenation during one-lung ventilation in dogs: the effects of positive end-expiratory pressure and blood flow restriction to the nonventilated lung. Anesthesiology 1981;55:381.
63. Chen L, Miller FL, Williams JJ, et al. Hypoxic pulmonary vasoconstriction is not potentiated by repeated intermittent hypoxia in closed-chest dogs. Anesthesiology 1985;63:608.
64. Piper P, Vane J. The release of prostaglandins from lung and other tissues. Ann N Y Acad Sci 1971; 180:363.
65. Stern S, Braun K. Pulmonary arterial and venous response to cooling, role of alpha adrenergic receptors. Am J Physiol 1970;219:982.
66. Benumof JL, Wahrenbock EA. Dependency of hypoxic pulmonary vasoconstriction on temperature. J Appl Physiol 1977;42:56.

67. Marshall C, Lindgren L, Marshall BE. Effects of halothane, enflurane, and isoflurane on hypoxic pulmonary vasoconstriction in rat lung in vitro. Anesthesiology 1984;61:304.
68. Bjertnaes LJ, Hauge A, Nakken KF, et al. Hypoxic pulmonary vasoconstriction: inhibition due to anesthesia. Acta Physiol Scand 1976;96:283.
69. Bjertnaes LJ. Hypoxia-induced pulmonary vasoconstriction in man: inhibition due to diethyl ether and halothane anesthesia. Acta Anaesth Scand 1978;22:570.
70. Domino KB, Borowec L, Alexander CM, et al. Influence of isoflurane on hypoxic pulmonary vasoconstriction in dogs. Anesthesiology 1986;64:423.
71. Foex P. The heart and the autonomic system. In Nimmo WS, Smith G, eds. Anesthesia. Boston: Blackwell Scientific Publications, Vol. 1, 1989:115.
72. Carlsson AJ, Bindslev L, Hedenstierna G. Hypoxia-induced vasoconstriction in the human lung. Anesthesiology 1987;66:312.
73. Benumof JL, Augustine SD, Gibbons JA. Halothane and isoflurane only slightly impair arterial oxygenation during one-lung ventilation in patients undergoing thoracotomy. Anesthesiology 1987; 67:910.
74. Buckley MJ, McLaughlin JS, Fort L III, et al. Effects of anesthetic agents on pulmonary vascular resistance during hypoxia. Surg Forum 1964;15:183.
75. Mathers J, Benumof JL, Wahrenbrock EA. General anesthesia and regional hypoxic pulmonary vasoconstriction. Anesthesiology 1977;46:111.
76. Sykes MK, Hurtig JB, Tait AR, et al. Reduction of hypoxic pulmonary vasoconstriction in the dog during administration of nitrous oxide. Br J Anaesth 1977;49:301.
77. Hurtig JB, Tait AR, Sykes MK. Reduction of hypoxic pulmonary vasoconstriction by nitrous oxide administration in the isolated perfused cat lung. Can J Anaesth 1977;24:540.
78. Saidman LJ, Trousdale FR. Isoflurane does not inhibit hypoxic pulmonary vasoconstriction. Anesthesiology 1982;57:A472.
79. Carlsson AJ, Bindslev L, Hedenstierna G. Hypoxia-induced vasoconstriction in human lung exposed to enflurane anesthesia. Acta Anaesthesiol Scand 1987;31:57.
80. Kaur AE, Mazzic VV, Bergofski CH. Effect of anesthesia and neuromuscular blockers on pulmonary vascular responses to hypoxia and hypercapnia. Anesth Analg 1972;51:402.
81. Fargas-Babjak A, Forrest JB. Effect of halothane on the pulmonary vascular response to hypoxia in dogs. Can J Anaesth 1979;26:6.
82. Sykes MK, Gibbs JM, Loh L, et al. Preservation of the pulmonary vasoconstrictor response to alveolar hypoxia during the administration of halothane to dogs. Br J Anaesth 1978;50:1185.
83. Sykes MK, Davies DM, Chakrabarti MK, et al. The effects of halothane, trichloroethylene, and ether on the hypoxic pressor response and pulmonary vascular resistance in the isolated, perfused cat lung. Br J Anaesth 1973;45:655.
84. Loh L, Sykes MK, Chakrabarti MK. The effects of halothane and ether on the pulmonary circulation in the innervated perfused cat lung. Br J Anaesth 1977;49:309.
85. Sykes MK, Hurtig JB, Tait AR, et al. Reduction of hypoxic pulmonary vasoconstriction during diethyl ether anaesthesia in the dog. Br J Anaesth 1977;49:293.
86. Sykes MK, Arnot RN, Jastrzebski J, et al. Reduction of hypoxic pulmonary vasoconstriction during trichloroethylene anesthesia. J Appl Physiol 1975; 39:103.
87. Sykes MK, Davies DM, Loh L, et al. The effect of methoxyflurane on pulmonary vascular resistance and hypoxic pulmonary vasoconstriction in the isolated perfused cat lung. Br J Anaesth 1976;48:191.
88. Marin JLB, Carruthers B, Chakrabarti MK, et al. Preservation of the hypoxic pulmonary vasoconstrictor mechanism during methoxyflurane anaesthesia in the dog. Br J Anaesth 1979;51:99.
89. Pavlin EG. Respiratory pharmacology of inhaled anesthetic agents. In: Miller RD, ed. Anesthesia. New York: Churchill Livingstone, 1981:363.
90. Tait AR, Chakrabarti MK, Sykes MK. Effect of cyclopropane on pulmonary vascular resistance and hypoxic pulmonary vasoconstriction in the isolated perfused cat lung. Br J Anaesth 1978;50:209.
91. Bjertnaes LJ. Intravenous versus inhalation anesthesia, pulmonary effects. Acta Anaesthesiol Scand Suppl 1982;75:18.
92. Susmano A, Passovoy M, Carleton RA. Comparison of the effects of two anesthetic agents on the production of hypoxic pulmonary hypertension in dogs. Am Heart J 1972;84:203.
93. Wetzel RC, Martin LD. Pentobarbital attenuates pulmonary vasoconstriction in isolated sheep lungs. Am J Physiol 1989;257:H898.
94. Bindslev L, Cannon D, Sykes MK. Effect of lignocaine and nitrous oxide on hypoxic pulmonary va-

soconstriction with dog constant flow perfused left lower lobe preparation. Br J Anaesth 1986;58:315.
95. Rees D, Gaines GY. One-lung anesthesia—a comparison of pulmonary gas exchange during anesthesia with ketamine or enflurane. Anesth Analg 1984;63:521.
96. Naeije R, Lejeune P, Leeman M, et al. Effects of propofol on pulmonary and systemic arterial pressure-flow relationships in hyperoxic and hypoxic dogs. Br J Anaesth 1989;62:532.
97. VanKeer L, Van Aken H, Vandermeersch E, et al. Propofol does not inhibit hypoxic pulmonary vasoconstriction in humans. J Clin Anesth 1989;1:284.
98. Marin JLB, Orchard C, Chakrabarti MK, et al. Depression of hypoxic pulmonary vasoconstriction in the dog by dopamine and isoprenaline. Br J Anaesth 1979;5:303.
99. Furman WR, Summer WR, Kennedy TP, et al. Comparison of the effect of dobutamine, dopamine, and isoproterenol on hypoxic pulmonary vasoconstriction in the pig. Crit Care Med 1982;10:371.
100. McFarlane PA, Mortimer AJ, Ryder WA, et al. Effects of dopamine and dobutamine on the distribution of pulmonary blood flow during lobar ventilation hypoxia and lobar collapse in dogs. Eur Clin Invest 1985;15:53.
101. Hales CA, Kazemi H. Hypoxic vascular response of the lung: effect of aminophylline and epinephrine. Am Rev Respir Dis 1974;110:126.
102. Haas F, Foster WM, Bergofsky EH. Direct effects of ouabain on the pulmonary vasculature and its enhancement of the vasoconstrictor response to hypoxia. Prog Resp Res 1975;9:273.
103. Miller JR, Benumof JL. Combined effects of sodium nitroprusside and propranolol on hypoxic pulmonary vasoconstriction. Anesthesiology 1982;57:267.
104. Bishop MJ, Kennard S, Artman LD, et al. Hydralazine does not inhibit canine hypoxic pulmonary vasoconstriction. Am Rev Respir Dis 1983;128:998.
105. D'Oliveira M, Sykes MK, Chakrabarti MK, et al. Depression of hypoxic pulmonary vasoconstriction by sodium nitroprusside and nitroglycerine. Br J Anaesth 1981;53:11.
106. Hales CH, Westphal D. Hypoxemia following administration of sublingual nitroglycerin. Am J Med 1978;65:911.
107. Porcelli RJ, Bergofsky EH. Adrenergic receptors in pulmonary vasoconstrictor responses to gaseous and humoral agents. J Appl Physiol 1973;34:483.
108. Benumof JL, Trousdale FR. Aminophylline does not inhibit canine hypoxic pulmonary vasoconstriction. Am Rev Respir Dis 1982;126:1017.
109. Reyes A, Sykes MK, Chakrabarti MK, et al. Effect of orciprenaline on hypoxic pulmonary vasoconstriction in dogs. Respiration 1979;38:185.
110. Reyes AR, Sykes MK, Chakrabarti MK, et al. The effect of salbutamol on hypoxic pulmonary vasoconstriction in dogs. Bull Physiopath Respir 1978; 14:741.
111. Chen L, Miller FL, Clarke WR, et al. Low-dose almitrine enhances hypoxic pulmonary vasoconstriction in closed chest dogs. Anesth Analg 1990; 71:475.
112. Nakanishi S, Hiramoto T, Ahmed MN, et al. Almitrine enhances in low dose the reactivity of pulmonary vessels to hypoxia. Respir Physiol 1988; 74:139.
113. Chen L, Miller FL, Malmkvist G, et al. The effect of almitrine on hypoxic pulmonary vasoconstriction in dogs subjected to thoracotomy. Anesthesiology 1985;63:A534.
114. Chen L, Miller FL, Malmkvist G, et al. High-dose almitrine inhibits hypoxic pulmonary vasoconstriction in closed-chest dogs. Anesthesiology 1987;67:534.
115. Romaldini H, Rodriguez-Roisin R, Wagner PD, et al. Enhancement of hypoxic pulmonary vasoconstriction by almitrine in the dog. Am Rev Respir Dis 1983;128:288.
116. Tucker A, Weir EK, Reeves JT, et al. Failure of histamine antagonists to prevent hypoxic pulmonary vasoconstriction in dogs. J Appl Physiol 1976;40:496.
117. Silove ED, Simcha A. Histamine-induced vasodilation in the calf: relationship to hypoxia. J Appl Physiol 1973;35:830.
118. Storstein O, Cudkowicz L, Attwood HD. Effect of histamine on the pulmonary circulation in dogs. Circ Res 1959;7:360.
119. Dawson CA, Delano FA, Hamilton LH, et al. Histamine releasers and hypoxic vasoconstriction in isolated cat lungs. J Appl Physiol 1974;37:670.
120. Hauge A, Melmon KL. Role of histamine in hypoxic pulmonary hypertension in the rat. II. Depletion of histamine, serotonin and catecholamines. Circ Res 1968;22:385.
121. Hoffman EA, Munroe ML, Tucker A, et al. Histamine H_1- and H_2-receptors in the cat and their roles during alveolar hypoxia. Respir Physiol 1977;29:255.
122. Hales CA, Kazemi H. Role of histamine in the hypoxic vascular response of the lung. Respir Physiol 1975;24:81.
123. Ahmed T, Oliver W Jr. Does slow-reacting substance of anaphylaxis mediate hypoxic pulmonary vasoconstriction? Am Rev Respir Dis 1983;127:566.

124. Nyhan DP, Clougherty PW, Goll HM, et al. Bradykinin actively modulates pulmonary vascular pressure-cardiac index relationships. J Appl Physiol 1987;63:145.
125. Hauge A. Role of histamine in hypoxic pulmonary hypertension in the rat. I. Blockade or potentiation of endogenous amines, kinins, and ATP. Circ Res 1968;22:371.
126. Levy SE, Simmons DH, Assali NS. Serotonin, pulmonary hypertension, and airway constriction in the anesthetized dog. Proc Soc Exp Biol Med 1971; 138:365.
127. Garcia JGN, Noonan TC, Jubiz W, et al. Leukotrienes and the pulmonary microcirculation. Am Rev Respir Dis 1987;136:161.
128. Morganroth ML, Reeves JT, Murphy RC, et al. Leukotriene synthesis and receptor blockers block hypoxic pulmonary vasoconstriction. J Appl Physiol 1984;56:1340.
129. McDonnell, TJ, Westcott JY, Czartolomna, et al. Role of peptidoleukotrienes in hypoxic pulmonary vasoconstriction. Am J Physiol 1990;259:H751.
130. Schnader J, Undem B, Adams GK III, et al. Effects of hypoxia on leukotriene activity and vasomotor tone in isolated sheep lungs. J Appl Physiol 1990; 68:2457.
131. Schuster DP, Dennis DR. Leukotriene inhibitors do not block pulmonary vasoconstriction in dogs. J Appl Physiol 1987;62:1808.
132. Leffler CW, Mitchell JA, Green RS. Cardiovascular effects of leukotrienes in neonatal piglets. Role in hypoxic pulmonary vasoconstriction? Circ Res 1984;55:780.
133. Gottlieb T, McGeady M, Adkinson NF, et al. Inhibition of hypoxic pulmonary vasoconstriction in ferret lungs by nordihydroguaiaretic acid (NGDA). Am Rev Respir Dis 1984;129:A343. Abstract.
134. Kadowitz PJ: Joiner PD, Hyman AL. The hypertensive effect of $PGF_{2''}$ on the pulmonary circulation of swine, lamb, dog. Prog Respir Res 1975;9:285.
135. Weir EK, Reeves JT, Grover RF. Meclofenamate and indomethacin augment the pulmonary pressor response to hypoxia and exogenous prostaglandin F_2. Physiologist 1974;17:355. Abstract.
136. Scherer RW, Vigfusson G, Hultsch E, et al. Prostaglandin $F_{2''}$ improves oxygen tension and reduces venous admixture during one-lung ventilation in anesthetized paralyzed dogs. Anesthesiology 1985; 62:23.
137. Chen L, Miller FL, Malmkvist G, et al. Intravenous $PGF_{2''}$ infusion does not enhance hypoxic pulmonary vasoconstriction during canine one-lung hypoxia. Anesthesiology 1988;68:226.
138. Gause GE, Tod ML, Cassin S. Hemodynamic effects of postpulmonary administration of prostaglandin D_2 in fetal animals. Proc Soc Exp Biol Med 1985; 179:373.
139. Cassin S, Tod M, Philips J, et al. Effects of prostaglandin D_2 on perinatal circulation. Am J Physiol 1981;240:H755.
140. Philips JB III, Lyrene RK, McDevitt M, et al. Prostaglandin D_2 inhibits hypoxic pulmonary vasoconstriction in neonatal lambs. J Appl Physiol 1983;54:1585.
141. Sprague RS, Stephenson AH, Lonigro AJ. Prostaglandin I_2 supports blood flow to hypoxic alveoli in anesthetized dogs. J Appl Physiol 1984;56:1246.
142. Tyler T, Leffler C, Wallis R, et al. The effects of prostaglandins of the E-series on pulmonary and systemic circulations of newborn goats during normoxia and hypoxia. Prostaglandins 1975;10:963.
143. Garrett RC, Foster S, Thomas HM III. Lipoxygenase and cyclooxygenase blockade by BW755C enhances pulmonary hypoxic vasoconstriction. J Appl Physiol 1987;62:129.
144. Marshall C, Kim SD, Marshall BE. The actions of halothane, ibuprofen, BW755C on hypoxic pulmonary vasoconstriction. Anesthesiology 1987;66:537.
145. Voelkel NF, Morganroth M, Feddersen OC. Potential role of arachidonic acid metabolites in hypoxic pulmonary vasoconstriction. Chest 1986;88(Suppl): 254S.
146. Rubin LJ, Hughes, JD, Lazar JR. The effects of eicosanoid synthesis inhibitors on normoxic and hypoxic pulmonary tone. Am Rev Respir Dis 1985;132: 93.
147. Lock JE, Olley PM, Coceani F. Hemodynamic effects of intravenous indomethacin in unsedated newborn lambs. Circulation 1978;58(Suppl II):44.
148. Hales CH, Rouse ET, Slate JT. Influence of aspirin and indomethacin on variability of alveolar hypoxic constriction. J Appl Physiol 1978;45:33.
149. Ali T, Duke K. Does indomethacin affect shunt and its response to PEEP in oleic acid pulmonary edema? J Appl Physiol 1987;62:2187.
150. Fritts HW, Jr, Harris P, Clauss RH, et al. The effect of acetylcholine on the human pulmonary circulation under normal and hypoxic conditions. J Clin Invest 1958;37:99.
151. Catravas JD, Hofman WF, Ehrhart IC. Prostanoid inhibition potentiates vasoconstrictor response to acetylcholine in dog lung. J Appl Physiol 1986; 61:1035.

152. McMurtry IF. Angiotensin is not required for hypoxic constriction in salt solution-perfused rat lungs. J Appl Physiol 1984;56:375.
153. Marshall C, Marshall BE. Endothelium-derived relaxing factor is not responsible for inhibition of hypoxic pulmonary vasoconstriction by inhalational anesthetics. Anesthesiology 1990;73: 441.
154. Kerr JH, Smith AC, Prys-Roberts C, et al. Observations during endobronchial anaesthesia. II. Oxygenation. Br J Anaesth 1974;46:84.
155. Marshall BE. Importance of HPV with atelectasis. Adv Shock Res 1982;8:1.
156. Torda TA, McCullough CH, O'Brien HD, et al. Pulmonary venous admixture during one-lung anaesthesia. Anesthesia 1974;29:272.
157. Capan LM, Turndorf H, Chandrakant P, et al. Optimization of arterial oxygenation during one-lung anesthesia. Anesth Analg 1980;59:847.
158. Katz JA, Laverne RG, Fairley HB, et al. Pulmonary oxygen during endobronchial anesthesia: effects of tidal volume and PEEP. Anesthesiology 1982;56:164.
159. Rogers SN, Benumof JL. Halothane and isoflurane do not decrease P_{AO_2} during one-lung ventilation in intravenously anesthetized patients. Anesth Analg 1985;64:946.
160. Bjork VO, Carlens E. The prevention of spread during pulmonary resection by the use of a double-lumen catheter. J Thorac Cardiovasc Surg 1950; 20:151.
161. Benumof JL. One-lung ventilation and hypoxic pulmonary vasoconstriction: implications for anesthetic management Anesth Analg 1985;64:821. Review.
162. Malmkvist G. Maintenance of oxygenation during one-lung ventilation: effect of intermittent reinflation of the collapsed lung with oxygen. Anesth Analg 1989;68:763.

CHAPTER

5

Physiology of the Lateral Position and One-Lung Ventilation

Edmond Cohen

Pulmonary surgery is usually performed with the patient in the lateral decubitus position. To understand the distribution of ventilation and perfusion in the lateral decubitus position and the degree of venous admixture or shunt (Q_S/Q_T, expressed as a percentage), the reader should be familiar with the physiology of the upright position (Figure 5-1).[1] For detailed discussion the reader is referred to Chapter 3 on Ventilation-Perfusion Relationship and Pulmonary Gas Exchange for an extensive review of the ventilation-perfusion relationship.

Basically, blood flow distribution to the lung is gravity-dependent and therefore is primarily directed to the dependent portion of the lung. The blood flow is directly dependent upon the relationship between the alveolar pressure (P_A), the pulmonary artery pressure (P_A), and the pulmonary venous pressure (P_V). The amount of blood flow depends on the pressure difference between the P_A and the P_V. There are several factors that influence the distribution of perfusion: One, the absolute pressure in the pulmonary artery and the pulmonary veins is greater in the dependent part because of the vertical hydrostatic gradient; the pressure in a column of liquid is greatest at the base. Second, the alveolar pressure is equal throughout the lung. The apex of the lung (zone 1) has poor perfusion, since the pressure in the alveolar is greater than that in the pulmonary artery. A collapsed alveoli is considered to be a dead space. In the more dependent area of the lung with the increment in pressure in the pulmonary artery and vein, the flow is intermittent (zone 2). As in an analogy to a waterfall, the upstream river (Pa) is flowing over a dam (P_A) to the downstream river (P_V). The P_A is intermittently obstructing the blood flow between the pulmonary artery and the veins. The blood flow, in addition to the pressure in the pulmonary artery and veins depends on the respiratory and the cardiac cycle. Zone 3, the most dependent part of the lung, is where most of the perfusion is directed; the vessels are most distended in this zone. The pressure in the pulmonary veins exceeds that of the alveolar pressure, which does not play any significant role in obstructing the blood flow.[2,3]

Ventilation is distributed mainly to the more compliant regions at the base of the lung. Because the alveoli at the apex of the lung (zone

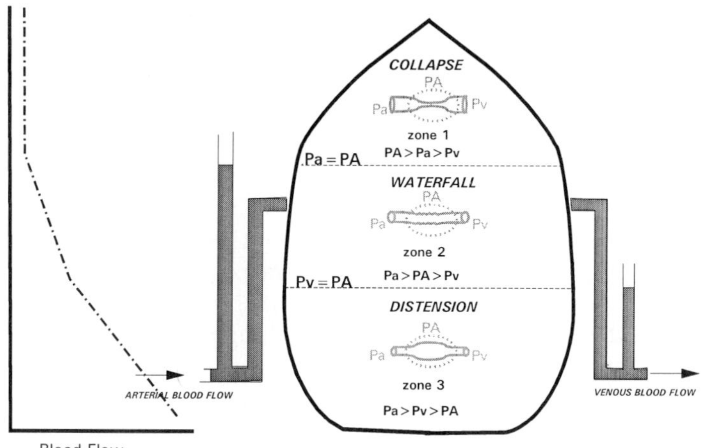

Figure 5-1. Schematic diagram showing the distribution of blood flow in the upright lung. In zone 1, alveolar pressure (P_A) is greater than the arterial pressure (P_{pa}) and no flow occurs because the alveolar pressure collapses the intra-alveolar vessels. In zone 2, arterial pressure exceeds alveolar pressure, and alveolar pressure exceeds venous pressure (P_{pv}). In zone 2, the arterial-alveolar pressure difference (P_{AO_2} − PaO_2) determines the flow. Since P_{pa} increases in zone 2 and P_A remains constant, the perfusion pressure increases, and flow steadily increases down the zone. In zone 3, pulmonary venous pressure (P_{pv}) exceeds P_A, and flow is determined by the arterial-venous pressure difference (P_{pa} − P_{pv}), which is constant in this part of the lung. However, the transmural pressure across the vessel walls increases in this zone such that the vessel caliber is greater (resistance decreases); flow increases as a result. (Adapted, with permission, from West[1–3])

1) are already distended by the negative intrapleural pressure at the apex, they are less compliant. In contrast, the alveoli at the base of the lung are less distended but more compliant. For the same increase in intra-alveolar pressure, the alveoli at the base of the lung receive the major portion of the tidal volume. This results in a good ventilation/perfusion matching, predominately in the dependent zone 3, since both perfusion and ventilation are primarily directed to the dependent portion of the lung.[4–7]

The Lateral Decubitus Position

Thoracic anesthesia is associated with the lateral position because surgery is usually performed in that position. Several factors influence the distribution of ventilation and perfusion in the lateral decubitus position. The induction of general anesthesia, paralysis, and opening the chest, cause major alterations in the distribution of perfusion (Q), ventilation (V), and the ventilation/perfusion ratio (V/Q ratio). When both lungs are being ventilated. The effect of the lateral position on the distribution of perfusion and ventilation will be considered before exploring each of these specific situations is discussed.

Distribution of Perfusion in the Lateral Position

The blood flow in the lateral position is similar to that of the upright position and is gravity-dependent. The relationship between PA, Pa, and Pv that exists in the lateral position is similar to that of the upright position. Blood flow distribution in the lateral position is essentially unchanged whether the patient is awake, anesthetized, or paralyzed. Pulmonary blood flow increases with lung dependency; it is greater in the dependent lung than in the nondependent lung. Therefore, when considering the V/Q relationships in a variety of clinical situations, the distribution of the perfusion is primarily towards the dependent part of the lung. It is the distribution of the ventilation that changes during the various clinical situations.

Two important concepts affect the distribution of blood flow in the lateral position as compared to upright. First, since perfusion is gravity-dependent, the vertical hydrostatic gradient is smaller in the lateral position as compared to the upright position (Fig. 5-2). Consequently, in the lateral position, there is less of zone 1 and more of zones 2 and 3. The decrease in zone 1 reduces the extent of the patient dead space.[8,9]

In the upright position the blood distribution to the lung is split; 55% goes to the right lung, which has three lobes, and 45% goes to the left lung, which has two lobes. In the right decubitus position the split is approximately 65% to the right dependent lung and 35% to the left lung. In the left lateral position the dependent left lung receives 55% of the total blood flow, whereas the right lung receives 45% (Fig. 5-3). It is reasonable to average blood flow regardless of which side is dependent; it can be assumed that 60% flows to the dependent lung and 40% flows to the nondependent lung.

Distribution of Ventilation in the Supine and Lateral Positions

An in-depth evaluation of the influence of position and paralysis on diaphragmatic movement

Figure 5-2. Schematic diagram showing how the lateral position affects the distribution of blood flow in the lateral position as compared to upright. Since perfusion is gravity-dependent, the vertical hydrostatic gradient is smaller in the lateral position as compared to the upright position. Consequently, more flow occurs in zones 2 and 3 than in zone 1. The reduction in zone 1 decreases the patient's dead space.[8,9]

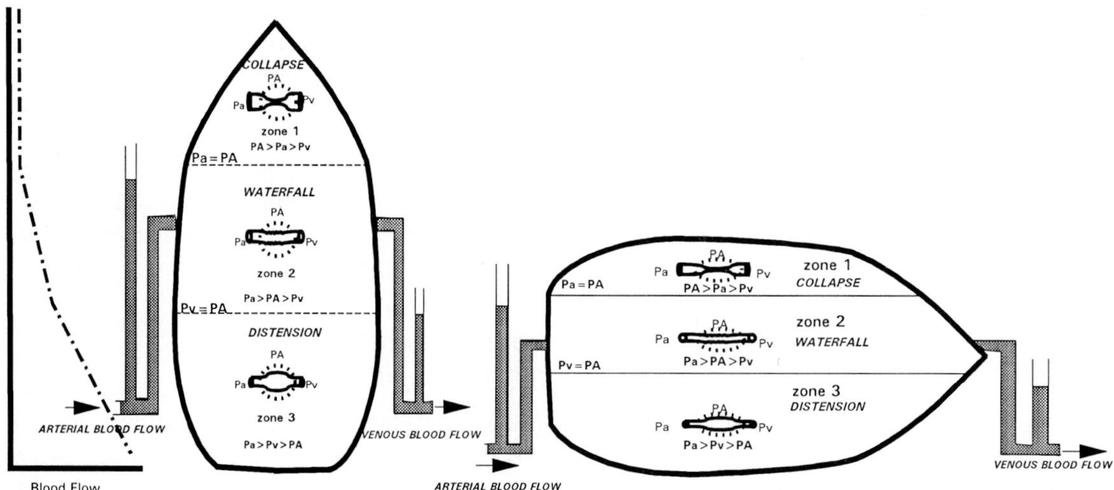

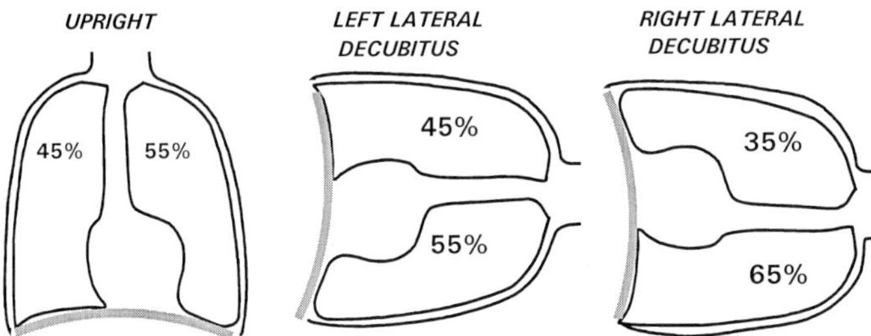

Figure 5-3. Schematic representation of the blood flow distribution in the upright and lateral positions. In the upright position the blood flow distribution is 45% to the left (smaller) lung as compared to 55% for the right (larger) lung. When the left lung is the nondependent lung, the distribution of the blood flow is 35% to the nondependent lung and 65% to the dependent lung. When the right lung is the nondependent lung the blood flow distribution between the nondependent and dependent is 45%/55%. When both lungs are nondependent, the average blood flow is 40%/60%.

and the changes in lung volumes was reported by Froese et al.[10] The position and the pattern of the diaphragm movements during both supine and lateral decubitus positions were assessed by fluoroscopy in healthy volunteers. The patients were studied while awake, supine, breathing spontaneously in the lateral position, or paralyzed. Two components, the change in diaphragmatic position and the change in pattern of displacement, have been evaluated in particular.

Figure 5-4 shows the regional diaphragm displacements during spontaneous breathing and paralysis in the supine position. Spontaneous ventilation in the awake subject is characterized predominately by movement of the dependent part of the diaphragm. Anesthesia induces a cephalad shift during end-expiratory breathing in the diaphragmatic position that is most pronounced in the dependent areas. In spite of this shift, diaphragmatic movement remains greatest in the dependent diaphragm. Two mechanisms enable the actively contracting diaphragm to generate more force in the dependent diaphragm. One, the dependent part of the diaphragm has a smaller radius of curvature both in the supine and lateral positions. Therefore, for the same diaphragmatic tension, more pressure is generated across the dependent part (Laplace Law). Two, the isometric force developed by a muscle increases as its resting length increases. Not only is the dependent part of the diaphragm more curved, but it is also more stretched and therefore develops greater force due to the length/tension relationship. In paralyzed subjects, most of the cephalad displacement occurs in the nondependent areas, with minimal movement of the most dependent level.

Figure 5-5 shows the regional diaphragmatic displacement during the lateral decubitus position in patients who are awake, anesthetized and spontaneously breathing, or paralyzed. In this position three levels of the diaphragm, upper, middle, and lower, were assessed in terms of percent of total displacement. Although the weight of the abdominal contents pushes the lower diaphragm into the thorax, the lower most dependent part of the diaphragm, still has the greatest displacement during spontaneous ventilation, whether in the awake or anesthe-

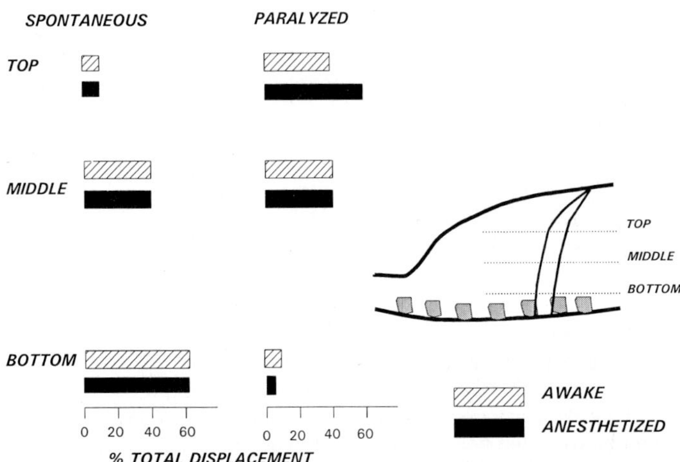

Figure 5-4. Regional diaphragmatic displacements during breathing in the supine position in awake, anesthetized patients who are breathing spontaneously and in similar patients who are paralyzed. Diaphragmatic displacement was analyzed at three levels: top, middle, and bottom. Regional displacement is expressed as a percent of the total value. (Reproduced with permission from Forese.[12])

Figure 5-5. Regional diaphragmatic displacements during breathing in the supine position in awake, anesthetized patients who are breathing spontaneously and anesthetized patients in the lateral position who are paralyzed. Diaphragmatic displacement was analyzed at three levels: top (T), middle (M), and bottom (B). Regional displacement is expressed as a percent of the total value. (Reproduced, with permission, from Forese.[12])

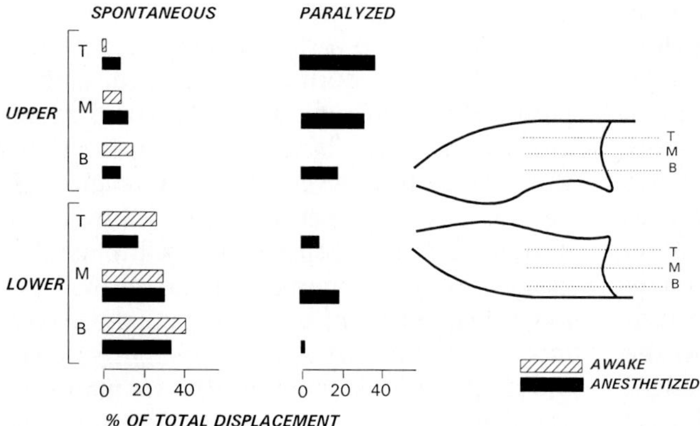

tized state. In paralysis the pattern of displacement is reversed, however, and displacement of the upper diaphragm is greater than that of lower part. When the diaphragm is paralyzed, its motion is no longer determined by active contraction. The relatively uniform pressure that is applied to the thoracic side of the diaphragm is opposed by the hydrostatic pressure gradient of the abdominal content. Therefore, the applied positive pressure ventilation displaces the diaphragm preferentially where abdominal pressure is least, that is, in the nondependent part.

In conclusion, the distribution of diaphragmatic displacement depends on whether the force develops as a result of active contraction of the diaphragm as a consequence of an external force acting on passive diaphragm.

The Lateral Decubitus Position, Awake, Spontaneously Breathing Patients

Chest Closed

The lateral position conserves adequate ventilation-perfusion matching, since most of the gravity-dependent blood flow is directed into the dependent lung and ventilation continues primarily to the dependent lung. The distribution of blood flow and ventilation is similar to that in the upright position (see above) but it varies by 90 degrees.

The nonparalyzed, dependent diaphragm retains the ability to contact and maintains an adequate volume of the dependent lung. The abdominal contents push the dependent hemidiaphragm further into the chest, as compared with the nondependent hemidiaphragm (Figure 5-6).

Figure 5-6. Pleural pressure (P_{pl}) in the awake, upright patient is most positive in the dependent portion of the lung, and therefore alveoli in this region are most compressed and have the lowest volume. In contrast, P_{pl} is most negative at the apex of the lung; here the alveoli are least compressed and have the largest volume. When these regional differences in alveolar volume are translated to a regional transpulmonary pressure-alveolar volume curve, the small, dependent alveoli lie on the steep portion of the curve (large slope), and the large nondependent alveoli are on a flat part (small slope). In this diagram, regional slope equals regional compliance. Thus, for a given and equal change in transpulmonary pressure, the dependent part of the lung receives a much larger share of the tidal volume than the nondependent part.

In the lateral decubitus position, gravity also causes pleural pressure gradients and therefore similarly affects the distribution of ventilation. The dependent lung lies on a relatively steep portion of the pressure-volume curve, and the nondependent lung lies on a relatively flat part. Thus in the lateral decubitus position, the dependent lung receives the majority of the tidal ventilation. V = alveolar volume; P = transpulmonary pressure; P_{AB}, pressure from abdominal content. (Modified, with permission, from Benumof JL: Physiology of the open chest and one-lung ventilation. In: Kaplan JA, ed. Thoracic anesthesia. 2nd ed. New York: Churchill Livingstone, 1991.)

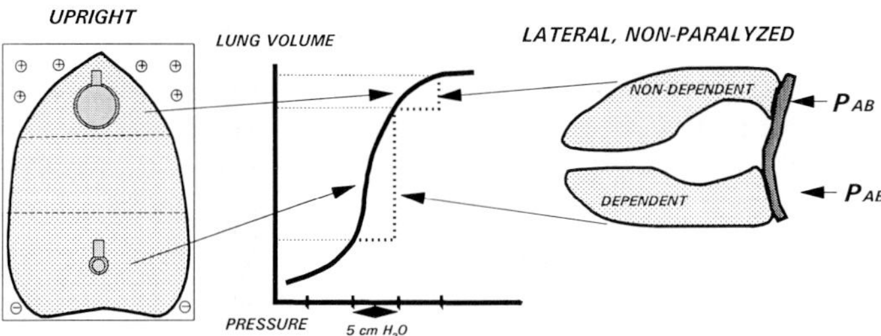

Figure 5-7 illustrates the movement of each hemidiaphragm in the supine and in the lateral nonparalyzed and paralyzed patient. In the nonparalyzed patient, active and efficient contraction of the diaphragm keep the dependent lung from reducing the functional residual capacity. The more sharply curved dependent lung hemidiaphragm contracts more efficiently to maintain volume exchange to the dependent lung as a result of an increase in the pressure of the abdominal contents pressure. In the lateral position, as in the upright position, gravity causes pleural pressure gradients that affect the distribution of ventilation. The dependent lung lies on a relatively steep portion of the pressure-volume curve, whereas the nondependent lung is on a relatively flat portion of the curve. Thus, for an equal change in transpulmonary pressure, the dependent lung receives the vast majority of the delivered tidal volume.[10, 11–13]

In conclusion, in the awake, spontaneously breathing patient in the lateral position, the tidal volume is preferentially delivered into the dependent lung where the gravity-dependent blood flow is primarily directed. The distribution of ventilation/perfusion ratios of the two lungs is not altered and is similar to that for a patient in the upright or supine position. The degree of shunt is not greatly affected; it depends on the age of the patient and the relationship between the closing capacity (CC) and the functional residual capacity (FRC).

Chest Open

Controlled positive pressure ventilation is the most common method used to (1) provide ade-

Figure 5-7. Schematic diagram showing the distribution of ventilation in the anesthesized nonparalyzed patient in the lateral decubitus position (top right) and in the anesthetized paralyzed patient in the same position (bottom right). Paralysis causes a loss of lung volume in both lungs; the nondependent lung moves from a flat, noncompliant portion to the steep, compliant part of the pressure-volume curve, and the dependent lung moves from a steep, compliant part to a flat, noncompliant part. Thus the anesthetized patient in a lateral decubitus position has the majority of the tidal ventilation in the nondependent lung (where perfusion is least) and the minority of the tidal ventilation in the dependent lung (where perfusion is greatest). V = alveolar volume; P = transpulmonary pressure; PAB = pressure from abdominal content. (Modified, with permission, from Benumof JL: Physiology of the open chest and one-lung ventilation. In: Kaplan JA, ed. Thoracic Anesthesia. 2nd ed. New York: Churchill Livingstone, 1991.)

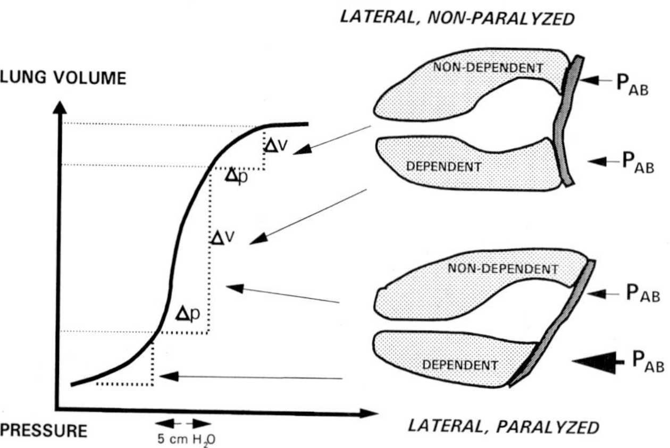

quate ventilation and (2) ensure gas exchange during open chest procedures. Several diagnostic procedures can be performed using thoracoscopy in an awake patient. A considerable number of procedures, such as lung biopsy, plural exploration and biopsy, random wedge resection, resection of a solitary lung lesion, and talc insufflation or pleuroabrasion, can be performed with video-assisted thoracoscopy (VAT), which has become increasingly popular.

In most circumstances, these procedures are carried out under general anesthesia. However, with caution, they can be performed using an intercostal block or a thoracic epidural. In such a case the patient breathes spontaneously to allow proper lung examination. The alternative is general anesthesia with a double lumen tube. The lungs are collapsed, since a thoracoscopic procedure is very difficult to perform with expanded lungs using positive pressure ventilation. The benefits and risk of general versus regional anesthesia should be carefully considered for each patient. The thoracoscope provides an adequate seal of the open chest to prevent a free, open-chest situation. In most cases, however, the surgeon often releases the seal intentionally to develop a pneumothorax and a collapsed lung and obtain an adequate surgical field.

Two important complications, mediastinal shift and paradoxic respiration, may occur in a patient breathing spontaneously with an open chest.

MEDIASTINAL SHIFT When the chest is closed, the inward recoil of the lung is balanced by the outward recoil of the chest wall. This results in equal negative pressures in each hemithorax. Only the weight of the mediastinum may cause some compression of the lower lung. When the chest is open, the negative pressure in the intact hemithorax compared relatively to the positive pressure in the open hemithorax, causes the mediastinum to move downward and push into the dependent hemithorax. During inspiration, the caudad movement of the dependent lung further increases the negative pressure, resulting in additional downward displacement of the mediastinum. During expiration, the cephalad movement of the dependent lung diaphragm creates a relative positive pressure in the dependent hemithorax, which pushes the mediastinum upward (Figure 5-8).[14,15]

This mediastinal shift impairs ventilation

Figure 5-8. Schematic representation of mediastinal shift in the spontaneously ventilating patient in the lateral decubitus position with an open chest. The open chest is always exposed to atmospheric pressure. During inspiration, negative pressure in the intact hemithorax causes the mediastinum to move downward. During expiration, relative positive pressure in the closed hemithorax causes the mediastinum to move upward (mediastinal shift). (Modified, with permission, from Tarhan and Moffitt.[15])

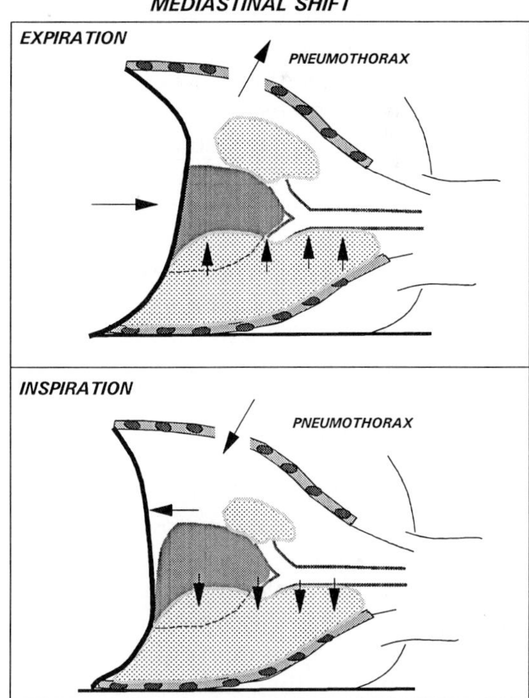

in the open chest, as the tidal volume in the dependent lung decreases by an amount equal to the resulting inspiratory displacement. In a young patient the mediastinal shift is marked, because the mobility of the mediastinal structure diminishes with age. Mediastinal movements are minimal during quiet respiration, whereas they are significant with increase respiratory effort; this may interfere with cardiac filling and cause hypotension. In fact, the clinical presentation is similar to shock. The patient may have hypotension and tachycardia, and be pale and cold. Assisting patient's breathing by applying positive ventilation by continuous positive airway pressure (CPAP), or in severe circumstances, by endotracheal intubation, eliminates the ventilatory and circulatory changes associated with mediastinal shift.

The mechanism involved in the mediastinal shift is believed to be reflex mediated. Manipulation of the mediastinum and dissection around the lung hilum provoke vagally mediated bradycardia, hypotension, and bronchoconstriction, with increased bronchial secretion. Infiltration of local anesthetic at the pulmonary plexus at the hilum, vagal nerve block at the neck, or the use of atropine can reduce the severity of these reactions.

PARADOXIC RESPIRATION When one hemithorax is exposed to atmospheric pressure, an inspiratory effort increases the negative pressure only of the dependent intact hemithorax. Gas is then drawn into the trachea and then into the lung on the intact hemithorax. In contrast, during expiration, the ascendent hemidiaphragm creates a positive pressure in the intact dependent hemithorax relative to the atmospheric pressure of the exposed, nondependent hemithorax. Gas is then displaced from the dependent lung into the nondependent lung, which paradoxically expands during expiration. This reverse gas flow into the nondependent lung is termed "paradoxic respiration." The gas, so-called "pendulum air," represents wasted ventilation and may compromise the adequacy of gas exchange, resulting in hypercarbia and hypoxemia (Figure 5-9).[16] The author's experience has shown that these changes are evident when spontaneous breathing occurs for more than one hour. A patient's paradoxical breathing can be controlled by giving positive pressure by face mask or by endotracheal intubation and mechanical ventilation.

Lateral Position, Anesthetized Patients

Chest Closed

The induction of general anesthesia and paralysis does not significantly change the distribution of blood flow but does have an important impact on ventilation. In the anesthetized paralyzed patient the dependent lung continues to receive most of the blood perfusion. The distribution of ventilation is altered, because most of the tidal volume switches to the nondependent lung; this results in a significant ventilation-perfusion mismatch. With the induction of general anesthesia, FRC decreases (see Fig. 5-7). In the lateral position, this reduction is more pronounced in the dependent lung for four reasons.

1. The loss of lung volume induced by anesthesia results in a lower volume on the pressure-volume curve in each lung. The dependent lung is no longer on the initially steep portion of the pressure-volume curve but on the lower, flatter part of the curve. Instead, the nondependent lung instead has steeper position on the compliance curve and receives most of the tidal volume.[17,18]
2. If anesthesia is associated with paralysis and mechanical ventilation, the diaphragm is no longer actively contracting and no longer offers any advantage to ventilation.

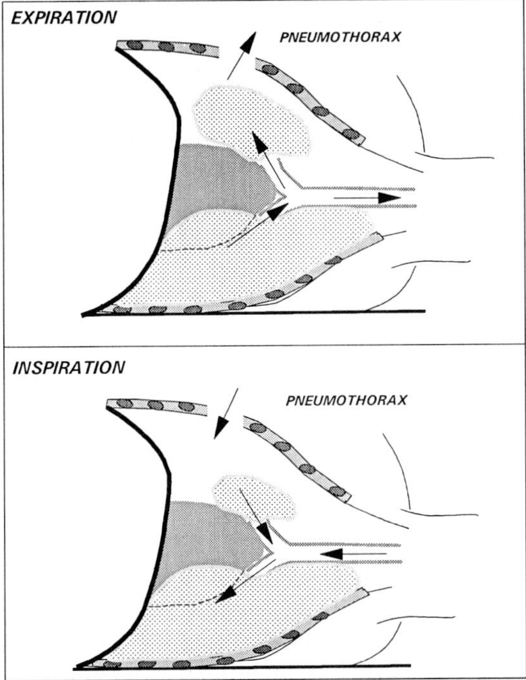

Figure 5-9. Schematic representation of paradoxic respiration in the spontaneously ventilating patient in the lateral decubitus position with an open chest. The open chest is always exposed to atmospheric pressure. During inspiration, gas moves from the nondependent lung in the open hemithorax into the dependent lung in the closed hemithorax, and air that moves from the environment into the open hemithorax causes the lung in the open hemithorax to collapse (paradoxical respiration). During expiration, the gas passes from the dependent lung to the nondependent lung and from the open hemithorax to the environment. Consequently, the nondependent lung expands during expiration. (Modified, with permission, from Tarhan and Moffitt.[15])

3. The mediastinum shifts downward and prevents the dependent lung from expanding.
4. The pressure of the abdominal content is larger in the dependent lung and interferes with expansion of that lung.

This reduction of volume of the dependent lung will have an impact on the ventilation-perfusion relationship and results in significant increase in shunting, since the nondependent lung is well ventilated but poorly perfused (V/Q ratio > 1), whereas the dependent lung is well perfused but poorly ventilated (V/Q ratio < 1).

Chest Open

The dependent lung continues to receive the vast majority of the perfusion, and opening of the chest wall causes further ventilation-perfusion mismatch. Hypoxemia may result because the upper lung is no longer restricted by the chest; it expands more freely then the dependent lung. Therefore, the nondependent lung is hyperventilated but underperfused.

Paralysis, which is essential with anesthesia and an open chest, affects the V/Q ratio during two-lung ventilation most unfavorably. Surgical retraction and compression of the nondependent lung may provide partial protection from hypoxemia by directing more blood to the dependent lung. The induction of general anesthesia and muscle relaxation results in a reduction in FRC, however. Diaphragmatic paralysis with a cephalad displacement of the diaphragm by pressure from the abdominal contents is more pronounced over the dependent part.[19,20] In addition, the mediastinal structures that press on the dependent hemithorax and the suboptimal positioning of the dependent lung on the operating table both contribute to a reduction in FRC. Both lungs are displaced to a lower resting volume on the sigmoid-shaped pressure-volume curve. The nondependent lung then lies on a more compliant portion of the curve and receives most of the tidal volume.

Physiology of One-Lung Ventilation

In the lateral position general anesthesia, paralysis, and compression by abdominal contents and mediastinal structures results in reduction of FRC. Therefore the dependent lung is no longer on the steep portion of the pressure-volume compliance curve and does not receive the majority of the tidal volume. During one-lung ventilation, the nondependent lung is excluded from the ventilation, and all the tidal volume is directed into the dependent lung. In this case, the distribution of perfusion is a significant determinant of the degree of shunting. The blood flow through the nondependent lung becomes a right-to-left shunt which will add to that in the dependent lung.[21,22] One-lung ventilation results in an increased ventilation-perfusion mismatch and a larger alveolar-arterial oxygen tension gradient.

In estimating the degree of shunt that is created by one-lung ventilation, it should be kept in mind that in the lateral position, an average of 40% of cardiac output (CO) perfuses the nondependent, nonventilated lung; the remaining 60% perfuses the dependent lung. In addition, the percent shunt through the nondependent lung depends on the hypoxic pulmonary vasoconstriction (HPV) response. The HPV response is a protective reflex in which vasoconstriction diverts blood away from the nondependent hypoxic lung to the ventilated lung and therefore reduces the degree of venous admixture.[10] When the HPV response is intact, the transpulmonary shunt through the nondependent lung is approximately about 23% of the CO (Figure 5-10).[23] The Q_S/Q_T during two-lung ventilation is assumed to be distributed equally between the two lungs (5% in each lung). In addition, uninhibited hypoxic pulmonary vasoconstriction is believed to reduce 35% of the total blood flow of the nondependent lung by 50%. One-lung ventilation at a given inspired F_IO_2 O_2 concentration (1) results in a much larger alveolar-to-arterial tension difference with a low P_AO_2 as compared with two-lung ventilation. This has been demonstrated in many studies where each patient served as his or her own control.[21,24–30]

Figure 5-10. Schematic representation of two-lung ventilation versus one-lung ventilation. The Q_s/Q_t during two-lung ventilation is assumed to be distributed equally between the two lungs (5% to each lung). Hypoxic pulmonary vasoconstriction (HPV) is assumed to reduce the 35% of the total flow perfusing the nondependent lung that is not shunt flow during two-lung ventilation by half to 17.5%. The total blood flow (obligatory shunt) through the nondependent lung is therefore 22.5%. (From Benumof JL. Special physiology of the lateral decubitus position, the open chest, and one-lung ventilation. In: Benumof JL, ed. Anesthesia for thoracic surgery. Philadelphia: WB Saunders, 1987:112.

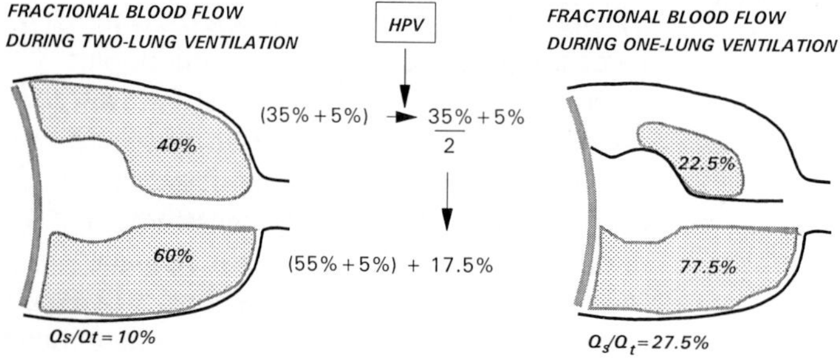

Several factors affect the distribution of perfusion and ventilation, resulting in a wide variety of alveolar to arterial O_2 partial pressure difference (1) P(A − a) O_2 due to the transpulmonary shunt.

Dependent Lung Atelectasis

Atelectasis of the dependent lung during one-lung ventilation is one of the many factors that can contribute to hypoxemia during anesthesia. The formation of an atelectatic area in the dependent lung has several causes.[31]

1. The increment of systemic vascular resistance resulting from the existence of a significant hypoxic compartment within the dependent lung interferes with the ability to ventilate the lung. That results in decreasing blood flow to the dependent lung; this blood is directed into the nondependent lung. The extent of disease in the lung determines the pulmonary vascular resistance and the degree of Qs/QT.[32,33]
2. Absorption atelectasis may occur in the dependent area of the lung that has a low V/Q ratio when exposed to high inspired oxygen concentrations.[34,35]
3. Loss of dependent lung volume due to the induction of general anesthesia and paralysis, compression from the mediastinal weight, and lung secretion.[9–11]
4. Finally, prolonged stay lateral decubitus position may cause fluid to transudate in the dependent lung; this leads to reduction in FRC and increased airway closure in the dependent lung.

Hypoxic Pulmonary Vasoconstriction

Hypoxic pulmonary vasoconstriction (HPV) is a protective autoregulatory mechanism that diverts blood flow away from the atelectatic portion of the lung by active contraction.[22,36,37] HPV is discussed in-depth in Chapter 4. HPV has the most significant influence on diversion of blood flow, although several factors may alter blood flow to the dependent lung. Therefore any factor that inhibits HPV has a negative effect on the distribution of blood flow during one-lung ventilation and impairs gas exchange. As shown in Chapter 4, when the percentage of lung that is hypoxic is intermediate, the shunt through the nonventilated lung is usually 20% to 30% of the CO as opposed to the expected 40 or 50% shunt without active HPV. Several factors listed below may inhibit HPV and thus lead to a further deterioration in arterial oxygenation:

- Low V/Q ratio or nitrogen-ventilated lung. Most of the blood flow reduction in the acutely atelectatic lung is due to HPV. Reexpansion and ventilation of a collapsed lung with nitrogen does not increase the blood flow to the lung, whereas ventilation with oxygen restores all blood flow to the precollapsed value.[39–41]
- Systemic vasodilators, such as nitroglycerin,[42–44] nitroprusside,[45–47] calcium antagonists, and beta$_2$-agonists,[48–50] inhibit HPV.
- Vasoconstricting drugs, preferably those that constrict the normoxic lung vessels.
- High pulmonary vascular pressure (smooth muscle cannot constrict to counter high vascular pressure) or low resistance (more areas of the lung are in zone 1 condition with a resultant increase in pulmonary vascular resistance/(1) PVR). HPV is maximal when pulmonary vascular pressure is normal.
- Either with low or high mixed venous oxygen saturation (SvO_2). HPV is maximal when SvO_2 is normal. With high SvO_2, reverse diffusion of oxygen occurs, which in-

creases the oxygen tension above the HPV threshold. Low SvO_2 decreases alveolar oxygen tension in the normoxic ventilated lung to raise HPV. This offsets the blood flow diversion that results from the HPV in the collapsed lung.[51–53]

Normocarbia has the least influence on HPV. Hypercarbia increases PVR and decreases HPV. Hypocarbia, which is achieved by hyperventilation of the dependent lung, therefore increase the period of positive pressure in that lung raises PVR and lowers HPV.

The effect of inhaled anesthetic on HPV discussed extensively in Chapter 3.[54–60] In brief, the average effect of a minimal alveolar concentration (1) 1-MAC dose of inhalational anesthetic is to reduce HPV response in 20%–30% of cases (Figure 5-11). According to Domino et al.,[61] administration of 1-MAC isoflurane anesthesia should cause a 21% decrease in HPV response, which would increase the expected blood flow through the nondependent lung from 20% to 24%. Figure 5-12 shows the percent pulmonary shunt and the proportion of atelectatic lung in humans undergoing anesthesia for thoracic surgery. In (1), the lateral position, the shunt is less than 5%; in (2), when the chest is open, it is slightly increased; in (3) when the upper lung is collapsed, the pulmonary shunt is not along the line of identity, and flow diversion is due to HPV response; and in (4), with the ligation of the pulmonary artery of the nondependent lung, the shunt returns to the expected value for the dependent lung.

Surgical Manipulation

Nondependent lung compression or retraction inhibits HPV response. Recent evidence shows that lung trauma may release the vasodilator prostaglandin, which inhibits HPV. Therefore

Figure 5-11. Schematic diagram showing the effect of 1-MAC isoflurane on shunt during one-lung ventilation (1 LV) of normal lungs. The two-lung ventilation, nondependent/dependent lung blood flow ratio is 40%/60% (left). When two-lung ventilation is converted to one-lung ventilation (as indicated by atelectasis of the nondependent lung), the hypoxic pulmonary vasoconstriction (HPV) response decreases the blood flow to the nondependent lung by 50%. The nondependent/dependent lung blood flow ratio is now 20%/80% (middle). According to Domino et al., administration of 1-MAC isoflurane should cause a 21% decrease in the HPV response. Consequently, the nondependent/dependent lung blood flow ratio would become 24%/76%, which represents a 4% increase in the total shunt across the lungs (right).

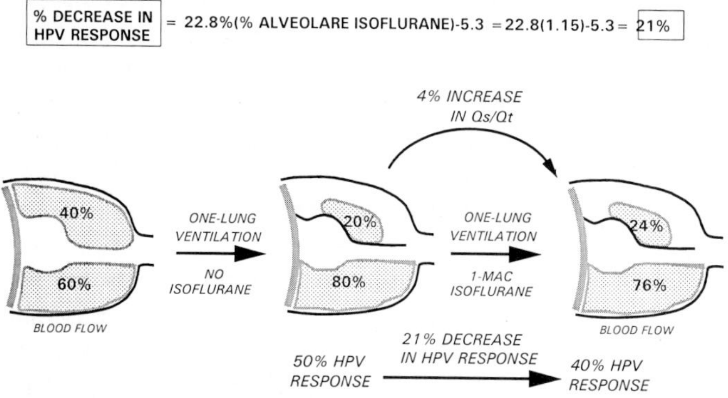

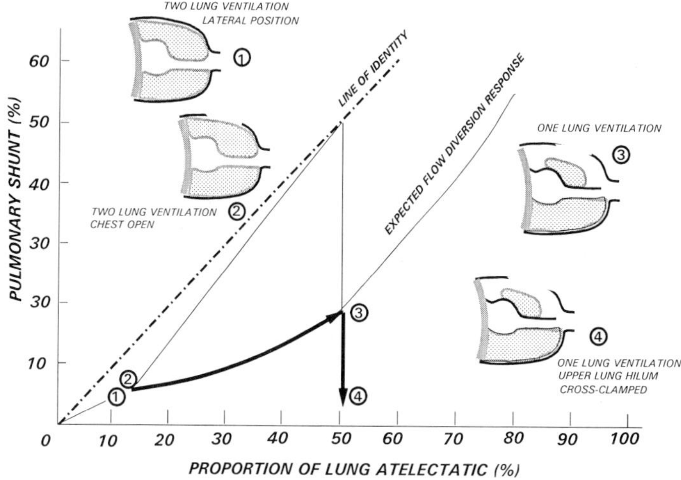

Figure 5-12. Pulmonary shunt measured in patient undergoing anesthesia for thoracic surgery. In 1, the shunt is less than 5%, and the patient is in the lateral position with two-lung ventilation. In 2, this increases only slightly when the chest is opened. In 3, the lung is collapsed, and the ventilatory exchange is maintained only through the dependent lung. The pulmonary shunt increases but not along the 45-degree line of identity that is expected in the absence of hypoxic pulmonary vasoconstriction (HPV). In 4, the upper lung hilum is cross-clamped, and the shunt returns to the value expected for the dependent lung. (From Kerr LH et al. Observation during endobronchial anesthesia. II. Oxygenation. Br J Anaesth 1974;46:84.)

surgical manipulation and lung dissection reduce the effectiveness of the HPV response.

Carbon Dioxide during One-Lung Ventilation

One-lung ventilation has less impact on $PaCO_2$ than it does on arterial oxygenation. Blood flow through the nondependent lung retains CO_2, since it does not take part in the gas exchange. Blood that flows through the over-ventilated, dependent lung compensates by giving up additional CO_2. In addition, the arterial-venous gradient in very small. The $PaCO_2$ is approximately 40 mm Hg, whereas the $PvCO_2$ is 45 mm Hg; this difference is only 5 mm Hg. Thus venous admixture due to increased shunt affects arterial oxygen more than arterial carbon dioxide. The ventilated lung cannot take up enough oxygen to compensate for the non-ventilated lung, and therefore the difference between P_AO_2 and PaO_2 is large.

References

1. West JB. Ventilation/blood Flow and gas exchange. 3rd ed. Oxford:Blackwell Scientific Publications, 1985.
2. West JB, Dollery CT, Naimark A. Distribution of blood flow in isolated lung: relation to vascular and alveolar pressures. J Appl Physiol 1964;19:713.
3. West JB. Blood flow to the lung and gas exchange. Anesthesiology 1974;41:124.
4. Hoppin FG Jr, Green ID, Mead J. Distribution of pleural surface pressure. J Appl Physiol 1969; 127:863.
5. West JB. Regional differences in gas exchange in the lung of erect man. J Appl Physiol 1962;17:893.
6. Milic-Emili J, Henderson JAM, Dolovich MB, et al.

Regional distribution of inspired gas exchange in the lung. J Appl Physiol 1966;21:749.
7. Wagner PD, Saltzman HA, West JB. Measurement of continuous distributions of ventilation-perfusion ratios: theory. J Appl Physiol 1974;36:588.
8. Svanberg L. Influence of posture on lung volumes, ventilation and circulation in normals. Scan J Clin Lab Invest (Suppl 25) 1957;9:1.
9. Rehder K, Sessler AD. Function of each lung in spontaneously breathing man anesthetized with thiopental-meperidine. Anesthesiology 1973; 38:320.
10. Froese AB, Bryan AC. Effects of anesthesia and paralysis on diaphragmatic mechanics in man. Anesthesiology 1974;42:242.
11. Wulff KE, Aulin I. The regional lung function in the lateral decubitus position during anesthesia and operation. Acta Anaesthesiol Scand 1972;16:195.
12. Rehder K, Wenthe FM, Sessler AD. Function of each lung during mechanical ventilation with ZEEP and with PEEP in man anesthetized with thiopental-meperidine. Anesthesiology 1973;39:597.
13. Benumof JL. Anesthesia for thoracic surgery. Philadelphia: WB Saunders, 1987.
14. Guz A, Noble MIM, Eislele JH, et al. The effect of lung deflation on breathing man. Clin Sci 1971; 40:451.
15. Tarhan S, Moffitt EA. Principles of thoracic anesthesia. Surg Clin North Am 1973;53:813.
16. Maloney JV, Schmutzer KJ, Raschke E. Paradoxical respiration and "pendelluft." Thorac Cardiovasc Surg 1961;41:291.
17. Werner O, Malmkvist G, Beckman A, et al. Gas exchange and haemodynamics during thoracotomy. Br J Anaesth 1984;56:1343.
18. Rehder K, Hatch DJ, Sessler AD, et al. The function of each lung of anesthetized and paralyzed man during mechanical ventilation. Anesthesiology 1972;37:16.
19. Nunn JF. The distribution of inspired gas during thoracic surgery. Ann R Coll Surg Engl 1961;28:223.
20. Benumof JL. Anesthesia for thoracic surgery; Philadelphia: WB Saunders, 1987:112.
21. Tarhan S, Lundborg RO. Carlens endotracheal catheter versus regular endotracheal tube during thoracic surgery: a comparison of blood tensions and pulmonary shunting. Can J Anaesth 1971;18:594.
22. Marshall BE, Marshall C. Continuity of response to hypoxic pulmonary vasoconstriction. J Appl Physiol 1980;59:189.
23. Benumof JL. Anesthesia for thoracic surgery; Philadelphia: WB Saunders, 1987:112.
24. Benumof JL. One-lung ventilation and hypoxic pulmonary vasoconstriction: implications for anesthetic management. Anesth Analg 1985;64:821.
25. Capan L, Turndorf H, Chandrakant P, et al. Optimization of arterial oxygenation during one-lung anesthesia. Anesth Analg 1980;59:847.
26. Cohen E, Eisenkraft JB, Thys DM, et al. Oxygenation and hemodynamic changes during one-lung ventilation: effects of $CPAP_{10}$, $PEEP_{10}$, an $CPAP_{10}/PEEP_{10}$. J Cardiothorac Anesth 1988;2:34.
27. Aalto-Setala M, Heinonen J, Salorinne Y. Cardiorespiratory function during thoracic anesthesia: comparison of two-lung ventilation and one-lung ventilation with and without PEEP. Acta Anaesthesiol Scand 1975;19:287.
28. Katz JA, Laverne RG, Fairley HB. Pulmonary oxygen exchange during endobronchial anesthesia. Anesthesiology 1982;56:164.
29. Tarhan S, Lundborg RO. Effects of increased respiratory pressure on blood gas tensions and pulmonary shunting during thoracotomy with use of the Carlens catheter. Can J Anaesth 1970;17:4.
30. Slinger PD, Hickey D, Gottfried S. Intrinsic PEEP during one-lung ventilation. Anesth Analg 1989; 68:S269.
31. Benumof JL. Anesthesia for thoracic surgery. Philadelphia: WB Saunders, 1987:120.
32. Craig JOC, Bromley LL, Williams R. Thoracotomy and contralateral lung. A study of the changes occurring in the dependent and contralateral lung during and after thoracotomy in the lateral decubitus position. Thorax 1962;17:9.
33. Kerr JH. Physiological aspects of one lung (endobronchial) anesthesia. Int Anesthesiol Clin 1972; 10:61.
34. Benumof JL. Respiratory physiology and respiratory function during anesthesia. In: Miller R, ed. Anesthesia. New York: Churchill Livingstone, 1986:1115.
35. Dantzker DR, Wagner PD, West JB. Instability of lung units with low V/Q ratios during O_2 breathing. J Appl Physiol 1975;38:886.
36. Benumof JL. Mechanism of decreased blood flow to atelectatic lung. J App Physiol 1979;46:1047.
37. Benumof JL. One-lung ventilation and hypoxic pulmonary vasoconstriction: implications for anesthetic management. Anesth Analg 1985;64:821.
38. Bjertanes LJ, Mundal R, Huage A, et al. Vascular resistance in atelectatic lungs: effect of inhalation anesthetics. Acta Anaesthesiol Scand 1980;24: 109.

39. Pirlo AF, Benumof JL, Trousdale FR. Atelectatic lung lobe blood flow: open versus closed chest, positive pressure versus spontaneous ventilation. J Appl Physiol 1981;50:1022.
40. Glasser SA, Domino KB, Lindgren L, et al. Pulmonary pressure and flow during atelectasis. Anesthesiology 1982;57:A504.
41. Carlsson AJ, Bindslev L, Santesson J, et al. Hypoxic pulmonary vasoconstriction in the human lung: the effect of prolonged unilateral hypoxic challenge during anesthesia. Acta Anaesthesiol Scand 1985;29:346.
42. Hill NS, Antman EM, Green LH, et al. Intravenous nitroglycerin. A review of pharmacology, therapeutic effects and indications. Chest 1981;79:69.
43. Kadowitz PJ, Nandiwada P, Grueter CA, et al. Pulmonary vasodilator responses to nitroprusside and nitroglycerin in the dog. J Clin Invest 1981;67:893.
44. Anjou-Lindskog E, Broman L, Holmgren A. Effects of nitroglycerin on central hemodynamics and VA/Q distribution early after coronary bypass surgery. Acta Anaesthesiol Scand 1982;26:489.
45. Parsons GH, Leventhal JP, Hansen MM, et al. Effect of sodium nitroprusside on hypoxic pulmonary vasoconstriction in the dog. J Appl Physiol 1981;51:288.
46. Sivak ED, Gray BA, McCurdy TH, et al. Pulmonary vascular response to nitroprusside in dogs. Circ Res 1979;45:360.
47. Hill AB, Sykes MK, Reyes A. Hypoxic pulmonary vasoconstrictor response in dogs and after sodium nitroprusside infusion. Anesthesiology 1979;50:484.
48. McFarlane PA, Mortimer AJ, Ryder WA, et al. Effects of dopamine and dobutamine on the distribution of pulmonary blood flow during lobar ventilation hypoxia and lobar collapse in dogs. Eur J Clin Invest 1985;15:53.
49. Furman WR, Summer WR, Kennedy PP, et al. Comparison of the effects of dobutamine, dopamine and isoproterenol on hypoxic pulmonary vasoconstriction in the pig. Crit Care Med 1982;10:371.
50. Bishop MJ, Cheney FW. Minoxidil and nifedipine inhibit hypoxic pulmonary vasoconstriction. J Cardiovasc Pharmacol 1983;5:184.
51. Domino KB, Glasser SA, Wetstein L, et al. Influence of PvO_2 on blood flow to atelectatic lung. Anesthesiology 1982;57:A471.
52. Benumof JL, Pirlo AF, Trousdale FR. Inhibition of hypoxic pulmonary vasoconstriction by decreased PvO_2: a new indirect mechanism. J Appl Physiol 1981;51:871.
53. Pease RD, Benumof JL. PAO_2 and PvO_2 interaction on hypoxic pulmonary vasoconstriction. J Appl Physiol 1982;53:134.
54. Benumof JL. Choice of anesthetic drugs and techniques. In: Benumof JL, ed. Anesthesia for thoracic surgery. Philadelphia: WB Saunders, 1987:209.
55. Domino KB, Borowee L, Alexander CM, et al. Influence of isoflurane on hypoxic pulmonary vasoconstriction in dogs. Anesthesiology 1986;64:423.
56. Lawler PGP, Nunn JF. A reassessment of the validity of the isoshunt graph. Br J Anaesth 1984;56:1325.
57. Benumof JL. Special physiology of the lateral decubitus position, the open chest, and one-lung ventilation. In: Benumof JL, ed. Anesthesia for thoracic surgery. Philadelphia: WB Saunders, 1987:113.
58. Benumof JL, Augustine SD, Gibbins J. Halothane and isoflurane only slightly impair arterial oxygenation during one-lung in patient undergoing thoracotomy. Anesthesiology 1987;67:910.
59. Carlsson AJ, Bindslev L, Hedenstierna G. Hypoxia pulmonary vasoconstriction in the lung. Anesthesiology 1987;66:312.
60. Carlsson AJ, Hedenstierna G, Bindslev L. Hypoxia-induced vasoconstriction in human lung exposed to enflurane anaesthesia. Acta Anaesthesiol Scand 1987;31:57.
61. Domino KB, Borowec L, Alexander CM, et al. Influence of isoflurane on hypoxic pulmonary soconstriction in dogs. Anesthesiology 1986;65:423.

SECTION

II

Preparation of the Patient for Surgery

CHAPTER

6

The Surgery-Anesthesia Relationship: A Surgeon's View

Paul A. Kirschner

"Thoracic surgery 'par excellence' is a branch of surgery where a full mutual understanding of the requirements and problems of the surgeon and anesthetist leads only to greater safety and well-being of the patient."[1]

The interrelationship between surgery and anesthesiology is nowhere more intimate than in thoracic surgery. The very organs that provide the vital bodily functions—respiration and circulation—are the ones being manipulated, indeed at times even compromised, by surgical procedures and often by anesthetic maneuvers as well. On the other hand, some manipulations may even improve these vital functions, either temporarily or permanently.

The anesthesiologist must be aware of surgical needs and requirements to provide a satisfactory and safe surgical field. The surgeon must temper his or her activities so as not to affect cardiopulmonary function deleteriously or interfere with anesthetic techniques. It is evident that close and ongoing communication between the surgeon and the anesthesiologist must take place before, during, and immediately following the operation.

Almost any lesion of the thorax and its contents may require some form of surgical intervention, whether diagnostic, therapeutic, reparative/reconstructive, or replacement (transplantation). Single lesions as well as combinations may occur. A short list of important diagnoses is presented in Table 6-1.

In this chapter the surgery-anesthesia relationship will be discussed under the following three headings:

1. Presurgical period.
2. Surgical period.
3. Postsurgical period.

Presurgical Period

From the moment a surgeon is consulted about a thoracic problem, an appropriate therapeutic program must be developed. In conjunction with the referring medical personnel in appropriate instances the surgeon must formulate a surgical plan and present it to the anesthesiologist. Although many issues are not much different from those involved in surgery in general, some are quite specific.

Table 6-1. Diagnosis of Thoracic Lesions

- **Lung**
  - Tumors
    - Benign (eg, hamartoma)
    - Malignant
      - Primary lung cancer
      - Metastatic tumors
    - Single or multiple lesions
      - Unilateral
      - Bilateral
    - Parenchymal ("peripheral")
    - Bronchial ("central")
  - Inflammatory lesions
    - Abscess
      - Pyogenic
      - Fungal
      - Bacterial, other (*Mycobacterium tuberculosis*)
      - Aspiration
      - Hematogenous
    - Bronchiectasis
      - Segmental and localized
      - Diffuse
    - Diffuse and scattered parenchymal lesions
      - Drug reactions
      - Interstitial lung disease
      - *Pneumocystis carinii* infection
      - Tuberculosis
      - Cancer
    - Emphysema
      - Blebs
      - Bullae
      - Presence or absence of pneumothorax
  - Traumatic lesions
    - Blunt injury
      - Contusion
      - Tracheobronchial disruption
      - Multiple injuries including thoracoabdominal trauma
    - Penetrating injury
      - Pneumothorax and hemothorax
      - Parenchymal damage
      - Multiple injuries including thoracoabdominal trauma
  - Congenital lesions
    - Sequestrations and cysts
    - Aerodigestive fistulae
- **Pleura** (visceral, parietal, pleural space)
  - Tumors
    - Localized masses (eg, fibroma)
    - Diffuse malignant mesothelioma
    - Metastatic tumors
  - Pleural space
    - Inflammatory (eg, empyema)
    - Pneumothorax (see above)
    - Hemothorax
    - Effusions (benign and malignant)
- **Musculoskeletal chest wall**
  - Tumors
    - Benign (eg, osteomas, chondromas)
    - Malignant
      - Primary
      - Direct extension from lung
      - Metastatic
  - Inflammatory lesions
    - Chondritis
    - Osteitis, including ribs and sternum
    - Combinations
    - Primary and secondary
    - Postoperative infections
  - Trauma
    - Rib fractures
      - Simple
      - Complicated
        - With pneumothorax
        - With hemothorax
        - Multiple with "flail" chest
  - Congenital
    - Pectus lesions
    - Other deformities of ribs and sternum
  - Diaphragm (muscular chest wall)
    - Hernia
      - Congenital
        - Bochdalek
        - Morgagni
        - Absence of diaphragm
      - Acquired: hiatal
        - "Sliding"
        - Paraesophageal
    - Paralysis (phrenic nerve)
      - Neoplastic
      - Traumatic (birth injury to brachial plexus)
      - Postoperative
      - Idiopathic
- **Mediastinum**
  - Tumors
    - Primary
      - Thymoma
      - Germ cell
      - Localized lymphoma
      - Cysts
    - Metastatic
      - Lymphadenopathy
      - Generalized lymphoma
  - Inflammatory (mediastinitis)
    - Pyogenic (esophageal perforations)
    - Chronic fibrosis
      - Idiopathic
      - Fungal (histoplasmosis)
  - Vascular obstruction (superior vena cava syndrome)
    - Benign
    - Malignant
- **Esophagus**
  - Congenital
    - Atresia
    - Web
  - Tumors
    - Benign
    - Malignant
  - Inflammatory
    - Esophagitis
    - Strictures
    - Ingestion of caustic substances
  - Perforation
    - Spontaneous (Boerhaave)
    - Iatrogenic (instrumental)
    - Foreign bodies

Long-range Evaluation

A number of questions concerning several topics should be asked about the patient.

Diagnosis

- Why has the patient been referred for surgery?
- Is the diagnosis proved, suspected, or unknown?
- Is the condition chronic, acute, or emergent?
- Do secondary diagnoses impact on the primary diagnosis?

Respiratory Tract

- What is the patient's age and general fitness?
- What is the background pulmonary function?
- What is the smoking history? Occupational/environmental exposure?
- Is there any previous or coexistent pulmonary disease? Systemic disease affecting pulmonary function? Is sputum, hemoptysis, infection, or fever present?
- Is the patient now taking, or has ever taken, any medications, including cancer chemotherapeutic agents and immunosuppressive drugs?
- Has there been previous thoracic surgery? Transplants? Radiotherapy? Chemotherapy?

Cardiovascular System

- What is the patient's background cardiovascular function?
- Coronary disease or myocardial infarction (previous or recent)?
- Previous myocardial revascularization?
- Congestive heart failure?
- Valvular disease, including previous valve surgery?
- Arrhythmias?
- Pacemaker?
- Congenital heart disease or surgery?
- Hypertension? Antihypertensive drugs?
- Chemotherapy affecting myocardial function?
- Pharmacologically active cardiovascular drugs, including digitalis, antiarrhythmics, beta-blockers, etc.?
- Involvement of great vessels—cavae, aorta, brachiocephalic vessels.
- Heart transplant?

Other Conditions

- Does the patient have neuromuscular disease (myasthenia gravis)? Diabetes?
- Is the patient receiving steroid therapy?
- Does the patient have pharmacoactive tumors: carcinoid [carcinoid syndrome] pheochromocytoma [hypertensive crisis] pleural fibroma [hypoglycemia], small-cell carcinoma [Cushing's syndrome], thyroid [hyperthyroidism])?
- Does the patient have hematologic problems, such as clotting disorders, anemia, leukopenia, or thrombocytopenia?

Airway Status

LARGE AIRWAYS.

- What is the condition of the mouth, lips, teeth, and tongue?
- Is there larynx/vocal cord paralysis?
- Has the patient had laryngeal surgery previously? A tracheostomy, prior or existing?
- Does the patient have a mediastinal tumor with tracheal, major bronchial and/or vascular compression, deviation, or invasion? Esophageal disease causing aspiration of secretions (tumor, reflux, aerodigestive fistula)?

SMALL AIRWAYS.

- Does the patient have COPD? Bronchial asthma?
- Is the patient taking bronchoactive medications, including some ophthalmic drugs (beta-blockers) chemotherapeutic agents (bleomycin)?

Short-range Evaluation

Factors having immediate bearing on the specific planned procedure include pulmonary function and medications.

Pulmonary Function

This information, a prerequisite for all types of thoracic surgery, begins with a history and clinical appraisal of normal activities (ie, walking, stair-climbing) and symptoms such as wheezing and coughing. Smoking history, if any, and environmental exposure (ie, dusts, fumes, chemicals, asbestos) should also be assessed.

Simple ventilatory studies of lung volumes and air flow are usually adequate. These include forced vital capacity (FVC), forced expiratory volume in first second (FEV_1) and the FEV_1/FVC ratio. In addition, measurement of airflow at various segments of the expiratory phase (FEF), maximum voluntary ventilation (MVV), and flow-volume loop determination aid in evaluation of large (FEV_1) or small ($FEF_{25\%-75\%}$) airway obstruction. Diffusion capacity (DLCO) and arterial blood gases are performed in special circumstances. The anesthesiologist routinely determines baseline arterial blood gases following the insertion of the arterial line before the induction of anesthesia.

The above determinations measure global pulmonary function. However, in certain situations there may be an anatomic-functional discrepancy. If substantial amounts of lung tissue must be removed, the important consideration is whether that resected lung tissue was functional. An example is removal of an entire but functionless atelectatic lung.

The reverse also is true, as in the situation where functionless lung tissue is restored to full or substantial function by the surgical procedure (eg, removal of an obstructing endobronchial tumor by bronchoscopy, bronchotomy, bronchoplasty, by decortication of an entrapped or imprisoned lung or lobe, or by bullectomy for giant bullous emphysema). Thus the impairment of global function may actually be an indication for rather than a contraindication to surgery.

To determine such variations in regional pulmonary function accurately, the function of each lung must be recorded separately. Effective, simple, noninvasive techniques include radionuclide quantitative ventilation and perfusion lung scans; ("radiospirometry"). A perfusion scan necessitates the intravenous injection of an insoluble radioisotope (^{99m}Tc-MAA), whereas the ventilation scan requires that the patient inhale an insoluble gaseous radioisotope (^{133}Xe). Peak radioactivity over each lung is proportional to the ventilation or perfusion in each lung. In the past such differential lung function was determined by bronchospirometry using specially designed, double-lumen endotracheal tubes, which have evolved into currently employed one-lung anesthetic techniques.

Medications

Both the surgeon and anesthesiologist must be aware of which drugs are "on board" at the time of surgery. Aspirin and other blood thinners such as dipyridamole, coumadin, and nonsteroidal anti-inflammatory agents should be discontinued preoperatively for long enough to obviate their effects on clotting and platelet function. On the other hand, steroid levels should be at least maintained, more often boosted (ie, "stress doses") to cover the demands of surgery, and they should be continued postoperatively for appropriate time periods. Cardiovascular drugs, including digitalis, nitrites, antihypertensive agents, beta-blockers, and others must sometimes be manipulated to minimize potentially adverse effects. Such unlikely drugs as ophthalmic drops (eg, timolol), which are beta-blockers, are absorbed systemically and may have such adverse effects as bronchospasm. In addition, intraoperative topical medications, such as neomycin, used by the surgeon must be made known to the anesthesiologist. Otherwise such harmful effects as respiratory depression from prolonged muscle relaxation may occur without warning. If the temperature of the irrigating fluid, in the chest in particular, is too hot or too cold, hemodynamic effects may result. Excessively hot solutions may cause bradycardia.

The presence of a pacemaker should also be noted. At times it may have to be temporarily inactivated preoperatively to allow for such surgical techniques as the use of an electrocoagulating apparatus. Bipolar cautery may be used safely. In addition, cardiac responses to anesthesia and surgical manipulation may be dampened or otherwise altered by pacemaker activity.

Surgical Period

Surgical Plan

This plan must be clearly presented to the anesthesiologist long enough in advance so that there are no last-minute surprises. The plan should include not only the main thoracic operation itself but also any additional procedures that may be performed at the same time, such as endoscopy, lymph node biopsy (scalene, mediastinoscopy, parasternal mediastinotomy), thoracoscopy, chest tube insertion, or even operation via other body cavities.

Such combinations of procedures may entail changes of position on the operating table, often with reprepping and redraping. Precautions must be taken to prevent dislodgement of monitoring lines, contamination of the sterile field, and production of any adverse hemodynamic effects resulting from the change of position on the operating table.

Thoracic Incisions

Posterolateral Incision

The most widely used approach to one hemithorax, this incision is suited for operations on the lung, pleura, diaphragm, esophagus, chest wall, and some mediastinal masses (Fig. 6-1).

The patient is placed in the lateral decubitus position. Monitoring lines and the endotracheal tube (single- or double-lumen) are first checked for correct position and secured before turning the patient. Hemodynamic alterations related to change of position of the

Figure 6-1. Posterolateral incision. The √ sign indicates the inferior border of the scapula.

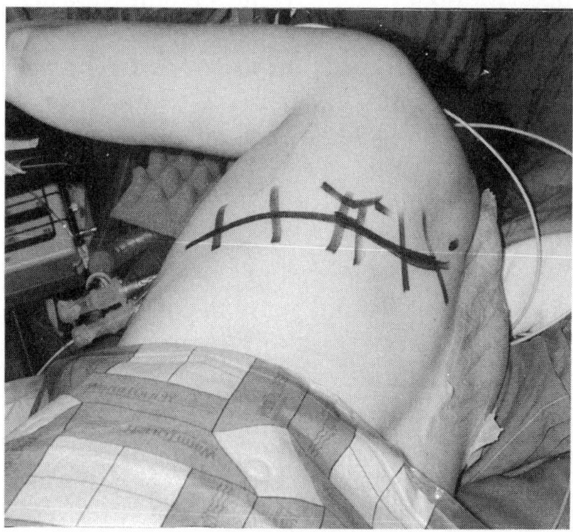

patient should be noted. Pressure points and the dependent axilla should be cushioned to prevent the possibility of brachial plexus injury and vascular compression. Draping should not interfere with the anesthesiologist's access to the monitoring lines and the endotracheal tube.

In the classical incision, the two musculofascial layers (latissimus dorsi-trapezius superficially and the serratus anterior-rhomboid deep) are divided in the line of the incision. In some situations depending on the surgeon's preference, varying degrees of muscle preservation can be achieved by appropriate undermining and retraction. Some surgeons claim that muscle-preserving incisions are less painful than muscle-cutting incisions, but this has not been the author's experience. In the author's view, trauma to the intercostal nerve caused by spreading the ribs is largely responsible for postthoracotomy pain.

The hemithorax is commonly entered through either an intercostal space of choice (usually the fifth or sixth) or the bed of a resected rib. In younger individuals (below age 30–40) with more flexible tissues, adequate exposure can be obtained by merely cranking open the rib spreader. In older patients, or when more exposure is required, the rib may be cut posteriorly with or without removing a small segment to avert a fracture at an undesirable random site; in effect a "controlled fracture" is produced. Despite a priori opinions, fracture of a rib does not necessarily increase postoperative pain. Indeed the reverse may be true; "springing" of the costovertebral joints is avoided, since a "hinge" at the point of controlled fracture is provided.

In conditions requiring wider exposure such as extrapleural pneumonectomy, the incision should be placed more inferiorly (seventh or eighth interspace) entering the chest through the bed of a subperiosteally resected rib. This allows more access to the deep posterior costophrenic sinus that extends down to the 12th rib but does not compromise access to the apex of the chest. Very rarely a double intercostal incision may be required. Muscle relaxants facilitate the opening of the chest by obviating any resistance by the chest wall musculature.

Anterolateral Incision

This incision is useful for certain special situations that do not require the wide exposure of the posterolateral approach. The patient is positioned about 30–40° off the horizontal, with the affected side elevated. The ipsilateral arm is raised, bent at the elbow, and the forearm is secured transversely in a horizontal position above the neck to an "ether screen" or similar support. As such, this arm is not suitable for venous or arterial access. In some circumstances the arm may be kept free and covered with sterile drapes so that it can be moved at will.

The skin incision varies in length depending on the procedure. At its maximum it may begin at the parasternal line anteriorly and continue as far as the posterior axillary line. The chest is entered through the third or fourth intercostal space. Rib resection is unnecessary because the anterior interspaces are wide. Sometimes a costal cartilage may have to be cut. Placing the skin incision in the inframammary fold in women and then elevating the breast to reach the intercostal space is of considerable cosmetic value.

A more limited version of this incision is useful for open lung biopsy in diffuse lung disease. If specific sites are required for biopsy rather than random samples the incision should be appropriately sized and placed.

Midaxillary Incision

Here a vertical incision is made in the midaxillary line, and the pectoralis major muscle is retracted anteriorly and the latissimus dorsi posteriorly (Fig. 6-2). The chest is entered through an intercostal space, usually the fourth or fifth, which is enlarged anteriorly and posteriorly as far as necessary. The long thoracic nerve must be protected.

Median Sternotomy Incision (Sternal Split)

This incision is used almost universally in cardiac surgery (Fig. 6-3). It is becoming increasingly valuable and useful in many general thoracic operations, including some major pulmonary resections especially simultaneous bilateral procedures. Usually the entire sternum is split longitudinally from the suprasternal notch down through and including the xiphoid process and extending into the soft tissues and fascia of the epigastrium. Variants of this approach include partial upper or lower sternotomy.

Another modification of the anterior bilateral thoracotomy approach is the transverse intercostal transsternal "clam shell" incision. An old incision, it has recently been used in bilateral lung transplantation, combined heart-lung transplantation, and some mediastinal tumors. The exposure afforded by the complete median sternotomy or the "clam shell" provides access to the entire anterior mediastinum and parts of the middle and more posterior recesses of the superior mediastinum and trachea and both pleural cavities.

Figure 6-2. Midaxillary incision.

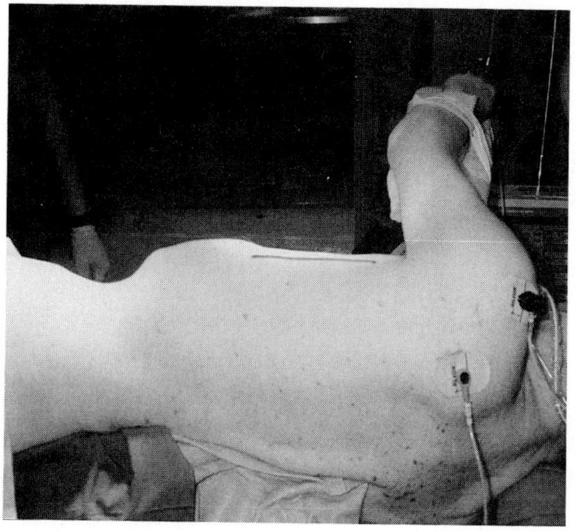

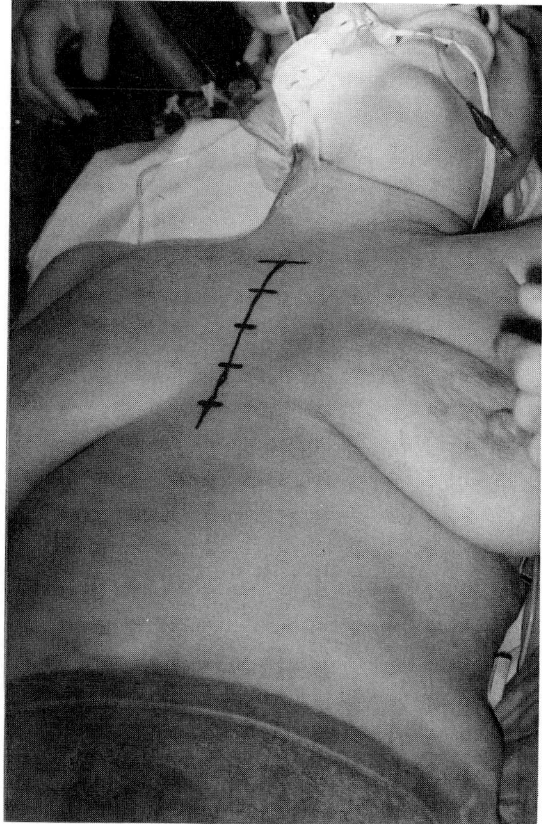

Figure 6-3. Median sternotomy (sternal split). Note that the incision extends from the suprasternal notch down through the xiphoid process into the epigastrium fascia.

The median sternotomy is eminently suitable for excision of most mediastinal tumors, particularly the thymus and thymoma, and a large variety of mediastinal masses and cysts. This method has been successfully used for closure of postpneumonectomy bronchopleural fistulae; by opening the pericardium, the origins of both main bronchi and the lower trachea can be exposed.

Opening the mediastinal pleurae provides access to both pleural cavities. A whole range of pulmonary resections can be performed, including total pneumonectomy. Such an incision is frequently used for bilateral pulmonary lesions including tumors, blebs, and bullae. The double-lumen tube provides alternating one-lung anesthesia for work on each lung in turn.

Among the advantages of the median sternotomy incision are better hemodynamic stability (by avoiding the sometimes deleterious positional changes of the lateral position), less postoperative incisional pain, and improved pulmonary ventilation. Patients with compromised pulmonary function and suitably located unilateral pulmonary lesions may benefit by a choice of the median sternotomy incision because of the lesser postoperative interference with chest wall mechanics and pulmonary function, and less postoperative pain.

Excessive sternal retraction may have two adverse effects. First is fracture of the posterior first rib, and second, brachial plexus injury. The former is manifested by postoperative pain in the upper interscapular region. The latter is evidenced by neurological changes in the distribution of the lower cords and nerves of the plexus, affecting hand and finger movement. These latter changes may be only slowly reversible and are occasionally permanent.

Poor exposure for left lower lobe resection is a disadvantage of the median sternotomy incision. The more posteriorly placed left lower lobe hilum poses difficulties, and dislocation and retraction of the heart for adequate exposure is necessary. Excessive cardiac retraction may cause hypotension and arrhythmia. If a double-lumen tube is situated in the left main bronchus, exposure of the left hilum may be even more of a problem because of the splinting action of the endotracheal tube.

Occasionally, patients undergoing cardiac surgery through a median sternotomy approach have coexisting pulmonary lesions or other conditions that require biopsy or resection. Such lesions are well-handled at the time of the cardiac surgery. Keeping the patient on cardiopulmonary bypass during this part of the operation provides a superb surgical field.

Combined Incisions

CERVICOTHORACIC INCISION. A cervicothoracic incision is suitable for cervicomediastinal goiter, "maximal" thymectomy,[2] some tracheal resections and reconstructions, "mediastinal" tracheostomy, and procedures on the great vessels. Such thoracic access is necessary in some emergency situations such as severe mediastinal bleeding during mediastinoscopy or transcervical thymectomy and trauma. The thoracic extension of the cervical incision may be a full or partial upper sternotomy or a "trap door" exposure to either side of the chest. As with any complicated cervicomediastinal lesion, monitoring lines and venous access for transfusion should be placed in the lower extremities.

ABDOMINOTHORACIC INCISION. Lesions of the lower esophagus, gastric cardia, spleen, and some types of diaphragmatic and hiatus hernias are best approached through an incision that exposes both the thorax and the abdomen (Fig. 6-4). Contrary to a priori considerations, this combined exposure is often better tolerated and leads to fewer postoperative respiratory complications than an inadequate abdominal incision. Many general surgeons who are unfamiliar with thoracic techniques misguidedly persist in avoiding thoracic entry.

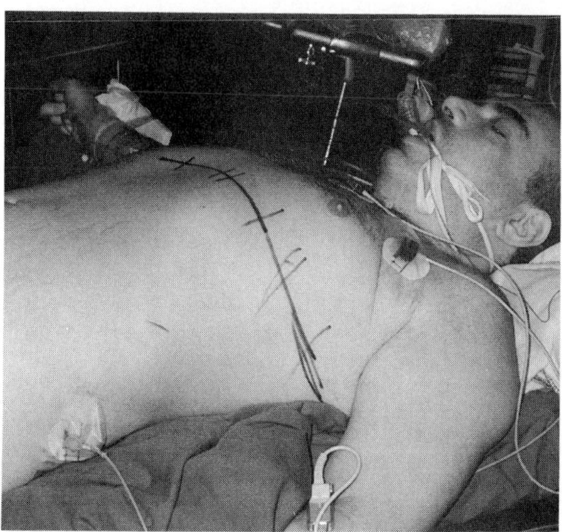

Figure 6-4. Abdominothoracic incision. Note that the abdominal extension of the incision can be carried more caudally, depending on the procedure.

"INDIRECT" THORACIC INCISIONS. Here "indirect" means access to the thorax through a nonthoracic portal. Examples of procedures that involve such indirect incisions are transcervical thymectomy and transhiatal esophagectomy. In both situations, the mediastinum is approached indirectly through the neck or abdomen. The same surgical and anesthetic precautions must be observed as when the thorax is entered directly. Pulmonary ventilation, control of hemorrhage and pneumothorax, use of one-lung anesthesia, and similar techniques are applicable.

Specific Surgical Procedures

Chest Wall Resections

These procedures include various types and degrees of resection and reconstruction. Diagnoses include primary or metastatic rib or cartilage tumors, sternal lesions, lung tumor invasion, and chest wall deformities such as pectus excavatum. One-lung anesthesia is usually unnecessary unless the operation includes resection of underlying lung or extensive intrapleural exposure.

The chief respiratory concern with such surgery is the postoperative maintenance of chest wall integrity to avoid the deleterious consequences of flail chest. Thus for large defects involving the anterolateral chest (unprotected by the scapulae), prosthetic repair of the defect with such various plastic materials as Marlex®, Goretex®, or Silastic® (alone or with added methyl methacrylate to give rigidity) is necessary. Chest wall resections located posteriorly beneath the scapulae are well tolerated without prosthetic repair except in unusually large resections. In cases of multiple fractured ribs with flail chest it occasionally becomes necessary to stabilize the rib fractures surgically if ventilation via an endotracheal tube is inadequate.

Pulmonary Resection

Pulmonary resection is used for a number of procedures, ranging from limited biopsy, through varying degrees of partial to complete lobectomy and total pneumonectomy (eg, enucleation of nodules, "wedge" resection, anatomical segmental resection, lobectomy, total pneumonectomy).

The single most important and valuable anesthetic technique is one-lung anesthesia. Properly used, it provides ample exposure by collapsing the ipsilateral lung. This allows for less retraction (fewer hands and retractors in the surgical field) and better anatomical exposure of lung parenchyma and hilar structures. Accurate placement of the double-lumen tube is essential. Malposition or double-lumen tube displacement may be discovered only after the chest is opened, in spite of all prethoracotomy maneuvers by the anesthesiologist, including fiberoptic bronchoscopy. Two major malpositions occur: one, inadvertent or persistent placement of the tube in the wrong bronchus and two, too distal placement resulting in lack of ventilation of the more proximal lobe (usually on the left side when a left double-lumen tube is used).

Surgeon-anesthesiologist cooperation can correct the problem in such a case. Especially on the right side, the surgeon can locate the tip of the tube by palpation of the main bronchus. By coordinating this tactile information with the anesthesiologist's manipulation of the tube, the tube can be correctly repositioned in the appropriate bronchus. This surgical maneuver may not be possible if there is extensive involvement of the hilum by tumor or other abnormal tissue.[3]

The other problem is the onset of oxygen desaturation when the ipsilateral lung is collapsed. If the double-lumen tube has been positioned too far distally on the left side, the left upper lobe may be occluded; then when the right lung is collapsed, ventilation via the left lower lobe alone may be insufficient to maintain adequate oxygenation. Gradual withdrawal of the tube in small increments then allows the upper lobe to ventilate.[4]

Desaturation may still persist, however, and in this instance the anesthesiologist may resort to continuous positive airway pressure (CPAP) to the nonventilated ipsilateral lung. CPAP causes varying degrees of inflation, however, which may defeat the purpose of one-lung ventilation for surgical exposure in some instances. Alternating periods of ventilation with lung collapse or high-frequency jet ventilation are other solutions to the problem.

Aside from providing a quiet well-exposed surgical field, the double-lumen tube effectively accomplishes lung separation; prevents spillage of blood, secretions, and pus; and prevents the passage of tumor fragments from the operated ipsilateral lung to the opposite side. The tube also allows for "open closure" of the bronchial stump, inspection of the bronchial lumen, and ideal working conditions for bronchotomy, bronchoplastic techniques, and bronchial anastomoses (see Bronchoplasty and Tracheal Resection, below).

Inflation on demand is another advantage to one-lung anesthesia. It is particularly valuable in the conduct of segmental resection, pulmonary decortication, development of incomplete fissures, and testing bronchial and parenchymal suture lines.

Rarely, traumatic rupture of the bronchus may occur because of excessively forceful attempts to pass or manipulate the double-lumen tube. This has been reported with older double-lumen tubes (of the Carlens and Robertshaw types with or without carinal hook); these tubes are made of rubber, are bulky, and may be difficult to pass.[5] Modern, disposable polyvinyl chloride (PVC) tubes, which are smaller and less traumatic, are most widely used. If rupture does occur, extensive mediastinal emphysema (pneumomediastinum) and air leak from the mediastinum is evident. The tear is usually in the membranous portion of the bronchial or tracheal wall. Such a tear must be exposed and surgically repaired.

An alternative to a double-lumen tube is a single-lumen endotracheal tube combined with a bronchial blocker such as a Fogarty arterial embolectomy catheter[6] or the Univent® tube, which is constructed with a blocker. Shortcomings of this tube include some limitations on guided unilateral aspiration for tracheobronchial toilet.

Bronchoplasty and Tracheal Resection

BRONCHOPLASTY ("SLEEVE" LOBECTOMY). This procedure consists of partial or complete cylindrical resection of main or lobar bronchi with reanastomosis. Most or all of the distal lobes or the entire lung are preserved. Bronchoplasty is used mainly for small, noninvasive or benign bronchial tumors and occasionally for highly selected localized bronchogenic carcinomas, as well as for nonneoplastic strictures and stenoses. The goal is to avoid excessive pulmonary parenchymal resection by restoring bronchial continuity, while at the same time preserving otherwise normal, functional lung.

One-lung anesthesia provides ideal working conditions for bronchoplasty. With the ipsilateral lung defunctionalized, the bronchus can be opened, resected, sutured or otherwise manipulated unhurriedly and with ease. Perhaps the only problem is working close to or including the carina where the presence of the tip of the bronchial lumen or the balloon of the bronchial blocker may interfere with the surgery (see Tracheal and Carinal Resection, below).

TRACHEAL AND CARINAL RESECTION. These resection procedures are performed for tumors and strictures involving the trachea proper, the carina, and the origins of the two main bronchi. The operation known as "sleeve" pneumonectomy entails carinal resection and reanastomosis of the remaining contralateral main bronchus to the trachea. Since at some point the surgical techniques interfere with axial ventilation (ie, through both lungs via the trachea), special, combined, anesthetic-surgical maneuvers must be used both to maintain distal ventilation and provide a satisfactory surgical field. Three methods can be used.

Existing Single-lumen Endotracheal Tube. In purely tracheal anastomoses, once the trachea has been transected and the segment containing the lesion has been removed, the existing endotracheal tube is passed through the gap into the distal tracheal segment. However, the very bulk of the tube may at times interfere with circumferential suturing.

High-frequency Jet Ventilation. This allows for the use of tubes of much more slender diameter and may permit passage of the jet ventilation tube across the gap into the distal segment, thereby facilitating suturing while maintaining ventilation.

"Across the field" Ventilation. Especially in the case of carinal resection or "sleeve" pneumonectomy, in which main bronchi are disconnected from the trachea, distal ventilation can be carried out by the passage, by the surgeon, of sterile anesthesia tubes through the open chest "across the field" into the open distal bronchi. These tubes are connected with a separate anesthesia circuit to maintain ventilation and anesthesia during the time of tracheobronchial discontinuity. This maneuver is an excellent example of surgeon-anesthetist interaction (see also Ch. 20).

Mediastinal Surgery

MEDIASTINOSCOPY (CARLENS PROCEDURE). This technique is the most common procedure for mediastinal biopsy. The patient is supine with a bolster under the scapulae. A single-lumen endotracheal tube is preferred to the double-lumen tube to avoid excessive bulk around the face, which interferes with head positioning, surgical access, and exposure. If thoracotomy and lung resection are to follow immediately, the single-lumen tube is then removed and replaced by the double-lumen tube after the mediastinoscopy has been completed.

Continuous monitoring of arterial blood pressure should occur via the *right* radial artery because the innominate artery is intermittently compressed against the manubrium and often occluded by the digital dissection and manipulation of the mediastinoscope. Such compression cuts off blood flow to both the right cerebrum (via the right common carotid artery) and the right upper extremity; attenuation of the pulse in the right arm is a warning sign. More than momentary periods of occlusion may cause right-sided brain ischemia with postoperative left-sided weakness or stroke. Continuous monitoring as described above is thus essential for recognition of damping of the arterial tracing.

The major intraoperative complication of cervical mediastinoscopy is hemorrhage from the azygos vein-vena cava area (venous) or innominate artery or aortic arch (arterial). Major bleeding requires immediate control via a median sternotomy incision. Minor bleeding or oozing from biopsy sites is well-handled through the mediastinoscope by temporary pressure with gauze followed by packing with absorbable hemostatic gauze (eg, Surgicel).

PARASTERNAL ANTERIOR MEDIASTINOTOMY (CHAMBERLAIN PROCEDURE). Single-lumen endotracheal anesthesia is used with the patient in the supine position. Incision is made on either side of the sternum in the second or third intercostal space or through the bed of the resected second or third costal cartilage. The location of the incision depends on the side of the pathology. The internal mammary vessels are controlled and divided, and the mediastinum is entered. A common additional step in this procedure is deliberate entry into the pleural cavity ("minithoracotomy") to facilitate biopsy of either the mediastinum or lung. Unless the lung proper is biopsied, creating a potential air leak, a chest tube is not necessary. It is sufficient to evacuate the pleural air as the incision is closed.

RESECTION OF MEDIASTINAL TUMORS. These tumors may produce certain circumstances that influence both anesthesia and surgery. Large tumors including thyroid masses (benign or malignant), lymphomas, and thymomas may be sufficiently sizable or invasive to produce varying degrees of tracheobronchial and vascular compression.

Tracheobronchial compression, even in the absence of symptoms, can be detected by x-rays and especially computed tomography (CT) scans, or be evident by flow-volume loops in the supine position as compared to the upright. Such compression can cause anesthetic problems.[7] A compromised airway may be adequate for a conscious patient who is able to recruit accessory muscles of respiration to maintain ventilation. With the combination of ventilatory impairment and skeletal muscle relaxation due to general anesthesia and paralysis, however, the now unsupported weight of the tumor may cause it to fall backward. This results in acute, complete closure of an already critically narrowed airway. Infants and young children are particularly prone to this complication because of their weak musculature and their small, soft, compliant airways. Fatalities have occurred.[7] Rapid intubation is necessary to avoid any prolongation of apnea. Even with an endotracheal tube in place, however, the lower trachea and carina below the tip of the endotracheal tube may still be compressed. The author has found that placing the patient in a lateral or semilateral position immediately after intubation allows the tumor to fall away from the airway, thereby relieving the compression.

In adults, problems caused by tracheobronchial compression are solved by intubation of the nonpremedicated, conscious patient using topical anesthesia. If only biopsy of a large tumor is performed, extubating the patient postoperatively may be difficult. If complete tumor removal is not possible, palliative partial resection to relieve the obstruction and to restore adequate ventilation may have merit.

Tracheomalacia (softening of the cartilaginous tracheal rings due to longstanding tracheal compression by thyroid and other tumors) has frequently been invoked as a cause for postoperative airway obstruction even after tumor removal. The author believes that the incidence of true tracheomalacia is highly overestimated. Surgical interference with the vagus and recurrent nerves with resultant vocal cord paralysis is the more likely scenario. In any case, prolonged postoperative intubation, and sometimes tracheostomy, may be required.

Superior vena cava obstruction syndrome is another ominous complication of mediastinal pathology. At times it may coexist with airway obstruction. Experience has shown that cervical mediastinoscopy can be used safely despite certain "a priori" objections. Special precautions must be taken. The patient should be positioned with the upper half of the body elevated to offset the effect of gravity on the peripheral venous pressure. The lower extremities should be used for vascular access in preference to the engorged neck and arms. Steroid therapy, with its antiedema action, can be helpful.

Open-lung Biopsy

Diffuse lung disease undiagnosed by simpler methods (eg, sputum examination, bronchoalveolar lavage, transbronchial lung biopsy) can be approached through a small, anterolateral, intercostal incision using endotracheal anesthesia. Random wedge biopsies using a stapler are usually sufficient. A chest tube is used routinely for pleural drainage and lung expansion.

Many patients who require open-lung biopsy have varying degrees of pulmonary insufficiency because of underlying lung disease; they may even be on ventilators. Surgery on almost any patient no matter how compromised is possible. Ultimate recovery from the surgery usually depends more on the underlying disease than on the surgery proper. Surgical complications include poor healing of the lung resection line (staple or suture) due to the underlying disease, steroid therapy (affecting wound healing), or both.

Thoracoscopy

CONVENTIONAL PROCEDURE. Inspection of the pleural cavity and its contents can be performed using slender telescopes inserted via small intercostal puncture sites. Additional cannulae can be inserted for biopsy purposes. Anesthesia can be intercostal nerve block or general endotracheal anesthesia.

The surgical prerequisite is a free pleural space, which is usually the case in instances of pleural effusion and pneumothorax. In patients with massive effusions, rapid evacuation of large volumes of pleural fluid should be avoided to forestall the occurrence of reexpansion pulmonary edema. The same precaution should be taken with large pneumothoraces.

VIDEO-ASSISTED PROCEDURE. Technological advances facilitate numerous procedures that involve varying degrees of pulmonary resection, even lobectomy, pleurectomy, pericardial window, and some mediastinal tumors. The application of a video camera for high-definition, magnified viewing of the pleural cavity with the aid of a television screen and the development of a seemingly endless array of instruments (eg, scissors, probes, biopsy forceps, staplers, retractors, forceps) has made this possible.

Anesthesia for video-assisted thoracoscopy is best handled by the double-lumen tube. Preexisting effusion or pneumothorax is not essential. If extensive visceroparietal adhesions obliterate the pleural space, however, the procedure cannot be performed. Lesser degrees of adhesion can be dissected free and sufficient working space in the pleural cavity can be provided. If any problems in collapsing the ipsilateral lung with one-lung ventilation arise despite a double-lumen tube, injection of carbon dioxide via the thoracoscope tube can ease the difficulty. Careful monitoring of gas pressure is essential to avert gas embolism.

Patients who undergo video-assisted thoracoscopy should be managed postoperatively as if they had had a major thoracotomy. Thoracoscopy does not require large incisions or the use of a rib spreader, however. Thus there is little postoperative pain or interference with chest wall mechanics, thereby minimizing the need for postoperative analgesics. Nevertheless, the patient should be managed overall with the same care as if a major thoracotomy had been performed.

Conditions That Require Emergency Surgery

MASSIVE HEMOPTYSIS. This condition is generally defined as expectoration of over 600 mL of blood in a 24-hour period. Much variation exists in the amount and rate of bleeding, however. Careful, discriminating judgment is necessary to determine whether or when surgical intervention is indicated. The most common causes of massive hemoptysis include:

1. Inflammatory disease (eg, abscess, bronchiectasis, tuberculosis, fungus infection).
2. Tumors (eg, carcinoma, carcinoid).
3. Cardiovascular disease (eg, mitral stenosis, pulmonary embolism, aortic aneurysm).
4. Iatrogenic (eg, bronchoscopic biopsy, needle biopsy, cardiac catheterization).

It is essential to understand that the problem in hemoptysis is primarily asphyxiation (suffocation) rather than exsanguination. The latter is the threat in gastrointestinal bleeding. Both suffocation and exsanguination may coexist in some cases, however. Hemoptysis is usually from a unilateral source. The patient may be aware of the side of bleeding. Chest x-rays are helpful. However sometimes bronchoscopy *during* the bleed is necessary to define the origin of the blood.

Rigid bronchoscopy, which permits better airway control and suctioning is more effective than flexible instrumentation in some cases of severe hemoptysis. Sometimes in severe unilateral bleeding, insertion of a double-lumen endotracheal tube or endobronchial blocker can be used to advantage by occluding the side of hemorrhage and at the same time protecting the uninvolved side from inundation. Surgery can then be performed with such airway control.

CHEST TRAUMA. This extensive subject can only be mentioned superficially here. Airway control, blood replacement, care of associated injuries, and appropriate thoracic surgery must be applied in an intelligent manner specific to each patient.

"BRONCHOPLEURAL" FISTULA. This fistula refers to any communication between the tracheobronchial tree (and lung parenchyma) and the pleural cavity. Thus a spectrum ranging from the tiny peripheral air leak in spontaneous pneumothorax to the open, unhealed main bronchus stump in the postpneumonectomy patient exists. The surgical-anesthesiological problem depends on the size of the fistula, the nature and volume of the passing material (air, bronchial secretions, pus, or blood), and whether the pleural cavity is drained (by tube or open incision). Any of these conditions are ultimately well-handled by a double-lumen endotracheal tube with defunctionalization of the side of disease.

However, the problem exists during induction of anesthesia and during the time needed to correctly position the endotracheal tube. If the pleural cavity has not been drained, provoking a tension pneumothorax or "spill-over" infection of the healthy lung from secretions or pus is a possibility.

A special situation exists when the fistula is very large—the complete diameter of the main bronchus—in which case that loss of ventilating gases through the defect is sufficient to prevent adequate gas exchange and oxygenation. Surgery-anesthesia coordination is essential in such instances.

Postsurgical Period

The surgery-anesthesia interaction does not end with the placement of the last skin suture and the application of the bandage. The patient now enters one of the most dangerous and treacherous phases of the entire procedure, which may be termed the period of "anesthesia follow-through." The problems encountered at this point must be addressed by both the surgeon and the anesthesiologist. They must remain vigilant and alert despite the natural tendency to relax when the actual operation is finished.

For example, after a lobectomy operation, the following precautions must be taken.

Position Change

The first maneuver involves turning the patient from the lateral decubitus to the supine position. Postural changes in blood pressure may occur. Whether other causes for hemodynamic instability such as hemorrhage exist must be determined before postural factors are held responsible.

Ventilation

Control of the airway is important at this point. The critical decision to extubate is based on the ability of the patient to breathe spontaneously and adequately. If so, the existent endotracheal tube, whatever the type, can safely be removed. Otherwise, provisions must be made for postoperative assisted ventilation. If a double-lumen tube has been in place, it should be exchanged for a single-lumen tube. Assisted ventilation should be maintained as long as necessary (hours to days). Such factors as depth of anesthesia, medication (eg, spinal or epidural morphine), marginal pulmonary function, hypothermia, neuromuscular disease (eg, myasthenia gravis), excessive secretions, bleeding, and airway obstruction, among others are determinants of such need. Premature removal of the endotracheal tube can result in fatality from respiratory failure. It is better to keep the patient intubated a little longer postoperatively than to have to reintubate hurriedly ("crash" reintubate) a patient in acute respiratory failure. Nevertheless, even a successfully extubated patient may occasionally require reintubation at any later time during the immediate postoperative period because of inadequate ventilation, excessive secretions, and the failure to maintain satisfactory blood gases. Reintubated patients may have to be converted to a tracheotomy status if prolonged intubation is necessary.

Chest Tube Drainage

Tubes are placed after lobectomy to facilitate the expansion of residual lung tissue by drainage of blood, fluid and air.

Bloody Drainage

Some bloody drainage is always evident. With change of position from the lateral decubitus to the supine, a sudden transient increase ("dumping") in drainage of up to 150 mL or more may occur as a result of intrathoracic fluid shift. This reaction should diminish promptly; a drainage rate of less than 50 mL per hour for the next four to six hours is acceptable. A higher rate should alert the surgical team to the possibility of active hemorrhage (see Hemorrhage, below). If no drainage occurs at all, obstruction or kinking of the tubes should be ruled out.

Air Leak

After lobectomy a variable amount of air leak frequently occurs despite careful surgical attention to exposed raw surfaces of the remaining lung tissue. This is more likely after segmental resection or procedures on emphysematous lungs. Usually the leak lessens when the patient is turned on to the back; the mediastinum shifts back to the midline, so that the residual lung tissue more easily fills the pleural space. Occasionally the air leak may be so profuse that the anesthetist has difficulty in ventilating the patient because of inability to maintain adequate tidal volume. A decision must be made whether to reopen the chest at this point (see Air Leak, below).

Pneumonectomy

In this situation the physics of the pleural space differs from the postlobectomy (or other partial lung resection) situation. The space is empty; no lung tissue is present. The goal is maintenance of the mediastinum in its preoperative position, usually the midline. A conventional drainage tube with underwater drainage is not ordinarily used after pneumonectomy with one exception because it causes displacement of the mediastinum to the ipsilateral side. This acute mediastinal shift produces severe arrhythmias, blood pressure gyrations, and shock. The exception is the placement of a drainage tube to monitor possible intrapleural bleeding. In this case the tube is kept clamped and not attached to a drainage system. It is opened only intermittently to evacuate measured amounts of bloody fluid that reaccumulates fast enough to displace the mediastinum to the contralateral side. This also results in adverse hemodynamic and respiratory dynamics, and hence shift of the mediastinum to either side is to be avoided.

When the postpneumonectomy patient is turned on to the back, the mediastinum that has sagged to the dependent side now moves back toward the midline. It is partially prevented from moving by the volume of air trapped in the closed, undrained hemithorax. The intrapleural pressure is now positive. A sterile large bore needle (14 or 15-gauge) is inserted into the hemithorax. This permits air to escape, thus equilibrating the intrapleural pressure with the atmosphere and allowing the mediastinum to assume a midline position (Fig. 6-5). If desired, a manometer can be attached to the needle to measure the pressure changes, but this is usually unnecessary.

Conditions That Require Immediate Chest Reopening

Hemorrhage

Copious, continuous bloody drainage through the chest tubes characterizes this condition, which is associated with hypotension and shock. If hemorrhaging is severe initially, the chest should be immediately reopened before the patient leaves the operating room. Often this decision is not made until a few hours postoperatively, however, when the bleeding shows no signs of abatement and the maintenance of hematocrit and hemodynamics is difficult despite multiple transfusions. In some cases, chest x-rays show evidence of bloody accumulation in the chest in the face of only small drainage volume caused by clogging of chest tubes by clots or kinking of the tubes. A pumping systemic artery (bronchial, intercostal, or from a severed adhesion) is the usual finding at reoperation. Rarely is the hemorrhage from a major pulmonary artery or vein.

Air Leak

The chest should be immediately reopened if the anesthesiologist cannot maintain tidal volume as mentioned previously. The airleak may be from a defective bronchial stump closure, raw lung parenchyma, surgically traumatized emphysematous lung tissue or ruptured bulla. It must be surgically repaired.

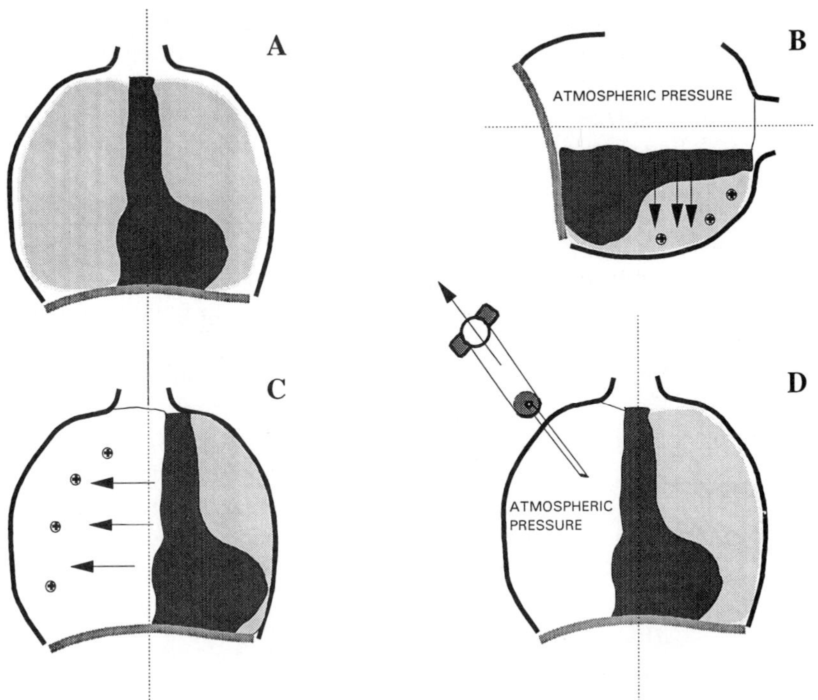

Figure 6-5. A. Presurgical supine position. B. Lateral position postpneumectomy. The mediastinum has sagged into the dependent hemithorax. C. Patient turned to the supine position postpneumectomy. The mediastinum moves back toward the midline and is partially prevented from moving by the volume of air trapped in the closed semidrained hemithorax. This will create a positive intrapleural pressure. D. A large-bore needle is inserted into the hemithorax to permit air to escape and to equilibrate the intrapleural pressure with the atmospheric pressure. This will allow the mediastinum to assume its midline position.

Lobar Torsion

Lobar torsion, a very rare condition, usually involves the middle lobe after a right upper lobectomy, although other lobes can also be affected. It is manifested by failure to ventilate that side. Bronchoscopy shows an obstructed, kinked bronchus, and x-rays reveal a large area of nonaerated lung on the affected side. The chest should be immediately reopened, and the lobe should be untwisted and fixed to adjacent tissues so that torsion does not recur. Unless this procedure is performed promptly, dangerous necrosis and gangrene of the twisted lobe necessitating resection is possible. This can be prevented at the initial operation by fixing the mobile middle lobe to the adjacent lower lobe before closing the chest.

Herniation of the Heart Out of the Pericardial Cavity

This rare situation may occur after radical intrapericardial pneumonectomy in two situations: one, if the large defect in the pericardium is not closed by suture or patch and two, if sutures give way. Although herniation can occur on either side, it usually involves the left side. The condition is manifested by severe sudden hypotension and shock when the patient is turned on the back. In some cases, ill-advised use of a chest tube with continuous suction drainage may lead to herniation. Chest x-rays often show the displaced heart.

A high index of suspicion expedites the diagnosis. The chest must be reopened immediately (1) to replace the herniated heart into the pericardial cavity and (2) to close the pericardial defect securely, usually with a prosthetic patch. Cardiac herniation does not occur after partial lung resection or cardiac surgery; the remaining lung tissue in the hemithorax prevents herniation.

Indications for Intraoperative and Postoperative Bronchoscopy

Intraoperative Indications

Eminently adaptable for use during the operative procedure, the chief value of the flexible bronchoscope is in helping to ascertain and correct the position of the double-lumen endotracheal tube. This instrument is sufficiently slender for traversing the lumen of the endotracheal tube, and it can detect obstructions due to tumor fragments, blood, and secretions and can inspect bronchial suture lines. The small suction channel and limitation of transbronchial instrumentation, such as use of biopsy forceps are drawbacks. It is passed easily with the patient in the lateral position.

Postoperative Indications

The rigid ventilating bronchoscope is more useful during the postoperative period. Adequate depth of anesthesia, removal of the endotracheal tube and the supine position are necessary for the passage of this bronchoscope. The large lumen allows for instrumentation, removal of free tumor fragments, and suction of blood and secretions. After removal of the rigid ventilating bronchoscope, it is often necessary to reintubate the patient. Spontaneous ventilation may be inadequate because of the enforced depth of anesthesia for the bronchoscopy.

Transportation

Transportation is a frequently neglected phase of postsurgical care. Depending on the institution and the local circumstances, transport of the patient for varying distances may be necessary (eg, up and down elevators to more remote areas where recovery rooms and intensive care units are located). Gurneys should be equipped with monitoring and resuscitation devices to cope with emergencies that may occur en route. Arrangements should always be made in advance for a bed in the recovery area.

References

1. Triscott, A. In: Nohl-Oser HC, Nissen R, Schreiber HW. Surgery of the lung. Part II: Notes on anesthesia for thoracic surgery, New York: Thieme-Stratton, 1981:24.
2. Jaretzki A III, Wolff M. Maximal thymectomy for myasthenia gravis (surgical anatomy and operative technique). J Thorac Cardiovasc Surg 1988;96:711.
3. Cohen E, Goldofsky S, Kirschner PA. Intraoperative manipulation for positioning of double-lumen tubes. Anesthesiology 1988;68:170.
4. Brodsky JB, Shulman MS, Mark JBD. Malposition of left-sided double-lumen endobronchial tubes. Anesthesiology 1985;62:667.
5. Guernelli N, Bragaglia RB, Briccoli A, et al. Tracheobronchial ruptures due to cuffed Carlens tubes. Ann Thorac Surg 1979;28:66.
6. Ginsberg RJ. New technique for one-lung anesthesia using an endobronchial blocker. J Thorac Cardiovasc Surg 1981;82:542.
7. Neuman GG, Weingarten AE, Abramowitz RM, et al. The anesthetic management of the patient with an anterior mediastinal mass. Anesthesiology 1984; 60:144.

CHAPTER

7

Preoperative Evaluation of Thoracic Surgical Patients

Steven M. Neustein
Edmond Cohen

Most thoracic operations involve resection of lung tissue for a wide range of pathologies, most commonly the presence of tumors. Preoperative evaluation, therefore, should focus on the severity of pulmonary disease, and involvement of the cardiovascular system.

Two important factors should be considered when evaluating patients for pulmonary resection. The first involves assessing the extent of resection that can be tolerated without creating a pulmonary cripple. The second is the expected status of the pulmonary vasculature following the resection. A fixed reduction in the cross-sectional area of the pulmonary vascular may lead to elevated pulmonary vascular resistance and pulmonary hypertension. Normally the pulmonary vasculature is compliant, allowing an increase in blood flow without an increase in pulmonary arterial pressure. Pulmonary hypertension can be exacerbated by factors that increase pulmonary vascular resistance, such as acidosis, hypoxia, and hypercarbia. The elevated pulmonary pressures may in turn lead to right ventricular failure.

Patients who present for a lung resection should receive an in-depth preoperative evaluation, including a thorough history, physical examination, and laboratory testing. The importance of each of these factors is discussed in detail in this chapter.

History

Cigarette Smoking

Most patients with carcinoma of the lung have a history of heavy cigarette use, which increases the risk of chronic lung disease and postoperative pulmonary complications. Harmful changes in respiratory air flow and closing capacity, which are related to the number of pack-years (packs per day multiplied by the number of years of smoking), may occur.[1] Such patients are at risk for postoperative atelectasis and hypoxemia. The importance of discontinuation of smoking before surgery is discussed in detail in Chapter 8, Preoperative Preparation of the Patient.

Cough

Cough is the most commonly occurring symptom in patients with bronchogenic carcinoma.

Cough, is usually present in cigarette smokers, which is necessary to clear the excessive amount of sputum that occurs as a result of smoking. A recurrent, productive cough lasting for 3 months for each of two consecutive years is indicative of chronic bronchitis. Bronchogenic carcinoma may lead to airway irritation and sputum production. If the cough is productive, the amount, consistency, and color of sputum should be ascertained. A productive cough calls for preoperative pulmonary toilet to reduce postoperative pulmonary complications. Purulent sputum which contains both mucus and pus, is usually yellow or green. A sputum culture can indicate if preoperative antibiotic therapy is warranted. Blood-tinged sputum or frank hemoptysis may be a sign of tumor invasion of the respiratory tract and may interfere with endobronchial intubation.

Dyspnea

In patients with chronic lung disease, dyspnea often develops only after major limitations of respiratory reserve. In patients with carcinoma, however, dyspnea may occur acutely and with less respiratory compromise. The degree of patient activity and the level of activity that leads to dyspnea should be ascertained. Patients with dyspnea are not able to complete an average sentence without pausing, and patients with severe dyspnea are likely to require postoperative ventilation. Severe exertional dyspnea often indicates impaired ventilatory reserve and a forced expiratory volume in 1 second (FEV_1) less than 1500 mL. Postural dyspnea with difficulty in breathing in the supine position may suggest tracheal compression from an anterior mediastinal mass.

Wheezing

Wheezing is often caused by chronic obstructive pulmonary disease (COPD) or emphysema, or may be due to airway obstruction from tumor. Tracheal involvement may lead to severe stridor and respiratory impairment. Wheezing may also be a result of bronchospastic disease, which may respond to bronchodilator therapy.

Chest Pain

Patients may complain of a constant, dull pain on the side of the tumor. Patients may also have pleuritic chest pain secondary to pleural effusion or from direct tumor extension.[2]

Extrapulmonary Symptoms

Symptoms may occur as a result of tumor growth beyond the lung. Spread to pleura or lymphatic obstruction may cause a pleural effusion, and spread to paraesophageal lymph nodes may lead to compression of the esophagus and dysphagia. Involvement of the paratracheal nodes may cause obstruction of the superior vena cava and a superior vena cava syndrome. Other symptoms may include chest wall pain resulting from chest wall invasion by the tumor, arm pain due to brachial plexus involvement, Horner's syndrome, and hoarseness caused by vocal cord paralysis from left recurrent laryngeal nerve impingement. Metastases, most commonly to brain, bone, liver, and adrenal glands, may also occur.

In addition, secretion of hormone-like compounds by the tumor can cause a paraneoplastic syndrome. Patients may have Cushing's syndrome, carcinoid syndrome, hypercalcemia, hypoglycemia, or syndrome of inappropriate antidiuretic hormone. Neuromuscular symptoms resembling myasthenia may occur. Clubbing of the distal phalanges may be present in patients with chronic hypoxemia and cyanosis.

Nonspecific systemic symptoms such as weight loss, weakness, and anorexia may also occur. Approximately 20% of patients may have fever.[2]

Physical Examination

A thorough physical examination is important. Like the history, it should focus on the cardiopulmonary systems. Pulmonary evaluation is essential.

Respiratory Rate and Pattern

The need to pause during a sentence is a sign of severe dyspnea. In the presence of diaphragmatic fatigue and respiratory dysfunction, inspiratory paradox, in which the abdomen and chest move in opposite directions at the same time, creating a rocking motion, may occur. Patients should also be evaluated for paroxysmal retraction (Hoover's sign), decreased diaphragmatic movement from hyperinflated lungs, asymmetrical chest movement from phrenic nerve dysfunction, hemothorax, pneumothorax, and pleural effusion.

The rate and pattern of breathing can help distinguish between restrictive and obstructive lung disease. For a constant minute volume, the work of breathing against air flow resistance (obstructive disease) is less when respiration is slow and deep. In contrast, work of breathing against elastic resistance (restrictive diseases such as pulmonary fibrosis or edema) is less when respiration is rapid and shallow (Fig. 7-1).

Cyanosis

If cyanosis is present, the arterial saturation is usually 80% or less ($PaO_2 < 50$ mmHg), and the concentration of desaturated hemoglobin is

Figure 7-1. Work done against elastic and airflow resistance. The total work of breathing is reported at different respiratory frequencies and is minimum at value about 15 breaths/min. For the same minute volume, the airflow resistance minimum work will be performed at higher frequencies (less compliance), and lower frequencies when the airflow resistance is increased. (Reprinted with permission from Nunn JF: Applied respiratory physiology. 4th ed. London: Butterworth-Heinemann, p. 127.)

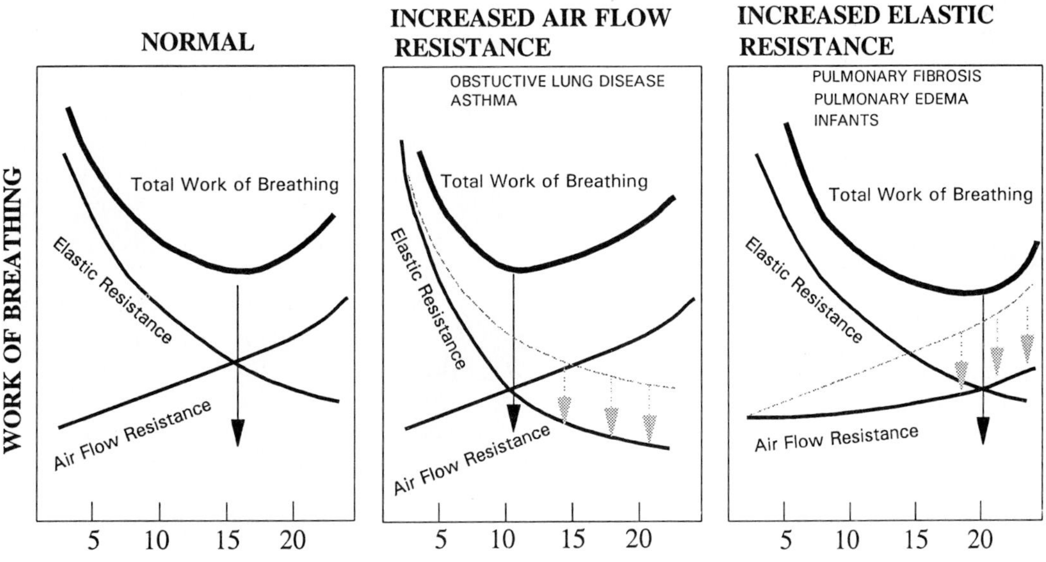

5 gm/dL. The presence of central cyanosis should be distinguished from peripheral cyanosis, which is cyanosis of the fingers, toes, or ears as a result of poor circulation (acrocyanosis).

Clubbing

Clubbing refers to the hypertrophy of the soft tissue of the distal phalanx of a digit. This condition may occur in the presence of primary or metastatic lung cancer, bronchiectasis, lung abscess, or mesothelioma. Clubbing is thought to be caused by a humoral substance that causes vasodilatation of the fingertips; however, its precise etiology is unknown.

Breath Sounds

Crackles (rales), which are usually due to the presence of fluid in the airways, may indicate sputum retention of pulmonary edema. Wheezing caused by air moving at high velocity through bronchi may be a sign of either airway obstruction or bronchospasm. Diminished breath sounds may indicate emphysema, bullae, pleural effusion, or pneumothorax.

In the presence of pulmonary hypertension, the splitting of the second heart sound may be fixed, and the pulmonary component of the second heart sound may increase in intensity.

Laboratory Testing

Electrocardiogram

The electrocardiogram should be evaluated for the presence of right atrial and ventricular hypertrophy. Lung hyperinflation in patients with COPD may lead to low voltage QRS complex and poor R wave progression from V_1 to V_6. Signs of right atrial and right ventricular hypertrophy, including an enlarged P wave (P pulmonale) in lead II (right atrial hypertrophy) and an R/S ratio greater than 1.0 in lead V_1 (right ventricular hypertrophy) may be present.

Chest Radiography

Patients with COPD usually have hyperinflated lungs. An increased anteroposterior chest diameter and an increased retrosternal air space may both be seen in the lateral chest x-ray.

In patients with bronchitis, increased vascular markings are usually evident. In patients with emphysema, these markings are reduced. In severe cases, bullae of the lung may be visible on chest x-ray.

The chest x-ray should also be evaluated for the presence of a deviated trachea or a mediastinal mass (Figs. 7-2–7-5), which may further complicate administration of the anesthetic. Computerized tomography (CAT) scans provide more intricate details of the chest anatomy, including the size of a mass or airway involvement.

Figure 7-2. Solitary left lung nodule.

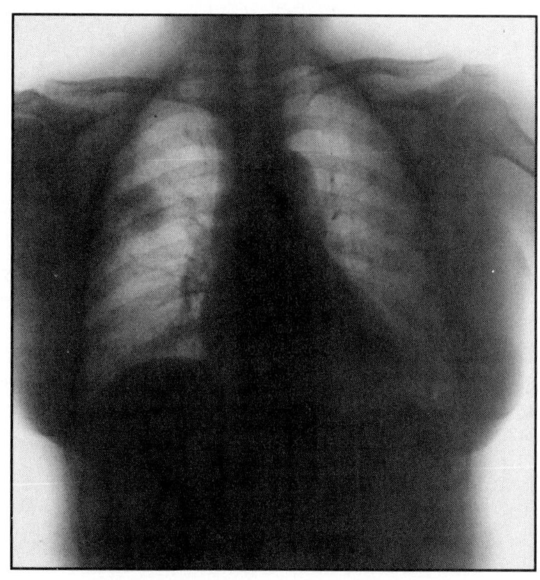

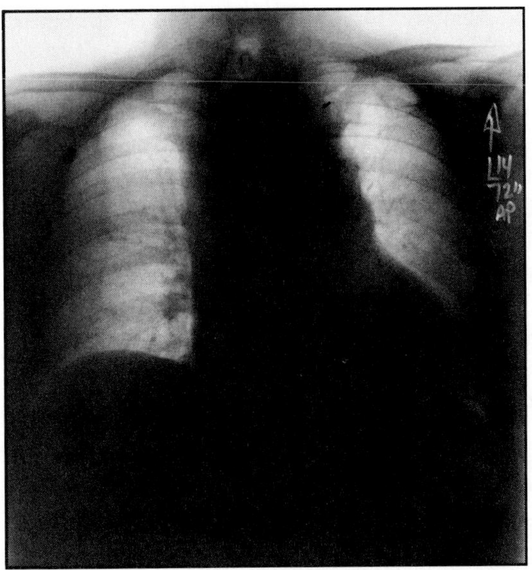

Figure 7-3. A large right lobe tumor with right main bronchus compression.

Figure 7-4. Postobstruction atelectatic left upper lobe from lung lesion invading the bronchus.

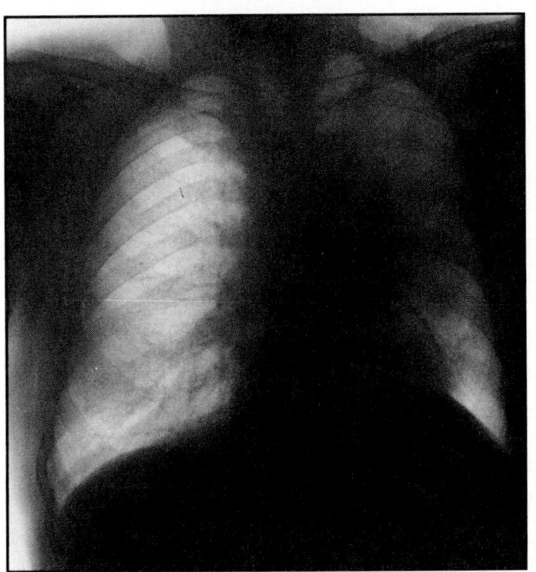

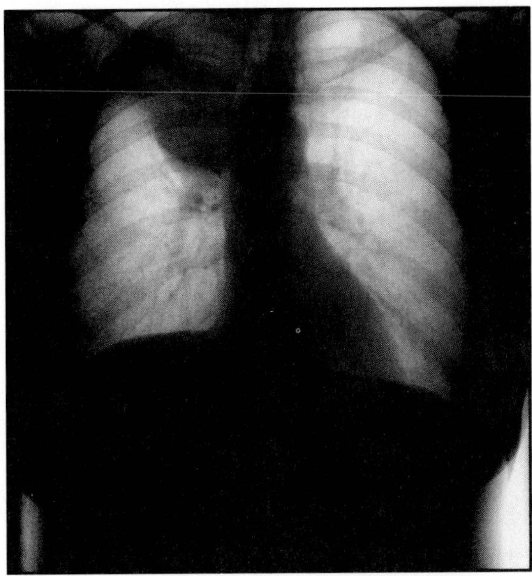

Figure 7-5. Mediastinal mass with right deviation of the trachea.

Arterial Blood Gas Determination

Patients who present for thoracic surgery should have a baseline arterial blood gas measurement. Patients with chronic bronchitis are often hypercarbic, hypoxemic, and cyanotic, and chronic respiratory failure may occur. A high $PaCO_2$ leads to an elevated bicarbonate level in the cerebrospinal fluid; chronic exposure of the medullary chemoreceptor results in a reduced ventilatory response to carbon dioxide. Administration of a gas mixture with an increased fraction of inspired oxygen (FIO_2) may lead to further hypoventilation caused by loss of the hypoxic drive to breathe.

Evaluation of Lung Resectability

It is important to estimate how much lung tissue can be safely removed in patients scheduled to undergo lung resection to avoid postoperative complications including dyspnea, pulmonary hypertension, cor pulmonale, and acute respiratory failure (Fig. 7-6). Pulmonary function tests (PFTs) and arterial blood gas determination are the initial steps of this determination. PFTs include measurements of forced vital capacity (FVC), forced expiratory volume in 1 second (FEV_1), and peak expiratory flow rate (PEFR). In chapter 2 PFTs are discussed in greater detail. If the $PaCO_2$ is above 40 mmHg, the maximum breathing capacity or FEV_1 is below 50%, or the residual volume/total lung capacity is greater than 50%, then split lung function tests should be performed (see Regional Pulmonary Function Tests, below). One of the potential limitations of PFTs is that individual results are compared with a large normal reference range; this can impair the sensitivity of the test.

Regional Pulmonary Function Tests

Arterial blood gas analysis and PFTs such as FEV_1 or FVC are measures of whole lung function; they do not indicate the contribution made by lung tissue that remains following the resection. These whole lung function tests may not adequately determine if patients have sufficient pulmonary reserve to undergo lung resection. In the case of a tumor that completely occludes a mainstem bronchus but does not affect the contraluminal side, the whole lung PFT results are an indication of the function of the lung that remains after pneumonectomy.

Evaluation of split lung function was originally performed with the double-lumen tube in awake, spontaneously breathing patients (differential bronchospirometry).[3] In fact, the double-lumen tube was originally introduced by Carlens for this purpose. This procedure is uncomfortable and technically difficult, however, and double-lumen tubes are no longer in clinical use for this purpose.

Interruption of blood flow was also attempted with the use of a specially designed pulmonary artery catheter.[4–5] With the blood flow to the diseased lung occluded, a mean pulmonary artery pressure greater than 30–40 mmHg or a PaO_2 less than 45 mmHg indicates that the patient is unable to tolerate pneumonectomy.[7] Since pulmonary artery catheterization is also invasive, relatively noninvasive methods of evaluating regional lung function have been developed and are now in clinical use.

One test entails injecting the intravenous injection of an insoluble radioisotope, usually ^{133}Xe. ^{99}Te or ^{131}I-MAP can also be used.[2] Xenon is distributed to the lungs according to the blood flow, is passed into the alveoli, and is exhaled. ^{99}Te and ^{131}I-MAA are not exhaled because of a larger molecular size and are lodged in the pulmonary microcirculation.[2] An external scintillation counter displays a rapid vascular-to-alveolar wash-in peak followed by an exponential alveolar-to-environmental wash-out peak. The regional fractional perfusion is determined by dividing the regional perfusion wash-in peak by the total perfusion wash-in count.

A second test measures regional ventilation. The patient takes a full breath of ^{133}Xe; this leads to a wash-in peak and then a wash-out peak. The calculation for regional fractional ventilation is similar to that for regional fractional perfusion, that is, regional counts are divided by total counts.

In a third test, the patient breathes into a closed system following the injection of ^{133}Xe. After 10 to 15 minutes, when the ^{133}Xe has equilibrated, the concentration of ^{133}Xe in the lungs and the closed system should be the same. At this time, the radioactivity count of each lung is proportional to the lung volume.

The predicted postoperative FEV_1 can be calculated by multiplying the preoperative FEV_1

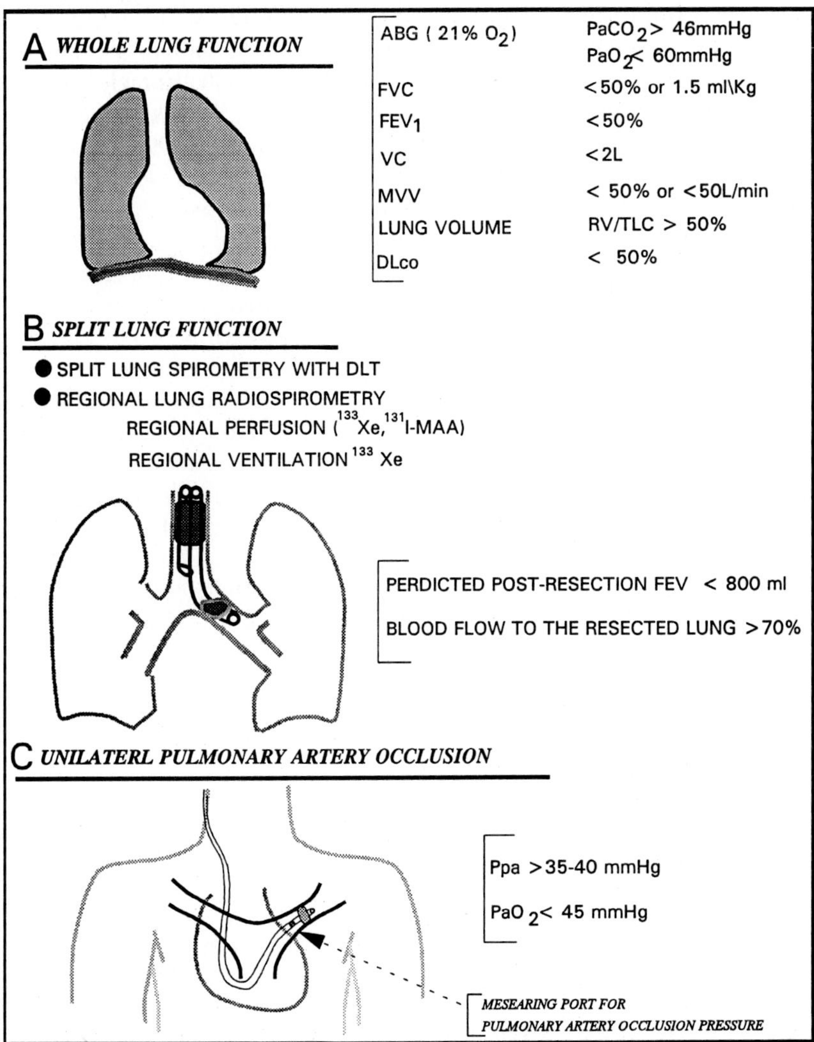

Figure 7-6. The order of tests to determine the cardiopulmonary function status of the patient and the extent of resection that will be tolerated by the patient. A. The whole lung function test is an analog to a basic screening test. B. The split lung function are regional tests to determine the extent of involvement of the diseased lung to be removed. C. Tests that mimic the postoperative cardiopulmonary function. These will be the decisive tests to determine whether the patient will be able to tolerate the planned resection.

by the percent of pulmonary function contributed by the uninvolved lung. The lowest predicted postoperative FEV_1 that allows adequate elimination of carbon dioxide is reported to be 800 mL.[8] Rather than requiring a fixed amount of postoperative lung volume for all patients, other researchers recommend that the predicted postoperative FEV_1 be at least 40% of the predicted postoperative FEV_1 based on age, sex, and size.[9,10]

If the split lung function criteria are not satisfied, and surgery is still planned, balloon occlusion of the pulmonary artery ipsilateral to the diseased lung can be performed. Simultaneous pulmonary artery and bronchus occlusion, which most closely mimic the conditions after pneumonectomy, can also be performed, but is considered too invasive for clinical use.[2]

Results concerning the usefulness of preoperative spirometry and radiography for predicting postoperative pulmonary complications have been conflicting.[11–19] This may in part be due to varying definitions of postoperative pulmonary dysfunction. In a recent study, Fogh et al,[20] who prospectively studied 125 patients undergoing major abdominal surgery, reported an 18% incidence of postoperative pulmonary complications (respiratory insufficiencies that required some form of treatment). These authors also investigated the predictive value of preoperative perfusion-ventilation scanning, spirometry, and radiography on postoperative pulmonary complications. They concluded that despite a correlation between test results and postoperative complications, the predictive value was too low to be of clinical use.

Exercise Testing

Exercise testing has been investigated as a method of preoperative evaluation. Such testing results in increased muscle consumption of oxygen, cardiac output, pulmonary artery blood flow. The rise in pulmonary blood flow may simulate the relative increase in pulmonary flow into a reduced vascular bed following lung resection. In a study of 460 thoracic surgery patients by Gaensler et al,[21] no association of the preoperative ability to walk 180 ft/min with postoperative morbidity was evident. Researchers have shown that two flights of stair climbing is not a more useful prediction of postoperative dysfunction.[22] In another report, patients scheduled for pneumonectomy underwent incremental exercising; investigators found a correlation between inability to perform exercise and postoperative morbidity and mortality.[14] Results of studies of only nonstrenuous amounts of exercise conflict.[23–25]

Combining exercise with pulmonary artery occlusion has been recommended as a better method of predicting postoperative complication.[26,27] Pulmonary vascular resistance during exercise above 190 dynes. sec. cm^{-5} may indi-

Table 7-1. The Patient With Cardiac Involvement, Undergoing Thoracotomy Should Have an Extensive Preoperative Evaluation of the Left and Right Ventricle. The Extent of the Coronary Involvement and the Patient Maximum Oxygen Consumption Ability Should be Investigated. The Pulmonary Circulation and the Right Ventricle Function Can be Evaluated by the Pulmonary Artery Balloon Occlusion Test to Mimic the Post Resection Pressure

Right Ventricle	ANGINA	Left Ventricle
Pulmonary Artery Balloon Occlusion		E.C.G. Exercise Testing
↓		↓
PVR Measurement During Exercise		Thallium Scan
↓		↓
MPAP <40 mmHg		Exercise Testing Vo_2 max
↓		↓
Acceptable CO, PVR		Coronary Angiogram
↓		↓
Surgery		Medical Treatment
	← CABG ←	
		Concomitant Operation

cate increased postoperative morbidity and mortality.[27]

The patient with cardiac involvement undergoing thoracotomy should have an extensive preoperative evaluation not only of the left ventricle but of the right ventricle as well. The extent of the coronary involvement (ECG, echocardiography, Thallium scan) and the patient's maximum oxygen consumption ability should be investigated. The pulmonary circulation and the right ventricle function can be evaluated by the pulmonary artery balloon occlusion test, with and without exercise, to mimic the post-resection pressure.

Exercise testing not only provides an overall assessment of cardiopulmonary function but may also allow separate evaluations of cardiac and pulmonary function (Table 7-1), which requires incremental exercising to maximal levels.[28] Oxygen consumption (Vo_2max) is evaluated during maximum voluntary ventilation (MVV) and peak heart rate. Above the anaerobic threshold (AT), both aerobic and anaerobic metabolism contribute to energy production, and lactate levels rise. Determination of the AT may allow differentiation between the two systems.

An approach that has been recently recommended is to begin with baseline resting PFTs, including pulmonary function spirometry both before and after inhaled bronchodilators, lung volumes, diffusing capacity (DLCO), and arterial blood gas measurement.[7] This method may predict the development of pulmonary hypertension following pulmonary resection.[7] Incremental exercising is performed to determine the Vo_2max and the AT. Smith et al. (Fig. 7-7) showed that when Vo_2 max was below 15 mL/kg/min all patients undergoing thoracotomy had postoperative pulmonary complications.

Figure 7-7. The relationship between extent of resection, maximal oxygen consumption grade exercise (Vo_{2max}), and postoperative pulmonary complications. (Reprinted with permission from Smith TP et al. Exercise capacity as a predictor of postthoracotomy morbidity. Am Rev Respir Dis 129:730–734, 1984.)

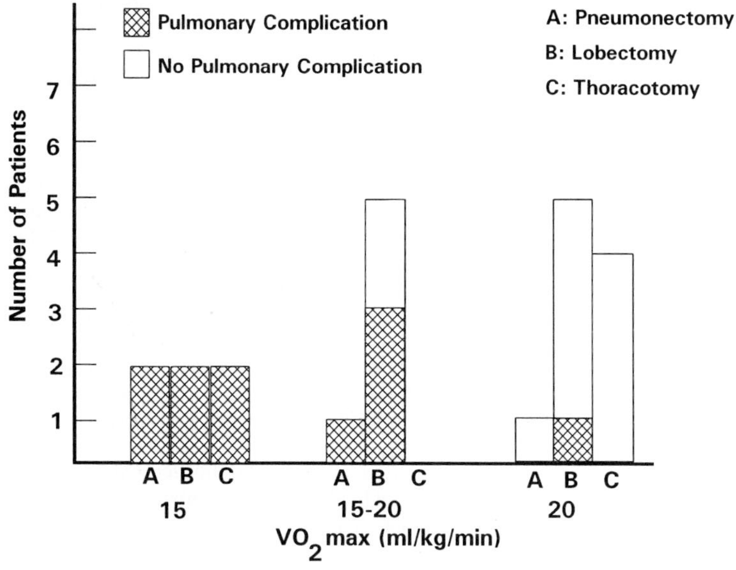

Table 7-2. Differentiation of Cardiac Versus Pulmonary Impairment by Exercise Testing

Measured Parameter	Cardiac	Pulmonary
$\dot{V}O_2max$	Decreased	Decreased
$\dot{V}_Emax/MVV$	50%	80–90%
$\dot{V}O_2max$/heart rate (O_2 pulse)	Decreased	May decrease
$\dot{V}O_2max/AT$	Decreased	Indeterminate
PaO_2/SaO_2	Maintained	Decreases
$PaCO_2$	Maintained or decreased	Often decreases
VD/VT	Normal = decreased	Often increases

Reprinted with permission from Boysen PG. Evaluation of pulmonary function tests and arterial blood gases. In: Kaplan JA, ed. Thoracic Anesthesia. New York: Churchill Livingstone, 1991:14.

During exercise continuous measurement of respired gases, airflow, pulse oximetry, and possibly arterial blood gas analysis from an indwelling arterial catheter occurs. The ability to reach the AT and maximal VO_2 with no drop in peripheral oxygen arterial saturation (SaO_2) as measured by pulse oximetry indicates adequate respiratory function. A decrease in oxygen saturation during exercise may suggest lung disease and has been correlated with increased postoperative morbidity.[29] If dyspnea prevents achievement of the AT and VO_2max then respiratory impairment is significant. Although patients with limited cardiac reserve use less than 50% of their MVV during exercise, patients with respiratory impairment use over 50% of their MVV. There is an increase in heart rate at low work levels or oxygen consumption. The ratio of VO_2/heart rate is often called "oxygen pulse." The differentiation of cardiac versus pulmonary dysfunction is presented in Table 7-2. The evolving role of exercising testing before lung resection has been given in a recent review.[30]

The usefulness of preoperative exercise testing for patients scheduled to undergo thoracotomies remains controversial. In a recent prospective study of 70 patients who underwent preoperative exercise treadmill testing, for VO_2max and VEmax had no predictive value.[31] The percentages of predicted VEmax and heart rate were associated with overall complications but not specifically those of the cardiopulmonary system. The researchers concluded that patients should not be refused thoracic surgery based on the results of exercise limitation.

References

1. Beck GJ, Doyle CA, Schacter FN. Smoking and lung function. Am Rev Respir Dis 1981;155:149.
2. Benumof JL. Preoperative cardiopulmonary evaluation. In: Benumof JL, Anesthesia for thoracic surgery. Philadelphia: WB Saunders, 1987:126.
3. Neuhaus H, Cherniak NS. A bronchospirometric method of estimating the effect of pneumonectomy on the maximum breathing capacity. J Thorac Cardiovasc Surg 1968;55:144.
4. Laros CD, Swierenga J. Temporary unilateral pulmonary artery occlusion in the preoperative evaluation of patients with bronchial carcinoma. Med Thorac 1967;24:269.
5. Uggla LG. Indication for and results of thoracic surgery with regard to respiratory and circulatory function tests. Acta Chir Scand 1956;111:197.
6. Olsen GN, Block AJ, Swenson EW, et al. Pulmonary function evaluation of the lung resection candidate: a prospective study. Am Rev Respir Dis 1975; 111:379.
7. Boysen PG. Evaluation of pulmonary function tests and arterial blood gases. In: Kaplan JA, ed. Thoracic anesthesia. New York: Churchill Livingstone, 1991:1.

8. Olsen GN, Block AJ, Tobias JA. Prediction of postpneumonectomy pulmonary function using quantitative macroaggregate lung scanning. Chest 1974;66:13.
9. Boysen PG, Block AJ, Olsen GN, et al. Prospective evaluation for pneumonectomy using the Tc^{99} quantitative perfusion lung scan. Chest 1977; 72:422.
10. Gass GD, Olsen GN. Preoperative pulmonary function testing to predict postoperative morbidity and mortality. Chest 1986;89:127.
11. Latimer RG, Dickman M, Day WC, et al. Ventilatory patterns and pulmonary complications after upper abdominal surgery determined by preoperative and postoperative computerized spirometry and blood gas analysis. Am J Surg 1971;122:622.
12. Schlenlaer JD, Hubay CA. The pathogenesis of postoperative atelectasis. Arch Surg 1973;107:846.
13. Stein M, Koota GM, Simon M, et al. Pulmonary evaluation of surgical patients. JAMA 1962;181:765.
14. Wiren JE, Lindell SE, Hellenkant C. Pre- and postoperative lung function in sitting and supine position related to postoperative chest x-ray abnormalities and arterial hypoxemia. Clin Physiol 1983; 3:257.
15. Stein M, Cassara E. Preoperative pulmonary evaluation and therapy for surgical patients. JAMA 1970; 211:787.
16. Appelberg M, Gordon L, Fatti LP. Preoperative pulmonary evaluation of surgical patients using the vitalograph. Br J Surg 1974;61:57.
17. Claque MB, Collin J, Flemming LB. Prediction of postoperative respiratory complication by simple spirometry. Ann R Coll Surg Engl 1979;61:59.
18. Graven JL, Evans GA, Davenport PJ, et al. The evaluation of the incentive spirometry in the management of postoperative pulmonary complications. Br J Surg 1974;1974:793.
19. Palmer KNV, Gardine JS. Effect of partial gastrectomy on pulmonary physiology. BMJ 1964;1:347.
20. Fogh J, Wille-Jorgensen P, Brynjolf I, et al: The predictive value of preoperative perfusion/ventilation scintigraphy, spirometry and x-ray of the lungs on postoperative pulmonary complications. A prospective study. Acta Anaesthesiol Scand 1987;31: 717.
21. Gaensler EA, Cusell DW, Lindgren I, et al. The role of pulmonary insufficiency in mortality and invalidism following surgery for pulmonary tuberculosis. J Thorac Cardiovasc Surg 1955;29:163.
22. Van Nostrand D, Kjelsberg MD, Humphrey EW: Preresectional evaluation of risk from pneumonectomy. Surg Gynecol Obstet 1968;127:306.
23. Reichel J: Assessment of operative risk of pneumonectomy. Chest 1972;62:570.
24. Berggren H, Ekroth R, Malmberg R, et al. Hospital mortality and long-term survival in relation to preoperative function in elderly patients with bronchogenic carcinoma. Ann Thorac Surg 1987;38:633.
25. Bagg LR. The 12-minute walking distance: its use in the preoperative assessment of patients with bronchial carcinoma before lung resection. Respiration 1984;46:342.
26. Uggla LG. Indication for and results of thoracic surgery with regard to respiratory and circulatory function tests. Acta Chir Scand 1956;111:197.
27. Fee JH, Holmes EC, Gerwirtz HS, et al. Role of pulmonary resistance measurement in preoperative evaluation of candidates for lung resection. J Thorac Cardiovasc Surg 1975;75:519.
28. Loke J. Distinguishing cardiac versus pulmonary limitation in exercise performance. Chest 1983; 83:441.
29. Markos J, Mullin JB, Hillman OR, et al. Preoperative assessment as a predictor of mortality and morbidity after lung resection. Am Rev Respir Dis 1989;139:902.
30. Olsen GN. The evolving role of exercise testing prior to lung resection. Chest 1989;95:218.
31. Boysen PG, Clark CA, Block J. Graded exercise testing and post-thoracotomy complications. J Cardiothorac Anesth 1990;4:68.

CHAPTER

8

Preoperative Preparation of the Patient

David Bronheim

The primary purpose of preoperative preparation in the patient undergoing surgery, thoracic or otherwise, is reduction of morbidity and mortality in the perioperative period. Thoracic surgery patients are at especially high risk for perioperative morbidity and mortality when compared to the general surgical population for two reasons. First, postoperative respiratory complications from any surgery are increased in patients with underlying respiratory disease, which is not surprising.[1] Unfortunately, concurrent lung disease is the rule rather than the exception in patients undergoing thoracic surgery. The majority have a significant smoking history, which causes a fourfold to sixfold increase in the incidence of postoperative pulmonary complications.[2] Chronic lung disease is also a common finding in patients who are scheduled for thoracic surgery. This concurrent diagnosis increases the incidence of postoperative pulmonary complications by a factor of approximately twenty.[1]

Second, as a consequence of thoracic surgery, overall pulmonary function may be impaired because of the resultant lung resection, trauma to unresected lung, atelectasis, and edema. Furthermore, pain associated with the common thoracotomy incision is frequently severe and results in patient resistance to deep breathing and coughing postoperatively. This may result in retained secretions, atelectasis, and pneumonia. Multiple studies have demonstrated the relationship between the site of surgery and postoperative respiratory complications.[3,4] To cite just one example, in 1500 patients with various degrees of pulmonary compromise, respiratory complications such as pneumonia and atelectasis occurred in 63% of those undergoing thoracic or upper abdominal surgery versus 15% to 19% in midabdominal surgery patients and 1% of lower abdominal surgery patients.[5] Several conditions show particular correlation with postoperative complications, including infection, dehydration, electrolyte imbalance, wheezing, obesity, cor pulmonale, malnutrition, and, as was stated before, cigarette smoking.

Multiple interventions have been attempted to decrease the postoperative morbidity and mortality associated with thoracic surgery. Fortunately, interventions before surgery and vigorous preoperative preparation have been demonstrated to decrease the incidence of postoperative pulmonary complications. These include smoking cessation, bronchodilator therapy, antibiotic therapy, maneuvers to loosen and remove secretions, and preoperative education in postoperative respiratory maneuvers.

Preoperative Interventions That Decrease Incidence of Postoperative Complications

Smoking Cessation

Approximately 33% of the adult patients presenting for surgery are smokers. Smokers who undergo major surgery have postoperative pulmonary complications at four to six times the rate of nonsmokers.[2] Smoking cessation for more than four to eight weeks before surgery is associated with a decrease in the incidence of respiratory complication by as much as 66%. Short-term smoking discontinuation for as little as 12–48 hours is associated with decreased carboxyhemoglobin levels, improvement in the hemoglobin dissociation curve (right shift of the curve with increased tissue oxygen availability), and a reduction in the usual nicotine-induced increase in heart rate. Several days of smoking cessation may improve ciliary transport and decrease airway irritability. One to two weeks of discontinuation may even be associated with a decrease in pulmonary secretions.[6–8] Unfortunately, no improvement in outcome has been demonstrated with short-term smoking discontinuation alone. Indeed, one study has even reported an increase in the incident of pulmonary complications in patients who stopped smoking shortly before surgery when compared to those who continue.[7] Withdrawal from smoking preoperatively may result in increased anxiety, increased pulmonary secretions, and perhaps even a higher incidence of postoperative deep vein thrombosis.[9,10]

Thus, although smoking cessation for more than four to eight weeks before surgery is advantageous and long-term smoking cessation benefits all smokers, the advantages of discontinuation of smoking shortly before surgery solely for the perioperative period remain less clear. Most physicians still recommend discontinuation of smoking at least 24 hours before surgery, however.

Bronchodilator Therapy

Bronchodilator therapy, as part of a general regimen that includes smoking cessation, antibiotic therapy for purulent sputum, postural drainage, and chest physiotherapy, may decrease postoperative morbidity and length of hospital stay, especially in those groups with the highest incidence of postoperative complications.[1,11,12] We recommend that all patients with some element of reversible airway disease be optimally prepared before anesthesia and surgery. A history of reversible airway disease is usually easily elicited from those who suffer from it. Physical examination may demonstrate anything from a completely asymptomatic patient to one with obvious shortness of breath, increased respiratory rate, and wheezing. The physician must assess to what degree symptoms are chronic, stable, and optimally treated, as opposed to acute and subject to treatment and reversal. In addition to history and physical examination, spirometry before and after bronchodilator therapy may provide supplemental data on the adequacy of therapy.

Patients with histories of asthma on chronic treatment who are asymptomatic and without wheezing or respiratory distress at the time of surgery should continue their usual regimens during the perioperative period. Aggressive therapy should be pursued if bronchospasm should occur either perioperatively or postoperatively. Patients with acute symptoms of bronchospasm preoperatively should first undergo aggressive therapy until an optimal respiratory baseline is reached for a period of weeks before surgery is electively scheduled.

An extensive literature exists on the therapeutic interventions for bronchospasm. Standard therapy usually consists of treatment with beta-agonists and methylxanthines. More recently, inhaled corticosteroids have been used. Anticholinergics and cromolyn sodium may be added to this regimen or used instead of these medications. Oral corticosteroids may be added chronically or intermittently in response to failure of these other modalities.

All these families of medications, with the exception of cromolyn sodium, are also used for acute therapy of bronchospasm. Individual drugs are discussed in more detail below.

Methylxanthines

Methylxanthines, initially in the form of caffeine in strong coffee,[13] were used as bronchodilators as early as 1859. Various theophylline preparation are widely used today in treatment of asthma and chronic obstructive pulmonary disease (COPD). The mechanism by which theophylline acts as a bronchodilator is not clear. Methylxanthines are phosphodiesterase inhibitors, and as such they have been thought to lead to the accumulation of cyclic adenosine monophosphate (cAMP) with resultant smooth muscle dilation. This effect occurs in vitro only at drug concentrations much higher than those demonstrated to cause bronchial muscle relaxation, however.[2,14,15] More recently, at concentrations within the therapeutic range, it has been noted that theophylline is a competitive antagonist of adenosine, an autocoid that reacts with specific receptors in the membranes of essentially all human cells. How adenosine affects bronchial smooth muscle tone remains unclear; however, both intravenous and inhaled adenosine are known to precipitate bronchospasm in asthmatics but to have little effect on normal subjects. Finally, methylxanthines may potentiate the inhibition of prostaglandin synthesis and may reduce the uptake and metabolism of catecholamines in nonneural tissue.

Besides bronchial smooth muscle relaxation, other effects may possibly be of therapeutic importance in patients with bronchospasm. These include an increase in mucociliary transport, inhibition of the release of mediators, suppression of airway edema, decrease in pulmonary hypertension, central stimulation of ventilation, and improved diaphragmatic contractility.[14] In patients with asthma and COPD, theophylline decreases both the frequency and severity of disease symptoms and can decrease steroid requirements in corticosteroid-dependent patients. Although intravenous aminophylline remains widely used as part of the standard therapy for acute asthma and status asthmaticus, it is unclear whether it adds any benefit to acute treatment with optimal doses of inhaled or subcutaneous beta-agonists.

Side effects are common and include nausea, vomiting, diarrhea, headaches, nervousness, tachycardia, seizures, and arrhythmias.[15,16] This association with arrhythmias should be borne in mind, as aminophylline when given acutely facilitates epinephrine-induced arrhythmias under halothane but not isoflurane anesthesia. This has not been proved with chronic treatment, however.

Usual dosages of oral maintenance therapy of theophylline are 7–12 mg/kg ideal body weight per day depending on age, individual tolerance, and subsequent plasma concentrations. In a patient not previously taking theophylline, intravenous therapy consists of a loading bolus of aminophylline, 6 mg/kg, followed by an infusion of theophylline, 0.13–0.80 mg/kg/h. The elimination half-life varies widely; fourfold differences are not uncommon. Drug half-life may be markedly increased in hepatic failure and congestive heart failure. It averages 3.5 hours in children and 8–9 hours in adults. Oral dosages and intravenous infusion should be titrated to plasma concentrations of 10–20 μg/mL.[14] Drugs such as cimetidine, propranolol, erythromycin, ciprofloxacin, steroids, and many others may decrease theophylline metabolism and increase serum drug levels, whereas smoking, phenobarbital, and phenytoin are known to increase metabolism and decrease blood levels. If side effects occur, oral dosages and intravenous infusions should be decreased even with a "therapeutic range." At serum concentrations greater than 20 μg/mL, the frequency and severity of adverse side effects increase. Despite what appears to be a narrow therapeutic window, serious toxicity reported occurred in only 30 of 36,000 patients who had serum concentrations monitored regularly in a nine-year period.[17]

Beta-adrenergic Agonists

Adrenergic receptors are present throughout the body, in areas such as the brain, heart, kidney, and bronchial smooth muscle. Activation of the β_2 adrenergic receptor in bronchial smooth muscle causes the formation of 3′5′-cAMP. cAMP causes bronchial smooth muscle relaxation by modulating the effects of intracellular calcium. Not surprisingly, sympathomimetic agents that activate the β_2-adrenergic receptor have proved efficacious in treatment of asthma and COPD. They have been widely used for this purpose for years.

The choice of a beta-agonist depends on the desired effects. Catechols produce peak bronchodilation within five minutes of inhalation as opposed to the noncatechols, which require 10 to 15 minutes. The catechols have shorter durations of action, however, making their prophylactic use less effective.

The β_2-selective drugs, especially when used by inhaler or via nebulized aerosols, tend to have less systemic effects and therefore may be better tolerated. In addition to their bronchodilatory effects, beta-agonists stimulate mucociliary clearance. They also inhibit the release of bronchoconstrictor mediators such as histamine, leukotrienes, kinins, and slow-reacting substance of anaphylaxis by mast cells.

Tachyphylaxis, possibly secondary to down regulation in the number of beta-receptors, occurs with chronic use of beta-adrenergic agents. Intravenous steroids may reverse this effect, with an onset in as little as one hour and a peak effect in six to eight hours. Finally, chronic, routine use of beta-agonists, as opposed to "as needed" administration, may be associated with increased mortality and increased bronchial hyperresponsiveness in patients with asthma. These findings have led to a much greater emphasis on the use of drugs on a chronic basis to prevent inflammatory responses as opposed to drugs with a bronchodilators property alone.

Several classes of sympathomimetic agents are currently available in the United States for clinical use (Table 8-1).

CATECHOLAMINES. The catecholamines, which include the naturally occurring epinephrine and the synthetic agents isoproterenol and isoetharine, are characterized by hydroxyl groups at position 3 and 4 of their phenolic moieties (Fig. 8-1). These agents are quickly metabolized by catechol-O-methyltransferase and monoamine oxidase, which explain their relatively short half-lives. When given orally they undergo metabolism by intestinal and hepatic sulfatases and are therefore largely ineffective when given by this route.

Epinephrine, a mixed alpha- and beta-agonist, is usually given subcutaneously in doses of 0.3–0.5 mL (1:1000 dilution) for treatment of acute bronchospasm in adults. It has duration of action of 1 to 2 hours. Cardiovascular beta-adrenergic effects such as tachycardia are common in response to subcutaneous administration. Although epinephrine is also use-

Table 8-1. Drugs for Treatment of Asthma and Chronic Obstructive Pulmonary Disease

Drug	Dose	Frequency
Beta-adrenergic bronchodilators		
Metaproterenol (Alupent)	2 puffs (1.3 mg) by metered dose inhaler (MDI)*	q3–4h
(Metaprel)	0.3 mL of 5% solution by nebulizer	q4h
	Syrup and tablets, 20 mg	tid to qid
Isoetharine (Bronkosol)	0.5 mL 1% solution by nebulizer	q4h
Isoproterenol hydrochloride (Isuprel)	25–200 ng/kg/min 0.5 by infusion	
	2 puffs (262 μg) by MDI*	q4h
	0.5 mL of 0.5% solution by nebulizer	q3–4h
Epinephrine solution	1 mg/ml (0.2–0.55 mL) SQ	0.5–4h
MDI	2 puffs (32 μg epinephrine base)	q3h
Albuterol (Proventil, Ventolin, and others)	2 puffs (180 μg) by MDI*	q4–6h
	Rotacaps, powder inhaler† (200 μg/capsule)	1–2 caps q4–6h
	0.5 mL of 0.5% solution by nebulizer‡	2.5 mg q1–4h
	Syrup or tablets, 2–4 mg	tid or qid
	Extended-release tablets (Repetabs, 4–8 mg)	q12h
Bitolterol mesylate (Tornalate)	MDI* (370 μg/puff)	2–3 puffs q4–6h
	Nebulized solution (2 mg/mL)	1.5–3.5 mg q4–6h
Pirbuterol (Maxair)	MDI (200 μg/puff)	2 puffs q4–6h
Terbutaline (Brethine, Bricanyl) (Brethaire)	Subcutaneous (1 mg/mL)	0.25 mg (may repeat once after 15–30 min; max. 0.5 mg in 4 h)
	Tablets	2.5–5 mg tid
	MDI* (200 μg puff)	2–3 puffs q4–6h PRN*
Theophylline	Extended-release capsules or tablets (Theo-Dur and others)§,‖	300–600 mg/day
Aminophylline	By infusion¶	6 mg/kg IBW, then 0.13–0.8 mg/kg/h
Anticholinergics		
Ipratropium bromide (Atrovent)	2 puffs by MDI* (36 μg)	q6h
Glyclopyrrolate (Robinul)	0.4–0.6 mg via nebulizer	q12h
Anti-inflammatory Drugs		
I. Corticosteroids		
Beclomethasone dipropionate (Beclovent, Vanceril)	MDI* (42 μg puff)	2–4 puffs bid to qid
Budesonide (Pulmicort)‡	MDI* (50,200 μg/puff) or Turbuhaler (100, 200, 400 μg/puff)	400–2400 μg divided bid to qid
Dexamethasone (Decodren)	MDI* 0.1 mg/puff	3 puffs tid to qid
Flunisolide (Aerobid)	MDI* (250 μg/puff	2–4 puffs bid to qid
Triamcinolone acetonide (Azmacort)	MDI* (100 μg/puff)	2–4 puffs bid to qid
Prednisone or prednisolone#	Oral tablets (5, 10, 20 mg); oral liquid (Liquid Pred, Pediapred, Prelone)	Acute: up to 80 mg/day for 7–14 days Chronic: up to 40 mg every day or every other day

Table 8-1 (Continued)

Drug	Dose	Frequency
II. Cromolyn (Intal)	Spinhaler, powder (20 mg/capsule)	1 capsule qid
	MDI (800 μg/puff)	2–4 puffs qid
	Nebulized solution (10 mg/mL)	20 mg qid
Nedocromil (Tilade)	MDI (10 mg/mL)	2 puffs

* Each puff should be separated by 1–3 minutes in patients in acute distress to improve deposition of the aerosol.
† Higher doses (up to 2–4 puffs every 5–15 min) can be used for acute attacks (limited by cardiac and other adverse effects).
‡ Higher doses (up to 2.5 mg every 15 min) can be used for acute attacks (limited by cardiac and other adverse effects).
§ Extended-release formulations may not be interchangeable.
‖ Begin with low dose and increase at 3–4-day intervals. Monitor clinical response and serum concentrations to determine if larger doses can be given safely.
§ No bolus necessary in patient on chronic preparation at initiation of treatment.
\# The glucocorticoid effect of 5 mg prednisone is equal to 0.75 ng dexamethasone; 4 mg methylprednisolone or triamcinolone; 20 mg hydrocortisone; or 25 mg cortisone. These medications may be used both orally and intravenously as available for treatment of asthma or COPD.

ful when given via inhaler or aerosol, it has largely been supplanted by more β_2-specific agents because of its side effects. Epinephrine continues to be used subcutaneously during therapy of acute bronchospasm, however.

Isoproterenol has been used for years as a metered dose inhaler and as an aerosol. More recently, longer lasting, more β_2-specific agents have largely supplanted it as well. Isoproterenol is still used in its intravenous form in pediatric patients with bronchospasm unresponsive to other agents and sufficiently severe to warrant consideration of endotracheal intubation and mechanical ventilation. In an intensive care setting, infusions of 50–100 ng/kg/min are initiated and titrated upward until heart rates exceed 200 beats/min, ectopy develops, or as occurs more commonly, bronchospasm resolves. The aggressive use of isoproterenol in the critical care setting has precluded endotracheal intubation and mechanical ventilation in many patients with severe status asthmaticus.[18,19]

Isoetharine, a mildly β_2-selective agonist with about one tenth the potency of isoproterenol and a duration of action of two to three hours is also available as an inhaler and aerosol. Like epinephrine and isoproterenol, it too has been largely replaced by more β_2-specific agents.

Bitolterol is an inactive compound that is hydrolyzed by lung esterases to the active compound called colterol, a catecholamine. When administered by inhaler or nebulizer, bitolteral has proven to be an effective $beta_2$ specific bronchodilator. Even when compared to metaproterenol and albuterol[20,21] it produces fewer systemic effects, perhaps because of the higher concentration of esterases in the lung as compared to cardiac tissue.[22]

RESORCINOLS. Resorcinols are beta-adrenergic agents in which the catechol ring is replaced with a 3,5-hydroxybenzene ring (Fig. 8-1). This change, along with increasing the size of the substitutions on the amine moiety, circumvent the catecholamine metabolic pathway, lengthen the effective duration of action of the resorcinols, and increase their β_2 specificity. There are three drugs in this group, metaproterenol, terbutaline, and fenoterol. Fenoterol is not available for clinical use in the United States, however.

Metaproterenol was the first of this new class of beta-agonists to be introduced. This drug is available as an inhaler, an aerosol, and in

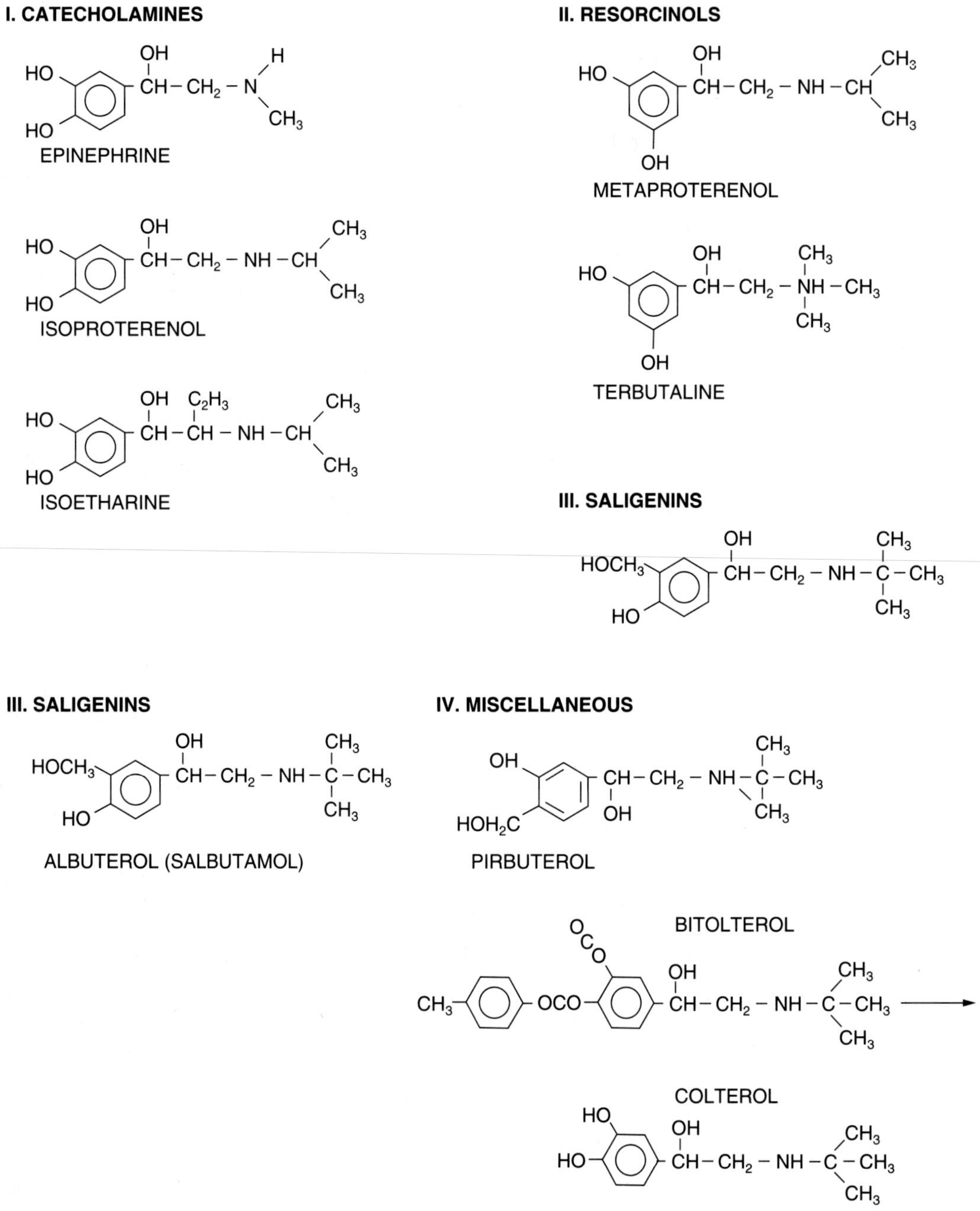

I. CATECHOLAMINES

EPINEPHRINE

ISOPROTERENOL

ISOETHARINE

II. RESORCINOLS

METAPROTERENOL

TERBUTALINE

III. SALIGENINS

III. SALIGENINS

ALBUTEROL (SALBUTAMOL)

IV. MISCELLANEOUS

PIRBUTEROL

BITOLTEROL

COLTEROL

Figure 8-1. Molecular structures of beta agonist bronchodilators.

an oral form. Although metaproterenol is less potent than isoproterenol, it produces fewer cardiovascular and neuromuscular side effects. Oral and inhaled forms are both efficacious, but when used by inhaler side effects are less frequent. The effective duration of action is four hours.

Terbutaline is only slightly less potent than isoproterenol but has far fewer cardiovascular side effects. It has been used subcutaneously, orally, and via inhaler and aerosol. When given subcutaneously, the duration of action of terbutaline is two to four hours, and it produces side effects equal to epinephrine.[23] Inhaled doses produce fewer side effects than the oral preparation and have an effective duration of action of six to seven hours.[24]

Fenoterol is available outside the United States as an inhaler, via aerosol, and as an oral agent. Its effective duration of action is six to eight hours and it is otherwise not clinically different from terbutaline. As previously noted, increased bronchial hyperresponsiveness and increased mortality has been associated with chronic, regular administration rather than "as needed" use of β_2-selective inhalers, particularly fenoterol.[25,26]

SALIGENINS AND SIMILAR COMPOUNDS. Saligenins differ from catechols due to substitution at the 3-hydroxy position (Fig. 8-1). In the United States, the only available saligenin is albuterol. It is a β_2-selective agent with a duration of action of four to six hours. Albuterol may be given orally, via aerosol or inhaler.[20,27] Pirbuterol differs structurally from albuterol in the substitution of a pyridine for benzene ring (Fig. 8-1). This agent is nine times more β_2 selective than albuterol and 15–20 times more than isoproterenol. It is presently available as an inhaler.[28]

Anticholinergics

Anticholinergic agents function as bronchodilators by inhibiting the action of acetylcholine at its receptor site, thus inhibiting the release of cyclic guanosine monophosphate, which normally produces bronchial smooth muscle contraction. Until isoproterenol was introduced in the 1940s, atropine was the only aerosol therapy available for bronchospasm. The subsequent use of atropine sulfate fell into disfavor because of its slower onset of action and systemic effects, including dry mouth, tachycardia, headaches, micturition difficulties, blurred vision, and constipation.[29,30]

Ipratropium bromide, a quaternary ammonium atropine derivative, has recently become available for clinical use. Because of its low lipid solubility, this agent is poorly absorbed across biological membranes. An effective bronchodilator when used as an inhaler or aerosol, it does not produce tachycardia or the usual anticholinergic side effects except dry mouth. Aerosol administration produces blood levels that are one thousandth of an equally effective oral dose. Eighty percent of its action is reached by 30 minutes, and maximal effect occurs at one-half to two hours. The duration of action is four to six hours.[31,32]

In clinical studies, ipratropium is active as a bronchodilator but has not proved quite as effective as beta-agonists in treatment of asthma.[33,34] The addition of ipratropium to beta-agonists may cause further bronchodilation.[35,36] In COPD, ipratropium has proven somewhat more effective than beta-agonists in producing bronchodilation.[37,38] Because of its lack of effect on heart rate and blood pressure, it is more useful in patients with underlying cardiac disease. In addition, recent data suggest that ipratropium may be more useful at preventing cholinergically mediated bronchospasm intraoperatively.[39]

Glycopyrrolate is widely used in the practice of anesthesia as a drying agent and as an antagonist to the cholinergic effect of reversal agents. Though not approved by the Food and Drug Administration as a bronchodilator, it too is a quaternary amide and has been shown to cause bronchodilation in patients with asthma for 8–12 hours with minimal side effects. Doses of 0.4–0.6 mg may be nebulized as an aerosol, but the optimal dose is as yet unknown. Ipratropium is recommended as a first choice until more data are available on its use as a bronchodilator.[40,41]

Cromolyn Sodium and Nedocromil

Although their mechanism of action remains the subject of debate, cromolyn sodium and nedocromil inhibit both immunological and nonimmunological mediator release from mast cells, macrophages, and eosinophils. In addition, these drugs reduce the nonspecific bronchial hyperreactivity seen in all asthmatics. These compounds have little oral absorption and are thus delivered to the airways by either spinhaler, as with cromolyn, or with metered dose inhaler or aerosol, as with both medications. Although these agents are somewhat less efficacious than bronchodilators in preventing bronchospasm and ineffective at treating active bronchospasm, use of these agents is recommended because of the low incidence of significant side effects. They are useful in preventing asthma symptoms but have essentially no role in treatment of acute bronchospasm. In fact, their use may even worsen acute bronchospasm.[42]

Corticosteroids

Corticosteroids, which possess glucocorticoid and mineralocorticoid properties to a varying degree, were proven efficacious in asthma as early as 1950, and since then they have been used in many diffuse inflammatory pulmonary processes.[43] The mechanism of action of corticosteroids is complex. In vivo, free steroid binds steroid receptors in cell cytoplasm throughout the body to form a steroid-receptor complex. After modification, this complex then binds chromatin in the nucleus. As a result, messenger RNA transcription is usually enhanced, and protein synthesis is subsequently affected.[44] Steroids have systemic effects, including regulating carbohydrate, protein, and lipid metabolism; electrolyte and water balance; vascular permeability; bone and muscular function; neural tissue excitability; and formed blood elements. Therefore, their chronic use has many potential complications.

As anti-inflammatory agents, corticosteroids inhibit both the early and late manifestations of the inflammatory reaction, including edema formation, fibrin deposition, capillary dilation, leukocyte migration and phagocytic activity, capillary and fibrinoblast proliferation, and collagen deposition. The ability of corticosteroids to inhibit leukocyte and macrophage recruitment and thus prevent the release of a large number of mediator factors largely explains their use in asthma and other inflammatory pulmonary processes. Steroids may also reverse the tachyphylaxis believed to be secondary to the down regulation of the beta-receptor associated with chronic beta-agonist use.[45,46] As therapy for asthma is now being more aggressively treated as an inflammatory process,[42] rather than just a spastic process, the use of steroids in their inhaled forms, where systemic absorption is low, has markedly increased.

Steroids may be given orally, intravenously, intramuscularly, topically, or by meter dose inhaler. They are remarkably effective in treatment of bronchospasm unresponsive to other medications, but their long-term use may lead to weight gain, a cushingoid appearance, adrenal suppression, cataracts, osteoporosis, hypertension, glucose intolerance, bruising, and growth suppression. Although beta-agonists, cromolyn sodium, and theophylline may be used in the absence of bronchospastic symptoms for prophylaxis, systemic corticosteroids are swiftly weaned over a course of days to weeks as tolerated. When complete weaning from oral therapy is not possible, alternate-day therapy with short-acting preparations has proved effective in minimizing the complications of long-term therapy. Fortunately, the chronic use of steroids by metered dose inhaler is effective in decreasing bronchospasm with little or no effect on the hypothalamic-pituitary-adrenal axis. This may decrease the need for intermittent therapy with oral or intravenous steroids and has allowed complete weaning of some chronic users from oral steroids. Doses of various corticosteroids are listed in Table 8-1. Those patients on long-term oral corticosteroid therapy with possible adrenal axis suppression should have stress-dose steroids added to their regimen through the perioperative period.

Antibiotic Therapy

In the presence of acute pulmonary or bronchial infection, elective surgery should be deferred until the infective process has cleared independent of the presence of underlying chronic pulmonary disease. Patients with COPD are not only at greater risk for the development of acute pulmonary infections but may have a chronic suppurative bronchitis with constant sputum production. Patients with chronic bronchitis and sputum production can usually give a reliable history about changing patterns of both sputum production and purulence. Acute infection may be heralded by an increase in sputum volume or purulence. Prospective studies examining the benefits of multiple preoperative interventions have demonstrated the beneficial effects of preoperative antibiotic therapy in patients with COPD.[1,12] Proper antibiotic therapy should be based on sputum Gram stains, cultures, and sensitivities. Common isolates in this population include *Streptococcus pneumoniae* and *Haemophilus influenzae.* Antibiotic regimens should be directed to these likely pathogens pending investigation. Treatment of the underlying infection usually decreases both sputum volume and viscosity and sometimes eliminates it completely.

Maneuvers for Loosening and Removing Secretions

Maneuvers for loosening and removing secretions in combination with bronchodilators, antibiotic therapy, and smoking cessation significantly reduce the incidence of postoperative pulmonary complications in patients with COPD.[1,12] Many different regimens are currently used to accomplish this goal.

Perhaps the most effective way to loosen thick secretions is hydration and humidification. Research has shown that the tracheal mucous transport velocity is increased by hydration and decreased by dehydration.[47] Ultrasonic nebulization and use of humidified air or oxygen usually ensure tracheobronchial humidification. In addition, systemic hydration should not be ignored.

Mucolytic agents such as acetylcysteine (Mucomyst) administered by nebulizer or expectorants such as guaifenesin, potassium iodide, and iodinated glycerol have been used for treatment of tenacious secretions. They are not without their own side effects, however.[48] Acetylcysteine may induce bronchospasm and expectorants may increase the absolute amount of sputum production. These agents have largely fallen out of favor for routine use but may benefit individual patients.

Removal of secretions may be further aided by postural drainage and chest physiotherapy in combination with deep breathing and coughing. These are frequently used as part of a standard regimen done several times a day in 15–30-minute sessions.[50–52] Intermittent positive-pressure breathing regimens, although widely used in the past, probably have no advantage over other modalities and do not warrant the additional costs.[53–55] Their use has been largely abandoned.

Preoperative Education in Postoperative Respiratory Maneuvers

The proper time to teach patients about deep breathing, coughing, and incentive spirometry is not in the early postoperative period when patients are obviously suffering from the postoperative consequences of surgery and anesthesia (eg, pain, nausea, vomiting, sedation) but rather during the preoperative period. The necessary time can be taken to ensure that patients are educated in the proper use of incentive spirometry and in the need for continued deep breathing and coughing despite anticipated postoperative discomfort. Patient preparation for what will be expected postoperatively, in combination with discussion of the plans for postoperative pain control before surgery, is more likely to lead to a less anxious patient who is more willing to cooperate in the management of pain and perform the necessary postoperative respiratory maneuvers.

Other Preoperative Measures

Optimization of Overall Medical Condition

In addition to all the preparation specific to patients undergoing thoracic surgery, all other medical conditions should be evaluated and treated to the extent possible before surgery. In this respect adequate preparation for thoracic surgery does not differ from preparation for any other surgery. Such therapy includes but is not limited to intervention for malnutrition, treatment of common concurrent cardiovascular diseases (eg, coronary artery disease, hypertension, cor pulmonale, congestive heart failure, arrhythmias), and management of fluid, acid-base and electrolyte abnormalities.

Preoperative Visit and Premedication

The value of the preoperative visit in minimizing preanesthetic anxiety and preparing the patient for surgery is well established in the practice of anesthesia.[56,57] This visit is used to confirm that the appropriate preoperative evaluation has been completed and that the patient's pulmonary and overall medical status has been optimized. The preoperative session is the appropriate time for explanation of the series of events leading up to the induction of anesthesia, including intravenous access, placement of invasive and noninvasive monitoring, and the planned use of a face mask. This is the best time to establish the subsequent plan for postoperative pain management and to educate the patient about the possible need for postoperative ventilatory support and intensive care, if appropriate. The preoperative visit provides an excellent opportunity to reinforce the expectations about postoperative respiratory maneuvers and incentive spirometry.

Premedication should be individualized in an attempt to make patients calm and cooperative on arrival to the operating suite. We have used benzodiazepines successfully, but almost any acceptable premedication regimen suffices. For patients with baseline hypoxia and hypercapnia, however, consideration should be given to avoiding preoperative sedation until actual arrival in the operating room suite where the patient may be more closely monitored.

Anticholinergics have been demonstrated to decrease the volume of secretions with little effect on viscosity.[58,59] This is especially useful where fiberoptic bronchoscopy is being planned. We have largely limited their preoperative use to patients with copious secretions because of the common complaint of excessive oral dryness that is associated with their use.

References

1. Stein M, Koota GM, Simon M, et al. Pulmonary evaluation of surgical patients. JAMA 1962;181:765.
2. Morton HJV, Comb DA. Tobacco smoking and pulmonary complications after operation. Lancet 1944;1:368.
3. Tisi GM: Preoperative evaluation of pulmonary function. Am Rev Respir Dis 1979;119:293.
4. Gracey DR, Divertie MB, Didier EP. Preoperative pulmonary preparation of patients with chronic obstructive pulmonary disease. Chest 1979;76:123.
5. Anderson WH, Dosett BE, Hamilton GE. Prevention of postoperative pulmonary complications. JAMA 1963;186:763.
6. Pearce AL, Jones RM. Smoking and anesthesia. Preoperative abstinence and perioperative morbidity. Anesthesiology 1984;61:576.
7. Warner MA, Tinker JH, Divertie MB. Preoperative cessation of smoking and pulmonary complications. Anesthesiology 1983;59A:60.
8. Davies JM, Latto IP, Jones JG, et al. Effects of stopping smoking for 48 hours on oxygen availability from the blood. A study on pregnant women. BMJ 1979;2:355.
9. Handley AJ, Teather D. Influence of smoking on deep vein thrombosis after myocardial infarction. BMJ 1974;3:230.
10. Marks P, Emerson PA. Increased incidence of deep vein thrombosis after myocardial infarction in nonsmokers. BMJ 1974;3:232.
11. Palmer KN, Sellick BA. The prevention of postoperative pulmonary atelectasis. Lancet 1953;1:164.
12. Veith FJ, Rocco AG. Evaluation of respiratory function in surgical patients: Importance of preoperative preparation in the prediction of pulmonary complications. Surgery 1959;45:905.
13. Salter H. On some points in the treatment and clinical history of asthma. Edinburgh Med J 1859; 4:1109.
14. Rall TW. Drugs used in the treatment of asthma. In: Gilman AG, ed. The pharmacological basis of therapeutics. 8th ed. New York: Permagon Press, 1990:618.
15. Hendeles L, Weinberger M. Theophylline. A state of the art review. Pharmacotherapy 1983;3:2.
16. Miech RP, Stein M. Respiratory pharmacology. Methylxanthines. Clin Chest Med 1986;7:331.
17. Darby LE. The incidence of theophylline toxicity in an outpatient setting. Pharmacotherapy 1990; 10:112.
18. Wood DW, Downes JJ, Scheinkopf H, et al. Intravenous isoproterenol in the management of respiratory failure in childhood status asthmaticus. J Allergy Clin Immunol 1972;50:75.
19. Hamstreet MP, Miles MV, Rutland RO. Effect of intravenous isoproterenol on theophylline kinetics. J Allergy Clin Immunol 1982;69:360.
20. Orgel HA, Kemp JP, Tinkelman DG, et al. Bitolterol and albuterol metered dose aerosols: comparison of two long acting beta$_2$-adrenergic bronchodilators for treatment of asthma. J Allergy Clin Immunol 1985;75:55.
21. Cockcroft W, Berscheid BA, Dosman JA, et al. Comparison of bitolterol mesylate and metaproterenol sulphate. Curr Ther Res 1981;30:817.
22. Kass I, Mingo TS. Bitolterol mesylate (Win 32784) aerosol. A new long-acting bronchodilator with reduced chronotropic effects. Chest 1980;78:283.
23. Amory DW, Burnham SC, Cheney FW, Jr. Comparison of the cardiopulmonary effects of subcutaneously administered epinephrine and terbutaline in patients with reversible airway obstruction. Chest 1975;67:279.
24. Geumei A, Miller WF, Paez PN, et al. Evaluation of a new oral β_2-adrenoreceptor stimulant bronchodilator, terbutaline. Pharmacology 1975;13:201.
25. Spitzer WO, et al. The use of beta-antagonists and the risk of death and near death from asthma. N Engl J Med 1992;326:501.
26. Cheung D, et al. Long-term effects of a long-acting beta α adrenoreceptor agonist; 5 almeterol on airway hyper responsiveness in asthmatics. N Engl J Med 1992;327:1198.
27. Tattersfield AE, McNicol MW. Salbutamol and isoproterenol: a double-blind trial to compare bronchodilator and cardiovascular activity. N Engl J Med 1969;281:1323.
28. Beumer HM. Pirbuterol aerosol versus salbutamol and placebo aerosols in bronchial asthma. Drugs Exp Clin Res 1980;2:77.
29. Cavanaugh MJ, Cooper DM. Inhaled atropine dose-

response characteristics. Am Rev Respir Dis 1976; 114:517.
30. Pak CCF, Kradjan WA, Lakshminarayan S, et al. Inhaled atropine sulfate: dose-response characteristics in adult patients with chronic airflow obstruction. Am Rev Respir Dis 1982;125:331.
31. Pakes GE, Brodgen RN, Heel RC, et al. Ipratropium bromide: a review of its pharmacological properties and therapeutic efficacy in asthma and chronic bronchitis. Drugs 1980;20:237.
32. Gross NJ. Ipratropium bromide. N Engl J Med 1988;319:486.
33. Ruffin RE, Fitzgerald JD, Rebuck AS. A comparison of the bronchodilator activity of SCH 1000 and salbutamol. J Allergy Clin Immunol 1977;59:139.
34. Marlin GE, Bush DE, Berend N. Comparison of ipratropium bromide and fenoterol in asthma and chronic bronchitis. Br J Clin Pharmacol 1978;6:547.
35. Lelcoe NM, Toogood JH, Blennerhassett G, et al. The addition of an aerosol anticholinergic to an oral beta-agonist plus theophylline in asthma and bronchitis. Chest 1982;82:300.
36. Rebuck AS, Chapman KR, Abboud R, et al. Nebulized anticholinergic and sympathomimetic treatment of asthma and chronic obstructive airways disease in the emergency room. Am J Med 1987; 82:59.
37. Poppius H, Salorinne Y. Comparative trial of a new anticholinergic bronchodilator, SCH 1000, and salbutamol in chronic bronchitis. BMJ 1973;4:134.
38. Tashkin DP, Ashutosh K, Bleeker ER, et al. Comparison of the anticholinergic bronchodilator ipratropium bromide with metaproterenol in chronic obstructive disease: a 90-day multicenter study. Am J Med 1986;81(Suppl 5A):81.
39. Wu SC, Hildenbrandt J, Isner PD, et al. Efficacy of anticholinergic and beta-adrenergic agonist treatment of maximal cholinergic bronchospasm in tracheally intubated rabbits. Anesth Analg 1992;75:777.
40. Gal TJ, Suratt PM, Lu J. Glycopyrrolate and inhalation: comparative effects on normal airway function. Am Rev Respir Dis 1984;129:871.
41. Walker FB, Kaiser DL. Prolonged effect of inhaled glycopyrrolate in asthma. Chest 1987;91:49.
42. Barnes PJ. A new approach to the treatment of asthma. N Engl J Med 1989;321:1517.
43. Carryer HM, Prickman LE, Maytum CK, et al. Effects of cortisone on bronchial asthma and hay fever occurring in subjects sensitive to ragweed pollen. Mayo Clin Proc 1950;25:482.
44. Munck A, Mendel DB, Smith LI, et al. Glucocorticoid receptors and actions. Am Rev Respir Dis 1990;141:S2–10.
45. Brodde O-E, Howe U, Egerszegei S, et al. Effect of prednisolone on β_2-adrenoreceptors in asthmatic patients receiving β_2-bronchodilators. Eur J Clin Pharmacol 1988;34:145.
46. Ellul-Micallef R, French FF. Effect of intravenous prednisolone in asthmatics with diminished adrenergic responsiveness. Lancet 1975;2:1269.
47. Chopra SK, Taplin GV, Simmons DH, et al. Effects of hydration and physical therapy on tracheal transport velocity. Am Rev Respir Dis 1977;115:1009.
48. Scheffner AL. The mucolytic activity and mechanism of action and metabolism of acetylcysteine. Pharmacother 1964;1:47.
50. May DB, Munt PW. Physiologic effects of chest percussion and postural drainage in patients with stable chronic bronchitis. Chest 1979;75:29.
51. Oldenburg FA Jr, Dolovich MB, Montgomery JM, et al. Effects of postural drainage, exercise and cough on mucus clearance in chronic bronchitis. Am Rev Respir Dis 1979;120:739.
52. Pavia D, Clarke FW. Is cough as effective as chest physiotherapy in the removal of excessive tracheobronchial secretions? Thorax 1981;36:683.
53. Gold MI. The present status of IPPB therapy. Chest 1975;67:469.
54. Gold MI. Is intermittent positive-pressure breathing therapy (IPBB Rx) necessary in the surgical patient? Ann Surg 1976;184:122.
55. Petty TL. A critical look at IPPB. Chest 1974;66:1.
56. Egbert LD, Battit GE, Turdorf H, et al. The value of the preoperative visit by an anesthetist. JAMA 1963;185:553.
57. Leigh JM, Walker J, Janaganathan P. Effects of preoperative anesthetic visit on anxiety. BMJ 1977; 2:987.
58. Lopez-Vidriero MT, Costello J, Clark TSH, et al. Effects of atropine on sputum production. Thorax 1975;30:543.
59. Aviado DM. Regulation of bronchomotor tone during anesthesia. Anesthesiology 1975;42:68.
60. Prokocimer PG, Nicholls E, Gaba DM, et al. Epinephrine arrhythmogenity is enhanced by acute but not chronic aminophylline administration during halothane anesthesia in dogs. Anesthesiology 1986;65:13.
61. Stint JA, Berger JM, Sullivan SF. Lack of arrhythmogenity of isoflurane following administration of aminophylline in dogs. Anesth Analg 1983;62:568.

SECTION

III

Intraoperative Management

CHAPTER

9

Intraoperative Monitoring

Steven J. Barker
Kevin K. Tremper

Maintenance of adequate oxygenation and ventilation is essential in anesthesiology and critical care medicine. Because the thoracic cavity contains organs that are heavily involved in these functions, intrathoracic procedures not surprisingly often make oxygenation and ventilation more difficult.

Monitoring of Oxygenation

The clinician has been able to quantitatively measure oxygen in arterial blood since the development of the first blood gas analyzer in the 1950s. This in vitro method of analysis remained the only quantitative assessment of oxygenation until the 1970s. The measurement of transcutaneous oxygen tension and the development of pulse oximetry, which followed a few years later, are two continuous, in vivo monitors of oxygenation in both tissue and arterial blood.

The currently available oxygen monitors are described below; the features that are most important in thoracic anesthesia are emphasized. The physical and engineering principles of each are discussed to the extent necessary to understand their sources of error. In addition, the physiology of measured oxygen variables are briefly reviewed; their clinical interpretation is crucial. Before the continuous in vivo oxygen monitors are discussed, the interpretation of oxygen tension from in vitro arterial blood gas analysis is considered.

Blood Gas Analysis: Arterial Oxygen Tension and Oxygenation

The in vitro blood gas analyzer measures arterial oxygen tension (PaO_2). Physicians often assume that an adequate PaO_2 indicates that the patient is well-oxygenated. However, an adequate PaO_2 is only the first step in the process of oxygen transport, whose purpose is to deliver oxygen to the mitochondria where it is actually used. PaO_2 is related to the arterial hemoglobin saturation (SaO_2) by the oxyhemoglobin dissociation curve shown in Figure 9-1. In the normal configuration, a P_AO_2 value of 60 mmHg produces an SaO_2 of 75%. Decreases in pH or increases in arterial carbon dioxide tension ($PaCO_2$), 2,3-diphosphoglycerate (2,3-DPG) or temperature shift the dissociation curve to the right. A rightward shift of the curve produces a lower SaO_2 value for a given PaO_2 (Fig 9-1), that is, the affinity of hemoglobin for oxygen

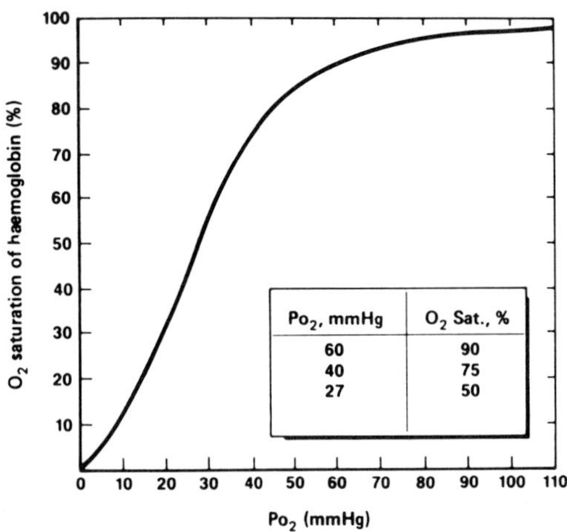

Figure 9-1. A plot of the oxyhemoglobin dissociation curve (hemoglobin saturation [Sao_2] versus arterial oxygen tension [Pao_2]). The curve is shifted to the right by decreasing pHa and increasing $Paco_2$, temperature, or 2,3-DPG. Sao_2 shows little variation with Pao_2 when Pao_2 is greater than 75 mmHg.

is lower. A right shift thus improve "unloading" of oxygen from the capillary blood into the tissues, but it requires a higher PaO_2 to achieve a given SaO_2. During one-lung anesthesia the maintenance of normal PaO_2 values is difficult, and a right-shifted dissociation curve may therefore be deleterious to oxygen delivery.

The arterial oxygen content (CaO_2) is the volume of oxygen (mL) carried by 100 mL of arterial blood. CaO_2 is related to SaO_2 and PaO_2 by the equation:

$$\text{(9-1)} \quad CaO_2 = (1.38(Hb)(SaO_2/100) + 0.003(PaO_2)$$

On the right side the first term represents the oxygen bound to hemoglobin (Hb), and the second term is oxygen dissolved in plasma. If normal values for Hb (15 g/dL) and PaO_2 (100 mmHg) are assumed, equation 9-1 yields a CaO_2 value of 21 mL/dL. That means that each 100 mL of arterial blood normally contains 21 mL of oxygen, 20.7 mL of which is bound to hemoglobin. If venous values are substituted into equation 9-1, the normal venous oxygen content (CvO_2) is 15.6 mL/dL. Therefore the amount of oxygen normally extracted from each 100 mL of blood as it passes through the tissues is the difference between CaO_2 and CvO_2 ($CaO_2 - CvO_2 = 5.4$ mL/dL).

The amount of oxygen delivered to the tissues is given by the product of CaO_2 and cardiac output Qt ($O_{2del} = Qt \times CaO_2$). If it is assumed that Qt = 5 L/min and CaO_2 = 21 mL/dL, then O_{2del} = 5 L/min × 21 mL/dL × 10 dL/L = 1050 mL/min. Cardiac output is measured in L/min, hence the multiplication by 10 dL/L; CaO_2 is measured in ml/dl. The oxygen consumption, VO_2, is the difference between arterial oxygen delivery and venous oxygen return (O_{2ref}):

$$\text{(9-2)} \quad VO_2 = O_{2del} - O_{2ret} = Qt \times (CaO_2 - CvO_2) = Qt \times ([1.38\ Hb][SaO_2 - SvO_2]/100) \times 10 = 13.8\ (Hb \times Qt)(SaO_2 - SvO_2)/100$$

In substituting for CaO_2 and CvO_2 (mixed venous oxygen content) from equation 9-1, the contribution of plasma-dissolved oxygen is neglected. Again, substituting normal values in this so-called "Fick Equation" for oxygen consumption gives:

$$VO_2 = 13.8(15)(5.0)(100 - 75)/100 = 259\ \text{mL/min}$$

PaO_2 relates to but does not solely determine the adequacy of tissue oxygenation. Its use in the evaluation of lung function, which is critical during thoracic anesthesia, will now be reviewed. The simplest measure of lung function in oxygen uptake is the alveolar-arterial oxygen difference, often called A-a DO_2 or A-a gradient. The alveolar oxygen tension (P_AO_2) is obtained from the alveolar gas equation:

$$(9\text{-}3) \quad P_AO_2 = F_IO_2(P_B - 47) - PaCO_2 \times F$$

F_IO_2 is inspired oxygen fraction, P_B is barometric pressure in mmHg, 47 mmHg is the vapor pressure of water at a body temperature of 37°C, $PaCO_2$ approximates alveolar carbon dioxide tension (P_ACO_2 and $PaCO_2$ are usually within 2 mmHg of each other), and F is a correction factor that reflects the fact that CO_2 production does not equal O_2 uptake. For F_IO_2 less than 0.5, F is approximately the reciprocal of the respiratory quotient (RQ), which is the ratio of CO_2 produced to O_2 consumed; therefore RQ is near 1.2.

Alveolar oxygen tension depends upon barometric pressure, F_IO_2, and $PaCO_2$ (equation 9-3). For $F_IO_2 = 0.21$ and $PaCO_2 = 40$ mmHg, the P_AO_2 at sea level is about 102 mmHg; at Denver (elevation: 1600 meters) it is 76 mmHg; and at 4000 meters (13,100 ft) it is 43 mmHg. As $PaCO_2$ rises to 60 mmHg at sea level, P_AO_2 falls to 78 mmHg; and at $PaCO_2 = 80$ mmHg, P_AO_2 reaches 54 mmHg. Carbon dioxide retention can clearly cause hypoxemia in individuals who are breathing room air. The combination of CO_2 retention and high altitude is particularly dangerous; for example, if $PaCO_2 = 80$ mmHg at Denver, $P_AO_2 = 27.5$ mmHg.

The problem with A-a DO_2 as a measure of lung function is that the normal range of values depends upon both P_B and F_IO_2. At sea level, when $F_IO_2 = 0.21$, the normal A-a DO_2 is 5–10 mmHg. For $F_IO_2 = 1.0$, the normal value ranges up to 100 mmHg. The arterial-to-alveolar oxygen ratio, PaO_2/P_AO_2, is an alternative parameter that is less dependent upon F_IO_2. This ratio is normally greater than 0.7 in healthy individuals at any F_IO_2, although it may be less during general anesthesia.

Arterial hypoxemia can be caused by alveolar hypoxia (low P_AO_2), right-to-left shunt, or pulmonary oxygen diffusion barrier. Once low P_AO_2 has been ruled out, shunt is by far the most common cause, particularly during anesthesia for thoracic surgery. Shunt may be absolute, with a ventilation-perfusion (V/Q) ratio of zero, or relative, with a V/Q ratio less than one. Relative shunt (low V/Q), which reflects poorly functioning or collapsed alveoli, is also called venous admixture. The total or physiologic shunt can be found from the shunt equation:

$$(9\text{-}4) \quad \frac{Qs}{Qt} = \frac{Cc'O_2 - CaO_2}{Cc'O_2 - C\bar{v}O_2}$$

Qs is the flow through the shunt, Qt is cardiac output, and $Cc'O_2$ is ideal pulmonary capillary oxygen content (usually determined by assuming $Pc'O_2 = P_AO_2$). For a given shunt fraction (Qs/Qt) and $C\bar{v}O_2$ value, this equation can be used to predict the PaO_2 as a function of F_IO_2, as shown in Figure 9-2. Note that at high shunt fraction (eg, $Qs/Qt = 0.5$) the P_AO_2 becomes relatively unresponsive to increases in F_IO_2. This may often occur during one-lung ventilation for thoracic surgery. The shunt equation also implies that in the presence of fixed shunt, a fall in $C\bar{v}O_2$ causes a fall in CaO_2. That means that if the venous blood being admixed with the pulmonary capillary blood has a lower saturation, the resulting arterial blood will also have a lower saturation. An increase in oxygen consumption (higher VO_2) can worsen hypoxemia in the presence of a fixed shunt by this mechanism.

Pulse Oximetry

Until the mid-1980s, sequential arterial blood sampling for in vitro PO_2 analysis was the only routine method of quantitatively assessing oxygenation in the operating room. This technique, described earlier, is usually accurate, but it is invasive, not continuous, and does not provide "real-time" data. During thoracic anesthesia, oxygenation status can change so rapidly that continuous, real-time monitoring of arterial oxygenation is essential. Of the several

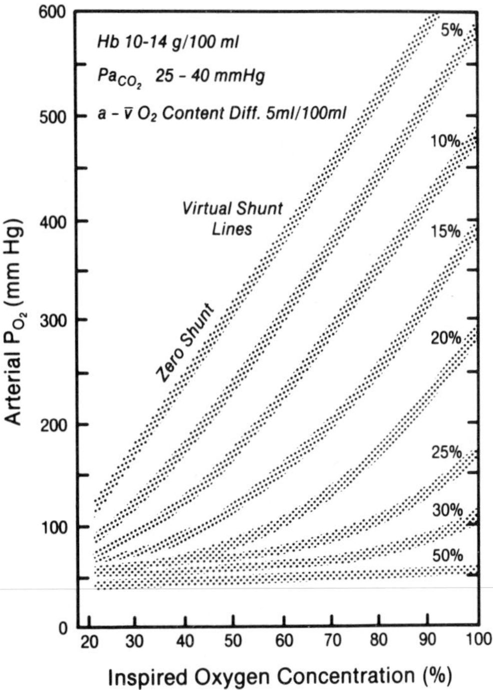

Figure 9-2. The isoshunt diagram, with the arterial oxygen tension (PaO_2) versus the inspired oxygen concentration (FIO_2) for various values of shunt fraction (Q_s/Q_t). For small values of shunt fraction, PaO_2 increases almost linearly with FIO_2. As the shunt increases, PaO_2 becomes less responsive to increasing FIO_2, until for a shunt of 50% or more the PaO_2 is virtually independent of FIO_2.

methods discussed below, no technique has had as much impact on the field of anesthesiology as pulse oximetry. The pulse oximeter is noninvasive (hence nearly risk-free) and continuous, and it has rapidly become standard for all anesthetics. A discussion of the physiology of saturation monitoring, the design principles of the pulse oximeter, and the most important sources of measurement error follows.

Saturation Monitoring

In the previous section arterial hemoglobin saturation (SaO_2) is used to determine oxygen content, but saturation is not defined. Oxygen saturation is the blood oxygen content divided by the oxygen capacity times 100; it is expressed as a percent. Oxygen content was originally measured volumetrically by the method of Van Slyke and Neills.[1] The oxygen capacity is defined as the oxygen content of blood after equilibration with room air (PO_2 = 159 mmHg). At the time this definition was made, the maximum blood oxygen content occurred during breathing of room air, because supplemental oxygen was not available. From the blood oxygen content formula (equation 9-1), this definition of saturation includes contributions from both hemoglobin-bound and dissolved oxygen. Adult blood can contain at least four species of hemoglobin: oxyhemoglobin (O_2Hb), reduced hemoglobin (Hb), methemoglobin (MetHb), and carboxyhemoglobin (COHb). Because COHb and MetHb, which are found in low concentrations except in pathologic states, these dyshemoglobins do not transport oxygen, and they do not contribute to the oxygen content or to the above definition of oxygen saturation.

When spectrophotometric methods for measuring concentrations of hemoglobin species became available, saturation could be more easily determined. The term functional hemoglobin saturation is defined as:

$$\text{(9-5)} \quad \text{Functional saturation} = SaO_2 = \frac{O_2Hb}{O_2Hb + Hb} \times 100\%$$

Fractional hemoglobin saturation, also called oxyhemoglobin fraction, is defined as:

$$\text{(9-6)} \quad \text{Fractional saturation} = HbO_2\% = \frac{O_2Hb}{O_2Hb + Hb + COHb + MetHb} \times 100$$

This ratio of oxyhemoglobin to total hemoglobin ($HbO_2\%$) is the saturation used in the calculation of oxygen content and delivery (equation 9-1).

Principles of Pulse Oximetry

The use of light absorbance to measure the concentrations of dissolved solutes is called spectrophotometry. This method was first used to determine the hemoglobin concentration of blood in the 1930s.[2] Theoretically it is based on the Lambert-Beer law, which relates the concentration of a solute to the intensity of light transmitted through the solution (Fig. 9-3):

$$I_{trans} = I_{in}e^{-DC\alpha_\lambda} \qquad (9\text{-}7)$$

where I_{trans} = intensity of transmitted light, I_{in} = intensity of incident light, D = distance light is transmitted through the liquid, C = concentration of the solute (hemoglobin), and α_λ = extinction coefficient of the solute

Figure 9-3. The Lambert-Beer Law, which shows how the concentration of a solute can be determined from a logarithmic relationship between the incident and transmitted light intensities and the solute concentration. (Reprinted, with permission, from: Tremper KK, Barker SJ. Pulse oximetry and oxygen transport. In: Payne JP, Severinghaus JW, eds. Pulse oximetry. Berlin: Springer-Verlag, 1986;19.

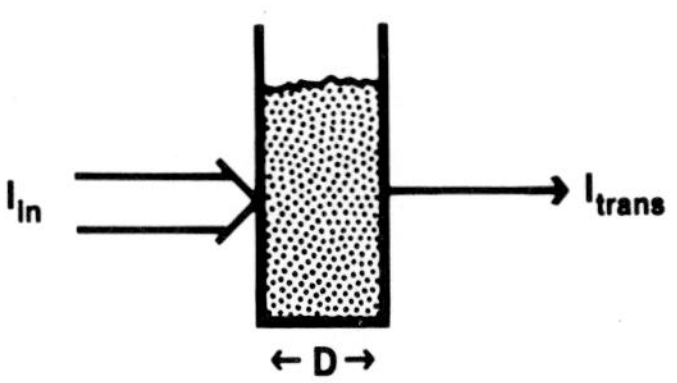

(a constant for a given solute at a specific light wavelength λ).*

Thus if a known solute is dissolved in a clear solvent in a transparent cuvette of known dimensions, then the solute concentration can be calculated from the incident and transmitted light intensities. The extinction coefficient α_λ is independent of the concentration, but is a function of the light wavelength used (Fig. 9-4).

Laboratory in vitro oximeters use this principle to determine hemoglobin concentration by measuring the intensity of light transmitted through a hemoglobin dispersion produced from lysed red blood cells.[3] For each wavelength of light used, an independent Lambert-Beer equation (equation 9-7) can be written. If the number of equations is equal to the number of solutes (ie, hemoglobin species), the concentration of each one can be found. To determine the concentrations of four species of hemoglobin at least four wavelengths of light are needed. For the Lambert-Beer equation to be valid, both the solvent and cuvette must be transparent at the light wavelengths used, the light path length must be known, and no other absorbers can be present in the solution. It is difficult to fulfill all of these requirements in clinical devices. Consequently, although such devices are theoretically based on the Lambert-Beer law, they require empirical corrections to improve their accuracy.

The term "oximeter" was coined by Millikan, who developed a lightweight, noninvasive, in vivo hemoglobin saturation monitor in the 1940s.[4] There are two primary, technical problems with in vivo oximetry: (1) there are many light absorbers other than hemoglobin are present in tissue and (2) tissue contains not only arterial blood, but also venous and capil-

* This law also states that the exponent DC for multiple solutes in solution is the sum of the absorbances of the various solutes times their respective concentrations (eg, $D(C_1\alpha_1 + C_2\alpha_2 + C_3\alpha_3)$).

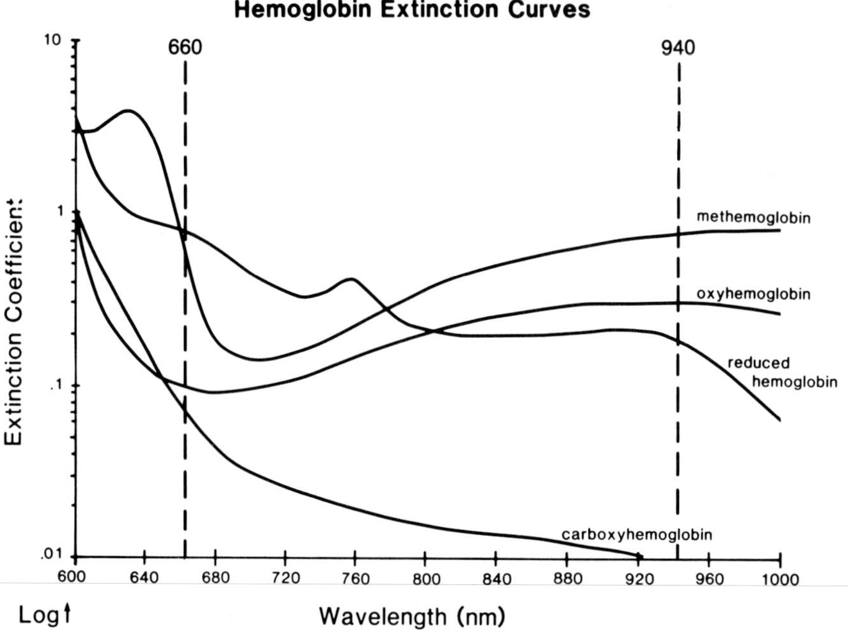

Figure 9-4. Hemoglobin light absorbance spectra—the extinction coefficient versus the wavelength of light for four different hemoglobin species: oxyhemoglobin (O_2Hb), reduced hemoglobin (RHb), methemoglobin (MetHb), and carboxyhemoglobin (COHb). The absorbance of COHb is similar to O_2Hb at red wavelengths, and MetHb has a high absorbance at both red and infrared wavelengths. (Reprinted, with permission, from: Barker SJ, Tremper KK. Pulse oximetry: applications and limitations. Int Anesthesiol Clin 1987;25:155.)

lary blood. Millikan approached these problems by first measuring the absorbance of the ear while it was compressed to eliminate the blood. After this bloodless baseline measurement, the ear was heated to cause hyperemia and thus "arterialize" the blood. The difference between this absorbance signal and the baseline value was related to the arterial blood. Millikan's device estimated saturation by transilluminating the ear using two wavelengths of light. The transmitted light was measured by a photodetector, effectively using the earlobe as a cuvette that contained hemoglobin. In the early 1950s a similar device was shown to detect intraoperative desaturations accurately, but because of technical difficulties with its use it was not adopted as a routine clinical monitor.[5]

In the mid-1970s, Takuo Aoyagi noted that the pulsatile component of the absorbance of light transmitted through tissue related to arterial hemoglobin saturation.[4] This eliminated the need to heat the tissue to obtain an arterial value. Aoyagi's oximeter used two wavelengths of light, one red and one infrared. This device relies on the detection of a pulsatile absorbance signal; hence it is referred to as a "pulse oximeter." Figure 9-5 schematically illustrates the absorbers in living tissue. At the top of the figure is the pulsatile, or AC component, which is attributed to the pulsating arterial blood. The base-

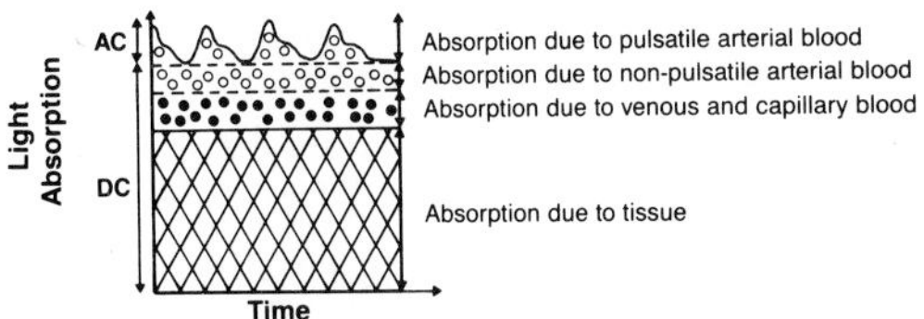

Figure 9-5. Diagram representing the light absorbances of living tissue. The AC or oscillatory signal is caused by the pulsatile component of the arterial blood, and the DC or constant component is caused by the nonpulsatile absorbers in the tissue. These include the nonpulsatile arterial blood, venous and capillary blood, and all of the solid tissues.

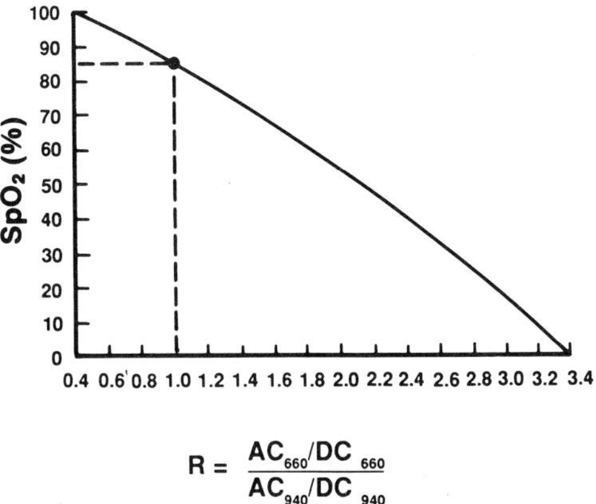

$$R = \frac{AC_{660}/DC_{660}}{AC_{940}/DC_{940}}$$

Figure 9-6. A pulse oximeter calibration algorithm. SpO_2 is plotted versus the ratio R of the pulse-added absorbance at the red wavelength (AC_{660}/DC_{660}) to the pulse-added absorbance at the infrared wavelength (AC_{940}/DC_{940}). This ratio varies from about 0.4 at 100% saturation to 3.4 at zero saturation. R has a value of 1.0 at a saturation of approximately 85%, which is important to the understanding of low signal-to-noise ratio performance.

line, or DC component, represents the absorbances of the tissue bed, including venous blood, capillary blood, and nonpulsatile arterial blood. All pulse oximeters assume that the only pulsatile absorbance between the light source and the photodetector is that of arterial blood. The pulse oximeter microprocessor first determines the AC component of the absorbance at each wavelength, which it divides by the corresponding DC component to obtain a "pulse-added" absorbance. This absorbance is independent of the incident light intensity. The device then calculates the ratio (R) of the pulse-added absorbances at the two wavelengths (usually 660 and 940 nanometers), which is empirically related to SaO_2:

(9-8) $$R = \frac{AC_{660}/DC_{660}}{AC_{940}/DC_{940}}$$

Figure 9-6 is an example of a pulse oximeter calibration curve, which relates R to the pulse oximeter saturation estimate, SpO_2. These curves are developed by measuring R in human volunteers and simultaneously sampling arterial blood for in vitro saturation (SaO_2) measurements. R varies from 0.4 to 3.4 over the saturation range of 0 to 100%. R values for saturations less than 70% result from extrapolation of experimental data. The pulse oximeter is therefore less accurate for values of SaO_2 less than 70%.

Sources of Error

Although the theory of the pulse oximeter is simple, the application of this theory to a clinically useful device engenders technical problems and limitations. One of these limitations is a consequence of Lambert-Beer law and the definitions of functional and fractional hemoglobin saturation (equations 9-5 and 9-6). Being a two-wavelength device, the pulse oximeter assumes that only two hemoglobin species, oxyhemoglobin (O_2Hb) and reduced hemoglobin (Hb), are present. If methemoglobin (MetHb) or carboxyhemoglobin (COHb) are also present, they will contribute to the pulse-added absorbance signal and be interpreted either as O_2Hb or Hb, singly or in combination. The effects of dyshemoglobins on the pulse oximeter can be understood by examining their absorbance spectra (Fig. 9-4). Note that COHb absorbs very little light at 940 nm (infrared), whereas at 660 nm (red) it absorbs as much as does O_2Hb. This is clinically illustrated by the fact that patients with carboxyhemoglobinemia appear red. The effects of COHb on pulse oximeter saturation values have been evaluated experimentally in animals.[6] SpO_2 is approximately given by:

$$([O_2Hb + 0.9 \times COHb]/\text{total Hb}) \times 100\%$$

In the case of methemoglobin, the extinction coefficient is high at both the red and infrared wavelengths (Fig. 9-4), yielding large pulse-added absorbances. Adding large absorbances to both the numerator and denominator of the ratio R in equation 9-8 tends to force this ratio toward unity. On the pulse oximeter calibration curve (Fig. 9-6) an R value of 1 corresponds to an SpO_2 of 85%. The effects of methemoglobinemia have also been evaluated experimentally and confirm the hypothesis that high MetHb levels drive SpO_2 toward 85%.[7] Although both COHb and MetHb cause significant SpO_2 errors, extinction coefficients for fetal hemoglobin (HbF) are similar to those of adult hemoglobin (1) HbA. Thus the presence of HbF does not cause an error in SpO_2.[8,9]

Any substance in the arterial blood that absorbs light at the red or infrared pulse oximeter wavelength may cause SpO_2 errors. This effect is clinically illustrated by intravenously injected dyes. Scheller et al evaluated the effects of bolus injections of methylene blue, indigo carmine, and indocyanine green on SpO_2 values in volunteers.[10] They found that methylene blue caused a fall in SpO_2 to approximately 65% for one to two minutes, whereas indigo carmine led to a smaller decrease. Indocyanine green had an intermediate effect.

Since the photodiode detectors in the pulse oximeter sensor respond to light of any wavelength, ambient light can contaminate the light-emitting diode (LED) signal.[11–13] Most pulse oximeters reduce this light interference by alternating turning on the red LED, the infrared LED, and then turning off both LEDs. The photodiode first detects a signal from the red LED plus ambient room light, followed by the infrared LED plus room light, and finally the room light alone. This sequence is repeated many times per second to subtract the room light signal in a quickly changing light background. Ambient light can cause erroneous SpO_2 values or prevent the pulse oximeter from obtaining any SpO_2 value despite this clever design. This problem is alleviated by covering the sensor with an opaque shield such as a dark towel.[14]

The most difficult problem in pulse oximeter design, however, is the management of low signal-to-noise ratios. One cause of this difficulty occurs when a small absorbance signal occurs due to a weak pulse and the device automatically increases its electronic amplification. Unfortunately, as the signal is amplified the background noise is also increased. In some situations, the noise may be amplified until it is interpreted as a pulse-added absorbance. Newer pulse oximeters have minimum signal strength limits below which they give an error message. Most devices also display an analog waveform as a visual indicator of signal quality, but the amplitude of this waveform may not relate to the pulse amplitude.

Whether a pulse oximeter displays an error message or an inaccurate SpO_2 value, a low pulsatile signal amplitude causes the device to fail to monitor saturation. Inadequate signal strength may be due to low cardiac output, cold extremities, or severe peripheral vascular disease. A recent study found the overall incidence of failure to generate an SpO_2 value in clinical use was approximately 1.2%.[15] In older patients with a higher incidence of peripheral vascular disease, this rate rose to 4.3%.[15] Another clinical study that compared various sensor sites showed that the finger sensor probe had the lowest overall failure rate (1.1%), followed by the earlobe sensor (2.5%–10%) and the nasal sensor (12%).[16]

The second major clinical source of low signal-to-noise ratio is patient motion artifact. This may be the most troublesome problem in the recovery room and intensive care unit. Most pulse oximeters make use of a variety of signal averaging techniques to minimize motion effects. Oximeters average multiple pulses to obtain the SpO_2 value, thereby diminishing the effect of spurious motion signals. Increasing the signal averaging time has a deleterious effect on the time response to acute saturation changes, however. Some manufacturers incorporate sophisticated algorithms to discriminate motion signals from arterial pulse signals by using the rate of SpO_2 change. For example, if the calculated SpO_2 value changes from 95% to 50% in 0.1 seconds, the new and presumably spurious saturation estimate is either dropped from the averaging or given a lower weighting factor. A novel approach taken by one manufacturer (Nellcor) involves a comparison of the pulsatile absorbance signal with the electrocardiogram (ECG) waveform. Absorbance pulsations that are not temporally related to the ECG R-wave are rejected; it is hoped that this removes the motion artifact. The effectiveness of this "C-Lock"* technique in eliminating motion artifact has not yet been established in clinical studies.

Another source of error with pulse oximeters involves the variability of the light wavelengths emitted by the LEDs. Although these diodes nominally give off monochromatic light at either 660 nm or 940 nm, each diode actually emits a spectrum of slightly different wavelengths. The peak or center wavelength can vary ± 10 nm from the specified value. The extinction coefficient curves in Figure 9-4 show that a small shift in the source wavelength significantly changes the measured absorbance. Since the oximeter software assumes an extinction coefficient at a specified wavelength, a change in that wavelength causes a systematic error in SpO_2 and results in a probe-to-probe variability in accuracy. Some manufacturers minimize this error by narrowing the acceptable wavelength tolerance on the LEDs used in their sensors. Others compensate for the error by designing the sensor to identify its specific LED wavelengths to the instrument by means of a pin-coded connector. The microprocessor then electronically corrects for shifted-center wavelengths.

Accuracy, Response, and Limitations

Most pulse oximeters have a specified accuracy of ±2% from 100% down to 70% saturation, ±3% from 70% saturation to 50%, and unspecified accuracy below 50% saturation.[17] This indicates that SpO_2 is within 2% above or below the actual SaO_2 value 68% of the time (±1 standard deviation). This corresponds to a 99% confidence interval (ie, 3 standard deviations) of ±6% from 100% to 70% saturation and ±9% from 70% to 50% saturation. These specifications are based on volunteer data collected under optimal conditions, but the accuracies found in clinical studies are comparable.[18–23]

The time response of pulse oximeters to sudden desaturation and resaturation, is an important characteristic of monitors during the rapid changes that can occur during thoracic anesthesia. Two recent experiments in adult volunteers evaluated the response of the devices under these conditions.[22,23] One study measured the time for 50% recovery of resaturation from an hypoxic state. The authors used a fast (3 second) time-averaging mode and found

* See Nellcor N-200 Pulse Oximetry Note #6: "C-Lock ECG synchronization—principles of operation," 1988.

a 50% recovery time ($T_{1/2}$) of 6 seconds for the ear sensor and 24 seconds for the finger sensor.[22] In the second study, the $T_{1/2}$ values for ear probes ranged from 9.6 to 19.8 seconds, whereas for the finger probes it ranged from 24 to 35.1 seconds.[23]

A number of clinical studies have shown that pulse oximetry is a far more sensitive detector of hypoxemia than visual observation by the most expert clinician. Arterial saturation monitoring provides limited information about the patient's oxygenation status, however, and clinicians must be particularly aware of these limitations in thoracic anesthesia. The hemoglobin saturation does not describe the oxygen content of the blood unless the total normal hemoglobin is known. The severely anemic patient with an arterial saturation of 100% can thus be suffering from tissue hypoxia.

In a study by Thys et al[23A], the pulse oximetry saturation readings ($SO_2[O]$) were compared to the calculated saturation ($SO_2[C]$) values during thoracic surgery. The pulse oximeter was found to have a sensitivity (ability to detect every incidence of hypoxemia with a $PaO_2 < 75$ mmHg) of 100%, a specificity of 91%, and a predictability of 70%. In addition, the accuracy of the pulse oximetry during episodes of low PaO_2 observed during thoracic surgery was investigated. Figure 9-7 shows the correlation between ($SO_2[O]$) and ($SO_2[C]$) for data with PaO_2 < 100 mmHg. The correlation was significantly better when the temperature was at least 36° C ($r = 9.56$ vs $r = 0.706$) or when the cardiac index was greater than 2.5L/min/M^2 ($r = 0.89$ vs $r = 0.41$). This suggests that, in a situation of poor perfusion (low cardiac index) or hypothermia (cold and vasoconstriction of the extremities), the accuracy of the pulse oximetry should be guarded with caution.

Furthermore, saturation monitoring does not give information about trends in PaO_2 until the latter falls below 70 to 80 mmHg. For all PaO_2 values above this range, SaO_2 lies within pulse oximeter error limits of 99%. A large "silent zone" of possible PaO_2 values from roughly 75 to 550 mmHg exists within which the pulse oximeter is effectively insensitive to changes. Since high FIO_2 values are often used during thoracic anesthesia, patients often have PaO_2 values within this zone. The detection of inadvertent endobronchial intubation is a good clinical example. A laboratory study has shown that in healthy animals who breathe gas mixtures of more than 30% oxygen, the pulse oximeter usually gives no indication of endobronchial intubation.[24] Metaphorically speaking, the pulse oximeter is a sentinel standing on the "cliff" of desaturation (Fig 9-1); it tells us when we are falling off the cliff, but does not tell us how close we are to the edge. Despite these limitations, pulse oximetry is a standard for all anesthetics. Its principles, interpretation, and sources of error should be well understood by every anesthesiologist.

Intra-arterial Blood Gas Sensors

The invention of the Clark polarographic oxygen electrode in 1956 and the Severinghaus-Stowe CO_2 electrode in 1958 led to the development of the in vitro blood gas analyzer, which became the "gold standard" for determining oxygenation and ventilation.[25] The chief shortcoming of this method, as previously mentioned, is that it does not provide continuous, real-time monitoring. Several attempts to miniaturize the electrodes for insertion through an intra-arterial cannula have been made.[26–28] Early miniature electrodes were hampered by their relatively large diameter, which required an 18-gauge or larger intra-arterial cannula. More recent PaO_2 versions fit through a 20-gauge cannula, but clinical results have been disappointing. Calibration drift problems and systematic underestimation of PaO_2 have so far

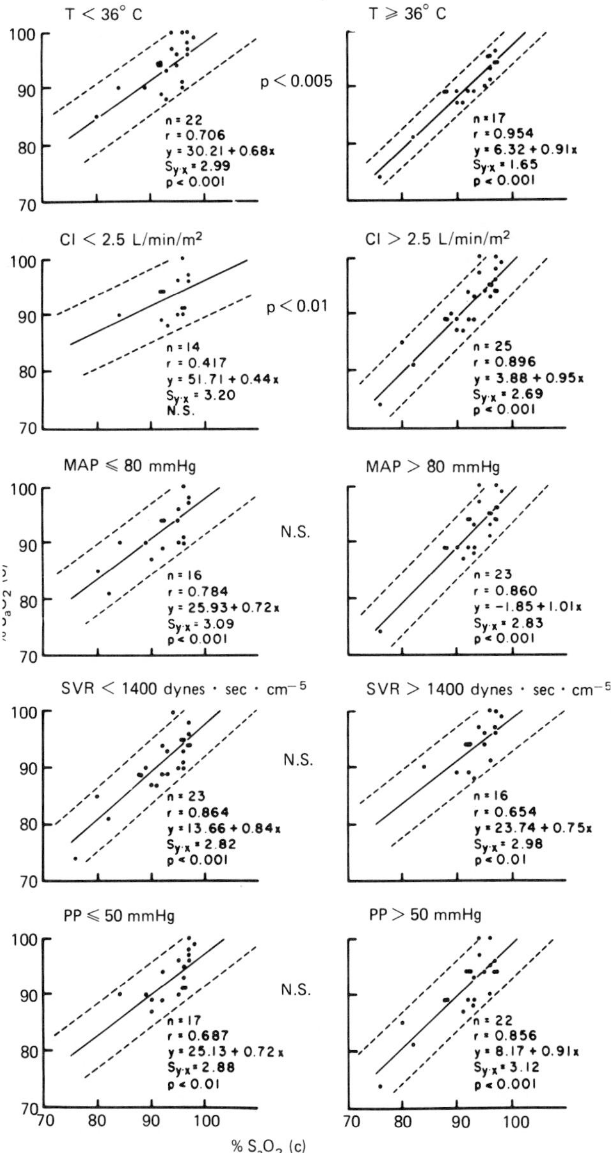

Figure 9-7. Correlation between SaO_2(C) and SaO_2(O) for data sets with $PaO_2 < 100$ mmHg. The measurements were divided according to temperature, cardiac index, mean arterial pressure, systemic vascular resistance and pulse pressure. The solid lines represent the regression slopes and the 95% confidence limit is represented by the interrupted lines. Note that with low temperature and low cardiac index the correlation between the pulse oximeter reading (%SaO_2[O]) and the calculated saturation (SaO_2[C]) is poor. Reprinted with permission from Thys DM, Cohen E, Girard D, Kirschner PA, et al. The pulse oximeter: a non-invasive monitor of oxygenation during thoracic surgery. Thorac Cardiovasc Surgeon 1986;34:382.

prevented these miniature polarographic electrodes from finding a permanent place in the operating room.

Another technology that shows greater promise as a practical intra-arterial blood gas monitor is based on photoluminescence quenching. In photoluminescence, light is shined on a luminescent dye and specific light frequencies are absorbed, exciting electrons to a higher energy state. These electrons then decay into a lower energy state by emitting photons of a frequency different from the original light. In some luminescent dyes this light emission is "quenched" by the presence of oxygen. When an excited electron falls into a lower energy state, the excess energy can be either emitted as a photon (luminescence) or absorbed by an oxygen molecule. The oxygen tension in the dye is related to the luminescent intensity by an empirical relationship known as the Stern-Volmer equation:[29]

$$\frac{1}{I} = \frac{1}{Io} + K(PO_2) \qquad (9\text{-}9)$$

where I is the intensity of the luminescent signal at the PO_2 being measured, Io is the intensity of the luminescent signal in the absence of oxygen, PO_2 is the oxygen tension, and K is the quenching constant.

The advantages of the photoluminescence quenching sensor, or "optode," as a PO_2 measuring device are its simplicity and size. The sensor, which can be easily miniaturized, consists of a thin fiberoptic strand with dye encapsulated at the tip. Figure 9-8 shows an optode that fits through a 22-gauge intravenous cannula.[30] Another advantage of this technology is that pH-and PCO_2-sensitive optodes are also available; a three-fiber optode can thus measure PO_2, PCO_2, and pH simultaneously.[31]

Although the first optical PO_2 sensor was developed by Lubbers in 1975,[32] the first intra-arterial measurements were not reported until 1984.[33] A period of refinement then began that led to further miniaturization and finally incorporation of the pH and PCO_2 optodes into the fiberoptic sensor. Mahutte et al[34] recently published a progress report on laboratory studies of intra-arterial optode sensors. Barker and Hyatt[35] reported the results of a clinical study of a three-component optode in the operating room. In this study, the fiberoptic sensor was inserted preoperatively through an 18-gauge radial artery cannula. Figure 9-9 shows a plot of optode PO_2 (PoO_2) and optode PCO_2 ($PoCO_2$) versus time during a thoracotomy requiring one-lung ventilation. The PoO_2 fell to less than 50 mmHg, even though the intermittent blood gas analyses (shown as "+" on Figure 9-9) failed to detect any PAO_2 values less than 150 mmHg. Greenblott et al[36] reported another case of continuous optode monitoring during thoracic anesthesia. In this case, the pulse oximeter failed to function during a period of hypoxemia that was accurately monitored by the optode.

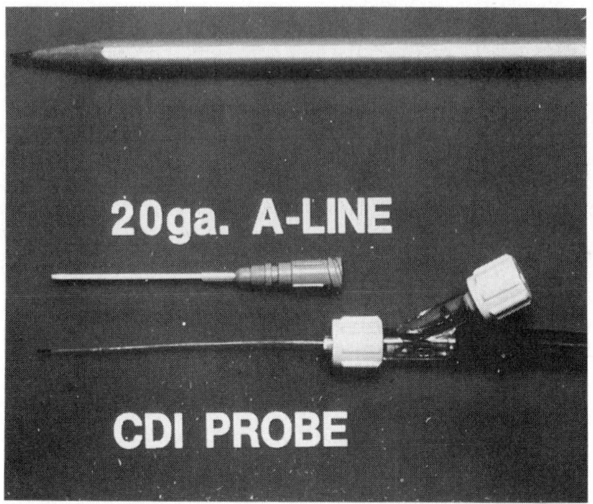

Figure 9-8. Photograph of a 0.5-mm diameter, three-component, fiberoptic optode blood-gas sensor and the 20-gauge arterial cannula through which it can be inserted. (Courtesy of 3M-Cardiovascular Devices, Inc.)

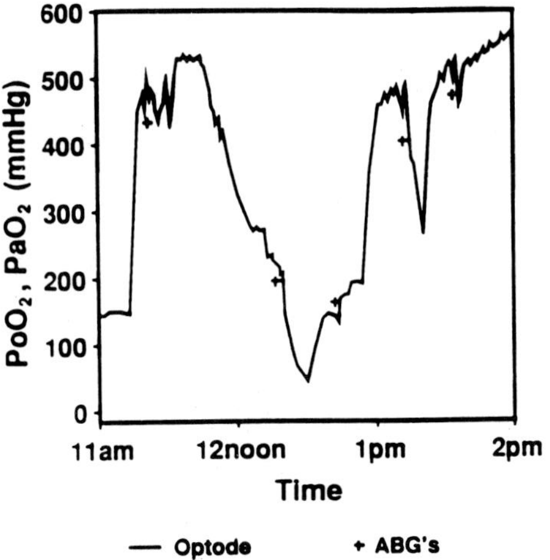

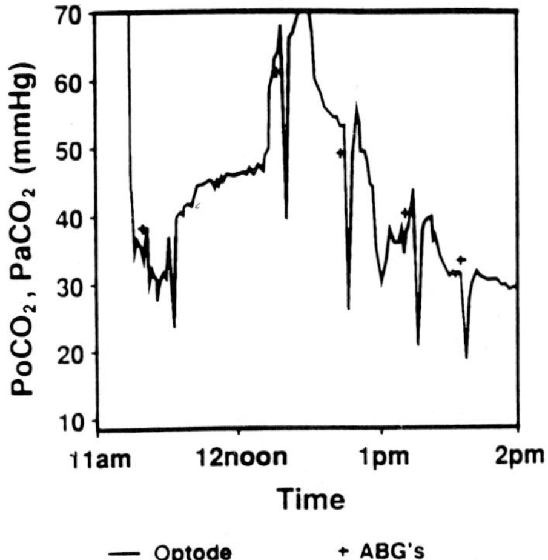

Figure 9-9. Continuous tracings of optode oxygen tension (Poo_2) and optode carbon dioxide tension ($Poco_2$) versus time during a thoracotomy requiring one-lung ventilation. In vitro blood gas analysis values are shown as (+) signs. Note the details of the hypoxemic, hypercarbic episode shown in the optode tracing but missed in the sequential blood gas analyses. (Reprinted from Barker SJ. Continuous measurement of intraarterial pHa, $PaCO_2$, and PaO_2 in the operating room. Anesth Analg 1991;73:43.)

Although optode sensors can perform accurately and reliably in an in vitro flow loop, their performance in vivo has been inconsistent. Possible formation of thrombus or platelet aggregates on the sensor or arterial wall effects yield both random and systematic errors as well as calibration drift. Once these problems are overcome the optode sensor will have a major impact in thoracic anesthesia.

Transcutaneous Oxygen Tension

Three methods of monitoring oxygenation at the level of the arterial have been discussed: intermittent blood gas analysis, pulse oximetry, and the intra-arterial optode. Ensuring adequate arterial oxygen content does not guarantee adequate tissue oxygenation; this depends upon perfusion as well as arterial oxygen content (equation 9-2). Transcutaneous oxygen tension ($PtcO_2$) is a noninvasive tissue oxygenation monitor that reflects changes in blood flow as well as arterial oxygenation.

In 1972 two European researchers reported that when a Clark electrode was heated and placed on the skin surface of a newborn infant, the PO_2 values obtained were very similar to arterial PO_2.[37,38] Over the next decade, transcutaneous oxygen monitoring became routine in the care of premature infants, who are at risk for both hypoxia and hyperoxia.[39,40] In the late 1970s investigators found that $PtcO_2$ values were significantly lower than PAO_2 values during conditions of hemodynamic instability.[41,42] Although this discovery lessened the usefulness of $PtcO_2$ as an arterial oxygen tension monitor, it provided the user with a valuable indicator of peripheral perfusion. Several animal studies of shock and resuscitation illustrated this blood flow dependence of $PtcO_2$.[43,44]

Transcutaneous PO_2 is the oxygen tension of heated skin. To obtain a measurable PO_2 at the skin surface with a fast response time, the skin temperature must be at least 43°C. This heating causes several changes in the various layers of the skin. The stratum corneum, composed of lipid in a protein matrix, is normally a very efficient barrier to gas transport. When heated above 41°C the structural characteristics of this layer change, allowing gases to diffuse through it readily.[45,46] In the epidermis, heating causes vasodilation of the dermal capillaries, which tends to "arterialize" the capillary blood. The perfusion of this hyperemic epidermal capillary bed also depends on adequate blood flow to the dermal vasculature. Consequently, a decrease in cardiac output leads to a decrease in skin blood flow and hence in oxygen delivery to the transcutaneous sensor.

Figure 9-10 illustrates the relation between PaO_2 and $PtcO_2$ during induced hypoxemia (hypoxemic hypoxia) followed by hemorrhagic shock (ischemic hypoxia) in an animal study.[43] During the shock state, $PtcO_2$ decreases with decreasing cardiac output even though P_AO_2 is relatively unchanged. This effect of cardiac output on the $PtcO_2$ – P_AO_2 relationship can be quantified in terms of the transcutaneous oxygen index:

(9-10) $PtcO_2 \text{ index} = PtcO_2/P_AO_2$

The $PtcO_2$ index has been used as an indicator of peripheral oxygen delivery, analogous to the alveolar-arterial PO_2 ratio for the assessment of pulmonary function.[47] Table 9-1 lists the mean values of the $PtcO_2$ index as a function of cardiac index found in adult patients in the intensive care unit. Under stable hemodynamic conditions the normal $PtcO_2$ index for adult patients was 0.8, but it fell to 0.49 when the cardiac index dropped to less than 2.2 L/min/m^2.

In the early work on newborn infants, $PtcO_2$ was found to be similar to PaO_2 (ie, the $PtcO_2$ index was approximately 1.0.[37,38] A review of the published $PtcO_2$ values on hemodynamically stable patients in various age groups reveals that the $PtcO_2$ index decreases progressively with age from premature infants to elderly patients (Table 9-1). Glenski et al found that the $PtcO_2$ index is relatively independent of probe location as long as the probe is on the central body rather than the extremities.[48] $PtcO_2$ is thus a noninvasive variable that

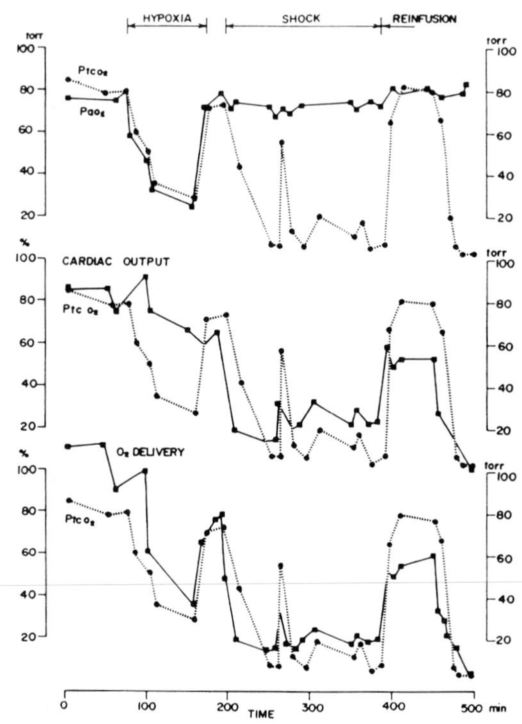

Figure 9-10. The effects of hypoxemia and hypovolemic shock on transcutaneous oxygen tension ($P_{tc}O_2$) in dogs. Top, $P_{tc}O_2$ and PaO_2 versus time during hypoxemia followed by hypovolemia and volume replacement. Middle, $P_{tc}O_2$ and cardiac output. Bottom, $P_{tc}O_2$ and oxygen delivery (arterial oxygen content times cardiac output). $P_{tc}O_2$ follows PaO_2 during hypoxemia but not during shock, it follows cardiac output during shock but not during hypoxemia, and it follows oxygen delivery during both hypoxemia and shock. (Reprinted, with permission, from: Tremper KK.[43])

Table 9-1. Changes in $PtcO_2$ Index ($PtcO_2/PaO_2$) with Age and Cardiac Output

Age*	
Premature infant	1.14
Newborn infant	1.0
Child	0.84
Adult	0.8
Older adult (65 years or older)	0.7
Cardiac Index (L/min/m^2)†	
>2.2	0.8
1.5 to 2.2	0.5
<1.5	0.1

* These values have a standard deviation of approximately 0.1.
† These data are from adult patients.

follows changes in PaO_2 under conditions of hemodynamic stability and decreases relative to PaO_2 as cardiac output falls below the normal range.

Several practical limitations must be considered when monitoring $PtcO_2$. Since the $PtcO_2$ electrode is heated above body temperature, electrode-sized skin burns are a possibility. Every time a $PtcO_2$ sensor is applied to the skin it produces a red, hyperemic area that usually disappears within 24 hours after electrode removal. No study has reported the incidence of burns from transcutaneous electrodes as a function of probe temperature and duration of application. The following guidelines are suggested based on the experience of frequent users of the technique. For premature infants an electrode temperature of 43.0 to 43.5°C should be used, and the electrode location should be changed every 2 to 4 hours. For older children and adults an electrode temperature of 44°C should be used, and the site should be changed every 4 to 6 hours. Personal intraoperative experience on adult patients, has shown that a 44°C electrode may be left in one location for as long as 8 hours with a very low incidence of blister formation (< 0.1%). Although electrode temperatures as high as 45°C have been used in the past, these are not needed for adequate function, and the incidence of burns is significantly increased.

As with any Clark electrode, the transcutaneous PO_2 sensor must be properly calibrated and maintained. The zero point on the $PtcO_2$ electrode (PO_2 = 0 mmHg) is usually stable and requires only monthly calibration. The high PO_2 calibration uses room air, and this should be rechecked prior to each skin application. Current $PtcO_2$ electrodes have miniaturized electrolyte reservoirs to bathe the electrodes and 12–25-micron-thick membranes to cover them. These small electrolyte reservoirs carry about one drop (0.05 mL) of electrolyte. Since the electrode is heated to 44°C, the electrolyte will evaporate more quickly than in the 37°C Clark electrode found in a blood gas analyzer. The electrolyte and membrane should therefore be checked daily; replacement is usually required at least once a week. Halothane is reduced at the cathode of the Clark electrode, thus causing an upward drift in the $PtcO_2$ value. Although a large drift results from direct exposure of the electrode to 3% halothane, the drift measured in patients under halothane anesthesia is clinically insignificant.[49]

Most of the clinical $PtcO_2$ data have been collected with a sensor on the chest or abdomen. Site-to-site variation in $PtcO_2$ values is significant; approximately 10% variation occurs even at adjacent locations. Lower values are found on the extremities in the absence of peripheral vascular disease. After placement on the skin surface, a $PtcO_2$ sensor requires 10 to 20 minutes to equilibrate before yielding a steady value. This may present a problem for intraoperative monitoring in short cases or when the sensor site must be changed during the procedure. The sensor should be placed in a location visible to the user. If the sensor becomes dislodged from the skin surface, it indicates the PO_2 of room air (approximately 159 mmHg at sea level). Furthermore, if the sensor is beneath the surgical drapes it may be under external pressure and produce falsely low $PtcO_2$ values.

In summary, transcutaneous PO_2 measures tissue oxygenation continuously and noninvasively. $PtcO_2$ values follow the trend of PaO_2 under conditions of adequate cardiac output, and decrease relative to PaO_2 during low cardiac output states. This can be an advantage to the experienced user, as it can aid in the diagnosis and treatment of low-flow shock conditions.

Pulmonary Artery Oximetry

Oxygen monitors that function at the level of the arterial blood and the peripheral tissues have been discussed. Now the monitoring of the venous blood oxygen is described. Mixed venous oxygen tension (PvO_2) and saturation (SvO_2) reflect the oxygen remaining in the blood after the oxygen transport process is completed. SvO_2 can be related to other cardiopulmonary variables by rearranging equation 9-2:

$$\frac{SvO_2}{100} = \frac{SaO_2}{100} - VO_2/[13.8(Hb)(Qt)] \qquad (9\text{-}11)$$

The mixed venous saturation varies with arterial saturation, oxygen consumption, hemoglobin, and cardiac output. A change in any of these variables affect SvO_2, and the astute clinician must determine which variables changing.

In 1973, researchers reported that a fiberoptic intravascular system accurately monitored mixed venous hemoglobin saturation in humans.[50] This device incorporated optical fibers into a pulmonary artery catheter to estimate the hemoglobin saturation by measuring reflected light. Light at red and infrared wavelengths was transmitted down one set of fibers while the reflected light from intact circulating red cells was transmitted back via other fibers to an external photodetector.[50]

The currently available systems use either two or three (670, 700, and 800 nm) wavelengths to calculate saturation. As shown previously, four wavelengths are required to calculate hemoglobin saturation from the Lambert-Beer law in the presence of MetHb and COHb. Although both the Abbott Critical Care (Oximetrix) and American Edwards systems can accurately estimate SvO_2 in the absence of dyshemoglobins, methemoglobinemia produces large errors in saturation measurement.[7]

Continuous SvO_2 monitoring can detect any acute change in the relationship between oxygen supply and demand (equation 9-11). Such monitoring is potentially helpful in cardiac surgery, major vascular surgery, massive trauma, or in the care of any other patients in whom this supply-demand relationship is in jeopardy. For example, Figure 9-11A is a plot of SvO_2 versus time for a patient whose SvO_2 varies rapidly to reflect changes in SaO_2 during a series of accidental extubations. Figure 9-11B is a similar plot for a patient whose SvO_2 rises in response to an increase in cardiac output resulting from a sodium nitroprusside infusion. These figures illustrate the dependence of SvO_2 on two of the four variables on the right side of equation 9-11:SaO_2 and Qt.

All four of the variables in equation 9-11 can change significantly during anesthesia for thoracic surgery. Some pathologic conditions cause SvO_2 to decrease (shock, hypoxemia, anemia), whereas others make it increase (sepsis, hypothermia, left-to-right arteriovenous shunt). SvO_2 is thus a nonspecific variable that can alert the clinician to many problems affecting the oxygen transport system. Once the decision to insert a pulmonary artery catheter has been made, the use of SvO_2 does not add any further risk and may yield significant benefits.

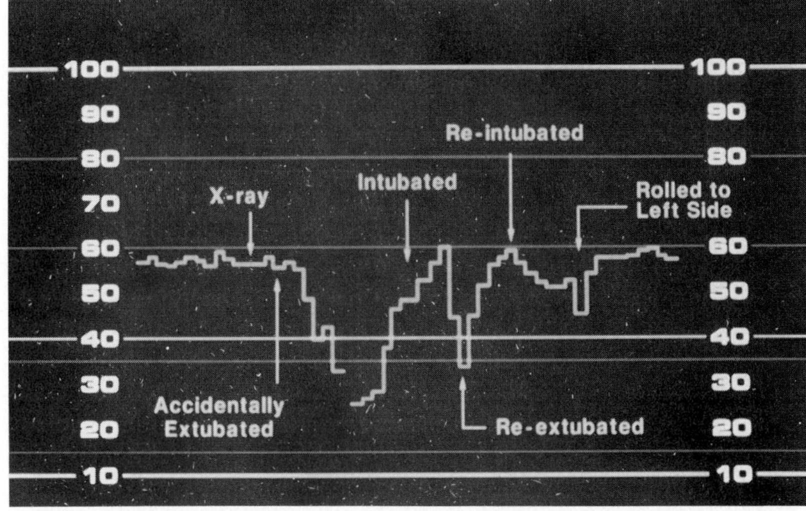

A

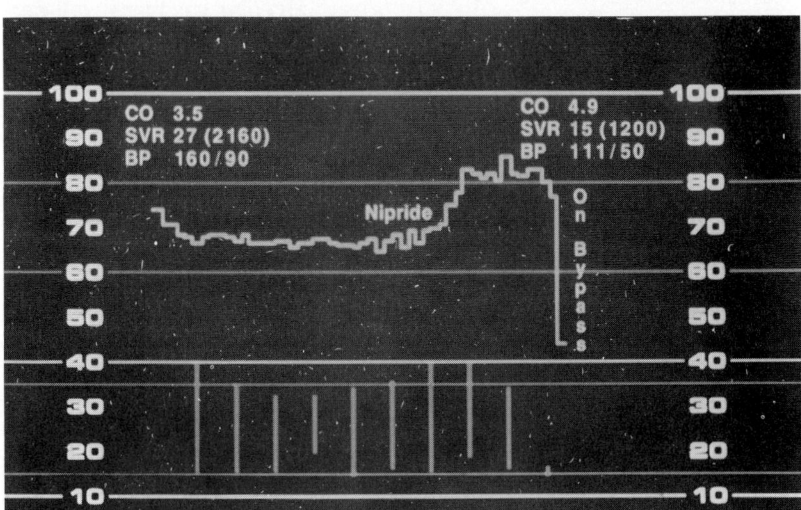

B

Figure 9-11. Plots of Svo_2 versus time showing two examples of the dependence of Svo_2 upon the four oxygenation variables: Sao_2, CO, Hb, and Vo_2. A, Svo_2 during accidental extubation and reintubation, showing the dependence upon SaO_2. B, Svo_2 during the beginning of a sodium nitroprusside infusion, showing the dependence upon cardiac output. (Courtesy of Abbott Critical Care, Inc.)

Monitoring of Ventilation

Carbon Dioxide Transport Physiology and the Concept of Dead Space

Two types of gas exchange must take place between the blood and the lungs to maintain homeostasis: oxygen must be absorbed and carbon dioxide must be eliminated. Oxygen transport and its associated monitoring has been discussed; now carbon dioxide transport and elimination, or ventilation, are described. Although auscultation and observation may detect ventilation, its adequacy must be confirmed by normal arterial blood carbon dioxide tension ($PaCO_2$ (ie, 35–45 mmHg). The normal arterial blood carbon dioxide content ($CaCO_2$) is 48 mL/100 mL blood. Carbon dioxide is carried in the blood in three forms: dissolved in plasma, bound to protein (hemoglobin), and transported as bicarbonate ion. The gas binds to hemoglobin by attaching to the terminal amino group on the globulin molecule, forming carbamino-hemoglobin. Since carbamino-hemoglobin contributes a small portion of the total carbon dioxide content of blood (ie, approximately 1.5 mL/100 mL blood), hemoglobin carbon dioxide saturation does not have the same importance as hemoglobin oxygen saturation. About 70% of the carbon dioxide is carried in the form of bicarbonate ion.

The usual venous carbon dioxide content ($CvCO_2$) is 52 mL/100 mL blood, which corresponds to a $PvCO_2$ of 44 mmHg. Systemic arterial blood thus captures approximately 4 mL of carbon dioxide per 100 mL of blood perfusing the tissue. The ratio of 4 mL/100 mL blood carbon dioxide acquired from the tissue to 5 mL/100 mL blood of oxygen released results in the usual respiratory quotient of 0.8. To remain at steady state with respect to carbon dioxide, the lungs must discharge 4 mL of carbon dioxide to the atmosphere for every 100 mL of blood flow. Because of the high solubility of carbon dioxide in water (approximately 20 times that of oxygen) and the body's ability to store the gas in the form of bicarbonate ion, the total amount of carbon dioxide in the body is approximately 100 times the amount of total oxygen.[51]

The rate at which carbon dioxide is removed from the lungs depends on the ventilation of well-perfused alveoli. To quantitate this relationship, the concept of "wasted ventilation," or dead space, must first be understood. Physiologic dead space is defined as the portion of each tidal volume that does not participate in carbon dioxide exchange.

$$V_T = V_{DS} + V_{ALV} \quad (9\text{-}12)$$

where V_T = tidal volume, V_{DS} = physiologic dead space volume, and V_{ALV} = "ideal" alveolar volume

V_{ALV} is "ideal" alveolar gas from well-perfused alveoli. The carbon dioxide tension in this alveolar gas ($P_{ALV}CO_2$) is nearly equal to $PaCO_2$. Bohr derived an equation for the ratio of V_{DS} to V_T based upon the simple assumption that the total carbon dioxide leaving the mouth equals the carbon dioxide leaving the ideal alveolar volume. Since the carbon dioxide concentration in the gas phase is proportional to the $PaCO_2$, the following expression can be written:

$$V_T \times P_{ME}CO_2 = V_{ALV} \times P_{ALV}CO_2 \quad (9\text{-}13)$$

$P_{ME}CO_2$ is the mixed expired carbon dioxide tension in a tidal volume. If a patient expires one V_T into a well-mixed bag, $P_{ME}CO_2$ is the carbon dioxide tension in that bag. Solving equation 9-12 for V_{ALV} and substituting into equation 9-13, the following equation is obtained:

$$V_T \times P_{ME}CO_2 = (V_T - V_{DS}) \times P_{ALV}CO_2 \quad (9\text{-}14)$$

Assuming that $P_{ALV}CO_2 = PaCO_2$, equation 9-14 can be solved for V_{DS}/V_T:

(9-15) $$\frac{V_{DS}}{V_T} = \frac{PaCO_2 - P_{ME}CO_2}{PaCO_2}$$

Using equation 9-15, the Bohr Equation, the physiologic dead space (V_{DS}) can be determined by measuring $P_{ME}CO_2$ and analyzing an arterial blood sample for $PaCO_2$. The assumption that there is no carbon dioxide in the inspired gas has been made.

Capnography

End-tidal Carbon Dioxide and its Relationship to P_ACO_2In the 1920s Aitken and Clarke-Kennedy made the first measurements of carbon dioxide concentration in expired gas during the course of the respiratory cycle.[52] This yielded the first expired carbon dioxide-versus-time waveform or "capnogram." The expired carbon dioxide tension at the end of expiration is called the end-tidal or end-expiratory carbon dioxide $P_{ET}CO_2$. To understand the capnogram and the relationship between $P_{ET}CO_2$ and $PaCO_2$, physiologic dead space (V_{DS}) must first be divided into its three components: apparatus dead space (V_{APPDS}) anatomical dead space (V_{ANDS}), and alveolar dead space (V_{ALVDS}).[51]

(9-16) $$V_{DS} = V_{APPDS} + V_{ANDS} + V_{ALVDS}$$

Apparatus dead space is the part of V_T contained within the breathing apparatus. For a circle system, APPDS is any part of the apparatus on the patient side of the "Y-connector." Anatomical dead space is the volume within the trachea and the conducting airways. Alveolar dead space consists of those alveoli that are ventilated but not perfused.

Figure 9-12 illustrates the relationship of each of these dead spaces to the capnogram. The first gas expired is that left within the breathing apparatus at the end of inspiration (V_{APPDS}). This gas has the same carbon dioxide tension as the inspired gas, which is usually zero. The anatomical dead space gas (V_{ANDS}) is expired next, and this should also contain little or no carbon dioxide. Finally the gas from the alveoli is expired, which includes both V_{ALVDS} and V_{ALV}. These two alveolar gases are mixed, and the resulting PCO_2 depends on the relative volume of each gas and the $PaCO_2$. As the alveolar gas reaches the airway, the expired carbon dioxide rises rapidly to this mixed value ($P_{ET}CO_2$), forming the alveolar plateau (Fig 9-12). When inspiration begins, the PCO_2 in the airway rapidly drops to zero, assuming the inspired PCO_2 is zero. If no alveolar dead space existed, then the $P_{ET}CO_2$ value would equal $PaCO_2$. If half of the alveolar volume were alveolar dead space and half well-perfused alveoli, then the $P_{ET}CO_2$ value would equal one-half the $PaCO_2$. The difference between $PaCO_2$ and $P_{ET}CO_2$ is thus proportional to V_{ALVDS}.

Figure 9-13 shows a normal capnogram, that is, the expired carbon dioxide tension as a function of time. During early expiration (phase I), the PCO_2 value is near zero, as V_{APP} and V_{AN} are expired. As alveolar gas begins to reach the carbon dioxide detector, the PCO_2 value rises to the alveolar plateau. This rapidly increasing portion (phase II) results from a mixture of V_{ALVDS}, V_{ALV}, and V_{AN}. The alveolar plateau (phase III) is achieved when only alveolar gas is being expired.

Alveolar dead space represents a ventilation-perfusion ratio (V/Q) of infinity (ie, no perfusion). In this model it is assumed that all alveoli are either well-perfused, with PCO_2 equal to $PaCO_2$, or they are unperfused, with no carbon dioxide exchange. In reality the lung is composed of many units having various V/Q ratios. The apparatus and anatomical dead spaces are called "series" dead spaces, because they are expired sequentially before the alveolar gas. The alveolar dead space is referred to as "parallel" dead space, because it is expired

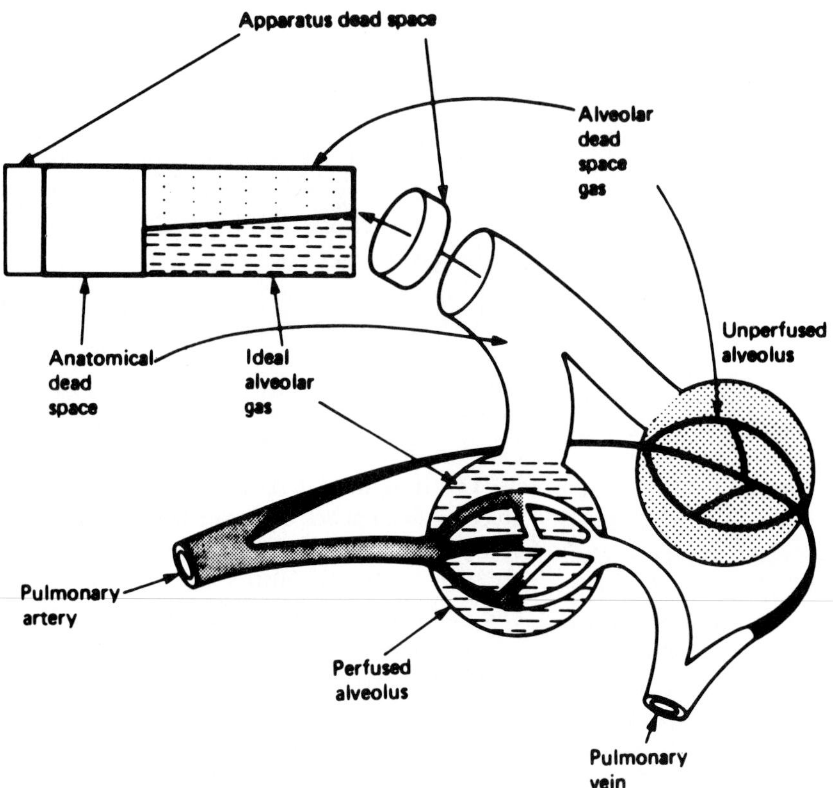

Figure 9-12. A schematic presentation of the origins of apparatus, anatomical, and alveolar dead spaces and their influence on the capnogram. Two representative lung units are shown: one is well-perfused and the other has no blood flow. The "series" dead space (apparatus and anatomical) is expired first and contains little CO_2. The "parallel" dead space (alveolar) is expired together with the ideal alveolar gas, and the proportions of each determine the height of the alveolar plateau, $P_{et}CO_2$. (Reprinted, with permission, from Nunn JF.[51])

at the same time as the ideal alveolar gas (Fig 9-11).

Interpretation of the Capnogram

A normal capnogram implies ongoing metabolism to produce carbon dioxide, circulation to transport this gas from the tissues to the lungs, and ventilation to remove it. Continuous capnography can detect sudden changes in all these vital functions noninvasively. Any deviations from the normal size or shape of the capnogram should be immediately investigated. For example, a depressed or absent capnogram may be a sign of ventilator disconnection, cardiac arrest, pulmonary embolism, or a dislodged, misplaced or obstructed endotracheal tube. The presence of a stable capnogram is the quickest and most certain way of verifying endotracheal intubation.

A decrease in $P_{ET}CO_2$ can be caused by any increase in V_{ALVDS}. During anesthesia such rises are often a result of pulmonary hypotension,

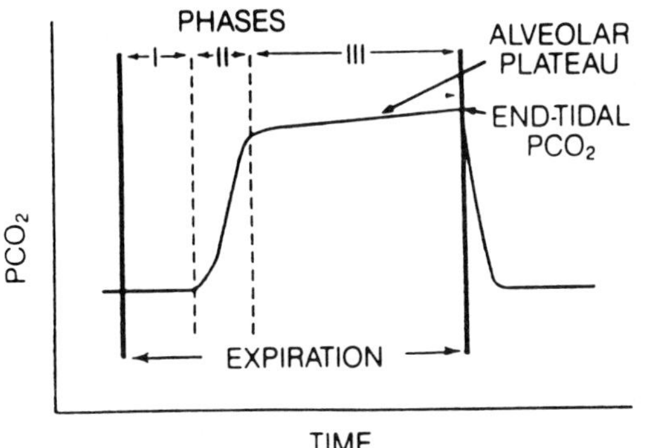

Figure 9-13. The normal capnogram, showing the three phases: I, II, and III. Phase I gas is pure "series" dead space that contains no CO_2. Phase II gas contains a mixture of anatomical dead space, alveolar dead space, and ideal alveolar gas and produces the rapidly rising portion of the capnogram. Phase III gas is a mixture of ideal alveolar and alveolar dead space gas and produces the alveolar plateau.

which increases the extent of West's zone I, the lung region of little or no perfusion. Common intraoperative causes of a larger zone I include pulmonary artery dilators (eg, volatile agents, atropine, nitroprusside), hypovolemic shock, upright or decubitus position, and mechanical obstruction of pulmonary arteries during surgical manipulation. This last possibility should always be considered during thoracic surgery. Increases in $P_{ET}CO_2$ reflect either rising metabolic rate (eg, malignant hyperthermia, thyroid storm, fever), the addition of carbon dioxide to the circulation (eg, sodium bicarbonate therapy, carbon dioxide insufflation for laparoscopy, release of tourniquet), or carbon dioxide rebreathing. Rebreathing is also detected as a nonzero baseline reading during the inspiratory phase of the capnogram.

The shape of the capnogram also contains important information about patients well-being. Infrared absorption, mass spectrometry, Raman spectrometry, and photoacoustic methods are among the capnographic technologies in current use. Detailed descriptions of the various techniques are beyond the scope of this book; the reader should referred to other texts.[53,54] Although these are not discussed here, the system configurations in current use must be understood to interpret capnogram shapes.

All clinical capnographs interface with the patient airway in one of two ways. In the sidestream configuration, an adaptor with a small sideport is connected in the airway at the endotracheal tube (Fig. 9-14). A capillary tube aspirates gas from the adapter into the instrument, where carbon dioxide analysis for occurs. The response time of the system is depends on the

Figure 9-14. A schematic illustration of the two clinically used capnograph configurations: sidestream and mainstream. Sidestream capnographs aspirate sample gas into the instrument through a length of thin tubing, whereas mainstream capnographs locate the infrared CO_2 detector in the airway at the end of the endotracheal tube.

Capnometers:

Side Stream

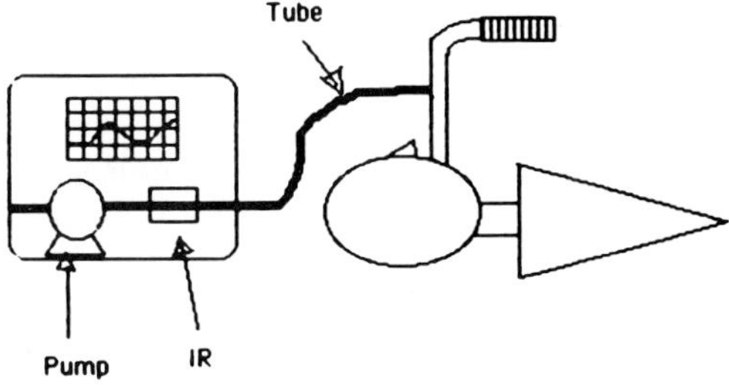

Main Stream

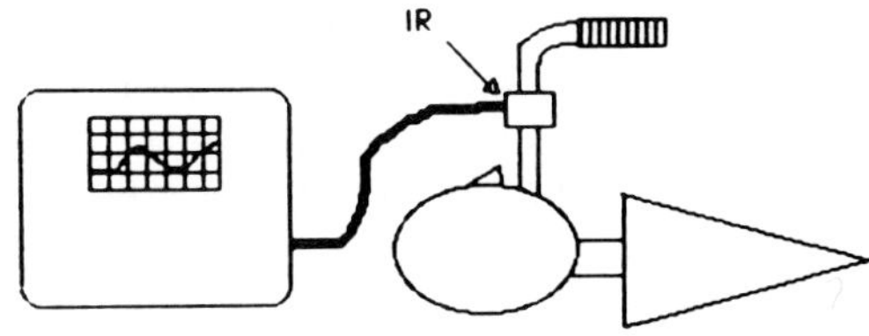

length and diameter of the tubing, the sampling flow rate (usually 150 cc/min), and the response of the carbon dioxide detector itself. Most sidestream capnographs use approximately 3 meters of tubing that is about 1 mm in diameter. This produces a sampling delay time of about 1 second. Reducing the diameter decreases the delay, but condensed water droplets tend to clog smaller tubing. A higher sampling flow rate also reduces delay but will cause errors by aspirating fresh gas, as well as expired gas, from the circuit. Multiport or time-shared mass spectrometers use much longer sampling tubes; hence the delay time is longer despite a relatively high flow rate.

In the mainstream capnograph, an infrared absorbance carbon dioxide detector is placed directly in the breathing circuit (Fig. 9-14). The patient actually breathes directly through the carbon dioxide analyzer, thus eliminating the aspiration system and its associated time delay. This does improve the time response of this system, it also has disadvantages. The entire optical system must be sufficiently small and light to attach to an endotracheal tube. This requirement generally limits the infrared absorption measurements to one wavelength, which makes the device more vulnerable to interference by nitrous oxide. Because the optical windows in the airway adapter are subject to water vapor condensation, they must be heated to minimize the problem. In addition, the delicate optical module is vulnerable to inadvertent damage in its exposed location.

In 1975, Smalhout and Kalenda published the first atlas of capnography, which described the clinical conditions that result in various capnographic patterns.[55] The normal capnogram has previously been described; it is illustrated in Figure 9-13. The phase I portion, produced by the expiration of the apparatus and anatomical dead space, should be a straight line near PCO_2 = 0 (the inspired carbon dioxide concentration). As shown in Figure 9-15, the phase II, or quickly rising portion of the capnogram, exhibits decreased slope in the presence of either chronic or acute reductions in expiratory flow (eg, emphysema, bronchospasm, obstructed endotracheal tube). This slope reduction reflects a mixture of parallel and series dead space gas with ideal alveolar gas. If the expiratory resistance is very high, the capnogram may never reach an alveolar plateau (phase III), and the $P_{ET}CO_2$ value may be substantially lower than the alveolar PCO_2. Without studying the exact shape of the capnogram, the clinician has no way of becoming aware of this situation.

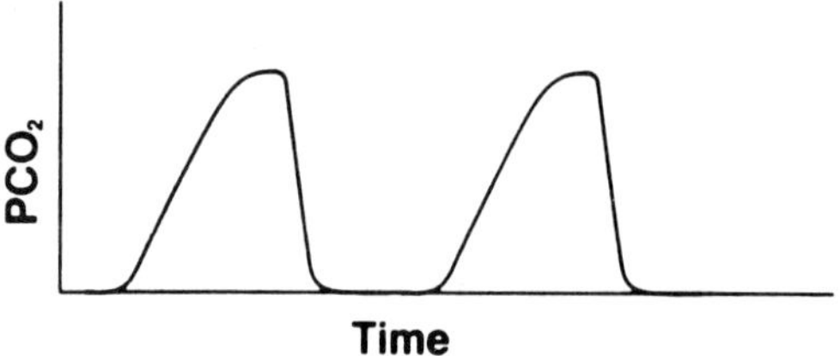

Figure 9-15. Expiratory obstruction capnogram seen in patients with asthma, bronchospasm, and chronic obstructive pulmonary disease. The decreased slope of the phase II portion is caused by slowed expiration and abnormal emptying of the various perfused and unperfused lung segments. In some cases, the phase III alveolar plateau may be entirely absent, and a greater than normal end-tidal to arterial CO_2 gradient occurs.

Figure 9-16 illustrates the "camel capnogram," which can result from either a physiologic or technical problem. If a patient is placed in the lateral decubitus position during general anesthesia, the nondependent lung has a higher V/Q ratio and thus contains more alveolar dead space (West's zone I). The nondependent lung tends to empty first, and it thus produces a lower phase III plateau on the capnogram. A second, higher plateau follows as the dependent lung empties because this lung has a lower V/Q ratio and less alveolar dead space. The camel capnogram is a common finding in the decubitus position. A similar capnogram

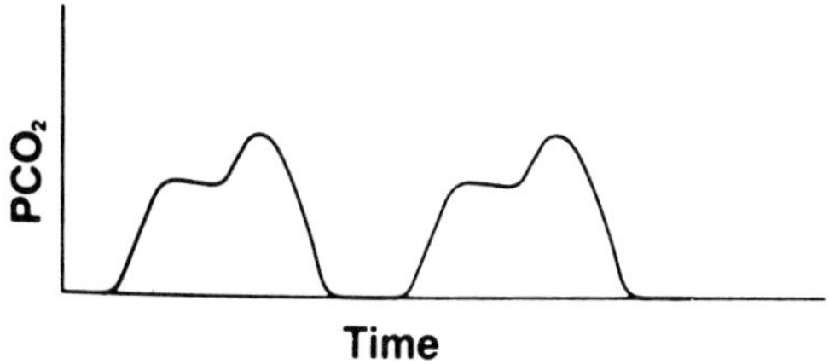

Figure 9-16. "Camel" capnogram caused by the lateral decubitus position or a tubing leak in a sidestream capnograph. In the decubitus position, the nondependent lung, which contains more alveolar dead space, tends to empty first. The delayed emptying of the dependent lung then produces the second alveolar plateau, which is higher than the first because this lung contains less alveolar dead space.

pattern can occur when the aspiration tubing of a side-stream analyzer leaks. The initial phase III plateau value is reduced because of the aspiration of room air through the leak into the sampling tube and the resulting dilution of the alveolar gas sample. The rise in carbon dioxide at the end of expiration (Fig. 9-16) is caused by the beginning of a positive-pressure ventilator breath, which increases the pressure in the aspiration tubing above the ambient level. This reverses the flow through the leak, allowing the gas contained in the tubing between the patient and the leak to reach the capnometer without being diluted.[56] This segment of undiluted alveolar gas causes the second phase III plateau in Figure 9-16.

As a patient regains neuromuscular function following paralysis under general anesthesia, there is a lack of coordination between the diaphragm and intercostal muscles. The capnogram illustrated in Figure 9-17 is called the "curare" capnogram. In paralyzed patients it is an early sign that the diaphragm is regaining neuromuscular function. A phase III Surgical manipulation of the chest or abdominal contents, which causes small amounts of gas to move in and out of the lungs, can also produce with multiple irregular peaks and valleys. A similar pattern may occur when a patient fights the ventilator.

Phase IV of the capnogram normally begins with an abrupt drop to the baseline PCO_2 value of zero at the start of inspiration. During anesthesia an undulating, gradual PCO_2 decrease, called cardiogenic oscillations is often seen (Fig. 9-18). These oscillations, which are synchronous with the heartbeat, are produced when the right heart pumps a stroke volume of blood into the lungs, causing a small amount of alveolar gas to be expelled.[57] Phase IV of the capnogram may also exhibit a decreased negative slope with a side stream capnometer due to the aspiration of fresh gas from the breathing circuit at the end of expiration. This pattern is often seen in pediatric patients when the expired minute volume is comparable to the aspiration flow rate of the capnometer. The problem is aggravated when the sampling site is located closer to the Y-piece of the circle system.

If phase I of the capnogram (inspiration) fails to return to a baseline PCO_2 value of zero, either carbon dioxide is present in the inspired gas or the capnometer has not been zeroed properly. When using a partial rebreathing or semiopen system (eg, Bain circuit), a nonzero

Figure 9-17. The "curare cleft" capnogram resulting from an incomplete neuromuscular blockade. The diaphragm, which recovers from muscle relaxants earliest, contracts slightly near end-expiration to produce a spontaneous small inspiration, causing the "cleft." This is followed by the positive-pressure inspiration from the mechanical ventilator, which ends the phase III plateau.

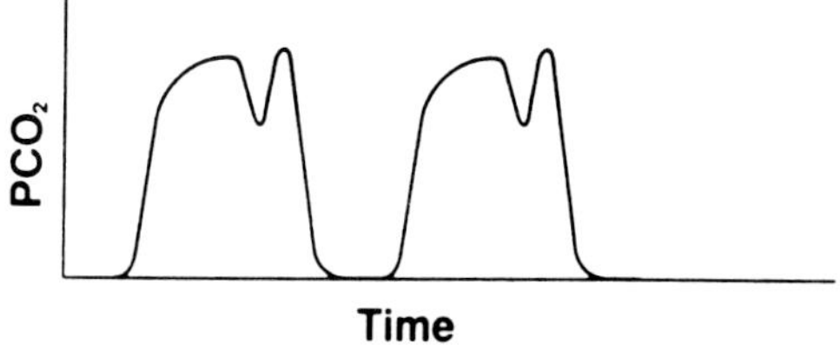

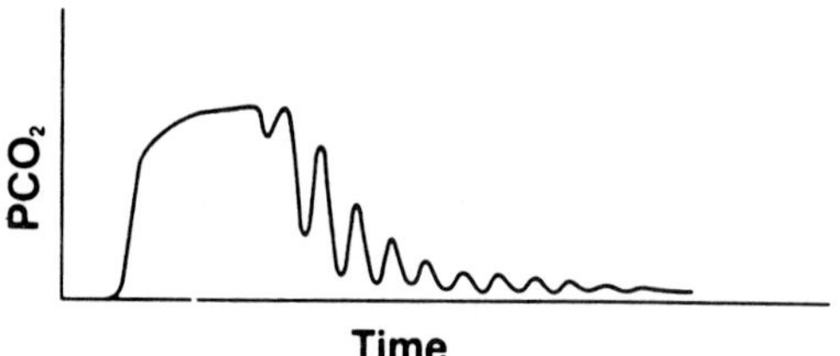

Figure 9-18. A cardiogenic oscillations capnogram exhibiting phase III oscillations that are synchronous with the electrocardiogram. These are often seen at slow respiratory rates and during hypovolemia. Each right ventricular systole pumps a bolus of blood that contains carbon dioxide into the lungs. In addition, heart movement can cause some gas movement in and out of the lungs at the end of expiration.

baseline value indicates that the fresh gas flow rate is inadequate. In a circle system, such a baseline reading implies that either the absorber is not removing all the carbon dioxide from the system or one of the valves is incompetent. A malfunctioning absorber may result from exhausted soda lime or "channeling" of gas through the absorber. An artifactual, non zero baseline value may be produced by water vapor condensation on the cuvette windows of a mainstream capnometer. Since the windows are heated to 44°C to "defrost" them, vapor condensation suggests either excessive gas humidification or contamination of the windows by secretions.

As stated previously, a high $P_{ET}CO_2$ value implies hypoventilation, whereas a low $P_{ET}CO_2$ suggests either hyperventilation or increased alveolar dead space. Complete absence of a capnogram is the result of no ventilation, no circulation, or a disconnect of the capnometer. A sudden cardiac arrest actually does not produce a zero capnogram until all of the carbon dioxide has been removed from the lungs. Experimental and clinical studies have shown that cardiac arrest produces an abrupt decrease in $P_{ET}CO_2$, and that effective cardiopulmonary resuscitation (CPR) restores $P_{ET}CO_2$ to a higher value than does ineffective CPR.[58,59] Unfortunately, an esophageal intubation may temporarily result in a similar depressed capnographic pattern.[60] However, the depressed capnogram seen in some esophageal intubations decreases in height with each breath until the carbon dioxide is removed from the stomach.

Capnography can provide the anesthesiologist with a wealth of information regarding the patient's ventilation, circulation, metabolism, and airway. Although capnography is now a minimum standard of care for all general anesthetics, it has particular importance during thoracic anesthesia because of the frequent changes in alveolar dead space, minute ventilation, and airway resistance. Although the $P_{ET}CO_2$ values provide much of this information, clinicians must learn to "read" the capnogram and monitor it continuously to realize its full potential.

Transcutaneous Carbon Dioxide Monitoring

Because of the influence of alveolar dead space, $P_{ET}CO_2$ does not provide a direct measure of $PaCO_2$, the defining variable for ventilation. Furthermore, the measurement of end-tidal carbon dioxide in patients who are not intubated is difficult and often impractical. Transcutaneous carbon dioxide tension ($PtcCO_2$) is a noninvasive monitor that provides helpful additional data and can be used on patients whether or not they are intubated.

Transcutaneous carbon dioxide monitoring was introduced shortly after $PtcO_2$ in the early 1970s. The technique uses a Severinghaus-Stowe electrode that is heated and placed on the skin surface, yielding continuous PCO_2 values, which follow changes in $PaCO_2$. The PCO_2 of heated skin is expected to be higher than the $PaCO_2$ for two reasons: one, tissue PCO_2 values are higher than those for venous PCO_2 and two, heated tissue should produce more carbon dioxide than normal. Indeed, the original $PtcCO_2$

values on awake volunteers were approximately 60 mmHg. Several methods were proposed to adjust $PtcCO_2$ values to closely approximate $PaCO_2$ values over the next decade.[61,62] The most commonly used correction is that proposed by Severinghaus, which divides the $PtcCO_2$ value by 1.33 and then subtracts 3.0 mmHg.[61] The Severinghaus adjustment is physiologically justified by the fact that heating the blood increases the PCO_2 by approximately 33%; tissue-to-blood metabolic gradient is 3 mmHg. $PtcCO_2$ with the Severinghaus adjustment has been shown to predict $PaCO_2$ to within $\pm$ 10%.[63]

As with $PtcO_2$, $PtcCO_2$ has been most extensively used in the care of neonatal patients. In contrast to $PtcO_2$, $PtcCO_2$ values are less sensitive to skin perfusion and do not change appreciably with age. Therefore the interpretation of $PtcCO_2$ measurements are much easier than their oxygen counterparts. In addition, the $PtcCO_2$ sensor also has a much shorter warm-up time after skin placement; it attains steady-state values within about 5 minutes. Like $PtcO_2$, the $PtcCO_2$ sensor requires calibration (a 2-point gas calibration) and regular maintenance.

The relative unpopularity of transcutaneous oxygen since the advent of pulse oximetry has meant that $PtcCO_2$ receives much less attention than it deserves. It should be remembered that $PtcCO_2$ does not have all of the disadvantages of $PtcO_2$. Furthermore, no CO_2 equivalent of the pulse oximeter exists. This noninvasive and risk-free monitor is especially useful in thoracic anesthesia, where the relationship between end-tidal and arterial PCO_2 can change rapidly.

Future Developments Oxygen and Carbon Dioxide Monitors

The current techniques for monitoring oxygenation and ventilation during thoracic anesthesia have been briefly described. To use these monitors effectively and safely, the clinician must know the basic engineering principles of each as well as the common sources of error. To treat a monitor as a "black box" that must yield valid data (if it provides any data) is an invitation to disaster. Every monitor that has been discussed is subject to conditions under which it will give erroneous data.

In addition, the wise clinician must understand the physiology behind the particular variable being monitored and the influence of other physiologic parameters on this variable. For example, mixed venous oxygen saturation (SvO_2) is a global variable of oxygen transport that depends explicitly on four other variables: SaO_2, Hb, Qt and $\dot{V}_2$. Transcutaneous oxygen tension ($PtcO_2$) depends on skin perfusion as well as arterial oxygenation. No single variable quantitates oxygen or carbon dioxide transport. Like the pilot of a complex airplane, the clinician must integrate data from the various monitors to arrive at a complete picture of a patient's status.

Cost-effectiveness is a consideration in all aspects of medicine today, and monitoring is no exception. The costs of any monitor are usually divided into two categories: (1) capital costs of acquiring equipment and (2) recurrent or disposable costs associated with the use of the monitor in each patient. An example of the first category is the purchase price of an SvO_2 analyzer; an example of the second is the cost of an SvO_2 pulmonary oximetry catheter. The capital costs are often amortized into the disposable costs to reduce or eliminate the financial impact of a large equipment purchase.

The recurrent cost is usually small for noninvasive monitors. So-called "disposable" pulse oximeter sensors are relatively inexpensive; they are often reused several times, but are sometimes discarded after one use. The primary cost of noninvasive monitoring is the instrument itself. Once the equipment has been purchased it should be used whenever it has any medical value. On the other hand, the disposable costs for invasive monitors can be significant, and cost-effectiveness should be considered before each use. The two best examples in thoracic anesthesia are the SvO_2 fiberoptic pulmonary artery catheter and the intra-arterial optode sensor. The unit cost of each of these disposables is approximately $200. Two questions must be answered before deciding whether this cost is justified. One, what are the additional costs of *not* using the invasive monitor? For example, how many additional blood gas analyses would be required if a continuous intra-arterial blood gas sensor is not used in a given patient? Two, what is the value of the new information provided by the monitor that could not be obtained in some other way? The second question is clearly the most difficult to answer objectively, and depends on the clinician's own perspective and prejudices. If the use of a monitor shortens the patient's hospital stay by one day, the use is unquestionably justified from the cost-effectiveness standpoint. Of course the clinician can never know a priori when this might be the case.

Monitoring oxygenation and ventilation in the near future will include the refinement and widespread availability of intra-arterial blood gas sensors. These instruments will have their greatest impact in cardiothoracic anesthesia, where most patients already have arterial cannulas in place for hemodynamic reasons. The access to continuous, real-time pHa, $PaCO_2$, and PaO_2 data will improve patient care in both the operating room and the intensive care unit. The current problems of accuracy, reliability, and cost must be solved before this can take place, however.

In the more distant future, noninvasive monitors that provide complete data on arterial oxygenation and ventilation should be available. Although the pulse oximeter is an excellent noninvasive oxygenation monitor, it does not provide trend information when the hemoglobin saturation is high (ie, for P_AO_2 values greater than 75 mm (Hg). Likewise, although the capnograph is also an excellent monitor, $P_{et}CO_2$ is not equal to $PaCO_2$, and the relationship between the two measurements can change rapidly during thoracic anesthesia. With the perfection of continuous, noninvasive blood pressure monitors and the development of a noninvasive blood gas monitor, the need for arterial cannulas will be small.

Finally, noninvasive monitors of regional oxygenation and perfusion will add another dimension to clinicians' abilities to maintain homeostasis during the stress of thoracic surgery. One such monitor, the "cerebral oximeter,"[64] is already on the market, and others will undoubtedly soon follow. In 2010 the anesthesiologist may be faced with regional PO_2, PCO_2, and perfusion data coming continuously from the brain, heart, kidneys, and liver; the question will be "Is this too much information?"

References

1. Van Slyke DD, Neill JM. The determination of gases in blood and other solutions by vacuum extraction and manometric measurement. Int J Biol Chem 1924;61:523.
2. Severinghaus JW. Historical development of oxygenation monitoring. In: Payne JP, Severinghaus JW, eds. Pulse oximetry. Berlin: Springer-Verlag, 1986;1.
3. Brown LJ. A new instrument for the simultaneous measurement of total hemoglobin, % oxyhemoglobin, % carboxyhemoglobin, % methemoglobin, and oxygen content in whole blood. IEEE Trans Biomed Eng 1980;27:132.
4. Severinghaus JW, Astrup PB. History of blood gas analysis. In: International anesthesiology clinics, Vol. 25. Boston: Little, Brown, 1987;167.

5. Stephen CR, Slater HM, Johnson AL, et al. The oximeter—A technical aid for the anesthesiologist. Anesthesiology 1951;12:541.
6. Barker SJ, Tremper KK. The effect of carbon monoxide inhalation on pulse oximeter signal detection. Anesthesiology 1987;67:599.
7. Barker SJ, Tremper KK, Hyatt J, et al. Effect of methemoglobinemia on pulse oximetry and mixed venous oximetry. Anesthesiology 1989;70:112.
8. Pologe JA, Raley DM. Effects of fetal hemoglobin on pulse oximetry. J Perinatol VII 1987;7:324.
9. Anderson JV. The accuracy of pulse oximetry in neonates: Effects of fetal hemoglobin and bilirubin. J Perinatol 1987;7:323.
10. Scheller MS, Unger RJ, Kelner MJ. Effects of intravenously administered dyes on pulse oximetry readings. Anesthesiology 1986;65:550.
11. Brooks TD, Paulus DA, Winkle WE. Infrared heat lamps interfere with pulse oximeters. Anesthesiology 1984;61:630. Letter.
12. Costarino AT, Davis DA, Keon TP. Falsely normal saturation reading with the pulse oximeter. Anesthesiology 1987;67:830.
13. Eisele JH, Downs D. Ambient light affects pulse oximeters. Anesthesiology 1987;67:864.
14. Siegel MN, Gravenstein N. Preventing ambient light from affecting pulse oximetry. Anesthesiology 1987;67:280.
15. Overand PT, Freund PR, Cooper JO, et al. Failure rate of pulse oximetry in clinical practice. Anesth Analg 1990;70:S289.
16. Barker SJ, Hyatt J, Rumack WA. Pulse oximeter failure rates: effects of manufacturer, sensor site, and patient. Anesth Analg 1992;74:S15.
17. Nellcor N100 Technical Manual. Hayward CA: Nellcor Corporation 1983.
18. Mihm FG, Halperin DH. Noinvasive detection of profound arterial desaturations using pulse oximetry device. Anesthesiology 1985;62:85.
19. Cecil WT, Thorpe KJ, Fibuch EE, et al. A clinical evaluation of the accuracy of the Nellcor N100 and the Ohmeda 3700 pulse oximeters. J Clin Monit 1988;4:31.
20. Boxer RA, Gottesfeld I, Singh S, et al. Noninvasive pulse oximetry in children with cyanotic congenital heart disease. Crit Care Med 1987;15:1062.
21. Fait CD, Wetzel RC, Dean JM, et al. Pulse oximetry in critically ill children. J Clin Monit 1985;1:232.
22. Kagle DM, Alexander CM, Berko RS, et al. Evaluation of the Ohmeda 3700 pulse oximeters: steady-state and transient response characteristics. Anesthesiology 1987;66:376.
23. Severinghaus JW, Naifeh KH. Accuracy of response of six pulse oximeters to profound hypoxia. Anesthesiology 1987;67:551.
23a. Thys DM, Cohen E, Girard D, Kirschner PA, et al. The pulse oximeter: a non-invasive monitor of oxygenation during thoracic surgery. Thorac Cardiovasc Surgeon 1986;34:380.
24. Barker SJ, Tremper KK, Heitzmann H. Comparison of three oxygen monitors in detecting endobronchial intubation. J Clin Monit 1988;4:240.
25. Severinghaus JW, Bradley AF. Electrodes for blood PO_2 and PCO_2 determination. J Appl Physiol 1958; 13:515.
26. Harris TR, Nugent M. Continuous arterial oxygen tension monitoring in the newborn infant. J Pediatr 1973;82:929.
27. Bratanow N, Polk K, Bland R, et al. Continuous polarographic monitoring of intra-arterial oxygen in the perioperative period. Crit Care Med 1985; 13:859.
28. Malalis L, Bhat R, Vidyasagar D. Comparison of intravascular PO_2 with transcutaneous and PaO_2 values. Crit Care Med 1983;11:110.
29. Gehrich JL, Lubbers DW, Opitz N, et al. Optical fluorescence and its application to an intravascular blood gas monitoring system. IEEE Trans Biomed Eng 1986;33:117.
30. Barker SJ, Tremper KK, Hyatt J, et al. Continuous fiberoptic arterial oxygen tension measurement in dogs. J Clin Monit 1987;3:48.
31. Shapiro BA, Cane RD, Chomka CM, et al. Evaluation of a new intra-arterial blood gas system in dogs. Crit Care Med 1987;15:361.
32. Lubbers DW, Opitz N. Die pCO_2/pO_2-optode: eine neue pCO_2 bzw. pO_2-Messonde zur Messung des pCO_2 oder pO_2 von Glasen und Flussigkeiten. Z Naturforsch [C] 1984;30:532.
33. Peterson J, Fitzgerald R, Buckhold D. Fiberoptic probe in vivo measurement of oxygen partial pressure. Anal Chem 1984;56:62.
34. Mahutte K, Sassoon SH, Muro JR, et al. Progress in the development of a fluorescent intravascular blood gas system in man. J Clin Monit 1990;6:147.
35. Barker SJ, Hyatt J. Continuous measurement of intra-arterial pHa, $PaCO_2$, and PaO_2 in the operating room. Anesth Analg 1991;73:43.
36. Greenblott G, Barker SJ, Tremper KK, et al. Detection of venous air embolism by continuous intra-arterial oxygen monitoring. J Clin Monit 1990;6:53.

37. Eberhard P, Hammacher K, Mindt W. Perkutane messung des sauerstoffpartialdrukes: methodik und anwendugen. Stuttgart Proc Medizin-Technik 1972. Abstract.
38. Huch A, Huch R, Meinzer K, et al. Eine schuelle, behitze Ptoberflachenelektrode zur knotinuierlichen Uberwachung des PO_2 beim Menschen: Elecktrodenaufbau und Eigenschaften. Stuttgart Proc Medizin-Tecknik 1972;26. Abstract.
39. Huch R, Huch A, Albani M, et al. Transcutaneous PO_2 monitoring in routine management of infants and children with cardiorespiratory problems. Pediatrics 1976;57:681.
40. Peabody JL, Willis MM, Gregory GA, et al. Clinical limitations and advantages of transcutaneous oxygen electrodes. Acta Anaethesiol Scand Suppl 1978;68:76.
41. Marshall TA, Kattwinkel J, Bery FA, et al. Transcutaneous oxygen monitoring of neonates during surgery. J Pediatr Surg 1980;15:797.
42. Versmold HT, Linderkamp O, Holzman M, et al. Transcutaneous monitoring of PO_2 in newborn infants. Where are the limits? Influences of blood pressure, blood volume, blood flow, viscosity, and acid base state. Birth Defects 1979;4:286.
43. Tremper KK, Waxman K, Shoemaker WC. Effects of hypoxia and shock on transcutaneous PO_2 values in dogs. Crit Care Med 1979;7:526.
44. Rowe MI, Weinberg G. Transcutaneous oxygen monitoring in shock and resuscitation. J Pediatr Surg 1979;14:773.
45. Baumgardner JE, Graves DJ, Neufeld GR, et al. Gas flux through human skin: effects of temperature, stripping and inspired tension. J Appl Physiol 1985;5:1536.
46. Van Duzee BF. Thermal analysis of human stratum corneum. J Invest Dermatol 1975;65:404.
47. Tremper KK, Shoemaker WC. Transcutaneous oxygen monitoring of critically ill adults, with and without low-flow shock. Crit Care Med 1981;9:706.
48. Glenski JA, Cucchira RF. Transcutaneous O_2 and CO_2 monitoring of neurosurgical patient: detection of air embolism. Anesthesiology 1986;64:546.
49. Tremper KK, Barker SJ, Blatt DH, et al. Effects of anesthetic agents on the drift of a transcutaneous PO_2 sensor. J Clin Monit 1986;2:234.
50. Martin WE, Cheung PW, Johnson CC, et al. Continuous monitoring of mixed venous oxygen saturation in man. Anesth Analg 1973;52:784.
51. Nunn JF. Respiratory deadspace and distribution of the inspired gas. In: JF Nunn, ed. Applied respiratory physiology. 2nd ed. Boston: Butterworth, 1977:213.
52. Ailken RS, Clark-Kennedy AE. On the fluctuations in the composition of the alveolar air during the respiratory cycle in muscular exercise. J Physiology (Lond) 1928;65:389.
53. Hutton P, Owen H. Capnography: your questions answered ... Paramus NJ: Datascope Corporation.
54. Gravenstein JS, Paulus DA, Hayes TJ. Capnography in clinical practice. Stoneham MA: Butterworth-Heinemann, 1989.
55. Smalhout D, Kalenda Z. An atlas of capnography. Utrecht, Netherlands: University Hospital, Institute of Anesthesiology, 1975.
56. Zupan J, Martin M, Bennett J. End-tidal CO_2 excretion waveform and error with gas sampling line leak. Anesth Analg 1988;67:579.
57. Fowler KT, Read J. Cardiac oscillation in expired gas tensions and regional pulmonary blood flow. J Applied Physiology 1961;16:863.
58. Trevino RP, Bisera J, Weil MH, et al. End-tidal CO_2 as a guide to successful cardiopulmonary resuscitation; a preliminary report. Crit Care Med 1985; 13:910.
59. Weil MH, Bisera J, Trevino RP, et al. Cardiac output and end-tidal carbon dioxide. Crit Care Med 1985; 13:907.
60. Ping STS. (Letter to the Editor.) Anesth Analg 1987; 66:483.
61. Severinghaus JW, Stafford M, Bradley AF. $TCPO_2$ electrode design calibration and temperature gradient problem. Acta Anaesthesiol Scand 1978;68:188.
62. Monaco F, Nickerson BG, Mcquitty JC. Continuous transcutaneous oxygen and carbon dioxide monitoring in the pediatric ICU. Crit Care Med 1982; 10:765.
63. Palmirano B, Severinghaus JW. Transcutaneous PCO_2 and PO_2: a multi-centered study of accuracy. J Clin Monit 1990;6:189.
64. McCormick PW, Stewart M, Goetting MG, et al. Regional cerebrovascular oxygen saturation measured by optical spectroscopy in humans. Stroke 22:1991;5:596.

CHAPTER

10

Invasive Cardiovascular Monitoring

David Reich
Daniel M. Thys

With the aging of the population and advances in surgical management, anesthesiologists are often confronted with older and sicker patients as candidates for thoracic surgery. Although the benefits of monitoring are difficult to quantify, it is nonetheless generally accepted that extensive monitoring is beneficial and possibly improves outcome in these patients. Ideally, only noninvasive monitoring would be used, because it is usually associated with few complications. In practice, however, the shortcomings of noninvasive monitoring become readily apparent and, as a result, anesthesiologists often resort to invasive monitoring. The aim of this chapter is the review of some of the more common monitoring techniques for thoracic procedures and the description of their indications and potential complications.

Blood Pressure

Blood pressure (BP) is the most commonly used method of assessing the cardiovascular system. The magnitude of the BP is directly related to the cardiac output (CO) and the systemic vascular resistance (SVR). This is somewhat like Ohm's law of electricity (voltage equals current times resistance), where BP is analogous to voltage, CO to flow, and SVR to resistance. Thus, an increase in the BP may reflect a rise in either CO, SVR, or both. Although the BP is one of the easiest cardiovascular variables to measure, it gives only indirect information about the patient's cardiovascular status.

Mean arterial pressure (MAP) is probably the most useful parameter to measure in assessing organ perfusion, except for the heart, where diastolic blood pressure (DPB) is most important. MAP is measured directly by integrating the arterial waveform tracing over time, or using the formula:

$$\text{MAP} = [\text{SBP} + (2 \times \text{DBP})]/3 \qquad (10\text{-}1)$$

SBP is systolic pressure. The pulse pressure is the difference between SBP and DBP.

Anesthesia for thoracic surgery is frequently complicated by blood pressure lability. As a result of several factors, including direct heart compression, impaired venous return due to retraction, dysrhythmias from mechanical stimulation of the heart, and lung manipulations that may impair right ventricular outflow and pulmonary venous return. Sudden loss of significant blood volumes may occur at almost any time. Since the thoracic surgical population includes many patients with labile hypertension and atherosclerotic heart disease, a safe and reliable method is required for the accurate measurement of BP during thoracic surgery.

Noninvasive Blood Pressure Monitoring

The Riva-Rocci occlusive cuff for the sphygmomanometric measurement of blood pressure was described in 1896, and the measurement of blood pressure during anesthesia for neurosurgical procedures was promoted by Harvey Cushing in 1903. A sphygmomanometer is an elastic bladder surrounded by an unyielding cuff that evenly distributes the pressure in the bladder to the encircled extremity. The elastic bladder is filled with air until a suprasystolic pressure is applied to the extremity, and then the air is slowly released. For accurate blood pressure measurement, two conditions must be met: (1) the cuff width must be 20% wider than the diameter of the extremity and (2) the bladder must be attached to a calibrated aneroid or mercury manometer. A cuff that is applied too loosely or tightly also results in inaccuracy.[1]

Methods of Sphygmomanometry

PALPATORY TECHNIQUE. One of the easiest methods of obtaining a SBP is to locate a pulse, inflate a proximal cuff until the pulse is absent, and then slowly deflate the cuff until the first pulse is palpated. Variations on this technique include using a Doppler probe or a pulse oximeter to determine when the first pulse is present. In children under 1 year of age, the limb can be observed for flushing that occurs once the cuff pressure is less than SBP.[2] Unfortunately, only the SBP can be accurately measured using this technique.

KOROTKOFF SOUNDS. Korotkoff sound auscultation is the most traditional and widespread method of BP determination for vascular patients outside of the operating room. As the cuff is deflated from a suprasystolic pressure, a stethoscope is placed over a distal artery. The sound of blood rushing into the empty arterial tree creates Korotkoff sounds once the cuff pressure is less than the systolic pressure.[3] The sounds disappear once the cuff pressure is less than the diastolic pressure.

An accurate determination of BP using the Korotkoff sounds requires that the cuff be deflated slowly. Otherwise the systolic pressure will be underestimated, and the diastolic pressure will be either over- or underestimated. Other potential inaccuracies are associated with this technique. Atherosclerosis may result in stiffening of the artery that prevents the cuff from completely occluding the artery, even at suprasystolic pressures ("lead pipe syndrome") causing overestimation of the systolic BP. Hypotensive states such as hypovolemic shock and vasopressor infusions may lead to hypoperfusion of the extremity with underestimation of the BP.[4]

Oscillometry

The oscillotonometer was introduced by von Recklinghausen in 1931. The device consists of a double-cuff system with a proximal cuff for occlusion of arterial inflow and a distal cuff to measure arterial pulsations. The distal cuff begins to pulsate when the proximal cuff deflates below systolic pressure, and maximal oscillations occur when the proximal cuff is at mean arterial pressure. The diastolic pressure is not easily determined by this method, however.[5]

Automated oscillometric BP devices, which differ from oscillotonometers in that they have only one cuff, are available from numerous manufacturers. A solenoid valve controls the deflation of the cuff, holding the cuff volume momentarily constant so that the amplitude of the oscillation may be recorded. As the cuff deflates from a suprasystolic pressure, the oscillations are measured at multiple cuff pressures for at least two cardiac cycles. A computer then analyzes the pattern of oscillations at different cuff pressures. Systolic pressure is defined at the point of rapidly increasing oscillation, and diastolic pressure is defined at rapidly decreasing oscillation. Mean arterial pressure is the cuff pressure associated with maximal oscillation.[6]

Automated oscillometric BP measurements compare favorably with invasively determined BP values in both adults and neonates.[7,8] The cycle times are prolonged when the oscillations are irregular (as in atrial fibrillation or patient movement) or slow (sinus bradycardia), however. Oscillometric devices usually remain accurate during hypotension but may fail when severe hypovolemia or vasoconstriction is present.

Plethysmography

The Peñaz principle involves the measurement of an arterial pressure waveform by unloading the arterial wall of the finger.[9] The Finapres device (Ohmeda; Englewood CO) consists of a finger pressure cuff and an infrared photoplethysmograph. A servo-control mechanism varies the pressure in the cuff to maintain constant infrared absorbance distal to the cuff. The pressure waveform generated in the finger cuff correlates with the arterial pressure waveform. Arterial pressure measured by the Finapres device corresponds to arterial pressure determined by both the auscultatory method[10] and direct intra-arterial measurement.[11]

Some clinicians are concerned that this instrument may result in digital nerve injury or ischemic injury. The Finapres device has been used for prolonged periods without adverse sequelae, however.[12] Moderate degrees of peripheral vasoconstriction are associated with some measurement inaccuracy;[13] severe vasoconstriction (as with high vasopressor doses) and severe peripheral vascular disease will hinder the use of this technique.

Bardoczky et al[14] compared a total of 1861 measurements of arterial pressure, including 938 pairs during one-lung ventilation, by invasive and photoplethysmography techniques. The photoplethysmography underestimated SBP during two-lung ventilation, and overestimated SBP during one-lung ventilation. The precision was good and the biases were small, but individual variations were wide. The researchers concluded that with arterial blood pressure determinations photoplethysmography can be useful in estimating variation and following radial arterial blood pressure trends during thoracic surgery. Photoplethysmography is an acceptable alternative to invasive blood pressure monitoring.

Advantages and Disadvantages of Noninvasive Blood Pressure Monitoring

Noninvasive BP measurement techniques are advantageous in that they are technically easy to perform, easily automated, generally accurate, and have a negligible risk of infection. Several risks still remain, however. Electrical macroshock with electrical devices is a potential hazard. Prolonged or too frequent cuff inflation may result in tissue ischemia or nerve damage. Ulnar nerve palsy may occur with an automated device that compresses the nerve against the ulnar groove.[15]

In addition, BP readings may be inaccurate or delayed for the reasons mentioned above. Thoracic surgery patients may be especially prone to these errors because of slower or irregular heart rates from associated cardiovascular disease and rigid peripheral arteries from atherosclerosis. Thus possibility exists that the patient may be inappropriately managed because of erroneous or delayed information.

Invasive Pressure Monitoring

General Principles

In invasive pressure monitoring, systemic arterial blood pressure is gauged by placing a catheter into a peripheral artery while other catheters placed in the central circulation measure central venous or intracardiac pressures. The transmission of forces generated in the cardiac chambers is represented by pressure waves in the arterial and venous tree. These forces must be transmitted to a device that converts mechanical energy into electronic signals so that they can be measured. The signals are then processed by an electronic analyzer and stored or displayed. Thus for a system for intravascular pressure measurement, an intravascular catheter, fluid-filled tubing and connections, an electromechanical transducer, an electronic analyzer, and electronic storage or display systems are necessary.

Systemic Arterial Pressure Monitoring

GENERAL INFORMATION. Although numerous methods of noninvasive blood pressure measurement are clinically available, they all involve the detection of flow past an occlusive cuff. These methods tend to underestimate systolic pressure and overestimate diastolic pressure, regardless of technique. In addition, no method, except the Peñaz photoplethysmography technique generates an arterial waveform. Direct intra-arterial monitoring remains the "gold standard" against which all noninvasive techniques are compared.[16]

Surgery is frequently complicated by wide swings in arterial pressure as a result of shifts in intravascular volume, the effects of anesthetic agents, underlying cardiovascular disease, and surgical manipulations. The beat-to-beat indication of arterial pressure and waveform that intra-arterial monitor provides is necessary. Multiple arterial blood gases may also be obtained.

The arterial waveform tracing provides much information beyond timely pressure measurements. The slope of the arterial upstroke correlates with dP/dt and thus is a source of information on myocardial contractility; an increase in systemic vascular resistance alone also results in an increase in the slope.[17] The acute changes in arterial pressure associated with dysrhythmias give a visual estimate of the hemodynamic consequences of the rhythm disturbances. In addition, the onset of a nodal rhythm with loss of the atrial systole is often recognized by a sudden reduction in arterial pressure. Hypovolemia is suggested when the arterial pressure shows large respiratory variations and a narrowed pulse pressure.[18]

SITES. The most consistent measurement obtained from different cannulation sites is the mean arterial pressure. Factors that influence the site of cannulation include the surgery site, the possible compromise of arterial flow due to patient positioning or surgical manipulations, and any history of ischemia or prior surgery of the limb. Another variable that may affect the cannulation site is the presence of a proximal arterial cutdown site. The proximal cutdown may cause damped waveforms or falsely low pressure readings resulting from stenosis or vascular thrombosis.[19]

Radial and Ulnar Arteries. The radial artery is most commonly cannulated for intraoperative monitoring because of its superficial location, easy accessibility, and the presence of collateral circulation. Assessment of the adequacy of the collateral circulation and the absence of proximal obstructions prior to cannulating the radial artery is advisable for monitoring purposes.

In the normal patient, the radial artery pressure tracing differs from the central aortic pressure in that the systolic pressure is higher and the diastolic pressure is lower. This is a result of resonance of pressure waves in the arterial tree.[20] Despite this distortion, the mean arterial pressure measured in the radial artery should be identical to the central aortic pressure.

The ulnar artery provides the majority of blood flow to the hand in about 90% of humans.[21] The radial and ulnar arteries are connected by a palmar arch that provides collateral flow to the hand in the event of radial artery occlusion. Many clinicians routinely perform an Allen's test prior to radial artery cannulation. If the test demonstrates that the hand is dependent on the radial artery for adequate filling, and other cannulation sites are not available, the ulnar artery may be selected.

The Allen's test is performed by occluding both the radial and ulnar arteries by compression and exercising the hand until it is pale. With the hand opened loosely, the ulnar artery is then released and the time required for the hand to regain its normal color is noted.[22] With normal collateral circulation, color returns to the hand in about 5 seconds. If the hand takes longer than 15 seconds to return to its normal color, cannulation of the radial artery on that side is somewhat controversial. The hand may remain pale if the fingers are hyperextended or widely spread apart even in the presence of a normal collateral circulation.[23] Variations on the Allen's test include using a Doppler probe or pulse oximeter to document collateral flow.[24,25]

Recently the value of the Allen's test has been challenged. Slogoff et al cannulated the radial artery in 16 patients with poor ulnar collateral circulation as determined using the Allen's test with no complications.[26] An incidence of zero in a sample of only 16 patients, however, does not guarantee that the true incidence of the complication is negligible. Mangano and Hickey reported a case of hand ischemia requiring amputation in a patient with a normal preoperative Allen's test.[27] Thus the predictive value of the Allen's test is questionable.

The lateral decubitus position may complicate radial artery pressure monitoring in thoracic procedures. The arm on the downward side may have diminished perfusion if the axilla is not properly protected by placement of an axillary roll. The "upward" arm could always be monitored to avoid this problem, but monitoring the "downward" arm may aid in the detection of a displaced axillary roll and potentially avoid a brachial plexus injury.

Brachial and Axillary Arteries. The brachial artery lies medial to the bicipital tendon in the antecubital fossa in close proximity to the median nerve. The complications from percutaneous brachial artery catheter monitoring are fewer than those following brachial artery cutdown for cardiac catheterization.[28] Brachial artery pressure tracings resemble those in the femoral artery, with less systolic augmentation than in radial artery tracings.[29] Two large studies of perioperative brachial arterial monitoring have documented the safety of this technique.[30,31] However, because the brachial artery is an end-artery, the risk of compromising the blood flow to the hand should be considered.

The axillary artery may be cannulated by the Seldinger technique near the junction of the deltoid and pectoral muscles. This has been recommended for long-term catheterization in the intensive care unit[32] and in patients with peripheral vascular disease.[33] Since the tip of the 15–20-cm catheter may lie in the aortic arch, the use of the left axillary artery is recommended to minimize the chance of cerebral embolization during flushing. Lateral decubitus positioning occasionally results in kinking of axillary catheters with damping of the pressure waveform.

Femoral Artery. The femoral artery is usually cannulated for monitoring purposes when other sites are not accessible or other pulses are not palpable. This artery can be cannulated using any of the above techniques. The use of this site remains controversial because of the high rate of ischemic complications and pseudoaneurysm formation following diagnostic angiographic and cardiac catheterization procedures.[34] However, the size of monitoring catheters is considerably smaller than diagnostic catheters, and the incidence of these complications should be much less. Researchers previously stated that the femoral area was intrinsically dirty and that catheter sepsis and mortality were significantly increased as compared to other monitoring sites. More recent evidence suggests that femoral artery cannulation is safe, but that long-term cannulation (> 4 days) is associated with an 8% to 17% incidence of catheter-related infections.[35]

The patient undergoing thoracic aortic reconstruction may require femoral arterial monitoring in addition to monitoring in one of the upper extremities. In these operations, distal aortic perfusion (using partial cardiopulmonary or left heart bypass) may be performed during aortic cross-clamping to preserve spinal cord and visceral organ blood flow. It is important to measure the distal aortic pressure at the femoral (or dorsalis pedis) artery to optimize the distal perfusion pressure. In repairs of aortic coarctation, simultaneous femoral and radial arterial monitoring may help determine the adequacy of the surgical repair by documenting the pressure gradient following the repair.

In patients with peripheral vascular disease, the femoral artery is a less desirable choice as a site for arterial monitoring. Obstruction of aortic inflow may decrease the arterial pressure in the femoral artery or the femoral artery may have atheromatous plaques that may embolize and cause distal ischemia.

Dorsalis Pedis Artery. The dorsalis pedis is a relatively small artery that may be cannulated when other sites are not available. Because of its small size, the incidence of failed cannulation ranges up to 20%, and the incidence of thrombotic occlusion is about 8%.[36] The dorsalis pedis arterial waveform tends to have higher systolic and lower diastolic pressures than simultaneously measured radial or brachial pressures.[37]

Superficial Temporal Artery. The superficial artery, a branch of the external carotid that passes anteriorly to the ear, has a variable course, that may be determined with a Doppler probe.[38] Since this artery may be quite tortuous and difficult to cannulate, this site is not recommended in patients with carotid occlusive or cerebrovascular disease. The tip of the catheter must be positioned carefully so that embolization via the internal carotid to the cerebral circulation does not occur.

INDICATIONS. The indications for invasive arterial monitoring, which are summarized in Table 10-1, include the following:

1. Major thoracic procedures involving large fluid shifts or blood loss.

Table 10-1. Indications for Intra-arterial Monitoring

- Major thoracic procedures involving large fluid shifts or blood losses.
- Thoracic surgery requiring single lung ventilation.
- Patients requiring frequent arterial blood gases.
- Recent myocardial infarction, unstable angina, or severe coronary artery disease.
- Decreased left ventricular function or significant valvular disease.
- Shock or multiple organ failure.
- Deliberate hypotension or deliberate hypothermia.
- Massive trauma.
- Right heart failure, chronic obstructive pulmonary disease, pulmonary hypertension, or pulmonary embolism.
- Inotropes or intra-aortic balloon counterpulsation.
- Thoracic aortic cross-clamping.
- Massive ascites.
- Electrolyte or metabolic disturbances (frequent blood samples).
- Inability to measure arterial pressure noninvasively (morbid obesity).

2. Thoracic surgery requiring single-lung ventilation.
3. Patients with pulmonary disease requiring frequent arterial blood gases.
4. Patients with recent myocardial infarctions, unstable angina, or severe coronary artery disease.
5. Patients with decreased left ventricular function (ie, congestive heart failure) or significant valvular heart disease.
6. Patients with multiple organ failure or in hypovolemic, cardiogenic, or septic shock.
7. Procedures involving the use of deliberate hypotension or deliberate hypothermia.
8. Cases of massive trauma.
9. Patients with right heart failure, chronic obstructive pulmonary disease, pulmonary hypertension, or pulmonary embolism.
10. Patients requiring inotropes or intra-aortic balloon counterpulsation.
11. Patients undergoing surgery of the aorta requiring cross-clamping.
12. Patients with massive ascites.
13. Patients with electrolyte or metabolic disturbances requiring frequent blood samples.
14. Inability to measure arterial pressure noninvasively (eg, morbid obesity).

CONTRAINDICATIONS. There are several contraindications to arterial cannulation.

Local Infection. Placement of an arterial cannula through cellulitic or purulent tissue is likely to result in catheter sepsis. If signs of infection develop at an existing arterial cannulation site, the catheter must be removed. A separate cannulation site free of infection should be found. Strict aseptic technique is necessary during the insertion and maintenance of arterial cannulae.

Coagulopathy. Coagulopathy may result in hematoma formation during arterial cannulation at peripheral sites such as the radial and dorsalis pedis arteries. However, the risk of massive hematoma formation causing vascular or neurologic compromise during axillary and femoral cannulation attempts is more significant. Thus in anticoagulated patients, it is recommended that more peripheral arterial cannulation sites be used when this form of monitoring is required.

Proximal Obstruction. Anatomical factors may lead to intra-arterial pressure readings that markedly underestimate the central aortic pressure. Thoracic outlet syndrome and congenital anomalies of the aortic arch vessels obstruct flow to the upper extremities. Aortic coarctation diminishes flow to the lower extremities. Arterial pressure distal to a previous arterial cutdown site may be lower than the central aortic pressure resulting from arterial stenosis at the cutdown site.

Raynaud's Syndrome. Radial and brachial arterial cannulation are contraindicated in patients with a history of Raynaud's syndrome or Buerger's disease (thromboangiitis obliterans). In the perioperative setting, this is especially important, because hypothermia of the hand is the main trigger for vasospastic attacks in patients with Raynaud's syndrome.[39] In patients with either of these diseases, large arteries, such as the femoral or axillary, are recommended for intraarterial monitoring if indicated.

Surgical Considerations. Several surgical maneuvers may interfere with intra-arterial monitoring. During mediastinoscopy, the scope intermittently obstructs the innominate artery by compressing it against the manubrium. In other procedures, the lateral decubitus position may compromise flow to the downward arm if an axillary roll is not properly positioned.

In situations where the arterial waveform damping is intermittent, as in mediastinoscopy, monitoring radial artery pressure on the affected side has advantages. The surgeon can be informed whenever compression of the innominate artery occurs. In situations where the damping may be prolonged, however, monitoring arterial pressure in a different extremity is best.

Central Venous Pressure Monitoring

GENERAL INFORMATION. A central venous pressure (CVP) catheter is used to measure the filling pressure of the right ventricle and to assess the intravascular volume and right ventricular function. The distal end of the catheter must lie in one of the large intrathoracic veins or the right atrium. Water manometers have been used, but an electronic system is preferred. This allows the observation of the right atrial waveform, which provides additional information. In any pressure monitoring system, a reproducible landmark (such as the midaxillary line) as a zero reference. This is especially important in venous monitoring because compared to arterial monitoring, small changes in transducer height result in proportionately larger errors.

The right atrial waveform has three upward deflections (A, C, and V waves) and two downward deflections (X and Y descents) (Fig. 10-1). The "A" wave, produced by the atrial systole, occurs after the P wave on the electrocardiogram (ECG) but before the first heart sound. This is followed shortly thereafter by the "C" wave, is produced as the tricuspid valve closes and bulges upward into the right atrium. As ventricular systole continues, the tricuspid valve is pulled away from the right atrium by the contracting ventricle. This causes the "X" descent. The "V" wave results from the filling of the atrium prior to the opening of the tricuspid valve at the end of systole. The "Y" descent occurs as the tricuspid valve opens, the myocardium relaxes, and blood begins to fill the ventricle.[40]

Figure 10-1. Top, the relationship of the central venous pressure tracing to the ECG in normal sinus rhythm. The text describes the events responsible for the A, C, and V waves and the X and Y descents. Bottom, the relationship of the central venous pressure tracing to the ECG during junctional (AV nodal) rhythm. The contraction of the atrium against the closed tricuspid valve results in the "cannon A waves."

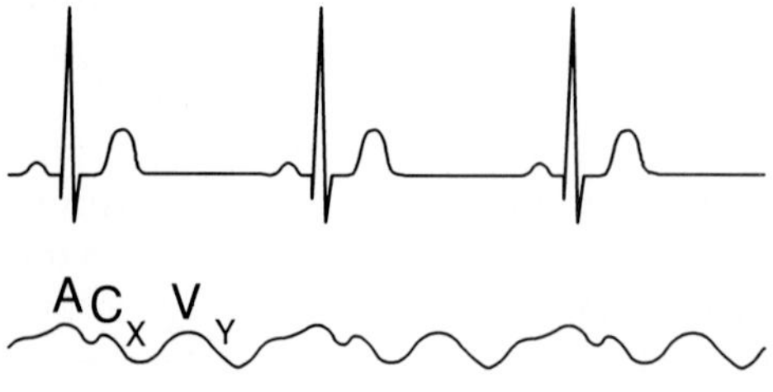

A C X V Y

The right atrial waveform may be useful in the diagnosis of pathological cardiac conditions. For example, onset of an irregular rhythm and the loss of the "A" wave suggests atrial flutter or fibrillation. Junctional (nodal) rhythm results in "cannon A waves" as the atrium contracts against a closed tricuspid valve. These waves may also be present in complete heart block and ventricular dysrhythmias. "Cannon V waves" occur if tricuspid regurgitation is significant. Large "V" waves may also appear on the right atrial waveform if the ventricle becomes noncompliant as a result of ischemia or right ventricular failure.[41]

INDICATIONS. CVP monitoring is performed primarily to obtain an estimate of intravascular volume. The accuracy and reliability of CVP monitoring depends on many factors, including the functional status of the right and left ventricles, the presence of pulmonary disease, and ventilatory factors such as positive end-expiratory pressure (PEEP). The CVP correlates with left heart filling pressures only in patients with good left ventricular function.[42] Elderly patients have a high incidence of coronary artery and pulmonary disease; therefore CVP is less likely to reflect left-sided filling pressures in this population accurately.[43] Indications for the intraoperative measurement of CVP are listed in Table 10-2.

CONTRAINDICATIONS

Absolute Contraindications. Superior vena cava syndrome is a contraindication to the placement of a CVP in the neck, subclavian area, or the upper extremities. Venous pressures in the head and upper extremities are elevated by the superior vena cava obstruction, and do not reflect right atrial pressure.

Relative Contraindications. Possible contraindications to CVP are listed below.

1. Infection at the site of insertion.
2. Coagulopathy, which predisposes to hemorrhagic complications of CVP placement, such as airway obstruction from a neck hematoma, hemothorax, or hematoma collection with subsequent infection.
3. Newly inserted pacemaker wires, which may be dislodged during the insertion of CVP catheters. This could result in a severe bradycardia, especially if the patient is pacemaker dependent.

Pulmonary Arterial Pressure Monitoring

GENERAL INFORMATION. The introduction of the flow-directed pulmonary artery catheter (PAC) has been a major advance in the monitoring of patients in the perioperative period. Since it was introduced in the 1970s,[44] its use has increased the amount of diagnostic information that can be obtained in critically ill patients. Patients with multisystem disease who undergo complex thoracic surgical procedures are likely to benefit from this "quantum leap" in monitoring.

Table 10-2. Indications for Central Venous Pressure Monitoring

- Major thoracic procedures involving large fluid shifts or blood losses in patients with good heart function.
- Intravascular volume assessment when urine output is unreliable or unavailable (eg, renal failure).
- Major trauma.
- Frequent blood sampling in patients who will not require an arterial line.
- Venous access for vasoactive or irritating drugs.
- Chronic drug administration.
- Inadequate peripheral intravenous access.
- Rapid infusion of intravenous fluids using large cannulae.

Specific information that can be gathered with the PAC includes pulmonary artery systolic pressure (PAS), pulmonary artery diastolic pressure (PAD), mean pulmonary arterial pressure (MPAP), pulmonary capillary wedge pressure (PCWP), mixed venous blood gases and saturation, and cardiac output (CO) by thermodilution. Special-purpose PACs for continuous mixed venous oximetry, pacing, and thermodilution right ventricular ejection fraction are also available. The PCWP and the PAD pressure are estimates of left atrial pressure, which in turn is an estimate of left ventricular end-diastolic pressure (LVEDP). However, the PCWP and the PAD pressures are not accurate measures of LVEDP in the presence of pulmonary vascular disease, PEEP,[45] or mitral valvular disease.[46]

LVEDP is an index of left ventricular end-diastolic volume, which is also known as left ventricular preload.[47] The relationship between LVEDP and end-diastolic volume is described by the left ventricular compliance curve. This nonlinear curve is affected by many factors, such as ventricular hypertrophy and myocardial ischemia.[48, 49]

The patency of vascular channels between the distal port of the PAC and the left atrium is necessary to ensure a close relationship between the PCWP and left atrial pressure. This condition is only met in the dependent portions of the lung (West's zone III) where the pulmonary venous pressure exceeds the alveolar pressure.[50] Otherwise the PCWP will reflect the alveolar pressure, not the left atrial pressure.

PEEP decreases the size of zone III, and it adversely affects the correlation between PCWP and left atrial pressures.[51] Interestingly, adult respiratory distress syndrome seems to prevent the transmission of increased alveolar pressure to the pulmonary interstitium. This preserves the relationship between PCWP and LVEDP during the application of PEEP.[52]

The lateral decubitus position may result in a change in the position of the distal end of a PAC relative to West's zone III. Most PACs are placed in the right pulmonary artery. Thus the left lateral decubitus position tends to place the tip of the PAC in zone I or II, with inaccurate PCWP results. Furthermore, collapse of the upward lung during one-lung ventilation causes complete collapse of the vascular channels due to hypoxic pulmonary vasoconstriction. Thus the PAC should be placed in the pulmonary artery of the nonoperative side whenever possible (Fig. 10-2); this is critical during pneumonectomies. Otherwise the tip of the catheter could be stapled or tied into the stump of the pulmonary artery on the operative side inadvertently. Transesophageal echocardiography and surgical palpation of the pulmonary artery can help to localize the location of the distal end of the PAC.

Cohen et al,[52A] reported a case of inadvertent transection of a pulmonary artery during a thoracotomy (Fig. 10-3). In that case the PA catheter was transacted during the resection of the left main pulmonary artery during a pneumonectomy. The PA catheter remained stapled to the suture line at the stump of the artery. It is important to emphasize the possible consequences that may follow if this event is unrecognized.

The PCWP waveform is analogous to the right atrial (CVP) waveform described previ-

Figure 10-2. During a left thoracotomy, the tip of the PA catheter is most likely in the ventilated lung (Zone 3). However, during a right thoracotomy, the tip of the PA catheter is most likely in the collapsed lung (Zone 1) and therefore measurements obtained from that catheter may be inaccurate.

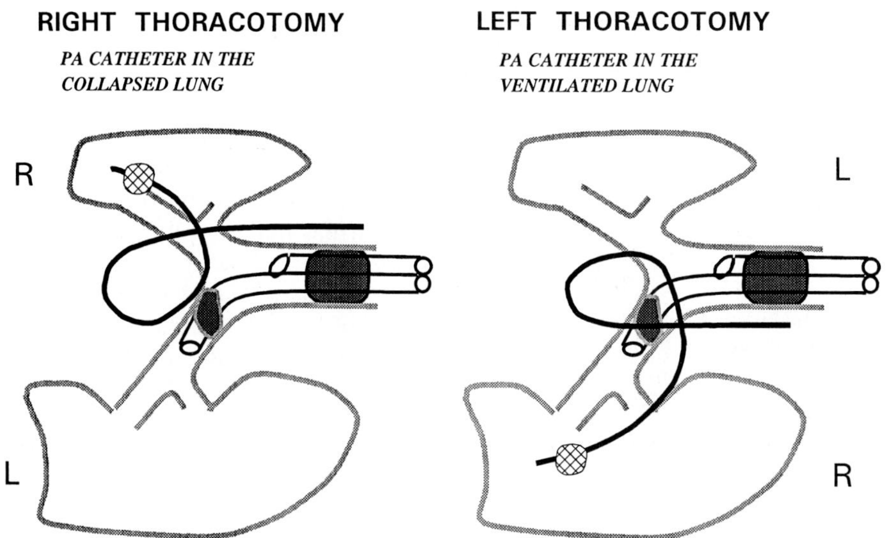

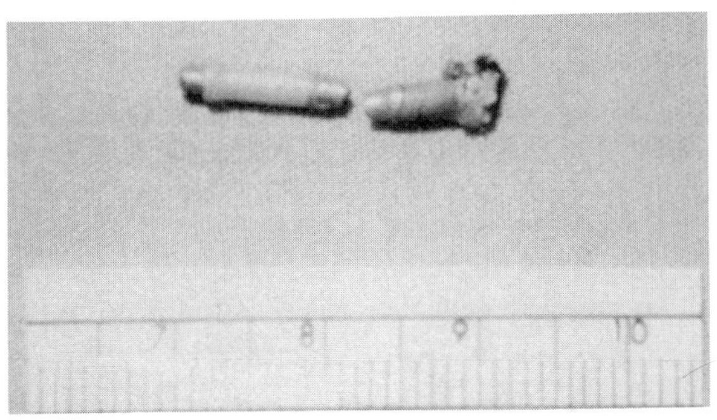

Figure 10-3. Photograph of the PAC specimen. The piece to the left results from the initial transection. The balloon can be identified as part of this piece. The fragment to the right was created during the resection of the staples. Reprinted with permission from Cohen E, Neustein SM, Kirschner PA. Inadvertent transection of a pulmonary artery during thoracic surgery. J Cardiothorac Vasc Anes 1993;7:339.

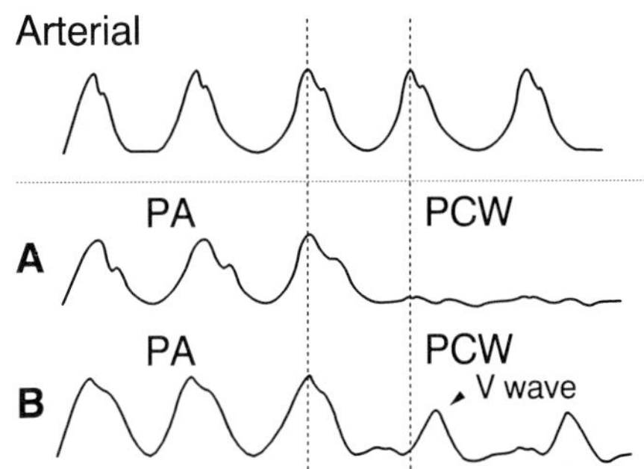

Figure 10-4. The relationship of the systemic arterial waveform, the pulmonary arterial (PA) waveform and the pulmonary capillary wedge (PCW) waveform are illustrated (A) in the normal situation, and (B) in the presence of "V" waves. Note the widening of the PA waveform and the loss of the dicrotic notch in the presence of V waves. In addition, note that the peak of the V wave occurs after the peak of the systemic arterial waveform.

ously. The "A," "C," and "V" waves are similarly timed to the cardiac cycle. "Cannon A" waves occur during nodal rhythm and complete heart block. (See above.) Large V waves have been described during mitral regurgitation and during episodes of myocardial ischemia (Fig. 10-4).[53]

The information gathered with the PAC allows the calculation of cardiac index, systemic and pulmonary vascular resistances, and ventricular function (Starling) curves. If simultaneous arterial and mixed venous blood samples are available, pulmonary shunt fraction, oxygen consumption, and lactate production can also be derived. In procedures where right ventricular failure is a possibility, such as pulmonary transplantation, the sudden appearance of right atrial V waves and elevation of pulmonary artery pressure is suggestive of right heart dysfunction.

INDICATIONS. The indications for pulmonary artery catheterization in the perioperative period remain controversial and vary in different institutions. A generally accepted list of indications for the PAC in the thoracic surgical population is given in Table 10-3.

Whether PAC monitoring improves outcome in critically ill patients is unresolved. Several studies support the idea that PAC monitoring improves patient outcome because of better management of alterations in cardiovascular status.[54, 55] A large prospective study of patients

Table 10-3. Indications for Pulmonary Artery Catheter Monitoring

- Major thoracic procedures involving large fluid shifts or blood losses in patients with poor heart function.
- Patients with recent myocardial infarctions or unstable angina.
- Patients in hypovolemic, cardiogenic, or septic shock or with multiple organ failure.
- Massive trauma.
- Patients with right heart failure, chronic obstructive pulmonary disease, pulmonary hypertension, or pulmonary embolism.
- Patients who require high levels of positive end-expiratory pressure.
- Hemodynamically unstable patients requiring inotropes or intra-aortic balloon counterpulsation.
- Patients undergoing surgery of the aorta who require cross-clamping.

undergoing elective coronary artery surgery did not identify differences in outcome between the CVP and PAC monitoring groups, however.[56]

CONTRAINDICATIONS

Absolute Contraindications. A PAC should not be used in the following situations:

1. Tricuspid or pulmonic valvular stenosis. The PAC would probably not be able to cross a stenotic valve; if it did so it would worsen the obstruction to flow.
2. Right atrial or right ventricular masses (eg, tumor, clot). The PAC may dislodge a portion of the mass, causing pulmonary or paradoxical embolization.
3. Tetralogy of Fallot. The right ventricular outflow tract is hypersensitive, and a PAC would probably induce a hypercyanotic episode due to "infundibular spasm."

Relative Contraindications. Possible contraindications to PAC use are listed below.

1. Severe dysrhythmias. Transient atrial and ventricular dysrhythmias are common during PAC placement in a normal patient. The risk of inducing a dysrhythmia in a patient prone to malignant dysrhythmias must be weighed against the potential benefits of the information gained from PAC monitoring.
2. Coagulopathy. The reasons relate to the potential complications involved in obtaining central venous access in the patient with coagulopathy. (See Central Venous Pressure Monitoring, above.)
3. Newly inserted pacemaker wires, which may be displaced by the PAC during insertion or withdrawal.

COMPLICATIONS. The complications associated with PAC placement include almost all of those detailed in the section on CVP placement (see Central Venous Pressure Monitoring, above). The only exception is atrial or ventricular perforation, which has never been reported with balloon-tipped catheters. Additional complications unique to the PAC are detailed below.

Endobronchial Hemorrhage. Iatrogenic rupture of the pulmonary artery has become more common since the advent of PAC monitoring in the intensive care unit and the operating room. Over 30 cases have been recorded in the medical literature.[57] The incidence of pulmonary artery catheter-induced endobronchial hemorrhage is 0.06%–0.20%.[58, 59] Hannan et al reported a 46% mortality rate in a review of 28 cases of pulmonary artery catheters' induced endobronchial hemorrhage, but the mortality was 75% in the anticoagulated patients.[60] Several risk factors are evident in these reports: advanced age, female sex, pulmonary hypertension, mitral stenosis, coagulopathy, distal placement of the catheter, and balloon hyperinflation.

When forming a therapeutic plan, the etiology of the hemorrhage is an important consideration. If the hemorrhage is minimal and a coagulopathy coexists, correction of the coagulopathy may be the only necessary therapy. Protection of the uninvolved lung is of prime importance. Tilting the patient toward the affected side or performing an endobronchial intubation both protect the contralateral lung.[61] Proposed strategies for stopping the hemorrhage include the application of PEEP, placement of bronchial blockers, rigid or flexible bronchoscopy, injection of clotted blood through the PAC, hyperinflation of the PAC balloon, and pulmonary resection.[62]

The etiology of endobronchial hemorrhage may be unclear, but the bleeding site must be unequivocally located before surgical treatment is attempted. Unless the site of hemorrhage is known the clinician is at a disadvantage. A chest x-ray usually indicates the general location of the lesion, and a small amount of radiographic contrast dye helps to pinpoint the lesion if active hemorrhage is present.

Pulmonary Infarction. Currently this is a rare complication of PAC monitoring. An early report suggested that the incidence of pulmonary infarction with PAC use was 7.2%.[63] Continuous monitoring of the pulmonary arterial waveform and deflating the balloon when not determining the PCWP to prevent inadvertent catheter wedging were not standard practice at that time. Distal migration of PACs may occur intraoperatively as a result of the action of the right ventricle. Retraction on the heart may cause inadvertent catheter wedging during thoracic surgery with diminished right ventricular chamber size. Embolization of thrombus formed on a PAC could also result in pulmonary infarction.

Measurements Using Special Catheters

MIXED VENOUS OXYGEN SATURATION. The addition of fiberoptic bundles to the PAC has enabled the continuous monitoring of mixed venous oxygen saturation using reflectance spectrophotometry. The cardiac output (CO) computer is modified to include a light-emitting diode and a sensor to detect the light returning from the pulmonary artery. A calculation of mixed venous oxygen saturation is based on the absorbance of various light wavelengths by the blood in the pulmonary artery.[64]

Principles. The Fick equation states that oxygen consumption equals the CO multiplied by the difference between the arterial and mixed venous oxygen contents:

$$\dot{V}O_2 = CO \cdot [CaO_2 - CmvO_2] \qquad (10\text{-}2)$$

The effect of dissolved oxygen is negligible in the mixed venous blood. Thus mixed venous oxygen saturation closely correlates with mixed venous oxygen content.

A reduction in mixed venous oxygen saturation indicates one of the following situations:

1. Decreased CO.
2. Decreased arterial oxygen content.
3. Increased oxygen consumption.
4. Reduced oxygen carrying capacity (ie, as with decreased hemoglobin).

Basically, one can understand the value of SvO_2 with the analogy O_2 (oxygen) = $ (dollar). The ***income*** is equal to the oxygen delivery (CO, Hb, and oxygen saturation), the ***expenses*** are equal to oxygen consumption, while the remainder ***balance*** is equal to SvO_2 (Fig. 10-5).

Limitations. In vivo continuous monitoring of mixed oxygen saturation has been complicated by artifacts due to the vessel wall, loss of light intensity due to clot formation on the catheter, and varying hematocrit. Gettinger et al[65] demonstrated that a three-wavelength system (Opticath [Oximetrix Inc, Mountain View CA]) was more accurate than a two-wavelength system (Swan-Ganz [American Edwards Laboratories, Santa Ana CA]).

Clinical Applications. The mixed venous oxygen saturation provides a global estimation of the adequacy of oxygen delivery relative to the needs of the tissues. If other variables remain constant, changes in mixed venous oxygen saturation correlate directly with changes in cardiac output. Continuous monitoring of the mixed venous oxygen saturation in the vascular surgical patient could be justified in patients with severe anemia (eg, bleeding Jehovah's Witnesses) or any condition in which a continuous assessment of CO is necessary. The use of mixed oxygen saturation PACs for thoracic anesthesia has been reported by several authors.[66,67]

In a study by Thys et al,[67A] the value of continuous monitoring of mixed venous oxygen saturation during thoracic anesthesia was investigated. Changes in SvO_2 measured

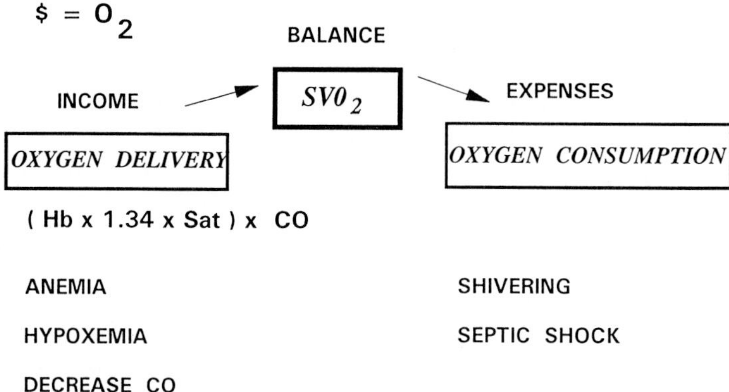

Figure 10-5. The value of SvO_2 can be understood with the analogy O_2 (oxygen) = $ (dollar). The *income* is equal to the oxygen delivery (CO, HB, and oxygen saturation), the *expenses* are equal to oxygen consumption), while the reminder *balance* is equal to SvO_2.

continuously with the fiberoptic pulmonary arterial catheter were found to be determined primarily by changes in oxygen saturation rather than by changes in cardiac output Fig. 10-6 and Fig. 10-7. In most instances the initiation of one-lung ventilation resulted in an increase in cardiac output to offset the hypoxemia. That increase in oxygen delivery was able to maintain SvO_2 relatively stable. A decrease in SvO_2, therefore, would indicate that the increase in oxygen delivery was smaller than when SvO_2 increased or remained unchanged.

Fig. 10-8 illustrates the simultaneous tracing of SvO_2 measurements, CO, and PaO_2 during two-lung ventilation and OLV. Fig. 10-8A: a reduction in SvO_2 is present with the initiation of OLV due to a decrease in PaO_2. Fig. 10-8B: Despite the reduction in PaO_2 with the initiation of OLV, SvO_2 increases secondary to a large increase in CO which maintained oxygen delivery.

RIGHT VENTRICULAR EJECTION FRACTION

Principles. The rapid-response thermistor PAC (American Edwards Laboratories, Santa Ana CA) incorporates three modifications from a standard pulmonary artery catheter:

1. A multihole injectate port located 21 cm from the catheter tip to aid complete mixing of the injectate in the right ventricle.
2. A thermistor incorporated into the catheter that responds approximately every 52 milliseconds (10 times more rapidly than a standard catheter).
3. Two ECG electrodes incorporated into the catheter that enable the CO computer to detect the R wave.

The technique described by Kay et al may be used for the determination of right ventricular ejection fraction (RVEF) by the thermodilution technique.[68] The catheter was floated so that the injectate port was 2 cm cephalad to the tricuspid valve in the right atrium.

With each injection, the end-diastolic temperature plateaus in the thermodilution curve are identified by the computer using the R-wave signal. RVEF is calculated from the exponential decay of the end-diastolic plateaus in the ther-

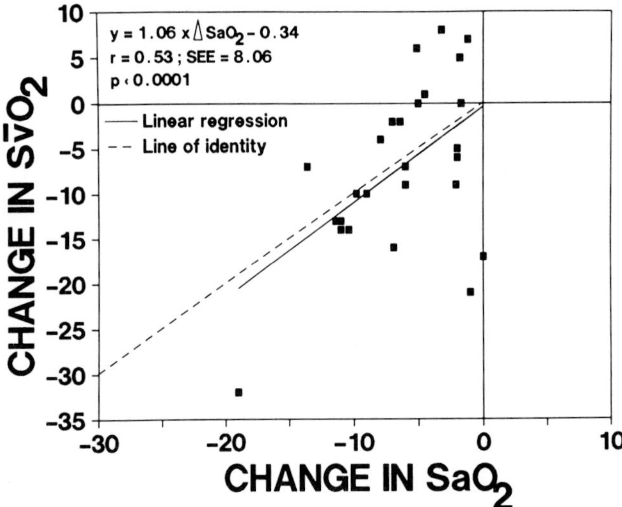

Figure 10-6. Correlation between the changes in SaO_2 (%) and $S\dot{V}O_2$ (%) after collapse of the non-dependent lung. SEE = standard error of the estimate. Reprinted with permission from Thys DM, Cohen E, Eisenkraft JB. Mixed venous oxygen saturation during thoracic anesthesia. Anesthesiology 1988;69:1007.

Figure 10-7. Correlation between the changes in cardiac index (CI; $1 \cdot min^{-1} \cdot m^{-2}$) and $S\dot{V}O_2$ (%) after collapse of the non-dependent lung. SEE = standard error of the estimate. Reprinted with permission from Thys DM, Cohen E, Eisenkraft JB. Mixed venous oxygen saturation during thoracic anesthesia. Anesthesiology 1988;69:1007.

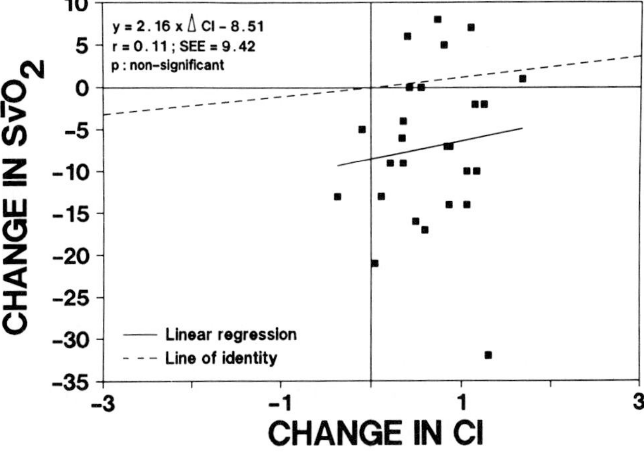

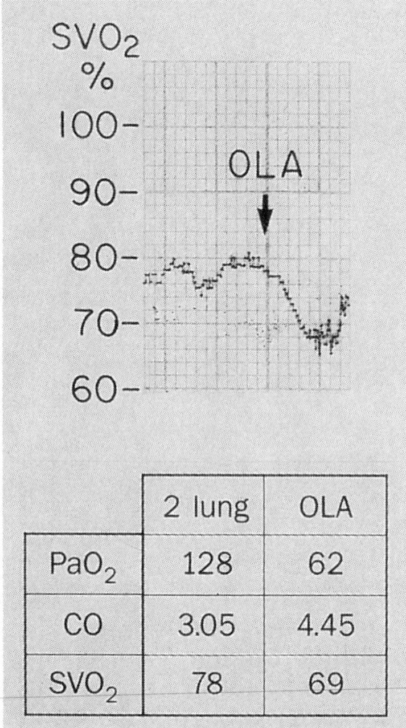

	2 lung	OLA
PaO_2	128	62
CO	3.05	4.45
SVO_2	78	69

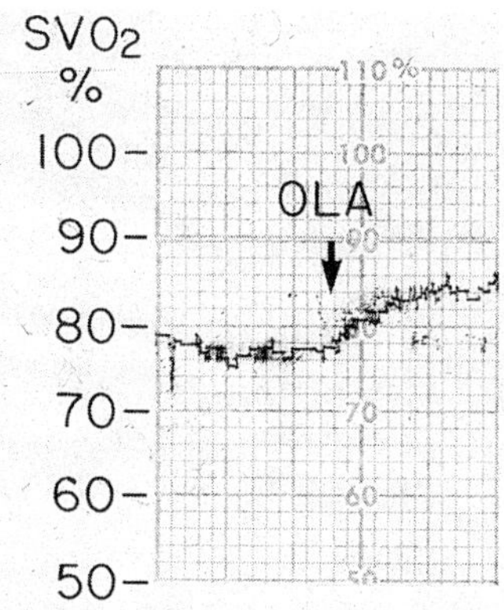

	2 lung	OLA
PaO_2	291	93
CO	4.37	7.73
SVO_2	82	87

Figure 10-8. The simultaneous tracing of SvO_2 measurements, CO, and PaO_2 during two-lung ventilation and OLV is illustrated. A. A reduction in SvO_2 is present with the initiation of OLV due to a decrease in PaO_2. B. Despite the reduction in PaO_2 with the initiation of OLV, SvO_2 increases secondary to a large increase in CO which maintained oxygen delivery.

modilution curve (Fig. 10-9). The difference in temperature between the baseline and the first end-diastolic plateau is defined as C_1, the difference between the baseline and the second plateau as C_2, etc. Residual fraction (RF), the portion of blood left in the ventricle at the end of systole, is calculated from the following equations:

(10-3) $RF_1 = C_2/C_1$

(10-4) $RF_2 = C_3/C_2$

(10-5) $RF_{mean} = (RF_1 + RF_2)/2$

The ejection fraction (EF) is calculated from the expression:

(10-6) $EF = 1 - RF_{mean}$

The heart rate (HR) is also measured by the computer from the catheter-ECG electrodes. The stroke volume (SV), right ventricular end-diastolic volume (RVEDV), and right ventricular end-systolic volume (RVESV) can be calculated using these data in the following equations:

(10-7) $SV = CO/HR$

(10-8) $RVEDV = SV/EF$

(10-9) $RVESV = RVEDV - SV$

Clinical Applications. The use of this type of RVEF monitoring can be justified in patients with severe right ventricular dysfunction due to infarction, pulmonary hypertension, left-sided

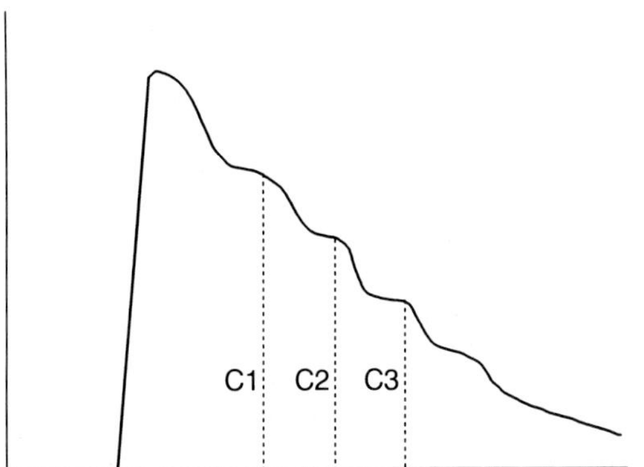

Figure 10-9. The thermodilution curve obtained from a rapid-response thermistor following the injection of a bolus of cold fluid into the right ventricle. The differences between the end-diastolic plateaus and the baseline temperature yield the constants C_1, C_2, and C_3, which may be used to calculate right ventricular ejection fraction. (See text.)

failure, or intrinsic pulmonary disease. This technique may be especially useful in thoracic procedures because of the additional strain placed on the right ventricle by increased afterload.

Limitations. Assumptions essential to the accuracy of this kind of RVEF monitoring include a regular ECG R wave-to-R wave (1) R-R interval to ensure consistent ejection fraction from beat to beat, "instantaneous" mixing of the injectate with the right ventricular blood, and absence of tricuspid regurgitation. Respiratory variations in pulmonary artery temperature may affect the accuracy of thermodilution measurements by changing the baseline temperature. The technique has been validated by comparison with radionuclide and angiographic determinations of RVEF.[69,70]

PACING CATHETERS

Electrode Catheters. The multipurpose PAC (Pacing TD Catheter [American Edwards Laboratories, Santa Ana CA]) contains five electrodes for bipolar atrial, ventricular, or atrioventricular (A-V) sequential pacing. This catheter may also be used for recording intracardiac ECG with appropriate filtering. The intraoperative success rate for atrial, ventricular, and A-V sequential capture has been reported to be 80%, 93%, and 73%, respectively.[71] Electrode detachment has been reported twice with the multipurpose catheter: with prolonged placement (60 hours)[72] and during catheter withdrawal.[73]

Wire Catheters. The Paceport and A-V Paceport catheters, recently introduced by American Edwards Laboratories (Santa Ana CA), both have lumens for the introduction of a ventricular wire (Paceport) or both atrial and ventricular wires (A-V Paceport) for temporary transvenous pacing. The incidence of atrial and ventricular pacing capture is expected to be higher with direct endocardial wire pacing, although data are not yet available. With thin pacing wires, the additional risk of atrial or ventricular perforation is also present.

Cardiac Output

INDICATOR DILUTION. The indicator dilution technique is based on the Fick principle but differs in one, a substance is injected into the circulation and two, its arrival is measured downstream. An amazing variety of substances, including water, methylene blue, tetanus antitoxin, and heavy water, have been injected into the circulation over the years in an attempt to measure CO.[74] The equation used to calculate CO by indicator dilution is known as the Stewart-Hamilton equation in recognition of the contribution of these two scientists to the development of the indicator dilution technique.

Principles. The indicator dilution theory is based on the observation that for a known amount of indicator introduced at one point in the circulation, an equal amount of indicator is detectable at some point downstream. Stewart and Hamilton established that the amount of indicator detected at the downstream point was equal to the product of CO and the change in indicator concentration over time. If the indicator is injected as a bolus, a recording of the indicator concentration over time produces a bell-shaped curve that is skewed to the left. The area under the curve represents the denominator in the Stewart-Hamilton equation. CO is thus equal to the amount of injected indicator divided by the area under the curve.

Thermodilution. The idea of a thermal indicator was introduced by Fegler in 1954,[75] who showed that the bolus injection of a cold solution in dogs resulted in a typical time-concentration curve. In addition, this study indicated that the principles developed by Stewart and Hamilton could be used for the determination of CO by injection of a thermal indicator. In his original publication Fegler concluded that the thermodilution method was more flexible than the dye dilution method and allowed a greater number of measurements to be made.

In 1968 Branthwaite and Bradley first reported the use of thermal indicator for the measurement of CO in humans.[76] These investigators mounted a thermistor on a long nylon catheter, guided this catheter into the pulmonary artery. They introduced a second, shorter catheter into the jugular vein and advanced until its tip was positioned near the junction of the superior vena cava and the right atrium. Curves of pulmonary artery temperatures were recorded following the injection of 10 cc of 5% dextrose at room temperature into the right atrium.

The need to place a thermistor in the pulmonary artery posed a problem. The reason for positioning the thermistor in the pulmonary artery rather than in a systemic vessel was that previous work had demonstrated that during the first passage of the cold bolus, considerable amounts of the indicator were absorbed by the heart and lung tissue. Since this indicator was then gradually released, the return to baseline of the thermistor temperature was prolonged, introducing substantial error into the CO calculations. With the subsequent development of the balloon-tipped, flow-directed, pulmonary arterial catheter, placement in the pulmonary artery became simple. In clinical practice, CO is now most commonly measured by the thermodilution technique.[77,78] When thermal indicator is used, the Stewart-Hamilton equation needs to be modified to take into account the particular characteristics of the indicator.

Early in the development of the thermodilution method, attempts were made to provide a continuous thermal signal and therefore continuous CO determinations. The initial experiments focused on the use of intravascular heating devices.[79,80] However, because heating blood is more dangerous than cooling it, the use of such devices was inherently more risky. As a result, very low amplitude heat signals were used, and separation of the introduced heat signal from background thermal variations became a major problem. More recently Philip et al have again explored the possibility of a continuous thermal signal.[81] With a very low power (5 W) sinusoidal thermal signal, the average increase in blood temperature was only about 0.02°C at typical flows. In both in vitro and in vivo conditions, the investigators obtained satisfactory correlations with conventional thermodilution over a wide range of COs.

DOPPLER TECHNIQUES: THE DOPPLER PULMONARY ARTERY CATHETER. A newly developed pulmonary artery catheter that incorporates an ultrasonic transducer is curved in such a way as to maintain contact with the wall of the pulmonary artery. Using the Doppler principle instantaneous stroke volume is calculated from the mean velocity of blood flow in the main pulmonary artery.[82] The accuracy of this technique is favorable when compared to an electromagnetic flow probe in tests using a bench model and an in vivo animal model.

The practicality of this device in clinical management is yet unproved. The high degree of accuracy, supported by clinical studies, is unlikely to result in changes in management. The additional cost may be prohibitive. However, the potential for research applications, such as investigations of right ventricular function and pulmonary vascular impedance, is promising.[83]

Transesophageal Echocardiography

PRINCIPLES. In echocardiography, the heart and great vessels are probed with ultrasonic waves, which are sound waves that are not audible to humans. The waves are sent into the thoracic cavity and is partially reflected by the cardiac structures. From these reflections, information on distance, velocity, and density of objects in the chest can be derived.[84] Images of the cardiac structures are constructed from the distance and density information. The flow within these structures is studied using the velocity information. With the development of transesophageal transducers, anesthesiologists have acquired the capability to apply echocardiography intraoperatively. Transesophageal echocardiography (TEE) is, however, not limited to anesthetized patients and is now widely used as a diagnostic tool in awake patients.[85]

CLINICAL APPLICATIONS

Thoracic Aortic Disease. Because of its posterior location, the thoracic aorta is difficult to image by transthoracic echocardiography. With TEE, however, most of the thoracic aorta is easy to visualize, with the exception of the arch vessels. As a result numerous investigators have explored the use of TEE in the diagnosis of thoracic aortic aneurysms and dissection. Erbel et al recently reported on the diagnostic accuracy of TEE in acute aortic dissection in 164 patients.[86] These researchers found that TEE had a 99% sensitivity and 98% specificity in diagnosing this condition. Other investigators have reported similar results, and many experts now consider TEE to be the diagnostic modality of choice in thoracic aortic pathology.[87–92] Images of the ascending aorta are obtained by advancing the esophageal probe with the ultrasonic array facing anteriorly. To visualize the descending aorta, the transesophageal probe is rotated 180 degrees. In thoracic aneurysms color flow Doppler helps to differentiate the true lumen from the false lumen, whereas in aortic dissection it may point to the site of an intimal tear.

The value of TEE during lung resection is expanding. TEE provides better imaging of the left atrium and the pulmonary veins than transthoracic echocardiography because of the proximity of the esophagus to the left atrium. TEE may therefore be useful in determining if there is cardiac involvement from a tumor originating in the pulmonary hilum. In addition, the extent of tumor invasion into the great vessels can be determined by TEE and may be the deciding factor for the extent and mode of resection. Neustein et al[92A] reported a case of left atrial invasion by a carcinoid tumor that changed the plan of the procedure to resection using a cardiopulmonary bypass (Fig. 10-10).

The limitation of the use of TEE during lung resection results from the difficulty to obtain a quantitative measurement of the right ventricle from the TEE image. In the left ventricle we can calculate the ejection fraction because it has a conical shape and formulas to calculate changes in volume are based on that assumption. The RV is wrapped around the LV and is mainly contracted to change its long axis. It is possible, however, to learn about the RV by the application of a pulse wave doppler to achieve a tracing of blood velocity over time. The slope of

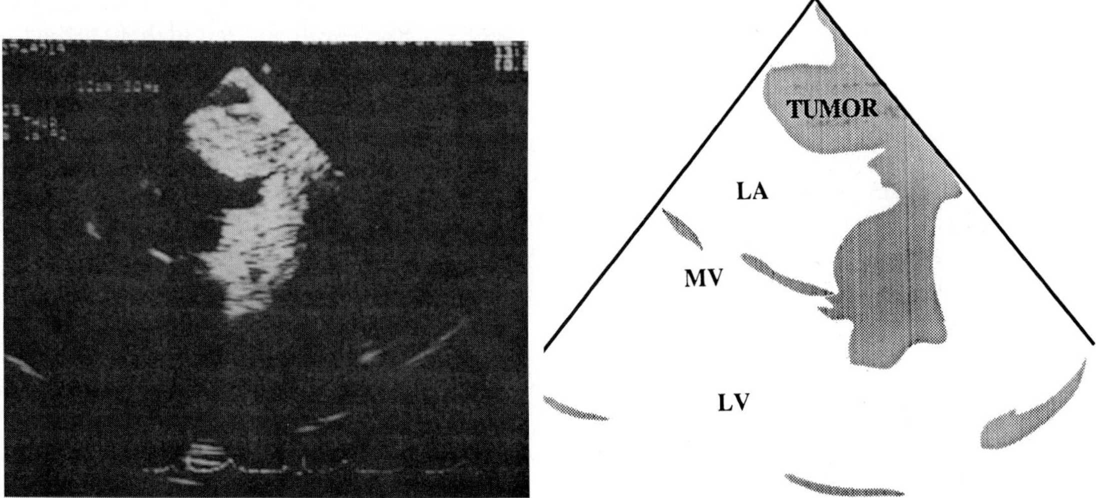

Figure 10-10. A. Longitudinal view transesophageal echocardiogram showing tumor invasion of the left atrium. B. Illustration of transesophageal echocardiogram seen in (A) in which the tumor is inside the left atrium (LA). The mitral valve (MV) and left ventricle (LV) are also illustrated. Reprinted with permission from Neustein SM, Cohen E, Reich D, Kirschner P. Transesophageal echocardiography and the intraoperative diagnosis of left atrial invasion by carcinoid tumor. Can J Anaesth 1993;40:665.

Figure 10-11. The application of a pulse wave doppler to achieve a tracing of blood velocity over time. The slope of the tracing, the maximal amplitude, and the relation to the ECG and the pulmonary artery pressures may provide some ideas of RV function.

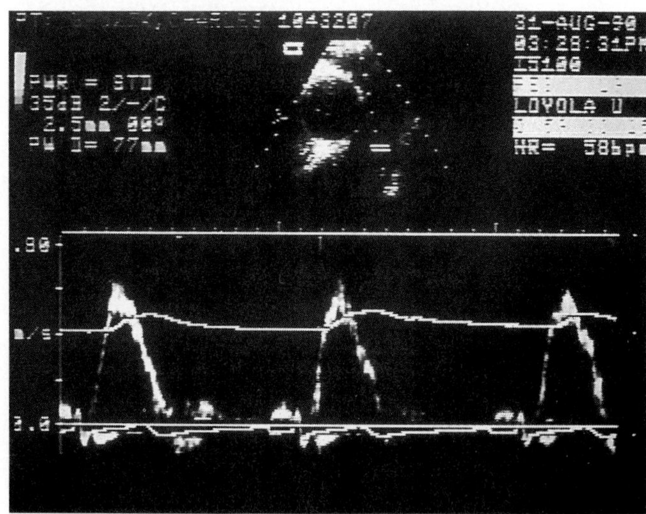

the tracing is the maximal amplitude and the relation to the ECG and the pulmonary artery pressures (Fig. 10-11). This may indirectly provide some idea of RV function.

COMPLICATIONS. TEE has been performed in many thousands of patients and has been remarkably free of complications thus far. Potential problems include damage to pharyngeal, laryngeal, esophageal, and gastric structures. Ruptures, tears, and hemorrhage are some possible complications. In two patients operated in the sitting position, vocal cord paresis has been attributed to the use of transesophageal echocardiography. O'Shea et al have evaluated the safety of transesophageal echo in animals by excising the entire esophagus after continuous TEE use of variable duration.[93] They observed no significant mucosal or thermal injury. In a study in humans, investigators found that the contact pressure between the transducer and the esophagus was low in five of six patients but markedly elevated (> 60 mmHg) in one patient.[94] Humphrey reported an unusual but interesting complication concerning a patient in whom manipulations of the transesophageal transducer led to the undetected displacement of an esophageal stethoscope into the stomach.[95] The errant stethoscope was discovered several weeks later was and was removed endoscopically.

References

1. Dripps RD, Eckenhoff JE, Vandam LD. Introduction to anesthesia, 7th ed. Philadelphia: WB Saunders, 1988:77.
2. Wallace CT, Baker JD, Alpert CC, et al. Comparison of blood pressure measurement by Doppler and by pulse oximetry techniques. Anesth Analg 1987; 66:1018.
3. Korotkoff NS. On the subject of methods of determining blood pressure. Bull Imperial Med Acad 1905;11:365.
4. Ramsey M. Noninvasive blood pressure monitoring methods and validation. In: Gravenstein JS, et al. eds. Essential noninvasive monitoring in anesthesia. Orlando: Grune & Stratton, 1980:37.
5. Hutton P, Prys-Roberts C. The oscillotonometer in theory and practice. Br J Anaesth 1982;54:581.
6. Ramsey M III. Noninvasive automatic determination of mean arterial pressure. Med Biol Eng Comput 1979;17:11.
7. Borrow KM, Newburger JW. Noninvasive estimation of central aortic pressure using the oscillometric method for analyzing systemic artery pulsatile blood flow: comparative study of indirect systolic, diastolic, and mean brachial artery pressure with simultaneous direct ascending aortic pressure measurements. Am Heart J 1982;103:879.
8. Friesen RH, Lichtor JL. Indirect measurement of blood pressure in neonates and infants utilizing an automatic noninvasive oscillometric monitor. Anesth Analg 1981;60:742.
9. Peñaz J. Photoelectric measurement of blood pressure volume and flow in the finger. Digest of 10th International Conference of Medical Biological Engineers, 1973:104.
10. Wesseling KH, van Bemmel R, van Dieren A, et al. Two methods for the assessment of hemodynamic parameters of epidemiology. Acta Cardiol 1978; 33:84.
11. Molhoek GP, Wesseling KH, Settels JJ, et al. Evaluation of the Peñaz servo-plethysmo-manometer for the continuous, noninvasive measurement of finger blood pressure. Basic Res Cardiol 1984;79:598.
12. Gravenstein JS, Paulus DA, Feldman J, et al. Tissue hypoxia distal to a Peñaz finger blood pressure cuff. J Clin Monit 1985;1:120.
13. Dorlas JC, Nijboer JA, Butijn T, et al. Effects of peripheral vasoconstriction on the blood pressure in the finger, measured continuously by a new noninvasive method (the Finapres). Anesthesiology 1985;62:342.
14. Bardoczky GI, Levarlet M, Engelman E, et al. Continuous noninvasive blood pressure monitoring during thoracic surgery. J Cardiothorac Vasc Anesth 1992;6:51.
15. Sy WP. Ulnar nerve palsy possibly related to the use of an automatically cycled blood pressure cuff. Anesth Analg 1981;60:687.
16. Van Bergen FH, Weatherhead DS, Treloar AE, et al. Comparison of indirect and direct methods of measuring arterial blood pressure. Circulation 1954; 10:481.

17. Bruner JMR, Krenis LJ, Dunsman JM, et al. Comparison of direct and indirect methods of measuring arterial blood pressure. Parts I, II, and III. Med Instrum 1981;15:11, 97, 182.
18. Kaplan JA. Hemodynamic monitoring. In: Kaplan JA, ed. Cardiac anesthesia. 2nd ed. Orlando: Grune & Stratton, 1987:183.
19. Ryan JF, Raines J, Dalton BC, et al. Arterial dynamics of radial artery cannulation. Anesth Analg 1973; 52:1015.
20. Remington JW, Wood EH. Formation of peripheral pulse contour in man. J Appl Physiol 1956;9:433.
21. Mozersky DJ, Buckley CJ, Hagood C, et al. Ultrasonic evaluation of the palmar circulation. Am J Surg 1973;126:810.
22. Allen EV. Thromboangiitis obliterans: methods of diagnosis of chronic occlusive arterial lesions distal to the wrist with illustrated cases. Am J Med Sci 1929;178:237.
23. Greenhow DE. Incorrect performance of Allen's test: ulnar artery flow erroneously presumed inadequate. Anesthesiology 1972;37:356.
24. Brodsky JB. A simple method to determine patency of the ulnar artery intraoperatively prior to radial artery cannulation. Anesthesiology 1975;42:626.
25. Nowak GS, Moorthy SS, McNiece WL. Use of pulse oximetry for assessment of collateral arterial flow. Anesthesiology 1986;64:527. Letter.
26. Slogoff S, Keats AS, Arlund C. On the safety of radial artery cannulation. Anesthesiology 1983;59:42.
27. Mangano DT, Hickey RF. Ischemic injury following uncomplicated radial artery catheterization. Anesth Analg 1979;58:55.
28. Barnes RW, Foster EJ, Janssen GA, et al. Safety of brachial artery catheters as monitors in the intensive care unit—prospective evaluation with the Doppler ultrasonic velocity detector. Anesthesiology 1976;44:260.
29. Pascarelli EF, Bertrand CA. Comparison of blood pressures in the arms and legs. N Engl J Med 1964; 270:693.
30. Barnes RW, Foster EJ, Janssen GA, et al. Safety of brachial arterial catheters as monitors in the intensive care unit: prospective evaluation with the Doppler ultrasonic velocity detector. Anesthesiology 44:260–264, 1976.
31. Gravlee GP, Wong AB, Adkins TG, et al. Comparison of radial, brachial, and aortic pressures after cardiopulmonary bypass. J Cardiothorac Anesth 1989; 3:20.
32. Gurman GM, Kriemerman S. Cannulation of big arteries in critically ill patients. Crit Care Med 1985; 13:217.
33. Yacoub OF, Bacaling JH, Kelly M. Monitoring of axillary arterial pressure in a patient with Buerger's disease requiring clipping of an intracranial aneurysm. Br J Anaesth 1987;59:1056.
34. Eriksson I, Jorulf H. Surgical complications associated with arterial catheterization. Scan J Thorac Cardiovasc Surg 1970;4:69.
35. Bedford RF. Invasive blood pressure monitoring. In: Blitt CD, ed. Monitoring in anesthesia and critical care medicine. New York: Churchill-Livingstone, 1989:93.
36. Youngberg JA, Miller ED. Evaluation of percutaneous cannulations of the dorsalis pedis artery. Anesthesiology 1976;44:80.
37. Husum B, Palm T, Eriksen J. Percutaneous cannulation of the dorsalis pedis artery. Br J Anaesth 1979; 51:1055.
38. Prian GW. New proximal approach works well in temporal artery catheterization. JAMA 1976;235: 2693.
39. Porter JM. Raynaud's Syndrome. In: Sabiston DC, ed. Textbook of surgery. Philadelphia: WB Saunders, 1985:1925.
40. Hurst JW, Schlant RC. Examination of veins. In: Hurst FW, Logue RB, eds. The heart. 4th ed. New York: McGraw-Hill, 1978:193.
41. Kaplan JA: Hemodynamic monitoring. In: Kaplan JA, ed. Cardiac anesthesia. Orlando: Grune & Stratton, 1987:185.
42. Mangano DT. Monitoring pulmonary arterial pressures in coronary artery disease. Anesthesiology 1980;53:364
43. Forrester J, Diamond G, Ganz W, et al. Right and left heart pressures in the acutely ill patient. Clin Res 1970;18:306.
44. Swan HJC, Ganz W, Forrester JS, et al. Catheterization of the heart in man with the use of a flow-directed balloon-tipped catheter. N Engl J Med 1970;283:447.
45. Lorzman J, Powers SR, Older T, et al. Correlation of pulmonary wedge and left atrial pressure: a study in the patient receiving positive end-expiratory pressure ventilation. Arch Surg 1974;109:270.
46. Manjuran RS. Relationship of pulmonary artery diastolic and pulmonary artery wedge pressures in mitral stenosis. Am Heart J 1975;89:207.
47. Lappas D, Lell WA, Gabel JC, et al. Indirect measurement of left-atrial pressure in surgical patients—

pulmonary capillary wedge and pulmonary artery diastolic pressures compared with left atrial pressure. Anesthesiology 1973;38:394.
48. Raper R, Sibbald WJ. Misled by the wedge? Chest 1986;89:427.
49. Nadeau S, Noble WH. Misinterpretation of pressure measurements from the pulmonary artery catheter. Can J Anaesth 1986;33:352.
50. West JB, Dellery CT, Nalmark A: Distribution of blood flow in isolated lung: relation to vascular and alveolar pressures. J Appl Physiol 1964;19:713.
51. Shasby DM, Dauber IM, Pfister S, et al. Swan-Ganz catheter location and left atrial pressure determine the accuracy of the wedge pressure when positive end-expiratory pressure is used. Chest 1980;80:666.
52. Teboul J-L, Zapol WM, Brun-Buisson C, et al. A comparison of pulmonary artery occlusion pressure and left ventricular end-diastolic pressure during mechanical ventilation with PEEP in patients with severe ARDS. Anesthesiology 1989;70:261.
52a. Cohen E, Neustein SM, Kirschner PA. Inadvertent transection of a pulmonary artery catheter during thoracic surgery. J Cardiothorc Vasc Anes 1993;7:337.
53. Schmitt EA, Brantigan CO. Common artifacts of pulmonary artery pressures: recognition and interpretation. J Clin Monit 1986;2:44.
54. Rao TLK, Jacobs KH, El-Etr AA. Reinfarction following anesthesia in patients with myocardial infarction. Anesthesiology 1983;59:499.
55. Moore CH, Lombardo TR, Allums JA, et al. Left main coronary artery stenosis: hemodynamic monitoring to reduce mortality. Ann Thorac Surg 1978; 26:445.
56. Tuman KJ, McCarthy RJ, Spiess BD, et al. Effect of pulmonary artery catheterization on outcome in patients undergoing coronary artery surgery. Anesthesiology 1989;70:199.
57. McDaniel DD, Stone JG, Faltas AN, et al. Catheter-induced pulmonary artery hemorrhage. J Thorac Cardiovasc Surg 1981;82:1.
58. Shah KB, Rao TLK, Laughlin S, et al. A review of pulmonary artery catheterization in 6245 patients. Anesthesiology 1984;61:271.
59. Dhamee MS, Pattison CZ. Pulmonary artery rupture during cardiopulmonary bypass. J Cardiothoracic Anesth 1987;1:51.
60. Hannan AT, Brown M, Bigman O. Pulmonary artery catheter-induced hemorrhage. Chest 1984;85:128.
61. Stein JM, Lisbon A. Pulmonary hemorrhage from pulmonary artery catheterization treated with endobronchial intubation. Anesthesiology 1981; 55:698.
62. Gourin A, Garzon AA. Operative treatment of massive hemoptysis. Ann Thorac Surg 1974;18:52.
63. Foote GA, Schabel SI, Hodges M. Pulmonary complications of the flow-directed balloon-tipped catheter. N Engl J Med 1974;290:927.
64. Krouskop RW, Cabatu EE, Chelliah BP, et al. Accuracy and clinical utility of an oxygen saturation catheter. Crit Care Med 1983;11:744.
65. Gettinger A, DeTraglia MC, Glass DD. In vivo comparison of two mixed venous saturation catheters. Anesthesiology 1987;66:373.
66. Thys DM, Cohen E, Eisenkraft JB. Mixed venous oxygen saturation during thoracic anesthesia. Anesthesiology 1988;6:1005.
67. Safran D, Journois D, Hubsch JP, et al. Surveillance continue de la SvO_2 au cours de l'anesthesie pour chirurgie pulmonaire. Ann Fr Anesth Reanim 1989; 8:682.
67A. Thys DM, Cohen E, Eisenkraft JB. Mixed venous oxygen saturation during thoracic anesthesia. Anesthesiology 1988;69:1005.
68. Kay HR, Afshari M, Barash P, et al. Measurement of ejection fraction by thermal dilution techniques. J Surg Res 1983;34:337.
69. Dhainaut JF, Brunet F, Monsallin J, et al. Bedside evaluation of right ventricular performance using a rapid computerized thermodilution method. Crit Care Med 1987;15:148.
70. Urban P, Scheidegger D, Gabathuler J, et al. Thermodilution determination of right ventricular ejection fraction: a comparison with biplane angiography. Crit Care Med 1987;15:652.
71. Zaidan J, Freniere S. Use of a pacing pulmonary artery catheter during cardiac surgery. Ann Thorac Surg 1983;35:633.
72. Macander PJ, Kuhnlein JL, Buiteweg J, et al. Electrode detachment: a complication of the indwelling pacing Swan-Ganz catheter. N Engl J Med 1986; 314:1711.
73. Heiselman DE, Maxwell JS, Petro V. Electrode displacement from a multipurpose Swan-Ganz catheter. PACE 1986;9:134.
74. Schreiner MS, Leksell LG, Neufeld GR. Evaluation of heavy water for indicator dilution cardiac output measurement. J Clin Monit 1989;5:236.
75. Fegler G. Measurement of cardiac output in anesthetized animals by a thermodilution method. Quart J Exp Physiol 1954;39:153.
76. Branthwaite MA, Bradley RD. Measurement of car-

diac output by thermal dilution in man. J Appl Physiol 1968;24:434.
77. Forrester JS, Ganz W, Diamond G, et al. Thermodilution cardiac output determination with a single flow-directed catheter. Am Heart J 1972;83:306.
78. Swan HJC, Ganz W, Forrester J, et al. Catheterization of the heart in man with use of a flow-directed balloon-tipped catheter. N Engl J Med 1970;283: 447.
79. Barankay T, Jansco T, Nagay S, et al. Cardiac output estimation by a thermodilution method involving intravascular heating and thermistor recording. Acta Physiol Hung 1970;38:167.
80. Khalil HH, Richardson TQ, Guyton AC. Measurement of cardiac output by thermal dilution and direct Fick methods in dogs. J Appl Physiol 1966; 21:1131.
81. Philip JH, Long MC, Quinn MD, et al. Continuous thermal measurement of cardiac output. IEEE Trans Biomed Eng 1984;31:393.
82. Segal J, Pearl RG, Ford AJ, et al. Instantaneous and continuous cardiac output obtained with a Doppler pulmonary artery catheter. J Am Coll Cardiol 1989; 13:1382.
83. Nishimura RA. Another measurement of cardiac output: is it truly needed? J Am Coll Cardiol 1989; 13:1393.
84. Konstadts S, Reich DL, thys DM, et al. Transesophageal echocardiography. In: Kaplan JA, ed. Cardiac anesthesia. 3rd ed. Philadelphia: WB Saunders, 1993:342.
85. Schiller NB, Maurer G, Ritter SB, et al. Transesophageal echocardiography. J Am Soc Echocard 1989; 2:354.
86. Erbel R, Rennollet H, Engberding R, et al. Detection of aortic dissection by transesophageal echocardiography. A multicenter cooperative study. Circulation 1988;78:II-297.
87. Mohr-Kahaly S, Erbel R, Steller D, et al. Aortic dissection detected by transesophageal echocardiography. Int J Card Imaging 1987;2:31.
88. Borner N, Erbel R, Braun B, et al. Diagnosis of aortic dissection by transesophageal echocardiography. Am J Cardiol 1984;54:1157.
89. Mohr-Kahaly S, Rennollet H, Wittlich N, et al. Follow-up of aortic dissection by transesophageal color Doppler echocardiography. Circulation 1987; IV-37.
90. Gussenhoven EJ, Taams MA, De Jong N, et al. Transesophageal echo in the diagnosis of thoracic aortic pathology. Circulation 1988;78:II-298.
91. Chan KL. Aortic disease in suspected aortic dissection—a transesophageal echo study. Circulation 1988;78:II-298.
92. Freeman WK, Khanderia BK, Oh JK, et al. Thoracic aortic pathology by transesophageal echocardiography. Circulation 1988;78:II-298.
92A. Neustein SM, Cohen E, Reich D, Kirschner P. Transesophageal echocardiography and the intraoperative diagnosis of left atrial invasion by carcinoid tumor. Can J Anaesth 1993;40:664.
93. O'Shea J, D'Ambra M, Magro C, et al. Transesophageal echocardiography: is it safe to the esophagus? An in vivo study. Circulation 1988;78:II-1756.
94. Urbanowicz JH, Kernoff RS, Oppenheim G, et al. Transesophageal echocardiography and its potential for esophageal damage. Anesthesiology 1990; 72:40.
95. Humphrey LS. Esophageal stethoscope loss complicating transesophageal echocardiography J Cardiol Thorac Anesth 1988;2:356.

CHAPTER

11

Positioning and Complications of the Supine and Lateral Positions

Leslie J. Weiss-Bloom

The patient who is undergoing thoracic surgery presents many challenges to the anesthesiologist. The initial positioning the patient on the operating table is of prime importance. The placement of both noninvasive and invasive monitoring devices and the induction of general anesthesia are also critical. These patients often have significant medical problems in addition to the ailment that brings them to the operating room. The importance of proper monitoring cannot be overemphasized, and the importance of a smooth and uneventful induction of anesthesia cannot be minimized. One remaining problem may be more difficult to solve. The anesthesiologist must supervise the movement of the anesthetized patient into the final operating position to allow the operating team optimal access to the surgical target.

This final position should give the surgeon good exposure and access to the pathologic lesion without causing any undue stress or pressure on the patient. To minimize complications relating to position on the operating table, the surgeon and the anesthesiologist may need to compromise. The surgeon prefers that the patient be in the position that allows the best operative exposure. The anesthesiologist must ensure that this position is obtained safely without compromising the cardiorespiratory stability or inducing neurologic or pressure-related injuries. On the other hand, if the position is not as the surgeon desires, then inadequate surgical exposure may unnecessarily prolong and complicate the procedure, which could lead to a suboptimal result. The surgeon must ensure that the planned approach to the pathologic lesion does not require that the patient be placed in a position that exceeds his or her tolerance; in some instances the operation may need to be delayed until the patient is hemodynamically stable.

These considerations should be contemplated before the patient arrives in the operating room. Decisions must also be made on an individual basis, as physiologic tolerances of various positions differ for each patient. The patient must be examined in advance to discover such limitations. Once general anesthesia has been induced, the concomitant attenuation of the pain response permits the patient to be positioned in such a way that might be intolerable for the patient if awake. A position-related injury is likely to occur in such an event. This devastating injury may significantly hinder the patient's recovery or result in a residual motor or sensory deficit.

The surgeon, circulating nurse, and anesthesiologist must combine efforts and skills to safeguard the patient. The anesthesiologist is ultimately responsible for the patient's well-being after induction of anesthesia. Therefore knowledge of proper positioning techniques is a prerequisite for caring for these patients.

Preoperative Assessment

The ability of the patient to sustain the optimal operating position without injury must be assessed during the preoperative visit. The anesthesiologist must confer with the surgeon in advance of this visit so he or she knows which position is planned for surgery. Preexisting anatomic limitations should be identified and evaluated. The neck of a patient with a cervical radiculopathy or the back of a patient with a lumbar radiculopathy of some patients must be examined to determine the allowable range of motion without neurologic symptoms. Any limitations should be carefully noted. The patient may need to wear a supporting brace (eg, cervical collar) to ensure that these limitations are not exceeded after induction of general anesthesia. The unfortunate patient with an unstable cervical radiculopathy may require an awake endotracheal intubation to ensure that no neurologic damage occurs to the cervical spinal cord or nerve roots during head and neck manipulation for direct laryngoscopy. If the patient is to be repositioned after general anesthesia is induced, then a cervical collar is still recommended to prevent extreme torsion of the head and neck.

One of the simplest methods of testing the patient's ability to tolerate the planned operating position is to have the patient assume this position while awake.[1] However, this generally reliable method of assessment has certain important limitations. The ability of the patient to achieve the desired position comfortably is reassuring. In a patient with a lumbar radiculopathy, the back and hips should be comfortably aligned in the proposed operating position while the patient is awake. After general anesthesia is induced, this same position may then be used, and the risk of aggravating the lumbar radiculopathy is minimized. The patient may be injured while being moved into the proposed position, however. In addition postoperative backache may occur despite proper positioning, since backache is a function of the duration that the patient is subjected to postural stress by being immobile on the operating table.[2] The patient may complain of back discomfort postoperatively even if positioned properly.

Physiology of Positioning the Anesthetized Patient

The patient is brought to the operating room and is guided onto the operating table in the supine position. Appropriate monitoring devices are placed, and the patient is made ready for the induction of general anesthesia. The head should be elevated approximately 10 cm and extended at the atlanto-occipital joint, described as the "sniffing position," to facilitate adequate visualization of the larynx and vocal cords for endotracheal or endobronchial intubation. The arms should be secured either on arm boards, which may need to be removed later or at the patient's sides. Once the patient is appropriately anesthetized, the position of the endotracheal tube is confirmed and secured, the corneas are protected, and all the monitoring devices are in place, the patient is ready to be moved into the final operating position.

If the patient is to be moved from the supine position, careful attention must be paid to hemodynamic monitoring. Several reflex mechanisms maintain hemodynamic stability in the healthy, awake patient. These including the baroreceptor or pressor receptor feedback mechanism, the central nervous system ischemic mechanism, and the chemoreceptor mechanism.[3] All of these reflexes act rapidly so that any change in arterial pressure will be counteracted within seconds.

The baroreceptors provide the most sensitive reflex protection against rapid swings in systemic blood pressure. These nerve endings located in the walls of large systemic arteries are most highly concentrated in the carotid arteries (carotid sinuses) and the aortic arch. Increased pressure causes stretching of these nerves with resultant increased impulse transmission via Hering's nerves to the glossopharyngeal nerves from the carotid sinuses or via the vagus nerves from the aortic arch. This inhibits the medullary vasoconstrictor center and excites the vagal center. Vasodilatation, decreased inotropy, and decreased chronotropy cause a reduction in systemic blood pressure. The baroreceptors are keenly sensitive to rapidly changing pressure.

The other two mechanisms guard against extreme hypotension. The central nervous system ischemic mechanism refers to the profound sympathetic stimulation that occurs in response to ischemia of the vasomotor center. The chemoreceptor mechanism is mostly concerned with respiratory control; it also plays a role in pressure control, however. Chemoreceptors are cells located in the carotid and aortic bodies that are stimulated by decreased oxygen supply and increased carbon dioxide and hydrogen ion concentration. Decreased systemic pressure with a concomitant decrease in blood flow excites these chemoreceptors, which then stimulate the vasomotor center. Vasomotor excitation raises the arterial pressure. The afferent limb of this reflex travels with the afferent limb of the baroreceptor reflex.[3]

Induction of general anesthesia attenuates and may abolish these protective reflexes. Therefore a change in arterial pressure, as would likely occur upon changing the patient's position, is not counteracted by the usual physiologic reflex responses, and, significant hypotension may occur. If this hypotension persists, vigilant monitoring and prompt treatment of hemodynamic aberrations are important to prevent untoward reactions. Careful, slow, steady movements of the patient, as opposed to quick and abrupt postural changes, may lessen any potential hemodynamic instability.[4]

These considerations must be remembered at the conclusion of the procedure as well when the patient is returned to the supine position. While being moved the patient remains at risk for hemodynamic instability. Special consideration should be given to the care of any chest tubes, if present. Sufficient slack should exist so that the tube does not become dislodged or kinked when turning the patient. Kinking may result in the accumulation of fluid within the chest and the development of either a tension pneumothorax or tension hemothorax.

The Lateral Decubitus Position

The lateral decubitus position is the most commonly used position for thoracic surgery. In this positon the posterior lateral incision, the most common thoracic incision, is performed (Fig. 11-1). The side named represents the side of the patient that contacts the plane on which the patient lies. For example, the right lateral decubitus position refers to the position where the right side of the patient touches the operating table and the patient's left side is exposed.

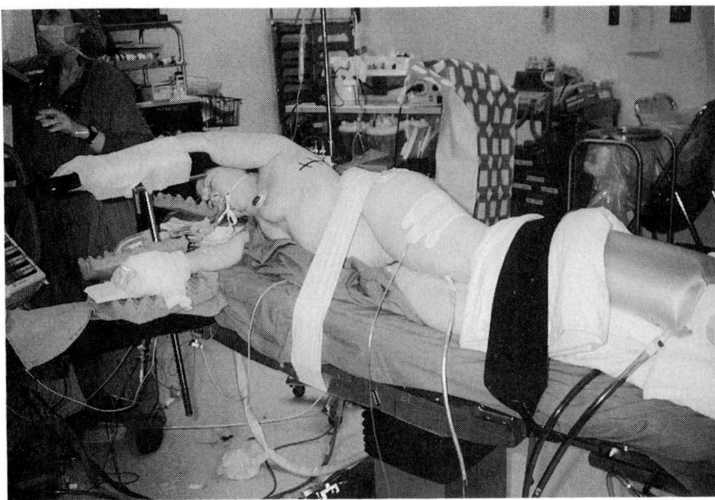

Figure 11-1. The lateral decubitus position, most commonly used for thoracic surgery. In this position, the most common thoracic incision, the posterior lateral incision, is performed.

The right lateral decubitus position is used for a left-sided thoracotomy.

Moving the Patient Into Position

Movement from the supine to the lateral decubitus position requires the coordinated efforts of at least four people. At least one person should be on each side of the patient, one at the feet, and the anesthesiologist at the head. The anesthesiologist must remain at the head to direct the others individuals so that all lifts and turns are synchronized. All movements must be designed so that all persons involved understands the plan and moves the patient slowly and smoothly in the desired direction. The movement of large patients and patients with joint instability requires more than four people.

Before directing any position change, the anesthesiologist must be confident that the endotracheal or endobronchial tube and all monitors are adequately secured. The fact that moving the patient's head and neck will almost certainly cause the endotracheal tube to move within the trachea must be appreciated. Flexing the head will result in cephalad movement of the trachea, causing the tip of an endotracheal tube to move closer to the carina. Extending the head will cause the tip to move further away from the carina. The friction generated by this movement of the tube within the trachea is a very potent stimulus, therefore an adequate level of anesthesia must be achieved prior to any position change. Unexpected, involuntary, patient movement at this point can cause accidental extubation, dislodgement of monitors or intravenous lines, or mechanical trauma. The use of muscle relaxants before the move is highly recommended.

The anesthesiologist should be at the patient's head to direct and coordinate the move, as well as to control the patient's head, neck, and airway. All persons involved in the move must act together. To position the patient in the right lateral decubitus position, the patient is lifted and first moved to his or her left. The right side of the patient should lie over the midline of the operating table. The shoulders and hips must remain in line to avoid torsion of the spinal cord with resultant neurologic damage.[5] The right arm should be abducted 90 degrees and placed on an arm board. The left side is then lifted until the patient's back is perpendicular to the operating table. The left arm may also be abducted 90 degrees and placed over the right arm with adequate padding between them (Fig. 11-2A, B). At this point, the anesthesiologist may proceed with an intrathecal injection (ie, intrathecal narcotic injection) if this procedure was previously planned. The hips and shoulders must then be secured in position. Thick tape can be used for this purpose. The importance of firmly securing the position cannot be overemphasized, because the operating table may need to be rotated during the procedure to aid the surgeon gain better anatomic exposure.

Assuring the Safety of the Patient in Position

Once the patient is on his or her side, care must be taken to ensure that each pressure point is protected and that no points that receive undue tension. The head must be supported so that the neck remains in the neutral position. Extreme flexion or rotation of the neck may result in postoperative stiffness and pain that can be quite severe, especially in the arthritic patient. Excessive lateral displacement of the head may impede jugular venous drainage. Head rotation also places the dependent eye in jeopardy of being in a weight bearing position (Fig. 11-3).

Additional precautionary measures must be taken to ensure that the pinna of the dependent ear lies flush with the pad below. Proper padding with a foam sponge distributes the weight evenly and avoids increased pressure to any particular part of the head. The head can be lifted and its position adjusted slightly at several points during the procedure to change its weight distribution. This helps to prevent the development of pressure alopecia.[6] Care must also be taken so that the head is not resting on any monitoring or intravenous lines.

The shoulders and arms of the patient in the lateral decubitus position must be carefully positioned to maintain adequate blood flow and avoid nerve damage. A rolled sheet should be placed just caudad to the dependent axilla to relieve the axilla and shoulder from bearing the weight of the thorax. This sheet also prevents the contents of the axilla from being compressed against the rib cage. It is imperative that this sheet is used to support the axilla and not be placed in the axilla.

The adequacy of placement and size of this axillary roll can be confirmed by comparing the contour of the radial arterial pressure waveform in the lateral decubitus position with the one obtained in the supine position. Axillary arterial compression appears as a damped tracing and represents compression of the axillary artery. If such compression occurs, then other structures within the axilla are likely to be squeezed together as well. For this reason, the radial arterial pressure monitoring line should be placed on the dependent side, unless this is otherwise contraindicated, to serve as a monitor of blood flow to the dependent arm. The pulse oximeter should not be relied upon for this purpose because its electronically adjusted waveform is an unreliable detector of changes in blood flow. If these precautions are used, the contents of the axilla should be relatively free of compression; however, some degree of venous or lymphatic compression may still exist. Ideally, the intravenous catheter should be placed in the nondependent arm.

An improperly placed axillary roll can have catastrophic consequences. Compression of the axillary artery may not be evident on the arterial waveform, because subtle changes may not be

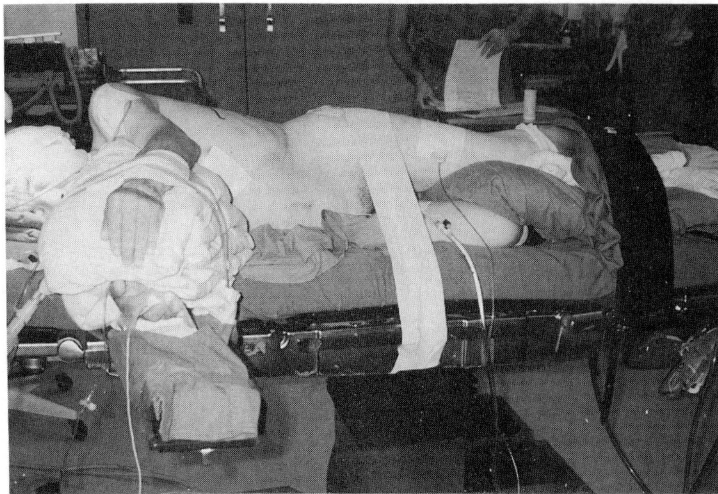

A

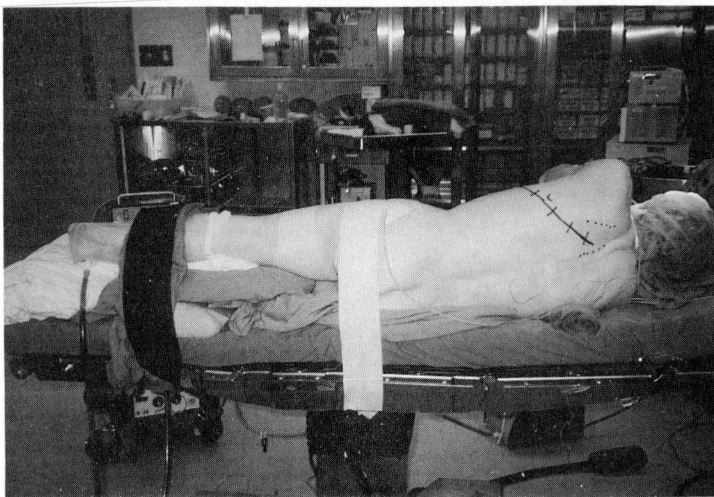

B

Figure 11-2. A front view of the right lateral decubitus position for left thoracotomy. Note that the shoulders and hips are in line to avoid spinal cord injuries. The left arm is abducted 90 degrees and placed on an arm board. The right arm is lifted until the patient's back is perpendicular to the operating table. A. The padding between the arms is from blankets or foam. B. The arm rests on a padded superior arm board. There is a wide adhesive strap to fix the patient's hips, and a safety table strap around the thighs. The superior leg is straight while the inferior is flexed. Finally, sheets or towels are placed to fill the waistline contour.

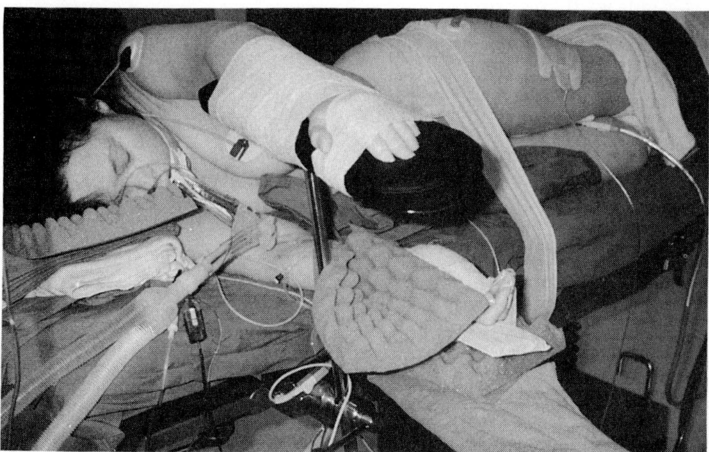

Figure 11-3. The head is protected to remain in neutral position in a straight line with the longitudinal axis of the body. Extreme flexion, extension or lateral rotation may result in stiffness, pain, or impede jugular venous return. The pinna of the dependent ear should be protected with a foam pad. No pressure should be applied to the taped eyes.

noticed. Compression for prolonged periods may result in ischemic damage to the poorly perfused arm. This condition can be assessed by making intermittent checks of capillary refill in the dependent hand. If capillary refill becomes prolonged and no other explanation is obvious (eg, vasoconstriction secondary to hypothermia), then the arm should be repositioned. A slight adjustment of the axillary roll often corrects the situation. The surgeon must be informed in advance of any movement to avoid unnecessary trauma caused by operating on a "moving target."

Even without compression of the axillary artery, an improperly placed axillary roll can result in severe compression of other structures. This danger is difficult to monitor, because damage may not become evident until the effects are considerable. Extensive swelling of the pectoral, deltoid, and other muscles around the shoulder can occur. This may result in an axillary compression syndrome with neurapraxia and require surgical decompression.[7] An improperly placed axillary roll can also result in suprascapular nerve injury. Ventral circumduction of the dependent shoulder can cause this nerve to be injured and lead to postoperative shoulder pain.[8]

The arms should be flexed at the shoulder not more than 90 degrees. This limit is necessary to avoid tension on the brachial plexus. Since the brachial plexus is anchored to the transverse processes of the cervical vertebrae in the neck and is located near mobile, bony structures, it is susceptible to stretch- and compression-related injuries during general anesthesia.[9] Injuries to the plexus usually result from excessive separation of the neck and shoulder. Paralysis of the musculature and loss of sensation in the upper limb is characteristic of such injuries.[10]

The arms may either remain straight or be flexed at the elbow (Fig. 11-4A, B). A supporting structure for them to rest on is required. Since the radial nerve is at risk for compression injury as it traverses the spiral sulcus of the humerus,

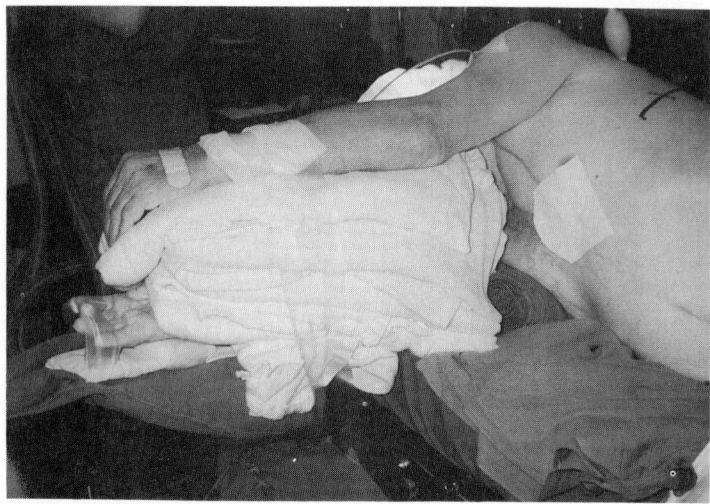

A

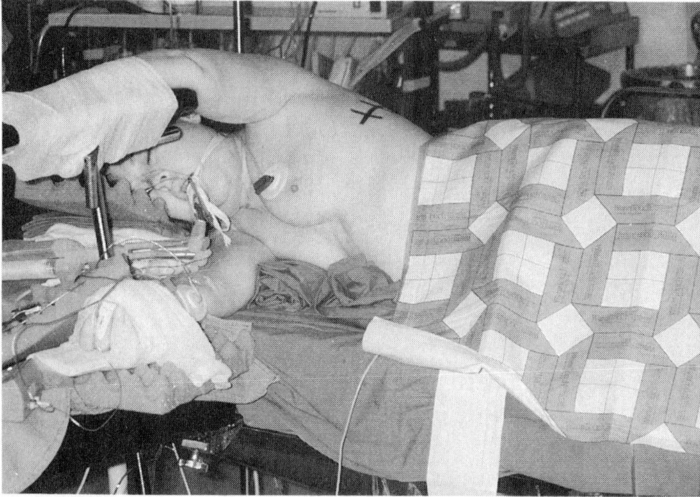

B

Figure 11-4. A detailed view of the upper body pressure points using a blanket for protection (A) or an arm board (B) between the arms. Note that all pressure points are padded. A foam pad is placed between the patient's arm and the metal bar of the arm board. This will avoid any pressure on the arms or potential ulnar nerve injury. An axillary roll is placed under the axilla to protect against excessive pressure or tension on the brachial nerve plexus and to maintain adequate blood flow to the dependent arm. (See text for more detail.)

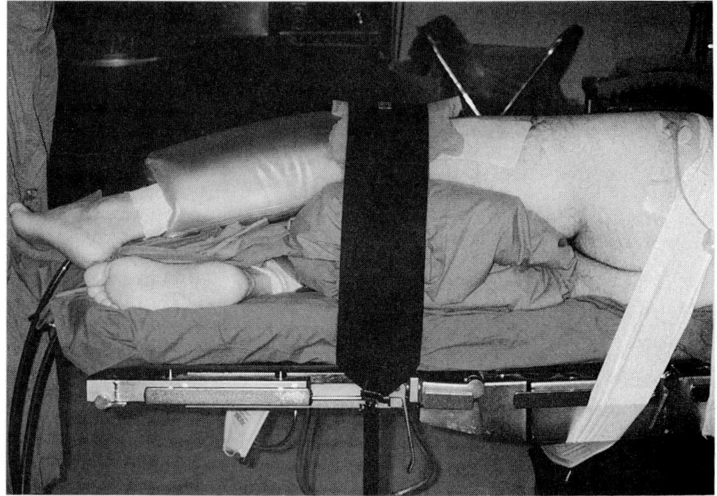

A

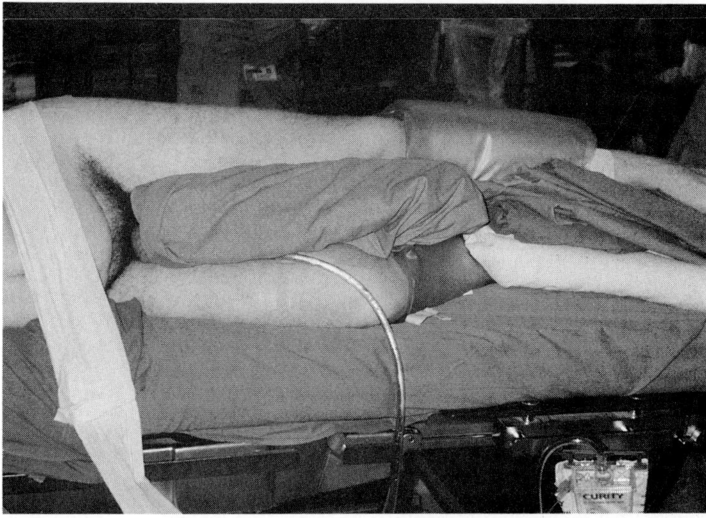

B

Figure 11-5. Anterior (A) and posterior (B) views of the lower body position with protection of the lower extremities. The dependent thigh is flexed; the upper leg is straight with padding between it and the lower leg. The presence of pulses in the lower extremities should be assured. The legs are well padded and protected from compression or direct contact with the metal part of the operating room table to avoid peroneal nerve injury (postoperative drop leg). Venodyne boots are placed on the legs to reduce the incidence of deep vein thrombosis and pulmonary embolism.

the level of the arm support to be at the same level as the table. Damage to the radial nerve at the level of the spiral sulcus results in the inability to straighten or extend the wrist (ie, wrist drop). Care must be taken to protect the ulnar nerve of the dependent arm if the arms are to be flexed at the elbows. The ulnar nerve is the most common nerve to sustain injury during anesthesia.[11] Compression injury to this nerve is likely if the medial epicondyle is placed near the edge of the table. To avoid this, the forearm must not be pronated. Postoperative ulnar neuropathy is manifested by inability to abduct or adduct the medial four digits and impaired flexion and adduction of the wrist. This condition is associated with a persistent, severe deficit. When the injury is due to compression at the cubital tunnel, the poor prognosis with either medical or surgical treatment is poor.[11]

Once the dependent arm is in proper position, the nondependent arm may be rested above it. Padding should be placed between the two arms. Proper function of the intravenous line should be confirmed once the arms are in their final position.

The legs should be positioned next (Fig. 11-5A, B). The dependent thigh should be flexed slightly at the hip and knee. The upper leg is left straight with padding between it and the lower leg. As in the pulse in the dependent limb should be verified as it was in the upper arm. Undue pressure in the groin can cause compression of the femoral triangle with resultant vascular compromise. Complications from compression of the dependent leg include transient paresthesias, massive swelling of the thigh with myonecrosis, acute renal failure secondary to myoglobinuria, and arterial insufficiency requiring below-the-knee amputation.[12] The presence of a pulse in the lower foot and proper padding between the legs to ensure that the weight of the upper leg is evenly distributed should reduce the risk of these devastating complications. The most common nerve to be injured in the leg is the common peroneal nerve. It may be compressed against a poorly padded operating table and the lateral aspect of the proximal fibula of the dependent leg.[13] This damage is manifested as postoperative foot drop.

Venodyne boots are wrapped around the legs. These boots are inflated and deflated periodically during the procedure. They have been found to reduce the incidence of deep vein

Figure 11-6. An inflatable sand bag is placed under the patient for positioning. When attached to suction, the sand inside the bag will harden and the bag will assume position around the patient's body.

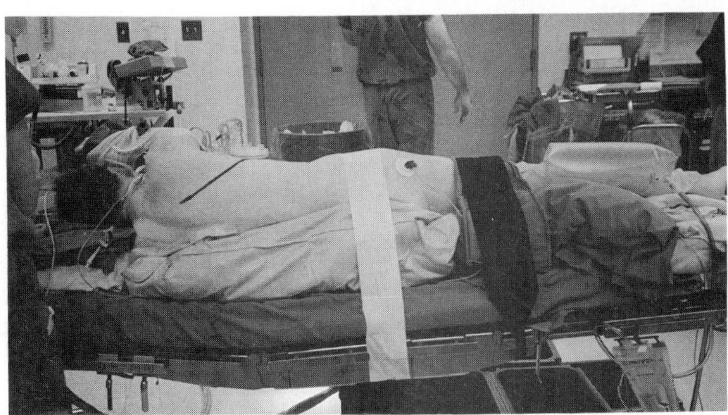

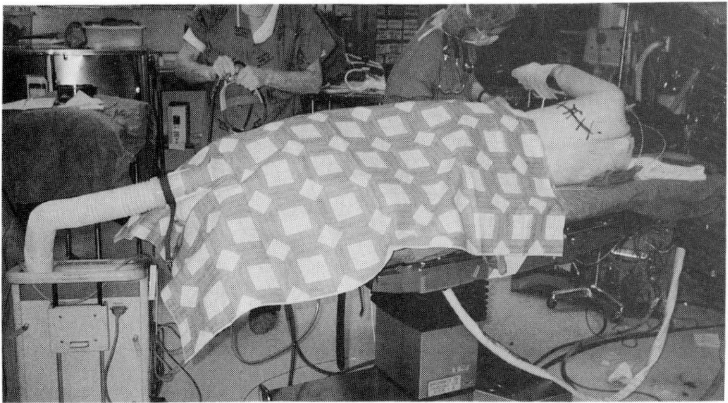

Figure 11-7. A warm air blanket that can be placed on the patient prior to draping. This device is efficient in conserving the patient's body temperature and rewarming during the thoracotomy.

thrombosis or pulmonary embolism. Proper position of the patient can be achieved with an inflatable sand bag. When attached to suction, the sand inside the bag will harden and the bag will assume position around the patient's body (Fig. 11-6). Finally, once the patient is in position, body temperature can be conserved with the use of a forced warm air blanket that can be placed on the lower part of the patient's body prior to placement of the drapes (Fig. 11-7).

Once in proper position the hips should be straight; they should be secured with a strap or with tape. The patient is now in the final operating position. Before the sterile preparation of the surgical field is begun, the correct placement of the endotracheal or endobronchial tube should be verified.

The Supine Position

In several instances (eg, median sternotomy, bilateral intercostal transverse sternotomy, anterior incisions) the thoracic surgeon requests that the patient be in the supine position during the surgery. Often the surgeon asks that a roll of sheets be placed under the patient's shoulders in order to facilitate operative exposure. The anesthesiologist must make certain that the patient's head is adequately supported and that the neck is not hyperextended in this position. Padding should be placed under the head to prevent such extension. Pressure alopecia is a concern during prolonged procedures, so the head should be placed on a foam sponge so that its weight is evenly distributed.[6] The arms may be either placed at the sides or on arm board extensions to the operating table. Proper precautions should be taken to guard against neurologic and pressure-related injuries. Once the patient is in the final operating position, proper placement of the endotracheal or endobronchial tube should be confirmed before he operation begins.

References

1. Martin JT. General aspects of safe positioning for the surgical patient. In: Martin JT, ed. Positioning in anesthesia and surgery. 2nd ed. Philadelphia: WB Saunders, 1987:9.

2. Brown EM, Elman DS. Postoperative backache. Anesth Analg 1961;40:683.
3. Guyton AC. Textbook of medical physiology. 6th ed. Philadelphia: WB Saunders, 1981:248.
4. Little DM Jr. Posture and anaesthesia. Can J Anaesth 1960;7:2.
5. Lawson NW. The lateral decubitus position: anesthesiologic consideration. In: Martin JT, ed. Positioning in anesthesia and surgery. 2nd ed. Philadelphia: WB Saunders, 1987:163.
6. Lawson NW, Mills NL, Ochsner JL. Occipital alopecia following cardiopulmonary bypass. J Thorac Cardiovasc Surg 1976;71:342.
7. Nambisan RN, Karakousis CP. Axillary compression syndrome with neurapraxia due to operative positioning. Surgery 1989;105:449.
8. Martin JT. Patient positioning. In: Barash PG, Cullen BF, Stoelting RK, eds. Clinical anesthesia. Philadelphia: JB Lippincott, 1989:656.
9. Lawson NW. The lateral decubitus position: anesthesiologic considerations. In: Martin JT, ed. Positioning in anesthesia and surgery. 2nd ed. Philadelphia: WB Saunders, 1987:174.
10. Moore KL. Clinically oriented anatomy. Baltimore: Williams & Wilkins, 1980:698.
11. Miller RG, Camp PE. Postoperative ulnar neuropathy. JAMA 1979;242:1636.
12. Smith JW, Pellicci PM, Sharrock N, et al. Complications after total hip replacement, the contralateral limb. J Bone Joint Surg 1989;71:528.
13. Lawson NW. The lateral decubitus position: anesthesiologic considerations. In: Martin JT, ed. Positioning in anesthesia and surgery. 2nd ed. Philadelphia: WB Saunders, 1987:177.

CHAPTER

12

Separation of the Lungs

Jay B. Brodsky

The development of the thoracic surgery has closely paralleled the evolution of a variety of anesthetic techniques that have allowed for effective separation of the lungs (Table 12-1). An understanding of how to use these techniques, the advantages of each specific method, their potential complications, and the physiologic changes that occur in single lung ventilation are the the basis for the safe practice of anesthesia in thoracic surgery.

Intentional separation of the lungs was first performed during surgery in 1931 when Gale and Waters advanced an uncuffed endotracheal tube into the bronchus.[1] The inflated cuff not only sealed off the airway of the intubated ventilated lung but also extended into the carina, thus obstructing the bronchus of the operated lung. Blocking the airway caused lung tissue distal to the obstruction to collapse which improved operating conditions for the surgeon.

All early techniques for separation of the lungs involved some method of bronchial blockade (Fig. 12-1). Selective airway blockade has been accomplished in many, often ingenious, ways. For example, Crafoord obstructed the bronchus by stuffing a gauze tampon through a rigid bronchoscope down into the airway.[2] A variety of rubber blockers with inflatable distal balloons were used in the past,[3–7] but these have now been almost completely replaced by plastic balloon-tipped catheters.[8–10] An endotracheal tube with a small, anterior channel containing another small tube with a bronchial balloon blocker is the most recent approach to bronchial blockade.[11–14]

In the past single-lumen bronchial tubes, both single-cuffed and double-cuffed, were often used in place of bronchial blockers. (In emergency situations, an uncut endotracheal tube advanced into the bronchus continues to be an excellent means of ventilating the patient with unilateral airway hemorrhage.) Like many of these tubes, Rovenstine's double-cuffed, single-lumen tube was a forerunner of the double-cuffed, double-lumen tubes now in use (Fig. 12-1). The tube was advanced into the bronchus of the lung to be ventilated.[15] When only the upper tracheal cuff was inflated, both lungs could be ventilated. When the lower cuff was inflated it blocked the trachea across the carina so only the intubated lung was ventilated; the nonintubated, operated lung collapsed. Other single-cuffed and double-cuffed single-lumen blocker tubes (Macintosh-Leatherdale, Bonica-

Table 12-1. Techniques for Separating the Lungs*

Technique
Uncut single-lumen endotracheal tube in bronchus (1)
Bronchial blockers
Gauze (2)
Rubber balloon catheters (3–7,44)
(Magill, Machray)
Urinary catheter (Foley)
Plastic balloon catheters (8–10,43)
Embolectomy (Fogarty)
Pulmonary artery catheter (Swan-Ganz)
Univent tube (11–14,47)
Single-lumen bronchial tubes (15–20)
Macintosh-Leatherdale
Gordon-Green
Bonica-Hall
Brompton
Double-lumen tubes
Rubber tubes
Carlens (21,22)
White (49)
Bryce-Smith (50,51)
Robertshaw (23,52,62)
Polyvinyl chloride (PVC) tubes
Robertshaw style (23,64,85,88)
Mallinckrodt
Sheridan
Portex Rusch
Carlens style
Mallinckrodt (53)
Separate tracheal and bronchial tubes (82–84)

* Numbers in parentheses indicate reference numbers.

Hall, Brompton Pallister) were once popular but are seldom used today.[16–18]

The Gordon-Green tube, which was intended for right bronchial intubation, deserves special recognition.[19] It incorporated a ventilation slot on the right bronchial cuff to allow right upper lobe ventilation. All tubes designed for right bronchial intubation that have subsequently followed, including the double-lumen tubes used today, have borrowed this concept.

A unique tube designed by Vellacot combined both bronchial blockade with the capability of two-lung ventilation (Fig. 12-2).[20] This single-lumen, right endobronchial tube could be used in patients who required right upper lobectomy when the affected lobe contained fluids that could contaminate the remainder of the right lung. In addition, the Vellacot tube could be used in patients who developed a bronchopleural fistula with empyema following right upper lobectomy. The tube was introduced into the right main bronchus with the aid of a bronchoscope. When inflated, the right bronchial cuff was intended to obstruct the right upper lobe bronchus, thus isolating that lobe. The left lung could be ventilated through an orifice in the left lateral wall of the tube's single lumen, located between the inflated bronchial and tracheal cuffs. This permitted ventilation of the left lung, while the right middle and lower lobes could be ventilated through the distal opening of the lumen in the right bronchus.

All these specially designed, older tubes have been replaced by the familiar, double-cuffed, double-lumen tube. Although the concept of a tube combining two lumens to ventilate both lungs independently was used as early as 1889,[16] the first double-lumen tube to be used clinically was introduced by Carlens in 1949.[21] This tube was originally intended to be used for differential bronchospirometry, but its potential was immediately recognized and it was used the following year during thoracic operations.[22]

Many refinements in tube and cuff design and material have occurred since the first Carlens tube was used. Currently, the most popular double-lumen tube is the plastic Robertshaw-style tube.[23]

Indications

Although many authors continue to list absolute and relative indications for lung separation, this author believes that there are no relative indications for these techniques. Lung separation should be used *whenever* it can be

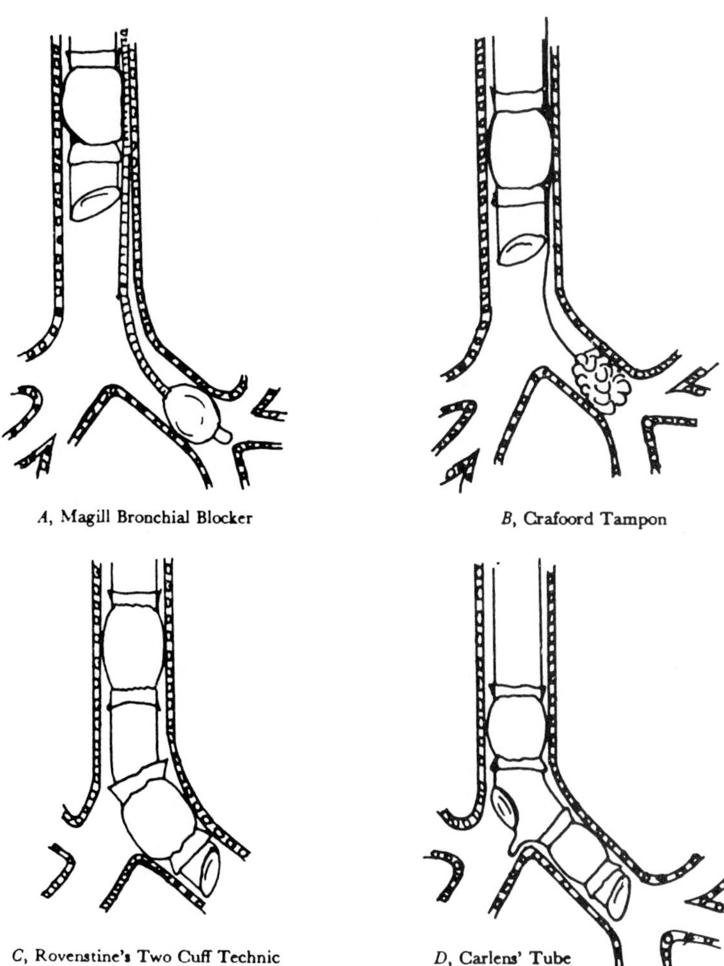

Figure 12-1. The development of anesthetic techniques for effective separation of the lungs. Magill (1936) used a catheter equipped with an inflatable cuff to block the diseased bronchus (A); Crafoord (1938) used a gauze tampon to block the airway (B); Rovenstine (1936) designed a single-lumen, double-cuffed endobronchial tube combining bronchial blockade and one-lung ventilation (C); and Carlens (1949) developed a double-lumen, double-cuffed endobronchial tube, which is the prototype for double-lumen tubes widely used today (D). (Reproduced, with permission, from Collins V, ed. Principles of anesthesiology. Philadelphia: Lea & Febiger, 1976:390.)

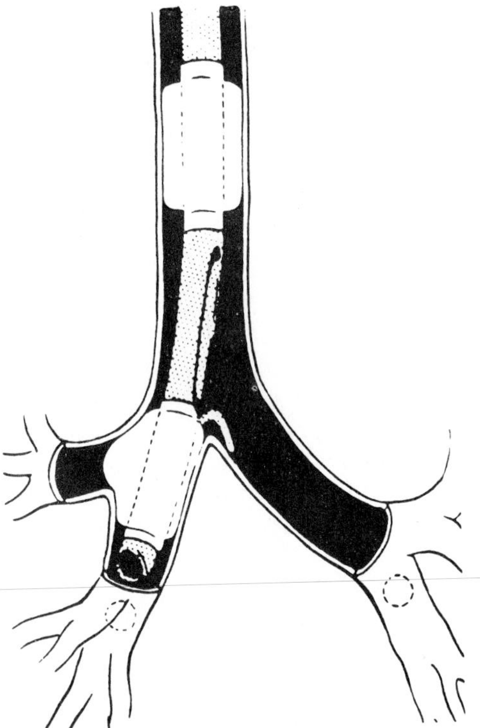

Figure 12-2. The single-lumen Vellacot tube (1954), which combined both bronchial blockade with two-lung ventilation. When properly positioned, the distal endobronchial cuff blocks the right upper lobe only.

Table 12-2. Indications for Double-Lumen Tubes

INTRAOPERATIVE
Contamination (infection, blood, tumor)
Special procedures
Bronchopleural fistula
Massive bronchopulmonary lavage (alveolar proteinosis, asthma, bronchitis)
Empyema drainage
Airway hemorrhage
Resection of bullae
Thoracoscopy (retrieval intrathoracic foreign bodies, pleural and lung biopsies, wedge resection, pleurodesis)
Ventilation-perfusion abnormalities
Protection of single functioning lung
Improvement of operating conditions (pulmonary, cardiac or major vascular, esophageal, gastric, and hepatic problems, vertebral column correction, chest wall deformities)
OUTSIDE THE OPERATING ROOM
Airway hemorrhage
Split-lung ventilation or selective application of peep* or cpap*
Bronchopleural fistula
Unilateral atelectasis
Pulmonary edema
Aspiration
Respiratory distress syndrome
Pneumonia
Pulmonary toilet
Differential bronchospirometry

* PEEP - positive end-expiratory pressure; CPAP - continuous positive airway pressure.

helpful, both in surgery and in situations outside the operating room in the critical care unit (Table 12-2). The use of modern, plastic double-lumen tubes and bronchial blockers, combined with the ready availability of fiberoptic bronchoscopes to help confirm accurate placement of the tubes, has made functional separation of the lungs not only safe but relatively easy for any anesthesiologist to perform.

The original indication for lung separation was the prevention of transbronchial spread of secretions from then prevalent tuberculosis and other pulmonary infectious processes.[22,24] Before the advent of antibiotics, aspiration of pus during pulmonary operations often resulted in death.[25] With the patient in the lateral decubitus position, the dependent lung must always be isolated when it is at risk to avoid aspiration of infected material, necrotic tissue, tumor, and blood from the nondependent, operated lung.[26] Even today, contralateral contamination remains a potentially serious complication of pulmonary surgery, as illustrated by a recent report in which aspiration of necrotic tumor material into the nonprotected, dependent lung occurred.[27]

Besides protection from contamination, there are many other clinical reasons to separate the lungs. Examples of procedures that could not be safely performed without isolation and selective ventilation include surgical closure of a bronchopleural fistula, massive bronchopulmonary lavage, drainage of a communicating empyema, control of a bronchial hemorrhage, surgery on giant bullae, cysts or persistent spontaneous pneumothoraces, and video-assisted thoracoscopy.[28–31] Selective, independent ventilation of one or both lungs with a double-lumen tube can also correct problems related to ventilation-perfusion abnormalities.[32] Patients with severe unilateral or bilateral pulmonary disease often benefit from independent selection of tidal volumes and selective application of positive end-expiratory pressure (PEEP).

For example, split-lung ventilation is useful in the treatment of bronchopleural fistula, a serious complication of acute lung disease, injury, or surgery and positive pressure ventilation. Selective ventilation allows alveolar ventilation to be maintained to the healthy lung, and reduced or discontinued ventilation to the diseased lung allows closure of the bronchopleural fistula and healing of the damaged lung.[33]

Split-lung ventilation has been life-saving for patients in whom conventional two-lung ventilation, with or without PEEP or continuous positive airway pressure (CPAP), actually worsened ventilation-perfusion mismatch. Lung separation and split-lung ventilation has been used successfully for critically ill patients with problems as diverse as pulmonary contusion,[34,35] pulmonary edema,[36] aspiration,[37] respiratory distress syndrome,[38] and pneumonia.[39] For patients with total unilateral collapse, sufficient CPAP or PEEP can be applied to the collapsed lung to reverse the atelectasis without subjecting the healthy lung to barotrauma.[40,41]

Today the most common reason to practice selective lung separation is to collapse the whole lung or portion of a lung intentionally to provide "a quiet" surgical field during intrathoracic operations. The advantages of selective one-lung ventilation for the surgeon are well documented.[42] During pulmonary operations a totally atelectatic lung is particularly helpful for hilar dissection and management of the bronchial stump. With a collapsed lung vigorous lung retraction is not needed, so the lung suffers less trauma and less impairment of gas exchange during and after the operation. Improving surgical conditions reduces operative time.

Not only is selective lung collapse useful for most pulmonary resections, it is often helpful during other thoracic operations. Non-pulmonary procedures where selective lung collapse can be beneficial include resection of a thoracic aortic aneurysm, repair of hiatal hernia, any transthoracic esophageal, gastric or hepatic operations, and procedures to correct vertebral column and chest wall deformities.

Bronchial Blockade

The bronchus to the lobe or lung can be obstructed with rubber balloon blockers, gauze, by specially designed single-lumen, single-cuffed or double-cuffed rubber or plastic bronchial blockers, with balloon-tipped embolectomy (Fogarty) catheters, pulmonary artery (Swan-Ganz) catheters[43] or even a urinary (Foley) catheter.[44] Lung tissue distal to the obstruction collapses after several minutes as gas is absorbed. If both lungs are ventilated with 100% oxygen prior to blockade, atelectasis is hastened.

In the majority of cases the indications for bronchial blockade are generally the same as those for double-lumen tubes—isolation of the lung and selective atelectasis to improve operating conditions. The choice between a double-lumen tube or a blocker is usually a matter of personal preference.

Proponents of bronchial blockade most often recommend this technique for rapid control of airway bleeding,[11,14,45,46] or to reduce the risk of airway trauma that might occur with the use of a larger double-lumen tube.[14] Although some anesthesiologists argue that double-lumen tubes are more difficult to position and have a greater chance of becoming malpositioned or causing tracheobronchial damage than bronchial blockers, these claims have not been substantiated.[47]

With all bronchial blocking techniques, dislodgement of the blocker during the procedure can completely obstruct the entire main bronchus or even both lungs if the blocker enters the carina. Of course, if the blocker moves from its optimal position, material from the diseased lung can then enter the carina and contaminate the healthy, dependent lung. All bronchial blockers, with the exception of the Univent tube, have another disadvantage: the lung or lobe that is being operated on cannot be suctioned or reexpanded during surgery.

Rubber Bronchial Blockers

Many different rubber bronchial blockers (Halton, Magill, Thompson, Moody, Stephen) have been used in the past.[4–7] Skill with a rigid bronchoscope was essential for any anesthesiologist wishing to use these blockers, since most required placement through a bronchoscope that had previously been positioned just proximal to the desired site of the obstruction. Passage down the bronchoscope obstructed the endoscopists view, so it was essential to measure the depth of the scope and the length of the blocker being inserted. The bronchoscope was removed after the blocker was properly positioned. Even for blockers designed to be passed without bronchoscopy, any pathologic distortion of anatomy made "blind" bronchial blocking both difficult and dangerous.

These blockers were safe only for left-bronchial blockade. The risk of displacement from surgical manipulation was always present, but was especially great during operations on the right lung because of the short length of the right bronchus. During surgery the blocker had to be removed or withdrawn immediately prior to clamping the bronchus, which increased the risks of aspiration. These procedures are seldom used today.[48]

Fogarty Catheter

Until pediatric double-lumen tubes become available, bronchial blockade using Fogarty catheters remains the only safe technique for lung separation in very small children. The smallest double-lumen tube now sold, size 28F, can be used for children 8–10 years of age. The distal balloons of Fogarty or Swan-Ganz catheters are most often chosen to block the airway in smaller children. 3–5F Fogarty embolectomy catheters can be used. Larger Fogarty catheters, 8–14F are sometimes used for adult patients.[9] The catheter must be placed under direct vision through a rigid bronchoscope or alongside a fiberoptic bronchoscope.[9,10]

In adults the styletted, distal 3 cm of the catheter is angled approximately 30 degrees to aid intubation of the appropriate bronchus. Following induction of general anesthesia, the catheter is "blindly" passed through the larynx into the lower trachea. The patient is then intubated with a standard endotracheal tube. The fiberoptic bronchoscope is then passed through the endotracheal tube, and the Fogarty catheter is advanced until its balloon is positioned at the desired level in the bronchus.

The tip is placed just inside the orifice of the left lower lobe for left lung blockade, because the balloon will occlude both lobar bronchi when inflated. For right lung surgery the tip is placed either just below the right upper lobe takeoff or in the anterior segment of the right upper lobe.[9] Once the catheter is in position the stylet is removed and the proximal end of the catheter is taped to the patient's face. After the patient is moved to the lateral decubitus position, the catheter position must be reconfirmed with the fiberoptic bronchoscope.

Whenever lung collapse or isolation is required, the balloon is inflated with sufficient air (usually 2–4 mL in adult patients) to produce total occlusion of the airway. Overinflation of the high pressure, low volume balloon represents a potential source for airway damage, although no such injuries have been reported with the use of a Fogarty catheter as a bronchial blocker.

The disadvantages of using a Fogarty catheter for bronchial blockade are similar to use of any bronchial blocker. During posterolateral thoracotomies, particularly with right lung blockade, the balloon is easily displaced into the carina where it can obstruct both lungs or allow contamination into the dependent, healthy lung. If problems occur during the operation, catheter position can only be reconfirmed and readjusted using a fiberoptic bronchoscope. The balloon must be deflated and blocker withdrawn slightly to avoid inclusion in the specimen before the affected bronchus can be resected.

Univent Tube

Recently, another approach to airway blockade, the Univent tube, has been used during pulmonary surgery with excellent results.[11–14] The Univent tube (Fuji Systems [Tokyo, Japan]) consists of a conventional endotracheal tube with an additional small anterior lumen containing a thin (2-mm internal diameter), movable tube (Fig. 12-3). The thinner tube has a distal low-pressure/high-volume balloon that serves as a bronchial blocker when inflated. The blocker tube can be advanced up to 8 cm beyond the tip of the endotracheal tube into the bronchus of either lung (Fig. 12-4). Since the smallest Univent tube currently available has an external diameter equivalent to a 9 mm conventional endotracheal tube, the tube may be too large for some adult patients and cannot be used at all in children.

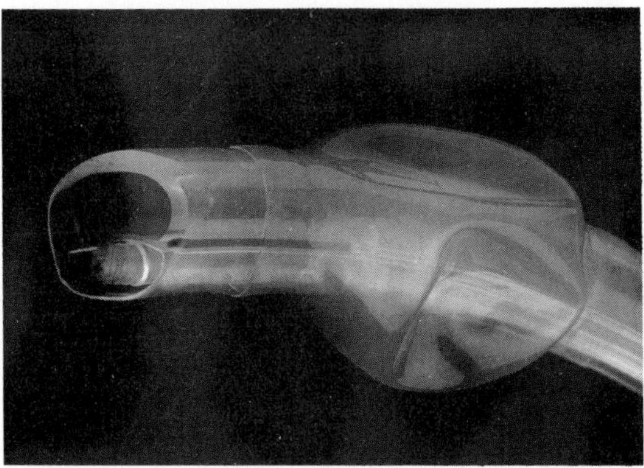

Figure 12-3. The moveable bronchial blocker is housed in a small channel within the anterior internal wall of the tube.

After the blocker balloon is tested for leaks and the balloon is deflated, the blocker tube is retracted into the small lumen in the body of the larger endotracheal tube. There are two methods for positioning the Univent tube. The first method is shown in Figure 12-5. Following the induction of anesthesia the Univent tube is inserted into the trachea (A). The tube is then turned 90 degrees towards the operative side (B). The blocker is pushed into the main bronchus (C). In most cases it will follow the lateral wall of the trachea and target the main stem bronchus. The blocker is inflated with 6–8 ml air to block the operative lung bronchus. The lung may be collapsed by having the surgeon gently squeeze the air out of the lung or by applying suction through the blocker lumen. The second method is illustrated in Figure 12-6.

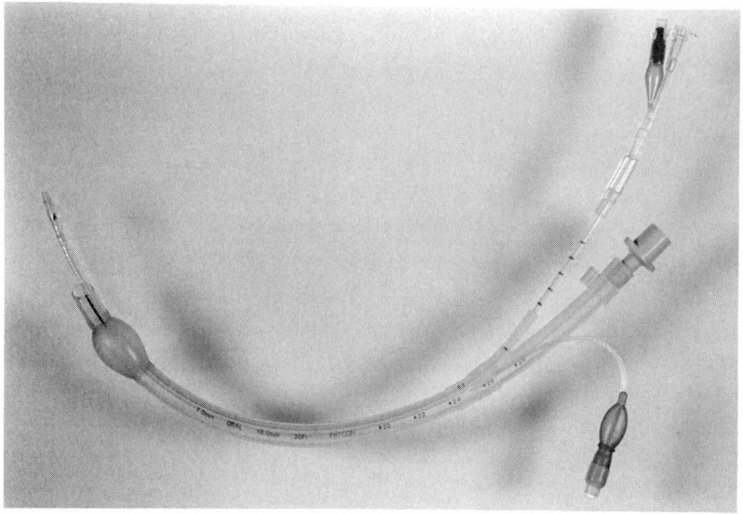

Figure 12-4. The Univent tube (Fuji Systems [Tokyo, Japan]), which consists of a conventional endotracheal tube with an additional anterior lumen that contains a thinner, movable tube. The smaller tube can be advanced up to 8 cm beyond the endotracheal tube. When inflated, a low-pressure/high-volume balloon on the distal tip of the smaller tube serves as a bronchial blocker.

The fiberoptic bronchoscope is used as a stylet. The Univent tube is positioned in the trachea and a fiberoptic bronchoscope is passed through tube lumen into the main bronchus of the operative lung (A). The fiberoptic bronchoscope is used as a stylet to advance the tube into the main bronchus (B). The blocker is then advanced into the main stem bronchus (C). The tube is then pulled back into the trachea while the blocker remains in the main stem bronchus (D). By inflating the bronchial balloon and capping the small bronchial tube's lumen, a segment, lobe, or entire lung can be isolated and collapsed. Position of the distal balloon can be confirmed either by fiberoptic bronchoscopy or direct palpation by the surgeon once the chest is opened. Recently Inoue[14A] developed a new style Univent tube which may decrease the need for fiberoptic guidance for positioning of the blocker. The new-style Univent (Fig. 12-7, A,B) has a small light source mounted on the front-most portion of the moveable blocker. In this case, following rotation of the tube toward the lung to be blocked, thoracotomy is performed and the lung is retracted down and forward to expose the main stem bronchus which is normally covered with the mediastinal pleura. The light source of the blocker is lit up and the blocker pushed downward while it is observed clearly by transillumination from the opened pleural cavity. Figures 12-8 A, B show a fiberoptic bronchoscopy view of the bronchial blocker of the Univent tube inserted into the right main stem bronchus. The bronchial cuff of the Univent tube is a clear color.

The Univent tube has several unique advantages over other blocker methods (Table 12-3). The same tube can be used for blockade of either the right or left lung. In addition, the Univent tube can selectively block lung segments as well as the entire lung, whereas double-lumen tubes can separate only the whole

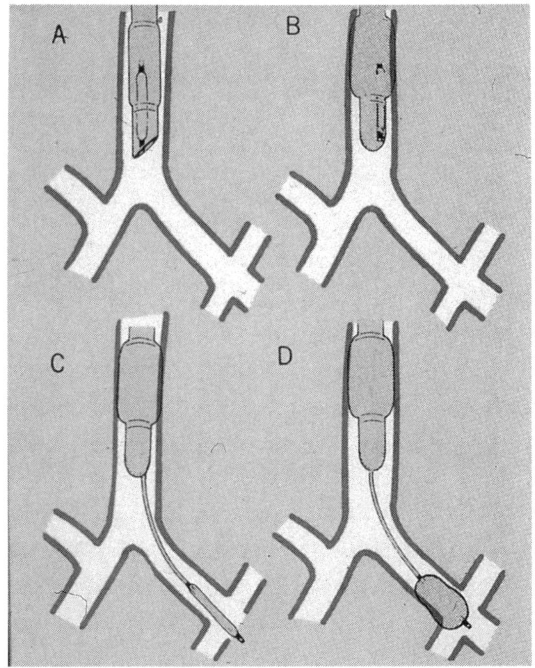

Figure 12-5. A. The Univent tube is inserted into the trachea. B. The tube is then turned 90 degrees toward the operative side. C The blocker is pushed to the main bronchus; and in most cases it will follow the lateral wall of the trachea and target the main stem bronchus. D. The blocker is inflated with 6–8 ml air to block the operative lung bronchus. The lung may be collapsed by having the surgeon gently squeeze the air out of the lung or by applying suction through the blocker lumen. (Courtesy of Fuji System Corporation, Tokyo, Japan.)

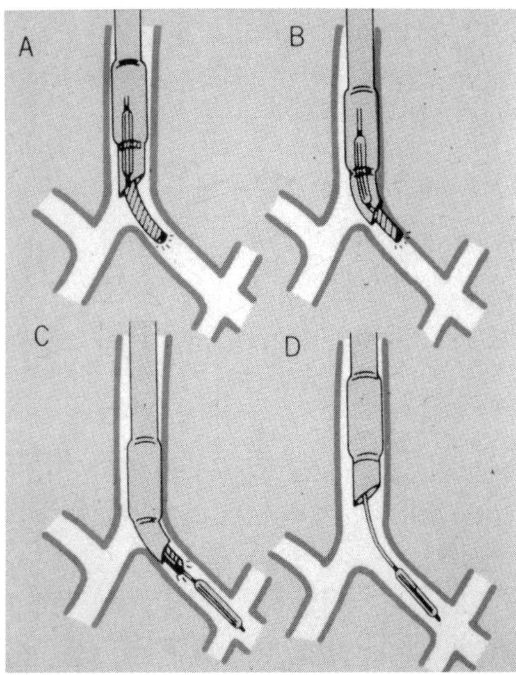

Figure 12-6. A. The Univent tube is positioned in the trachea and a fiberoptic bronchoscope is passed through tube lumen into the main bronchus of the operative lung. B. The fiberoptic bronchoscope is used as a stylet to advance the tube into the main bronchus. C. The blocker is then advanced into the main stem bronchus. D. The tube is then pulled back into the trachea while the blocker remains in the main stem bronchus. (Courtesy of Fuji System Corporation, Tokyo, Japan.)

lung. Furthermore, the blocker is attached to the main tube, therefore displacement of the bronchial balloon is less likely to occur. Lung tissue distal to the obstruction can be suctioned or reexpanded during the operation through the small axial lumen in the Univent blocker's tube unlike in other bronchial blocker techniques. Suction, pulmonary lavage, oxygen insufflation, or even jet ventilation can be performed through this lumen.[11–14] Two-lung ventilation can be reinstituted easily at any time by deflating the balloon and withdrawing the blocker tube into the body of the main tube. If postoperative ventilation is required, reintubation is therefore unnecessary.

The manufacturer of the Univent tube claims that fiberoptic bronchoscopy is not needed to position the Univent tube accurately, but in one study, "blind" placement was successful in only one of eight patients.[47] Because

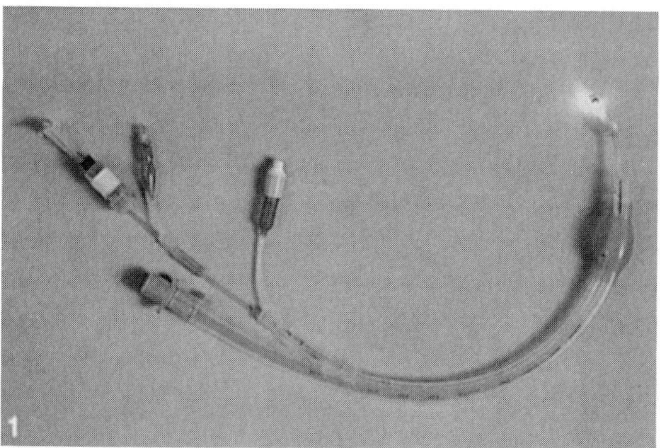

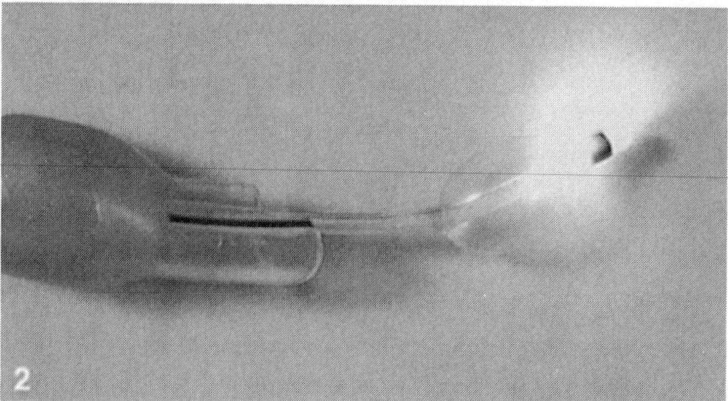

Figure 12-7. A. New style Univent with a small light source on the blocker. The power supply is attached to the rear end portion of the blocker. B. The light source is a visible laser. (Reprinted with permission from Inoue H. New-style Univent with a light source on the blocker. J Cardiovasc Surg 1993;34:1.)

the bronchial tube is so thin, the blocker balloon requires at least 5 mL of air to block the bronchus and achieve an airtight seal.[47] This is more than twice the volume required by the bronchial cuff of a polyvinyl chloride double-lumen tube. This relatively large volume increases the risk of balloon herniation into the carina, and overdistension of the balloon may cause pressure damage the airway.[47a] In the study cited, a satisfactory bronchial seal was never obtained in three patients, and the blocker herniated into the trachea, partially obstructing the ventilated lung in two patients. In several of the patients, the blocker had to be replaced with a double-lumen tube to provide satisfactory operative conditions.

Double-Lumen Endobronchial Tubes

Today double-lumen tubes are the most popular method for separating the lungs in adults. Modern double-lumen tubes are safe, easy to use, and require no special training. Bronchoscopy is not routinely needed for placement of double-lumen tubes, whereas bronchial blockers

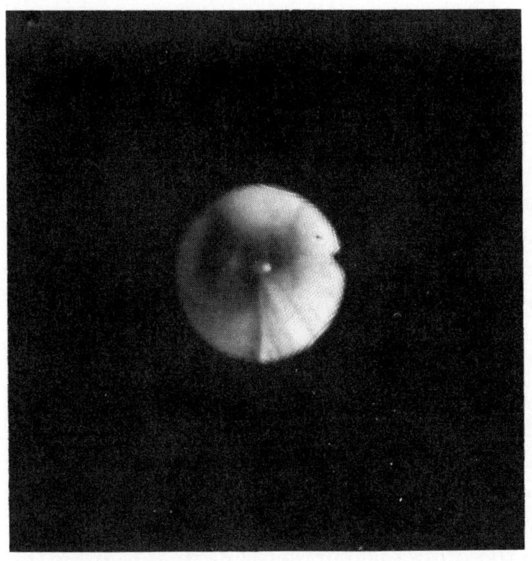

A

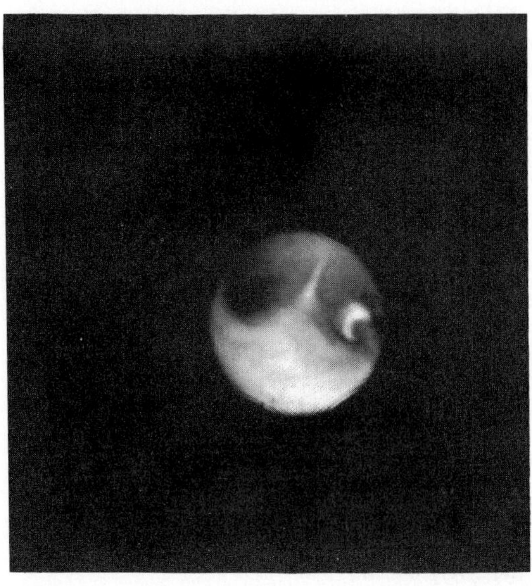

B

Figure 12-8. Fiberoptic bronchoscopy view of the bronchial blocker of the Univent tube inserted into the right main stem bronchus. The bronchial cuff of the Univent tube is of a clear color. See Color Plates 1 and 2.

almost always require skill with a bronchoscope. Double-lumen tubes allow each lung to be independently ventilated, collapsed, and reexpanded at any time. Either lung can be suctioned or examined with a fiberoptic bronchoscope if necessary during the procedure. If hypoxemia occurs during one-lung ventilation, CPAP can be applied to the nonventilated lung to improve oxygenation only when using a double-lumen tube.

Types

Carlens, who designed the original double-lumen tube for intubation of the *left* bronchus only,[21,22] recognized the danger of right upper lobe obstruction from the endobronchial cuff whenever a tube was placed in the right main bronchus. White introduced a similar tube with a fenestrated *right* endobronchial lumen to be used for right bronchial intubation.[49] He borrowed the concept of a fenestrated right bronchial cuff from the Gordon-Green single-lumen right endobronchial tube.[19] Like Carlens, White recognized the dangers of right bronchial intubation and recommended very careful auscultation over the right upper lung field to confirm apposition of the ventilation slot in the cuff to the right upper lobe orifice.

To aid in positioning, both the Carlens and White tubes have a hook to engage the carina. This carinal hook makes passage through the glottis difficult and is a potential source of airway injury. In addition, the rubber walls of the Carlens and White tubes are very thick, so their lumens are narrow relative to their large external circumference; hence resistance to airflow may be very high during one-lung ventilation. Furthermore, the oval cross-sectional shape of each lumen interferes with passage of suction catheters.

Table 12-3. Advantages and Disadvantages of Univent Tubes (Bronchial Blockers)

Advantages
Can block whole lung or lung segments
Can be used for right or left lung
Displacement is less likely than with other blockers
Collapsed lung can be reexpanded
Blocker tube contains a small axial lumen
CPAP suction
Pulmonary lavage
Oxygen insufflation
High-frequency jet ventilation
Reintubation with endotracheal tube unnecessary
Disadvantages
Requires bronchoscopy for accurate placement
Too large for small adults; unavailable for children
Blocker cuff requires more 5 mL air to block main bronchus
Possible airway trauma from overinflation
Failure to block the airway
Herniation of cuff into carina
Relatively Expensive

The first double-lumen tube without a carinal hook, the Bryce-Smith tube, was originally intended to reduce the trauma associated with the Carlens tube. Unlike the Carlens and White double-lumen tubes, the lumens of the Bryce-Smith tube are round to facilitate passage of suction catheters. A left-sided model was first described in 1959,[50] and a similar tube designed for right bronchial intubation was introduced by Bryce-Smith and Salt in 1960.[51] Both the left- and right-sided models are still available.

The Bryce-Smith tube combined the advantages of several different tube shapes and properties. The proximal limbs were intentionally left long so they could be cut to suit the individual patient. Like White's double-lumen tube, the right bronchial lumen slot for ventilation of the right upper lobe was copied from the Gordon-Green tube. The right Bryce-Smith tube was initially intended to be used in place of the only double-lumen tube then available, the left Carlens tube. At first, Bryce-Smith and Salt believed that a right double-lumen tube should be used only when left-sided intubation was not possible.[51] Because the shape of the airway made intubation of the right bronchus "distressingly simple" and easy to perform, however, they went on to recommend that their right-sided double-lumen tube be used routinely rather than as an alternative to left double-lumen tubes.[51] Bryce-Smith and Salt advised preliminary bronchoscopy when gross distortion of the trachea was present. Although they did not believe that bronchoscopy was essential for safe placement of their tube, they thought it might help assess those individual variations in airway anatomy within the range of normal variability. Bryce-Smith and Salt recognized certain complications that could arise using their right double-lumen tube.[51] Overinflation of the bronchial cuff could cause it to herniate over the right upper lobe ventilation slot, so careful inflation of the cuff was necessary. They reduced the risk of this complication by sealing the cuff at a distance above the slot. Bronchial cuff herniation over the distal lumen tip was still possible, however. These investigators also stated that if the tube was not passed far enough into the right main bronchus, right upper lobe obstruction by the distal portion of the tube or its cuff or carinal obstruction might still occur. They corrected this by advancing the tube. Adjustment of tube position was considered a major advantage of their tube. Such modification was not possible with a Carlens or White tube, because the carinal hooks prevented advancement into the bronchus.[51]

Inadequate depth of insertion was a much more common occurrence than cuff obstruction of the right upper lobe from a tube advanced too deep into the bronchus, as was true for all bulky, rubber double-lumen tubes.

Robertshaw introduced his famous double-lumen tube in 1962.[23] This tube not only lacks a carinal hook, but it also has a more gentle curve, thinner walls, and larger D-shaped internal lumens so resistance to airflow during one-lung ventilation is less than in other rubber double-lumen tubes.[52] Both right- and left-sided tubes are available. The right-sided tube has a slotted bronchial cuff for right upper lobe ventilation and an additional inflatable area just above the slot for a more effective seal of the right bronchus.

Almost all modern double-lumen tubes resemble Robertshaw tubes but are constructed of a polyvinyl chloride (PVC) plastic material instead of rubber. Four PVC double-lumen tubes are available in the United States (Broncho-Cath [Mallinckrodt, Argyle NY] Endobronchial Tube [Rusch NY], Broncho-Trach [Sheridan, Argyle NY] and Portex) (Fig. 12-9). Mallinckrodt offers the option of a Carlens style, PVC double-lumen tube with a carinal hook.[53]

Properties

All double-lumen tubes, whether constructed of rubber or plastic, are basically two air channels linked together. The shorter tube ends in the trachea and the longer tube ends in either the left or right main bronchus. Two pilot balloons are connected to inflatable cuffs on the outside walls of the tracheal and bronchial lumens. These balloons indicate when the cuffs are expanded, but they do not measure the volume of air required to provide an airtight, watertight seal of the airway or the pressure generated on the airway mucosa when the cuffs are inflated. Leakage of gas during positive-pressure ventilation is prevented by the tracheal cuff located just above the opening of the shorter lumen. When inflated, the tracheal cuff also serves as an anchor that limits, but does not prevent, tube movement. Separation of gas flow to each lung and protection from aspiration into the dependent lung is achieved when the bronchial cuff is inflated.

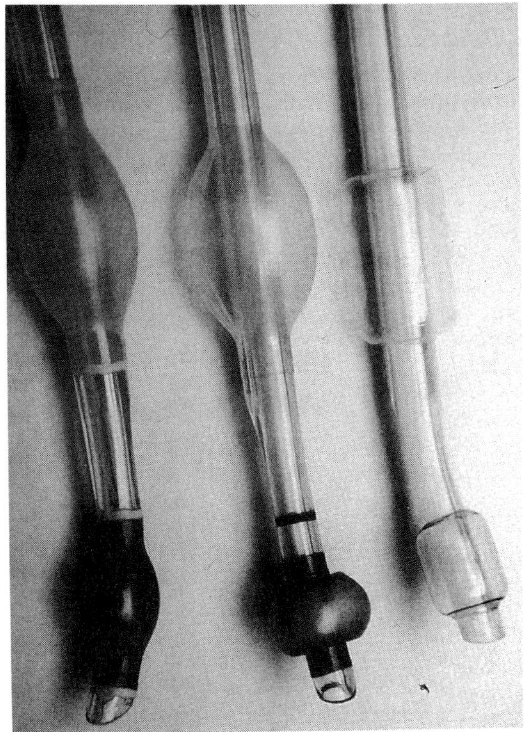

Figure 12-9. The three different designs of left double-lumen tubes studied with tracheal and bronchial cuffs inflated. Rusch on the left, Mallinckrodt in the middle, Sheridan on the right. The difference in the shapes of the distal (bronchial) cuffs is evident. (Reproduced with permission from Shinger PD, Chripko D. A clinical comparison of bronchial cuff pressures in three different designs of left double-lumen tubes. Anesth Analg 1993;77:305.)

In tubes designed for the right main bronchus, the lateral aspect of the bronchial cuff or the tube wall itself is fenestrated so that gas exchange with the right upper lobe bronchus is possible. This slot does not ensure adequate ventilation of the right upper lobe since the slot must open directly into the right upper lobe bronchial orifice. Because of normal anatomic variation, ventilation of the right upper lobe with a right-sided double-lumen tube is not possible in many adults.

At the oral end, both the tracheal and bronchial lumens are connected to the anesthesia circuit by one of a number of devices that permit inspired gas to be diverted into either or both lumens. Each lumen can be opened to the atmosphere independently, so that gas may escape, allowing the unventilated lung to collapse, while continuing to ventilate the other lung. A suction catheter can be passed down one lumen while still ventilating the other lung. PVC double-lumen tubes are available with a diaphragm on each connector which allows the introduction of a suction catheter or a fiberoptic bronchoscope into the lumen of the ventilated lung *without* causing that lung to collapse. Many special adaptors have been designed to facilitate lung collapse, passage of suction catheters, bronchoscopes, or the application of PEEP or CPAP.[54–60]

Rubber versus Polyvinyl Chloride

Originally all double-lumen tubes were constructed of relatively inflexible, bulky, red rubber. Although reusable, latex tubes are expensive and have a limited shelf life. Although the manufacturers of both rubber and PVC double-lumen tubes claim that their products have a shelf life of at least five years if kept under optimum conditions, rubber tubes are more likely to deteriorate sooner (Table 12-4).[61]

Using rubber double-lumen tubes in hospitals where thoracotomies are not frequently performed was not economically advantageous.[61] Furthermore, rubber double-lumen tubes are easily damaged during cleaning and resterilization, and this damage can result in tube tip irregularities that increase the risk of airway injury whenever these tubes are used.

Rubber Robertshaw tubes, which are still preferred by some anesthesiologists, may have advantages over plastic double-lumen tubes in special situations. For example, as discussed in a later section (see Left-sided versus Right-sided Tubes), the incidence of right upper lobe obstruction with a rubber Robertshaw tube is significantly less than with a right-sided, PVC double-lumen tube.[62] When right bronchial intubation is required, a rubber double-lumen tube may be the better choice (Fig. 12-10). A left-sided, rubber double-lumen tube may also be safer than a PVC tube for massive bronchopulmonary lavage.[63] With PVC tubes, any event that causes even the slightest movement

Table 12-4. Comparison of Double-Lumen Tubes

Type	Advantages	Disadvantages
Carlens; White	Carinal hook aid for positioning Reusable	Carinal hook causes trauma Narrow lumens Asymmetric cuff inflation Low-volume/high-pressure cuffs Oval lumens
Robertshaw	No carinal hook Wider lumen than Carlens tube Right- and left-sided tubes available Reusable	Low-volume/high-pressure cuffs Asymmetric cuff inflation Narrower lumens than PVC* tubes
Robertshaw-style, PVC* (Mallinckrodt, Sheridan, Rusch)	Clear lumens High-volume/low-pressure cuffs Widest lumens Blue bronchial cuff	Single use Expensive Narrow right ventilation slot

*PVC - polyvinyl chloride.

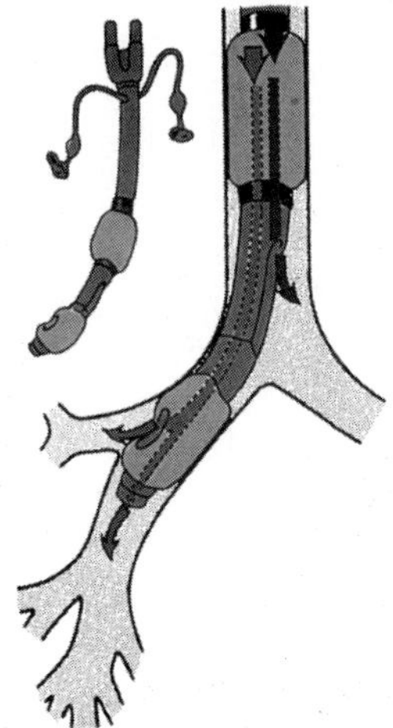

Figure 12-10. When right bronchial intubation is required, a rubber double-lumen tube may be the better choice. See Color Plate 3.

of the tube could partially displace the tube into the carina, with loss of the airway seal. The results may be catastrophic if the lavage fluid is aspirated into the nonlavaged lung. The distance from the proximal edge of the bronchial cuff to the proximal edge of the tracheal cuff in 39F and 41F PVC double-lumen tubes is only 3.4 cm. In contrast the distance in medium and large red rubber Robertshaw tubes is 5.3 and 5.8 cm, respectively (Fig. 12-11). The smaller distance in the PVC tube leaves little margin for error in tube placement during lavage, since the proximal cuff cannot be placed more than 3 cm into the left main bronchus.

In almost all other instances, however, disposable, PVC double-lumen tubes have replaced the older rubber tubes. Most anesthesiologists have found that PVC double-lumen tubes are easier and safer to use than rubber double-lumen tubes.[64, 65]

A major advantage of modern double-lumen tubes is the clear, nonirritating PVC composition, which allows continuous observation of moisture during ventilation and secretions or blood from either lung. The bronchial and tracheal cuffs of PVC double-lumen tubes have high-volume/low-pressure properties, in contrast to the low-volume/high-pressure cuffs of rubber double-lumen tubes, when properly used, should reduce the danger of ischemic pressure damage to the respiratory mucosa. In addition, when compared to rubber tubes of equivalent size, PVC double-lumen tubes have thinner tube walls; therefore they have significantly larger internal lumens relative to their external diameter. Thus the resistance to airflow during one-lung ventilation is less with PVC tubes.

PVC double-lumen tubes are available in four adult sizes (35F, 37F, 39F, and 41F). Their external circumferences are approximately 38, 40, 44, and 45 mm with internal lumen diameters of approximately 5.0, 5.5, 6.0, and 6.5 mm (Table 12-5).[64] Suction catheters or a fiberoptic bronchoscope easily pass through their D-shaped lumens. A 28F double-lumen tube is made for larger children, but no tube is currently available for small children and infants. Prototype pediatric double-lumen tubes have been used successfully in isolated cases, however.[35]

All bronchial cuffs on PVC double-lumen tube are dyed blue for easy identification during bronchoscopy. The cuff material is relatively thin and easily torn by the patient's teeth.

The difference between rubber and plastic double-lumen tubes size is best illustrated in patients with tracheostomies. Bulky rubber double-lumen tubes cannot be safely used in such patients since tubes small enough to fit through the stoma usually have too narrow an internal lumen for one-lung ventilation.[66, 67] Large, conventional PVC double-lumen tubes can be used, but length of these tubes makes management awkward.[68] A PVC double-lumen tube suitable for tracheostomies has been developed.[69] Our own PVC double-lumen tube (Sheridan [Argyle NY]) is constructed in propor-

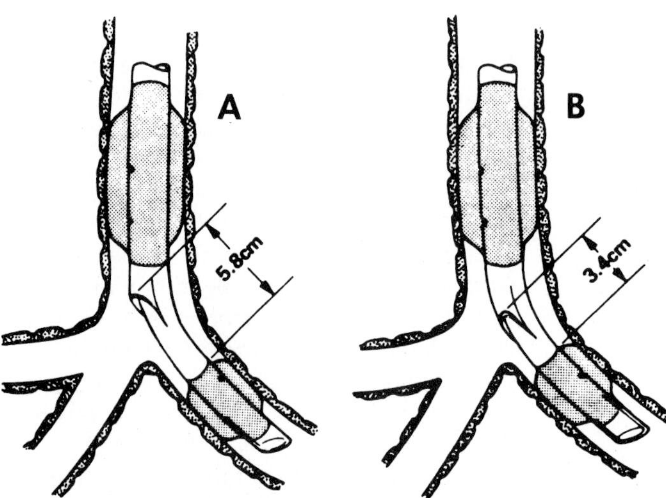

Figure 12-11. Two sketches showing that the distance from the proximal edge of the endobronchial cuff to the proximal edge of the tracheal lumen is only 3.4 cm in 39F and 41F polyvinyl chloride double-lumen tubes as compared to 5.3 and 5.8 cm in medium and large rubber Robertshaw tubes. The smaller distances in the plastic tubes leaves little margin for error in placement during bronchopulmonary lavage procedures. Even slight movement of the tube can cause loss of the airway seal. (Reproduced, with permission, from Shulman MS, Brebner J, Cain J, et al. Bronchopulmonary lung lavage. Anesthesiology 1983;59:597.)

tion to the shorter length of the upper airway in patients with tracheostomies (Fig. 12-12).

Both cuffs have pilot balloons with self-sealing valves. Manufacturers advise against leaving three-way stopcocks or other devices in the inflation valve for extended periods, since the resulting stress can crack the valve housing, allowing the cuff to deflate. The proximal tracheal and bronchial lumens are also clearly identified. Printed depth marks indicate the distance from the distal tip of the bronchial lumen. The distal ends of both lumens have radiopaque markings for radiographic identification.

Selection By Tube Size

As a rule, *the largest tube that can pass atraumatically through the glottis should be selected.* The average diameter of the left bronchus is 15 mm (range: 10–18 mm) in men and 12 mm (range: 9–15 mm) in women.[70] Therefore, a 41F, left-sided, PVC double-lumen tube easily fits most men; a 39F tube should be chosen for most women.[26] Whenever the size tube that can be accommodated is in doubt, the diameter of the bronchus can be directly measured from posteroanterior and lateral chest x-rays and the tube selected accordingly.[71]

Large tubes are preferred, because many of the complications associated with double-lumen tubes can be reduced or avoided by using bigger tubes.[72] With larger tubes, less air is required for the bronchial cuff to seal the airway; therefore the dangers of airway trauma from overinflation and cuff herniation into the carina are reduced. In addition, thinner double-lumen tubes can be advanced further into the bronchus, thus increasing the risks of obstruc-

Table 12-5. Maximal Circumference (mm) of Selected Double-Lumen Tubes*

Tube	Size			
	35F	37F	39F	41F
Mallinckrodt (polyvinyl chloride)	38	40†	44†	45†
Robertshaw (rubber)	—	44	49	55
Carlens (rubber)	—	49	52	55

* From Burton NA, et al. Advantages of a new polyvinyl chloride double-lumen tube in thoracic surgery. Ann Thorac Surg 1983; 36:78.

† 37F, 39F, and 41F polyvinyl chloride tubes correspond to small, medium, and large, Carlens and Robertshaw rubber tubes, respectively.

tion of the upper lobe bronchus.[73] Larger tubes have less resistance to air flow during one-lung ventilation than tubes with thinner lumens. However, a smaller double-lumen tube may be needed to pass through a narrow larynx or advance past the carina into the bronchus in the presence of intrinsic or extrinsic airway obstruction.[74]

Left-sided versus Right-sided Tubes

Many, anesthesiologists, such as this author, prefer a left-sided, double-lumen tube for both right and left thoracotomies.[75,76] On the other hand, some anesthesiologists always recommend intubating the bronchus of the operated lung,[77] whereas others always advise intubating the nonoperated lung.[62]

In humans, intubation of the right main bronchus is so easy because the length and anatomic configuration of the bronchial tree differs between the right and left lung. The average length of the right main bronchus is only 2.3 cm (males) and 2.1 cm (females). The left bronchus is longer, averaging 5.4 cm (males) and 5.0 cm (females)[70] (Table 12-6). The short length of the right bronchus increases the risk of upper lobe obstruction whenever a right double-lumen tube is used.

Figure 12-12. A specially designed, 41F polyvinyl chloride double-lumen tube (Sheridan [Argyle NY]) shown next to a regular tube. The special tube is constructed in proportion to the shorter length of the upper airway for use in patients with tracheostomies.

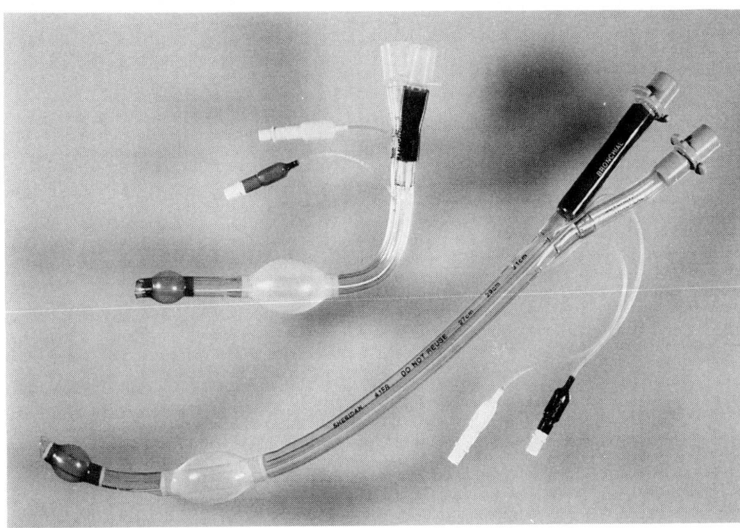

Table 12-6. Size Relationship Between Polyvinyl Chloride (PVC) Double-Lumen Tubes and Fiberoptic Bronchscope (FOB)*

Outside Diameter FOB (mm)	Tube Size
<4.5	35F, 37F, 39F, 41F
4.9	39F, 41F
>5.6	Will not fit 41F

*Information from: Slinger PD. Fiberoptic bronchoscopic positioning of double-lumen tubes. J Cardiothorac Anesth 1989; 3:486.

The rationale for intubating the operative (right or left) lung follows. A malpositioned tube usually presents with upper lobe atelectasis from bronchial cuff obstruction of the upper lobe bronchus.[72] Whenever the double-lumen tube is in the bronchus on the side of the operated lung, a poorly placed tube is evident as soon as the chest is opened or when selective deflation is attempted during surgery.[75,78,79] With the lumen in the bronchus on the operative side, the surgeon can manually determine tube position and guide the anesthesiologist if a change in placement is necessary during surgery.[80] Since the intubated lung is always visible, fiberoptic bronchoscopy is never needed to confirm placement. The dependent lung is safely ventilated through the tracheal lumen while the inflated bronchial cuff continues to protect the dependent lung from contamination.

Other anesthesiologists take a different approach and always intubate the dependent (right or left) lung. They argue that a double-lumen tube in the bronchus of the operative lung complicates airway management, especially during pneumonectomy. The risk of tube displacement from surgical retraction and manipulation increases.[62] Without the presence of a double-lumen tube to keep the bronchus patent, the weight of the mediastinum could possibly obstruct the dependent main bronchus.

No matter which bronchus is intubated, the ventilated lung is never visualized. The anesthesiologist must always be watch for dependent lung upper lobe obstruction, especially during left thoracotomy using a right-sided double-lumen tube. Signs of upper lobe atelectasis include a decrease in lung compliance, a drop in oxygen saturation, and a decrease in mediastinal movement during ventilation of the dependent lung.[73]

Unfortunately, the length of the bronchial cuff of a right-sided double-lumen tube may be longer than the length of the entire right main bronchus, or the ventilation slot may not open directly into the upper lobe orifice. Therefore even with the proximal edge of the cuff positioned just below the carina, the upper lobe may still be obstructed. If the lobe is not obstructed, the bronchial cuff may be in the carina, partially obstructing ventilation to the dependent lung. It is estimated that as many as 10% of the adult population cannot be safely intubated with any right-sided double-lumen tube that is currently available.[76]

The author uses a left-sided double-lumen tube whenever possible. Such a tube can isolate and separate either lung during right or left thoracotomy, with less risk than any potential benefit from a right-sided double-lumen tube. Even during left pneumonectomy, the bronchial cuff can be deflated and the tube withdrawn under the surgeon's guidance before the bronchus is clamped. A right-sided tube must be used at certain times, however. Right bronchial intubation may be necessary in the presence of a left endobronchial tumor or when the left main bronchus is obstructed for any reason. A thoracic aortic aneurysm can distort the airway making placement of a left-sided double-lumen tube difficult. Forced advancement of such a tube has actually ruptured an aneurysm compressing the bronchus.[81]

When a right-sided double-lumen tube is indicated, a rubber Robertshaw tube (Leyland [London]) is a better choice than a right-sided PVC tube (Mallinckrodt [Argyle NY]).[62] The rubber tube has a right upper lobe ventilation slot approximately twice as long as the PVC tube. In addition, the rubber tube is also shorter and thicker; this prevents it from being advanced as deep into the bronchus as the thinner, longer PVC tube.

Bronchoscopic confirmation showed that the right upper lobe was obstructed in two of 20 (10%) patients intubated with the rubber tube as compared to eight of nine (89%) patients intubated with the PVC double-lumen tube.[62] The incidence of right upper lobe obstruction is still clinically unacceptable and far too high to justify the use of right-sided double-lumen tubes for routine thoracotomies. Because the risk of upper lobe collapse is great whenever a right-sided double-lumen tube is used, other options should be considered. Use of a left-sided double-lumen tube or bronchial blockade are feasible alternatives.

Selective intubation of the right bronchus with a special cuffed tube inserted through a standard endotracheal tube has been recommended as another possible solution (Fig. 12-13).[82,83] The right lung can be independently ventilated through this bronchial tube while the left lung is ventilated through the tracheal tube. When left lung deflation is required, ventilation through the tracheal tube is discontinued. The trachea is first intubated with a large single-lumen tube. Any standard endotracheal tube can be used providing it does not have a Murphy eye lateral opening. After ventilating both lungs, the lubricated right bronchial tube is inserted into the tracheal tube and blindly advanced. A longitudinal blue line on the anterior surface of the bronchial tube provides a reference for proper orientation during insertion. An external mark on the bronchial tube indicates when its distal cuffed tip has passed the end of the tracheal tube. At this point, both tubes can be connected to a ventilator, and both lungs can be ventilated while the remainder of the intubation sequence proceeds.

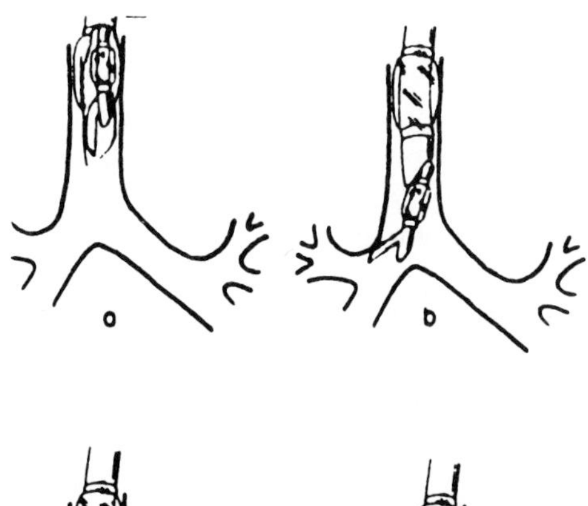

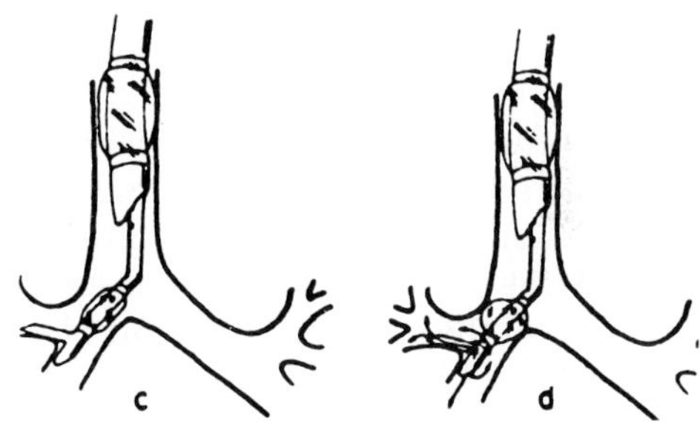

Figure 12-13. A diagrammatic representation of a technique for selective ventilation of the right lung. In A, a conventional endotracheal tube is placed in the trachea; in B, a bronchial tube is advanced through the endotracheal tube and directed towards the right main bronchus; in C, further advancement is stopped by engagement of the lateral branch of the upper lobe bronchus by the bifurcated tip of the bronchial tube; and in D, the cuff is inflated and the right lung is ventilated through the bronchial tube while the left lung is ventilated through the tracheal tube. (Reproduced, with permission, from Nazari S, Trazzi R, Moncalvo F, et al. Selective bronchial intubation for one-lung anaesthesia in thoracic surgery. Anaesthesia 1986; 41:519.)

For intubation of the right bronchus the smaller, longer tube is pushed down a few more centimeters until an increase in resistance occurs, indicating it is in correct position. The bronchial tube almost always enters the right main bronchus. No guidance is needed because of the less acute angulation of the right bronchus. When properly positioned, bifurcated distal tip of the tube engages the lateral branch of the right upper lobe bronchus, thus impeding further advancement. In this position the possibility of obstructing the upper lobe bronchus is minimized. The bronchial tube can also be used for left bronchial intubation but an angulated stylet is necessary. The bronchial tube is fixed in position with an external movable ring. Tube position is checked by auscultation while ventilating the intubated lung only.

One advantage of this technique is that an endotracheal tube is always present. Safe two-lung ventilation can be easily reestablished if problems occur. Laryngoscopy is not necessary for insertion of the bronchial tube. Bronchial intubation can be performed at any time, even while the patient is in the lateral decubitus position. In the majority of cases the right lung is easily intubated blindly, but fiberoptic bronchoscopy is occasionally needed.[84] When one-lung ventilation is no longer indicated, the bronchial tube can be removed and ventilation to both lungs continued through the tracheal tube.

Margin of Safety

The "margin of safety" is the length of the tracheobronchial tree over which a tube can be moved without obstructing a conducting airway.[76] The length of the bronchus between the most distal and proximal acceptable positions of the bronchial lumen defines the margin of safety for a double-lumen tube. When the tip of the bronchial lumen is at the proximal edge of the orifice to the upper lobe, a double-lumen tube is in the most distal acceptable position, since further advancement into the bronchus would obstruct the upper lobe. When the bronchial cuff is just below the carina in the bronchus, a double-lumen tube is in the most proximal acceptable position since if the cuff were more proximal it would begin to obstruct the trachea. The margin of safety varies with the individual patient and the specific double-lumen tube chosen.

The average margin of safety for three PVC left-sided tubes is 16–19 mm (Mallinckrodt, Rusch, and Sheridan), and for right tubes it is even less. For the right-sided Mallinckrodt tube the margin of safety is 8 mm and for the right-sided Rusch PVC tube, only 1–4 mm.[76]

Manufacturers of double-lumen tubes changed tube design to improve the margin of safety. For example, shortening the bevel of the tip of the bronchial lumen, which effectively brings the tip closer to the endobronchial cuff, would increase the margin of safety by 4–6 mm for PVC double-lumen tubes. Narrowing of the bronchial cuff by 5–8 mm would further reduce the chances of obstructing the upper lobe (Fig. 12-14).[85]

Figure 12-14. The Mallinckrodt left-sided DLT new design to improve the margin of safety. The bronchial curve is tighter to increase the chance of left main bronchus intubation and reduce the incidence of dislocation. The cuff is located closer to the tip, is shorter in length, and the tip is of square design. These all decrease the chance of left upper lobe occlusion.

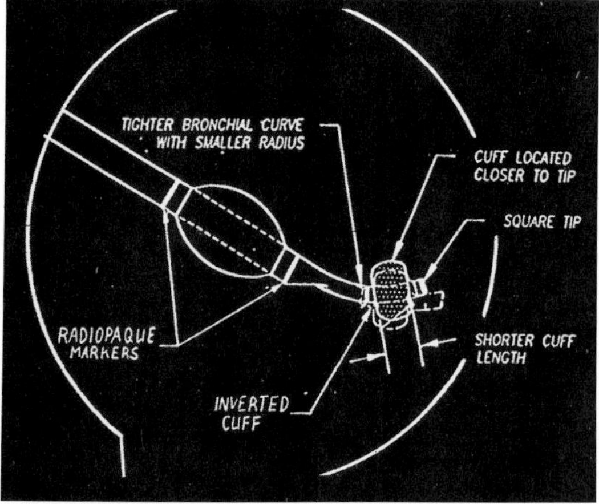

A left-sided PVC double-lumen tube with a radiopaque hook and a greater margin of safety is available from Mallinckrodt. Unlike a rubber Carlens tube, this tube possesses all the advantages of other PVC tubes but the carinal hook is 38 mm from the distal tip of the bronchial lumen. When the tube is properly positioned with its hook engaging the carina, ventilation of the upper lobe is assured, since the average length of the left main bronchus is approximately 50 mm. The margin of safety is therefore increased.[53] If the hook is improperly seated, however, upper lobe obstruction is more likely to occur. The hook itself increases the risk of airway trauma.

As previously discussed, right-sided double-lumen tubes are potentially more dangerous to use than left-sided tubes, because even when the bronchial cuff is immediately below the carina, the margin of safety is so small that the cuff still obstructs the right upper lobe bronchus in over 10% of patients.[76] PVC double-lumen tubes designed with a longer right upper lobe ventilation slot or a narrower bronchial cuff would reduce the chances of right upper lobe obstruction.

Positioning Double-Lumen Tubes

Preoperative examination of the chest roentgenogram helps to choose the appropriate tube size and alerts the anesthesiologist to the presence of compression or traction distortions of the trachea and bronchus that may interfere with double-lumen tube placement.[14,71] However, the single study that considered examination of the chest radiographs immediately before surgery found them *not* particularly helpful in predicting which patient would experience problems with double-lumen tube intubation.[86] Although preoperative chest x-rays revealed that 30% of patients had tracheal deviation or elevation of one or both hila with altered angularities of the main bronchi, intubation difficulties occurred only in patients with gross abnormalities.[86] If bronchial obstruction is suspected, a computerized tomography (CT) scan gives more information. Bronchoscopy immediately before intubation also provides helpful information about the presence of anatomic distortion or obstructions that may interfere with tube placement.[51,87]

Auscultation

The most frequently used method for positioning double-lumen tubes is "blind" advancement into the bronchus followed by careful auscultation. Several procedures can be used to perform "blind" bronchial intubation. This author prefers the following method for determining the position of double-lumen tubes because it is simple and follows a logical order.

Since a left-sided PVC double-lumen tube is preferred for either right or left thoracotomy, only the steps for positioning a left-sided double-lumen tube are described (Fig. 12-15).[75]

Before intubation, both cuffs are inflated and checked for leaks and are then deflated. The patient is preoxygenated and general anesthesia is induced. A Macintosh laryngoscopy blade is preferred since it provides the largest area through which to pass a double-lumen tube. The curved mid-portion of a conventional Macintosh blade produces a blind area (a "crest-of-the-hill" effect). A modified Macintosh blade, IV-MAC (Improved Vision-Macintosh), has a concave mid-portion which reduces the blind area by more than 50 percent.[87a] The IV-MAC blade is particularly useful in thoracic surgery since it optimizes visual exposure while still allowing maximal space for passage of a double-lumen tube. The tip of the double-lumen tube is advanced just past the vocal cords. At this point the stylet in the bronchial lumen is removed to avoid tracheobronchial trauma.

The tube is then rotated between 90–125 degrees toward the bronchus to be intubated and is advanced until moderate resistance is encountered. The usual depth of insertion for a PVC tube in adults (males and females) is about 29–30 cm (range: 28–32 cm) as measured from the patient's lips.[87b]

After advancing the tube into the bronchus, both the tracheal and bronchial cuffs are inflated with air. The bronchial cuff should be inflated first while ventilating the patient through the bronchial lumen with the tracheal lumen clamped. As the cuff is slowly inflated, the absence of the audible leak at the proximal open port of the tracheal lumen occurs when an airtight seal is achieved. When the appropriate-sized double-lumen tube is used, only 1–2 mL of air should be sufficient to seal the airway.[88] The syringe should be removed from the valve to avoid accidental deflation of the cuff.

The patient is then ventilated through both lumens. Moisture should appear in both lumens and the chest wall should show bilateral movement. The chest must be carefully auscultated for the presence of bilateral breath sounds, particularly over the left upper chest.

The tracheal lumen is the first to be clamped. Breath sounds should be heard only over the intubated (left) lung. If bilateral sounds are audible, the bronchial lumen is still not positioned deeply enough in the left bronchus or the bronchial cuff is not adequately sealing the airway. If breath sounds are heard only over the right lung, the left-sided tube is in the right bronchus. In this case, both cuffs are deflated and the tip of the tube is withdrawn above the carina. The tube is rerotated to the left and advanced. Bending and turning the patient's head and neck to the right (the side opposite the bronchus to be intubated) before readvancing the tube helps.[88b] Both cuffs are then reinflated.

Once the double-lumen tube is in the left bronchus, the left lumen is clamped and the patient is ventilated through the tracheal lumen. Breath sounds should now be heard only over the right lung. If ventilating the patient presents difficulties (very high pressures required or no breath sounds heard), only the bronchial cuff should be deflated and ventilation through the tracheal lumen should continue. If the tube is still not deep enough in the right bronchus, bilateral breath sounds are now audible, and if the tube is too deep in the left bronchus, breath sounds are heard only over the left lung.

The entire left lung must be carefully auscultated. The bronchial cuff of any double-lumen tube, especially that of smaller tubes, can be advanced past the orifice of the upper lobe bronchus. In this situation, clamping the bronchial lumen and ventilating through the tracheal lumen produces breath sounds over the entire right lung *and* the left-upper lung. The left lower lobe is not ventilated. More commonly, the inflated bronchial cuff is just at the orifice of the upper lobe bronchus and obstructs it.[73] When ventilating the left side with the tracheal lumen clamped, only the left lower lobe inflates. If the bronchial cuff is deflated the left upper lobe reexpands, and breath sounds are suddenly audible over the upper chest.

The tube should be advanced or withdrawn in 0.5–1.0-cm increments depending on these auscultatory signs, and all the previous steps should be repeated.

Fiberoptic Bronchoscopy

A 4 mm diameter fiberoptic bronchoscope is used by many anesthesiologists to confirm the position of the double-lumen tube visually following "blind" placement by auscultation.[89,90] Although no consensus as to whether fiberoptic bronchoscopy should be routinely used has been reached, the ability to recognize normal and abnormal double-lumen tube positions with a fiberoptic bronchoscope is a skill all an-

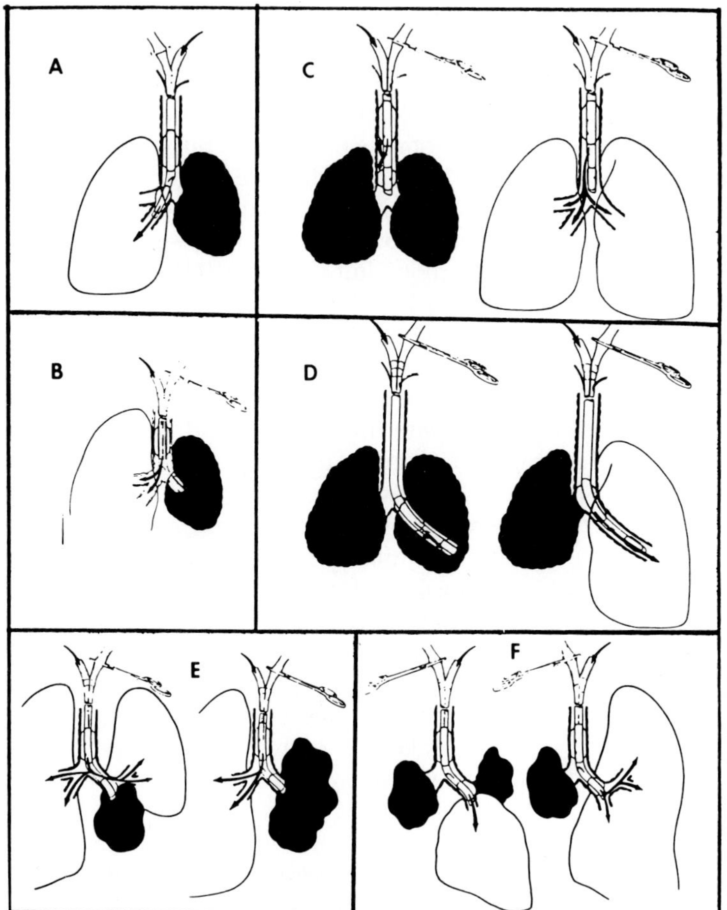

Figure 12-15. Illustration of the steps for positioning a left-sided double-lumen tube. After induction of anesthesia the tube is advanced into the left main bronchus. Both the tracheal (right) and endobronchial (left) cuffs are inflated with air and the right lumen is occluded. A shows that if breath sounds are present only over the right lung while ventilating through the left lumen, a right-sided intubation has occurred. B shows that once the tube is in the left bronchus, the left lumen is occluded and breath sounds should be heard only over the right lung. At this point it is difficult to ventilate through the right lumen, and only the left cuff is deflated. C illustrates that if the tube is not far enough into the left bronchus, breath sounds are now present over both lungs while ventilating through the right lumen. In D, breath sounds are now heard only over the left lung because the tube is too deep. E indicates that the left cuff may be past the orifice of the left upper lobe bronchus. Occluding the left lumen and ventilating through the right produces breath sounds over the entire right lung and the left upper lung. The left lower lobe will not be ventilated. F shows that the left cuff may obstruct the left upper lobe bronchus. Ventilating through the left with the right lumen occluded requires very high inspiratory pressures and breath sounds are present only over the left lower lung. Deflating the left cuff allows the left upper lobe to immediately reexpand. (Redrawn, with permission, from references 73 and 75.)

esthesiologists who manage thoracic surgical cases should possess.[91] Color photographs taken through a fiberoptic bronchoscope of properly and improperly placed double-lumen tubes, which have been recently published, are quite helpful in recognizing tube positioning problems.[91]

In order to properly perform fiberoptic bronchoscopy the reader should be familiar with the fiberoptic presentation of the main carina and the left and right bronchial carina (Fig. 12-16). Otherwise, a bronchial carina can

Figure 12-16. Fiberoptic presentation of the main carina and of the right and left bronchial carina. See Color Plate 4. (Reprinted with permission from Ovassapain A. Fiberoptic airway endoscopy in anesthesia and critical care. New York: Raven Press 1990.)

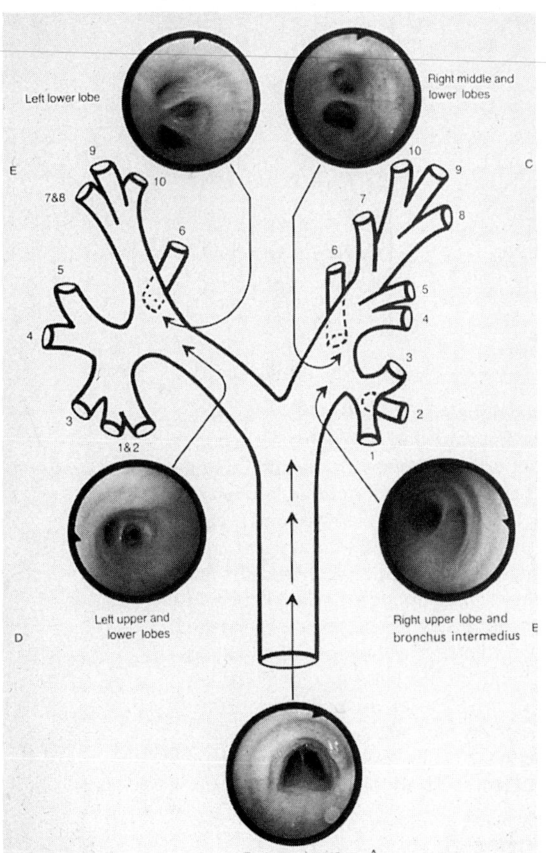

be mistaken for the main carina and vice versa. A double-lumen tube is in optimal position when view down the tracheal lumen of the blue bronchial cuff immediately below the carina in the appropriate bronchus is unobstructed.[72] An overinflated bronchial cuff herniating into the carina is easily recognized. Figure 12-17 shows a fiberoptic positioning of left-sided double-lumen tube. Unfortunately, if the cuff is immediately below the carina, any head movement or manipulations by the surgeon during the operation can easily displace the cuff into the carina. The safest position for a double-lumen tube is with the proximal end of its bronchial cuff to be several millimeters below the carina.

Observation through the tracheal lumen by fiberoptic bronchoscopy confirms only that the tube is in the correct bronchus. Verification that the upper lobe bronchus is not obstructed can only be obtained by bronchoscopy through the smaller bronchial lumen. Figure 12-18 shows a fiberoptic positioning of right-sided double-lumen tube.

The diameter of the bronchoscope must be at least 1 mm smaller than the lumen of the tube through which it is inserted. A silicon-based lubricant that does not interfere with vision may be necessary for smooth passage of larger fiberoptic bronchoscopes in smaller tubes. A bronchoscope with an outside diameter of 5.6 mm is too big for even the largest PVC double-lumen tube (Table 12-6). A 4.9-mm diameter bronchoscope can be used only for larger (39F and 41F) tubes. In order to see down both lumens of smaller (35F) tubes, a bronchoscope with a diameter of 4.5 mm or less and a working length of more than 50 cm is needed. Thinner instruments with 3.6–4.2-mm outside diameters pass through all double-lumen tubes, are more maneuverable, and cause less obstruction of gas flow than larger bronchoscopes. In choosing a fiberoptic bronchoscope, tip flexibility of 120° or more and a suction channel are

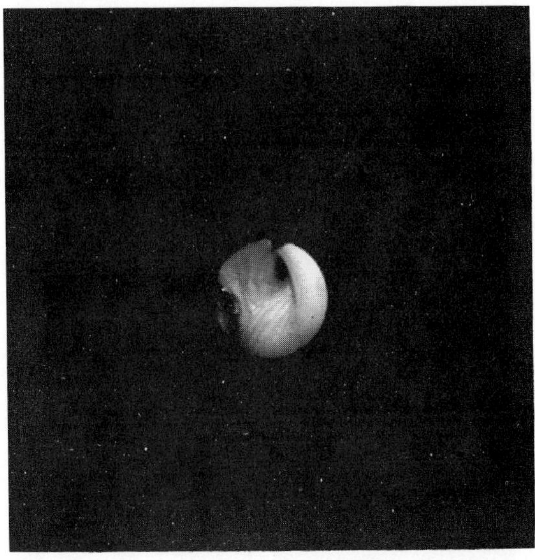

Figure 12-17. Endoscopic view of the left sided double-lumen tube positioning. The tip of the blue cuff of the bronchial lumen is visible at the carina. The right main stem bronchus orifice is fully open and is unobstructed by the bronchial cuff. This represents the proper position of the left sided tube. See Color Plate 5.

very useful properties to consider.[91] See Chapter 17 for more information on fiberoptic bronchoscopy.

If fiberoptic bronchoscopy is relied on solely for accurate double-lumen tube placement, it is important to have a portable disinfectant system in the operating room. The bronchoscope must be readily available throughout the entire procedure should any placement-related problems occur.

When properly used, fiberoptic bronchoscopy is the most accurate way to verify double-lumen tube position. However, the recommendation that fiberoptic bronchoscopy be a standard of care for placing a double-lumen tube should be challenged.[77] Bronchoscopy alone is not sufficient, since careful auscultation should always be performed.[92] Bronchoscopy down the tracheal lumen identifies bronchial cuff position as it relates to the carina, but it does not reveal other potential problems such as a twisted or obstructed bronchial lumen or an early take-off of the upper lobe bronchus with obstruction by the bronchial cuff.[73]

Auscultation is simple and follows a logical sequence that allows for rapid, accurate, double-lumen tube placement. However, reliance on breath sounds alone may not be possible in all situations. For instance, auscultation is impractical once the patient is prepped and draped in the lateral decubitus position. In addition, auscultation may not be reliable in the presence of very severe unilateral or bilateral pulmonary disease.

This author believes that an understanding of double-lumen tubes eliminates the need for routine verification by fiberoptic bronchoscopy in the vast majority of cases. Fiberoptic bronchoscopy sometimes may be time-consuming, expensive if institutional charges for

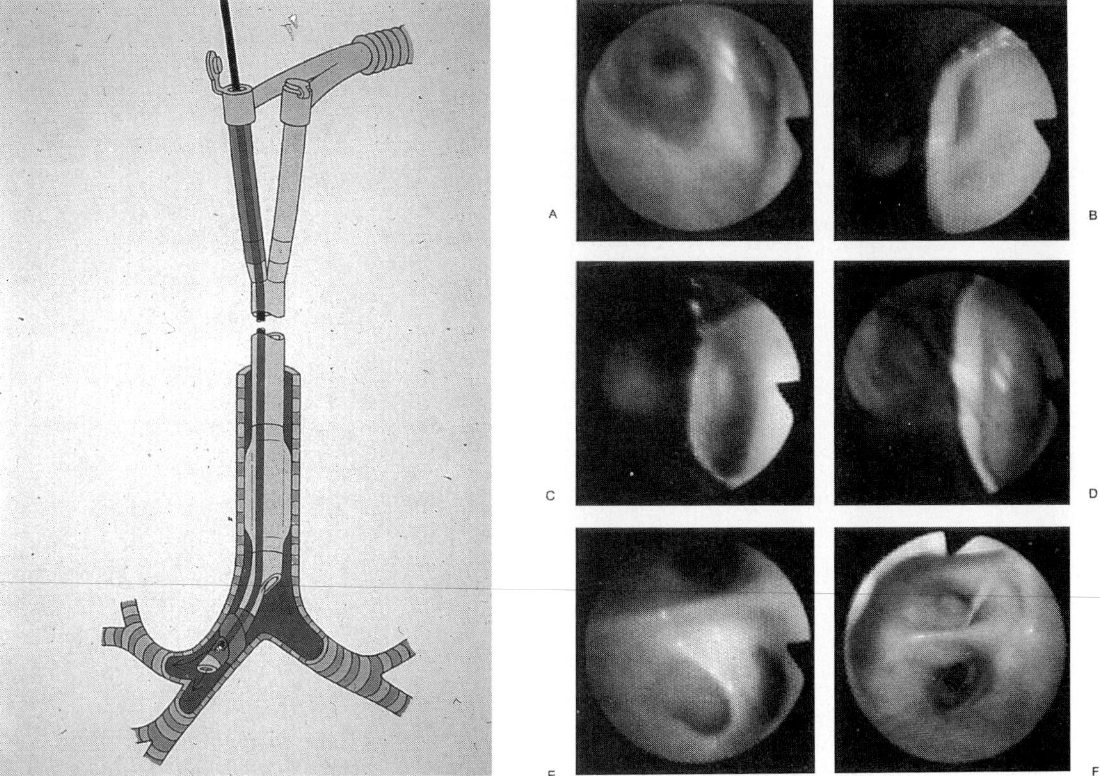

Figure 12-18. Endoscopic view of right-sided endobronchial tube positioning. A. Right upper lobe bronchus orifice and bronchus intermedius. B. The tip of the fiberscope at the upper level of the bronchial cuff slit showing the side opening of the bronchial tube and tracheal wall. C. As the fiberscope and tube are advanced, the opening of the right upper lobe bronchus comes into view. D. The bronchial cuff slit positioned against the right upper lobe bronchus orifice. The distal border of the orifice at the level of the distal border of the bronchial slit. E. The fiberscope is advanced through the bronchial cuff slit into the right upper lobe bronchus showing three segments of the right upper lobe. F. The fiberscope is advanced beyond the distal opening of the bronchial lumen to visualize the right middle and lower lobe bronchial orifices. See Color Plates 6 and 7. (Reprinted with permission from Ovassapain A. Fiberoptic airway endoscopy in anesthesia and critical care. New York: Raven Press 1990.)

its use must be considered, and is itself a potential source of airway trauma.

Although most often used to verify tube position, fiberoptic bronchoscopy can also be used to position the double-lumen tube.[87] The bronchoscope is placed through the tracheal lumen after the tracheal cuff is beyond the vocal cords. The trachea and carina are then inspected as the double-lumen tube is advanced into the appropriate bronchus. Direct visualization helps recognize anatomic abnormalities or pathology that may hinder placement and thus may reduce the risk of trauma from "blind" rotation and insertion.[81,87]

A small fiberoptic bronchoscope can be placed in the bronchial lumen as a stylet and the double-lumen tube advanced over it directly into the bronchus if desired. Ventilation can continue even while the bronchoscope is in place if the fiberoptic bronchoscope is inserted through a swivel adaptor. Once the appropriate bronchus has been intubated, the bronchoscope is withdrawn from the bronchial lumen. It is then be passed down the tracheal lumen to position the double-lumen tube more accurately.

A double-lumen tube, like a conventional endotracheal tube, can be placed over a fiberoptic bronchoscope for tracheal (and bronchial) intubation when visualization of the glottis by direct laryngoscopy is not possible.[93]

Radiography

Some anesthesiologists depend on chest radiographs or fluoroscopy to confirm double-lumen tube placement.[94] The radiopaque markers at the distal ends of both lumens and the tracheal carina must be clearly visible. This may be practical in the ICU where chest x-rays are taken routinely, however in the operating room this method is time-consuming, expensive, and often difficult to perform with the patient in the lateral decubitus position. It is impractical if intraoperative changes in tube position occur, especially in acute, life-threatening situations.

Capnography

Capnographic monitoring of each lung has also been used to determine double-lumen tube placement.[95] Two end-tidal carbon dioxide analyzers are connected to the proximal ends of both lumens, and the correct position of the tube is identified by the simultaneous and synchronous needle movement of the two analyzers. The wave forms from each lung can also be compared. If either lumen is clamped, no needle oscillation of the appropriate carbon dioxide analyzer is evident. Of course, when one lung is intentionally collapsed, no end-tidal carbon dioxide from that lung can be monitored. Thus changes in tube position cannot be recognized using capnography in many cases.

Spirometry

Presently Side Stream Spirometry (Datex Division Instrumentarium Corp., Helsinki, Finland) can provide close monitoring of the patient's pulmonary function by displaying breath-by-breath pressure and volume loops (see Fig. 12-19). This device may help to determine the correct positioning of the DLT or to detect intraoperative displacement. After the double-lumen endotracheal tube is "blindly" placed and both cuffs are inflated, the common connector is attached to a flow sensor.[95a] Displays representing pressure-volume and flow-volumes are recorded with both lungs inflated and with each lumen clamped. The pattern of the flow-volume loop is determined by the mechanical properties of the total respiratory system (the lung and thorax, the bronchial tube and the ventilator) but is reproducible for any given patient. When the double-lumen tube is accurately positioned, the curve is very similar during two- and one-lung ventilation. Figure 12-20 shows pressure-volume loops during two-lung and one-lung ventilation with obstruction and following adjustment of the DLT position.

Other Positioning Tests

Because a double-lumen tube is easily displaced, its position must always be rechecked after the patient is turned to the lateral decubitus position. A tube can be moved any time the surgeon manipulates the hilum or carina or causes any other anatomic distortion.[80] Head movement can result in changes in cuff position,[96] and flexion of the neck can cause a double-lumen tube to move distally by as much as 3 cm, thus increasing the chance of upper lobe obstruction. Extension of the neck can cause a bronchial cuff to move out of the bron-

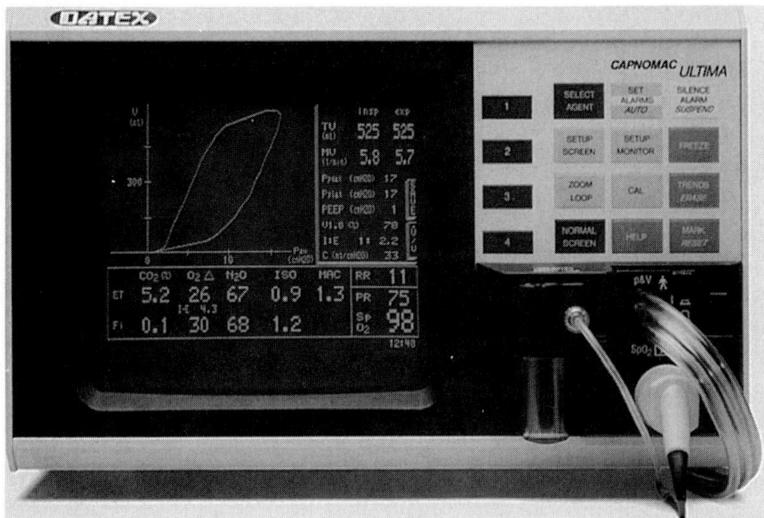

Figure 12-19. Side Stream Spirometry (Datex Division Instrumentarium Corp., Helsinki, Finland).

chus and into the carina, which results in obstruction of the opposite lung.

The anesthesiologist must always be alert for signs of dislodgement, because ventilation of the dependent lung through either the tracheal or bronchial lumen is never directly visualized. During one-lung ventilation, changes in the peak inspiratory pressure, end-tidal carbon dioxide, oxygen saturation, and mediastinal movement during inspiration must be continuously assessed as tube position can change at any time.[97]

When first placing a double-lumen tube, a simple test can be used. The tube can be withdrawn a few millimeters after it is first positioned. If the seal of the inflated bronchial cuff is maintained without requiring additional air, some leeway against accidental movement with herniation of the bronchial cuff into the carina during operation is assured.[86] If the seal is adequate, the tube should be readvanced the initial distance down the bronchus.

The surgeon can also help if the tube is not accurately placed initially or if it becomes dislodged during surgery. During left thoracotomy a left-sided double-lumen tube that is positioned too deeply produces upper lobe atelectasis, which is obvious when the chest is opened. The tube can be withdrawn in 1-cm increments until the left upper lobe reexpands. During right thoracotomy the bronchial cuff of a left-sided double-lumen tube may obstruct the left upper lobe; the surgeon can palpate the left bronchus through the mediastinum. The tube can then be withdrawn with digital guidance from the surgeon until it is just proximal to the left upper lobe bronchus. Even if the tip of the tube is accidently withdrawn into the trachea, the surgeon can compress the right bronchus while the anesthesiologist advances the double-lumen tube back into the left bronchus.[80]

Bronchial Cuff Tests

Periodic attention to the bronchial cuff, usually by digital examination of the pilot balloon to

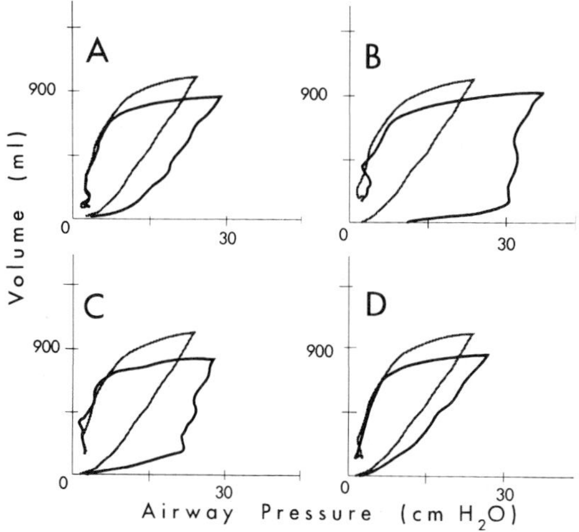

Figure 12-20. Pressure-volume loops during two-lung (stippled curve) and one-lung (solid curve) ventilation. A. Initial. B. Obstruction. C. Decreased obstruction as tube is withdrawm. D. Return to control state with further withdrawal. (Reproduced with permission from Simon BA, Hurford WE, Alfille PH, Haspel K, Behringer EC. An aid in the diagnosis of malpositioned double-lumen tubes. Anesthesiology 1992;76:862.)

the bronchial cuff, is always important. Underinflation of the cuff or loss of pressure from cuff rupture can result in failure to collapse the operated lung or contamination of the dependent lung. Overinflation of the cuff can cause airway damage or cuff herniation into the carina with tracheal obstruction. If nitrous oxide is used, caution is advised since it can lead to cuff distension.

Jenkins described an "air seal" technique for determining the precise end-point for cuff inflation.[98] This test is is also useful for continuing assessment of cuff integrity during surgery. The proximal end of the tracheal lumen is fitted with an airtight connector, which in turn feeds into a piece of rubber or plastic tubing. The distal end of this tubing is immersed in a bottle containing water. When ventilation occurs only through the bronchial lumen, any leaking gas around the bronchial cuff escapes into the trachea and is indicated by bubbling in the indicator bottle. The bronchial cuff is initially inflated with just enough air to stop the bubbling. The absence of bubbles after several inflations is a simple and sensitive indicator of functional separation of the lungs. It is important that the indicator bottle be positioned well below the height of the patient's carina to prevent siphoning of the indicator fluid from the bottle into the lungs. At least one double-lumen tube adaptor that incorporates a T-piece connected to an oxygen flowmeter and an underwater seal to test for bronchial cuff patency has been described.[54]

After the double-lumen endotracheal tube is first positioned and both cuffs inflated, the ventilatory circuit can be directly attached only to the lumen to the ventilated lung. A latex finger cot or a finger cut from a small latex glove is fitted snugly over the open lumen to the nonventilated lung. If lung separation is incomplete, the rubber "balloon" will inflate with each ventilation. Once the airway is completely sealed the balloon will cease to inflate.[98a]

To reduce the risk of bronchial wall injury, bronchial cuff pressure can also be monitored. A 10-mL syringe barrel can be taped upright to a pole near the patient's head.[99] A long length of intravenous tubing is attached to the syringe and run downward for a desired distance (for example, 25 cm for a pressure of 25 cm H_2O). The final 10 cm is coiled and taped perpendicular to the pole. The end of the tubing is clamped, and the syringe barrel is filled to the top with water. When the clamp is released, the tubing is filled with water to the last turn in the coil, and then the tubing is reclamped. After the double-lumen tube is positioned its cuffs are inflated with air until no leak is apparent. The end of the extension tubing is then plugged into the bronchial cuff's pilot balloon port and the clamp is released. The intracuff pressure then equals the height of the water column.

Diffusion of nitrous oxide into the cuff displaces air from the cuff and pushes the water up along the tubing coils, but the height of the water column and the pressure exerted by the bronchial cuff are essentially unchanged. A cuff leak may not be apparent.

Cuff pressure can be monitored by a sphygmomanometer gauge connected by a rubber hose to the pilot balloon of the bronchial cuff.[100] The gauge displays intracuff pressure and a three-way stopcock inserted in the rubber hose allows deflation of excessive intracuff gas volume if intracuff pressure rises. Plastic syringes connected directly to the pilot balloon can be used to vent pressures.[101] Usually, digital monitoring of the pilot balloon is sufficient to detect a cuff leak.[101a]

Complications

Some of the complications associated with double-lumen tubes (Table 12-7) are identical to those of conventional endotracheal tubes, and some are unique to just double-lumen tubes. These complications can be minimized or even completely eliminated if the properties of double-lumen tubes are understood. Special attention must also be paid to the selection of tubes of appropriate size for the particular patient.

Positioning

The most common positioning problems with double-lumen tubes are insufficient passage into the bronchus, intubation of the wrong bronchus, and advancement too far into the correct bronchus.[86]

Rubber double-lumen tubes are associated with a high incidence of these positioning difficulties. Complications occur in as many as 20–30% of patients intubated with Carlens and Robertshaw tubes.[64,86,102,103] These problems usually manifest themselves as failure to isolate the lung and cross-leakage during ventilation and the inability to deflate the operated lung when selective atelectasis is desired. Another frequently encountered problem with rubber double-lumen tubes is the initial selection of a tube that is too large to pass through either the vocal cords or into the bronchus.[86] When smaller tubes are substituted and intubation ac-

Table 12-7. Complications with Double-Lumen Tubes

Complications
Placement
Carinal hook unable to pass through glottis
Inability to advance tube into bronchus
Tube too large
Intrinsic or extrinsic airway obstruction
Positioning
Tube not far enough into bronchus
Herniation of bronchial cuff into carina
Inability to ventilate nonintubated lung when both cuffs inflated
Tube down wrong bronchus
Tube too deep in correct bronchus
Upper lobe obstruction
Failure to collapse lung
Position of tube changes during surgery
Surgical manipulation
Movement to lateral decubitus position
Head flexion or extension
Inadequate taping; patient poorly secured
Interference with operation
Bronchial lumen
Pneumonectomy
Carinal surgery
Trauma
Airway injury
Laryngitis, mucosal injury, arytenoid dislocation
Tracheobronchial rupture
Overinflation or too rapid inflation of cuffs
Use of nitrous oxide, causing cuff distention
Tube advanced with stylet still in place
Forceful insertion of too large a tube
Movement of double-lumen tube with cuffs inflated
Preexisting airway pathology
Hypoxemia
Malpositioned double-lumen tube
Upper lobe collapse
Carinal obstruction
Rupture of thoracic aneurysm
Displacement of mediastinal mass
Double-lumen tube sutured to pulmonary vessel (hemorrhage on attempted extubation)

complished, the airflow resistance during one-lung ventilation markedly increases.[86]

In one prospective study of the use of rubber Robertshaw double-lumen tubes in 59 patients, difficulties with intubation of the trachea occurred in seven cases, and problems with tubes inserted insufficiently far into the bronchus occurred in eight others.[86] When the tube is not inserted far enough into the bronchus, and the endobronchial cuff is hyperinflated, the bronchial lumen ventilates the intubated lung normally but the overdistended bronchial cuff can produce a valvular obstruction with gas trapping in the nonintubated lung. Besides failure to collapse the nonintubated lung, undetected gas trapping can progress to cardiorespiratory collapse or cause severe barotrauma.

In five other patients, the right bronchus was intubated with a left-sided tube. A left-sided, rubber double-lumen tube was advanced too far down the left bronchus in only one of the 59 patients, in contrast PVC double-lumen tubes where advancement of a left-sided tube too far into the bronchus is perhaps the most commonly encountered positioning problem encountered.[73]

Most clinicians find that PVC double-lumen tubes are easier to use than rubber tubes.[65] However, to avoid complications the tubes have to be used correctly. In an often quoted study, PVC double-lumen tubes were initially placed "blindly" by auscultation. Fiberoptic bronchoscopy was used after the patients were placed in the lateral decubitus position.[72] At that time the double-lumen tube was described as being "in less than optimal position" in 11 of the 23 patients (48%), that is, the cuff was not immediately below the carina. All but one man in this series were intubated with 39F tubes and the women with 37F tubes. The problems encountered in this study (upper lobe obstruction and carinal cuff herniation) could have been avoided if larger double-lumen tubes had initially been used and if the bronchial cuffs had not been overinflated.

The clinical experience of the author and others[92] has indicated that with proper selection of appropriately sized tubes and careful auscultation, the incidence of mechanically significant tube malposition is much less than 48%. Clinically significant problems occurred in only 4% of a large series of patients in which the double-lumen tube was positioned using only auscultation.[64]

Trauma

Double-lumen tubes, particularly those with carinal hooks, can injure the airway at any time, especially during intubation and extubation. Airway trauma ranges from ecchymosis of the mucous membranes to arytenoid dislocation and torn vocal cords. Laryngeal, tracheal, and distal airway trauma has been reported with both red rubber and PVC double-lumen tubes; these complications are relatively uncommon, however.[64, 103]

Tracheobronchial rupture, a more serious injury, has been reported with both rubber and PVC double-lumen tubes.[104–107] Overdistension of either the tracheal or bronchial cuffs, resulting in pressure damage to the airway, or asymmetric cuff distension (more common with rubber tubes), pushing the distal lumen tip into the bronchial wall, are the presumptive causes. Forceful insertion of a tube too large for the mainstem bronchus is another cause of airway perforation.[71] Factors that increase the risks of airway rupture include direct trauma during intubation, advancement of the tube into the airway with the stylet still in place, too rapid inflation and overinflation of the cuff, and preexisting respiratory tree pathology.[108–110] Such conditions as congenital abnormalities of the bronchus, weakness of the bronchial wall from tumor infiltration or from infection, and distortion of the airway by enlarged mediastinal lymph nodes or extrabronchial tumors increase the chances of bronchial rupture.[109]

The usual site of injury is the membranous wall of the distal trachea or main bronchus. Air leak, subcutaneous emphysema, airway hemorrhage, and cardiovascular instability from tension pneumothorax are signs of damage. With an incomplete laceration, air may dissect into the adventitia, thus producing an aneurysmal dilatation of the membranous wall. Nitrous oxide further distends the wall. The injury may not evident until hours later when rupture into the mediastinum or pleural space occurs.[111]

At the completion of surgery the integrity of the intubated bronchus should be tested by hand ventilation for leaks; only the tracheal cuff should be inflated. If airway laceration is suspected bronchoscopy should be performed before extubation to search for signs of trauma. Immediate recognition and surgical intervention is essential for a favorable prognosis.[112]

Airway rupture has been reported with PVC double-lumen tubes from overinflation of the bronchial cuff.[105–107] Although designed as high-volume/low-pressure cuffs, all PVC double-lumen tube bronchial cuffs develop dangerously high pressures when distended with volumes of air greater than necessary to seal the airway.[88,113] In an in vitro model, the bronchial cuffs of 41F Mallinckrodt and Rusch PVC double-lumen tubes needed less than 2 mL of air to seal the bronchus; and the 41F Sheridan PVC double-lumen tube required approximately 4 mL of air (Fig. 12-21).[88] Only 3 mL was required for the rubber double-lumen tube, which is not surprising since the lumen of the larger rubber tube almost completely fills the airway.

Inflation with larger volumes of air than necessary produces very high pressures in the bronchial cuffs of PVC tubes on the airway mucosa. These volumes approach those levels seen with the high-pressure cuffs on rubber tubes. At 4 mL, all PVC double-lumen tube cuffs generated pressures identical to those of low-volume/high-pressure rubber cuffs.

If larger than usual volumes of air are needed to effectively seal the bronchus during surgery, two explanations are possible. A cuff leak may be present. More likely, the tube may need to be advanced deeper into the bronchus, since a cuff herniating into the carina requires much larger volumes to even partially seal the intubated bronchus.

Bronchial rupture has been reported even when small volumes of air were initially used to inflate the cuff. If nitrous oxide is administered during long procedures, both cuffs must be deflated periodically to avoid excessive pressure from nitrous oxide distension of the cuff on the mucosa.[107] Initial cuff inflation with a gas mixture similar to that used to ventilate the patient prevents intraoperative cuff distension.

The bronchial cuff should also be deflated before placing the patient in the lateral decubitus position to decrease the chances of injury during movement. During surgery, many anesthesiologists deflate the bronchial cuff when the operated, non-dependent lung is ventilated to reduce the risk of mucosal injury. This maneuver may itself be dangerous, however since it allows material to be aspirated from the operated lung to the dependent lung.[27]

Hypoxia

The most common problem during one-lung ventilation is hypoxemia. When a lung is selectively collapsed, arterial oxygen tension may drop precipitously due to the blood that continues to perfuse the nonventilated lung. Malposition of the double-lumen tube may contribute significantly to the development of hypoxemia. Upper lobe obstruction with atelectasis in the intubated lung or carinal herniation of the bronchial cuff resulting in partial or com-

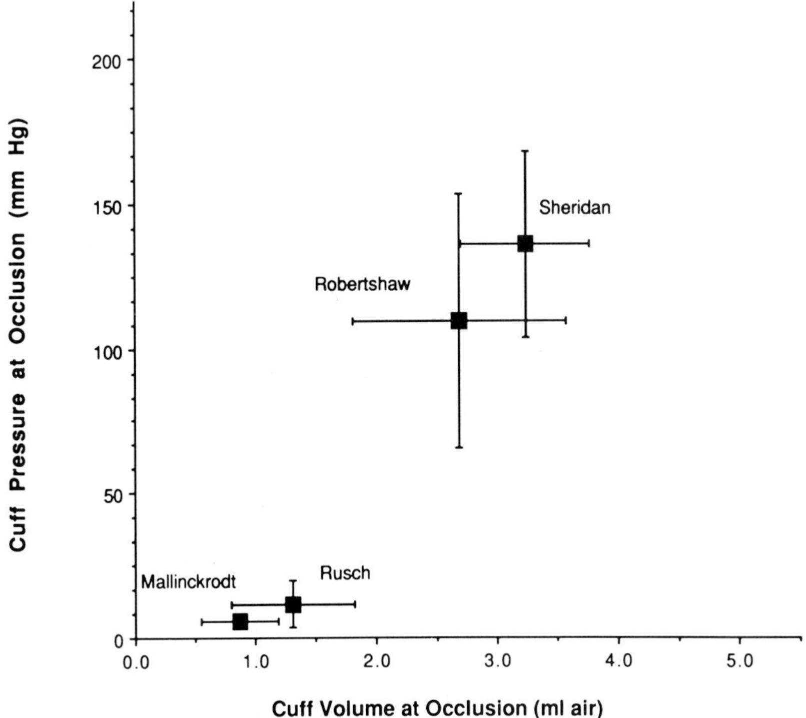

Figure 12-21. Graphical representation of the bronchial cuff pressure at the volume necessary to occlude a model of the left bronchus. Average values for occlusion pressure (mmHg) and occlusion volume (mL air) are shown ± 1 sd. There were no significant differences in either pressure or volume between the polyvinyl chloride Mallinckrodt and Rusch tubes, but both these tubes had occlusion pressures and volumes that were significantly lower ($P < .05$) than those of the plastic Sheridan and rubber Robertshaw tubes. (Reproduced, with permission, from Brodsky JB, Adkins MO, Gaba DM: Bronchial cuff pressure of double-lumen tubes. Anesth Analg 1989;69:608.

plete obstruction of ventilation to the nonintubated lung have been discussed.

Others Problems

Attempted passage of a double-lumen tube in the presence of a mediastinal mass can compress or displace the mass, leading to obstruction of major vessels and cardiac arrest. Wells et al described a case of cardiac arrest following satisfactory placement of a double-lumen tube.[114] Passage of a semi-rigid, rubber double-lumen tube displaced a large intrapulmonary cyst, which in turn compressed the pulmonary outflow tract. Until the obstruction was relieved, the patient was refractory to resuscitation. The authors postulated that early replacement of the large rubber tube with a thinner, softer plastic double-lumen tube may have been all that would have been sufficient to decompress the pulmonary artery and permit resuscitation.

Distortion of the upper airway by an aortic aneurysm makes "blind" placement of the double-lumen tube hazardous, especially if a left tube is chosen.[81]

At least one death has been attributed to the suturing of a double-lumen tube to a pulmonary blood vessel during surgery. After some resistance to extubation the tube was removed and this was followed by rapid exsanguination.[115] Excessive resistance to extubation should make the anesthesiologist consider the possibility of the inadvertant suturing of the airway or vessel to the bronchial portion of the double-lumen tube.

References

1. Gale JW, Waters RM. Closed endobronchial anesthesia in thoracic surgery. J Thorac Surg 1931; 1:432.
2. Crafoord C. On the technique of pneumonectomy in man. Acta Chir Scandinav 1938;81(Suppl 54):1.
3. Magill IW. Anaesthetics in thoracic surgery with special reference to lobectomy. Proc R Soc Med 1936;29:643.
4. Halton J. A method of controlling bronchial secretions in thoracic surgery. Lancet 1943;1:12.
5. Moody JD, Trent JC, Newton GW. An endobronchial balloon for the control of bronchial secretions during lobectomy and pneumonectomy. J Thorac Surg 1947;16:258.
6. Stephen EDS. Problems of "blocking" in upper lobectomies. Anesth Analg 1952;31:175.
7. Machray R. Anaesthesia for the surgical treatment of chest disease. Tuberculosis Index 1958;13:172.
8. Vale R. Selective bronchial blocking in a small child. Br J Anaesth 1969;41:453.
9. Ginsberg RJ. New technique for one-lung anesthesia using an endobronchial blocker. J Thorac Cardiovasc Surg 1981;82:542.
10. Oxorn D. Use of fiberoptic bronchoscope to assist placement of a Fogarty catheter as a bronchial blocker. Can J Anaesth 1987;34:427.
11. Inoue H, Shohtsua A, Ogawa J, et al. Endotracheal tube with movable blocker to prevent aspiration of intratracheal bleeding. Ann Thorac Surg 1984; 37:497.
12. Kamaya H, Krishna PR. New endotracheal tube (Univent tube) for selective blockade of one lung. Anesthesiology 1985;63:342.
13. Karande SV. A new tube for single lung ventilation. Chest 1987;92:761.
14. Herenstein R, Russo JR, Moonka N, et al. Management of one-lung anesthesia in an anticoagulated patient. Anesth Analg 1988;67:1120.

14a. Inoue H. New-style Univent with a light source on the blocker. J Cardiovasc Surg 1993;34:1.

15. Rovenstine EA. Anesthesia for intrathoracic surgery: the endotracheal and endobronchial techniques. Surg Gynecol Obstet 1936;63:325.
16. Mushin WW, Rendell-Baker L, eds. The principles of thoracic Anaesthesia, past and present. Springfield, IL: Charles C Thomas, 1953:103.
17. Macintosh R, Leatherdale RAL. Bronchus tube and bronchus blocker. Br J Anaesth 1955;27:556.
18. Green R, Gordon W. Right lung anaesthesia. Anaesthesia for left lung surgery using a new right endobronchial tube. Anaesthesia 1957;12:86.
19. Pallister WK. A new endobronchial tube for left lung anaesthesia, with special reference to reconstructive pulmonary surgery. Thorax 1959;14:55.
20. Vellacot WH. A new endobronchial tube for bronchopleural fistula repair. Br J Anaesth 1954;26:442.
21. Carlens E. A new flexible double-lumen catheter for bronchospirometry. J Thorac Surg 1949;18:742.
22. Bjork VO, Carlens E. The prevention of spread during pulmonary resection by the use of a double-lumen catheter. J Thorac Surg 1950;20:151.
23. Robertshaw FL. Low resistance double-lumen endobronchial tubes. Br J Anaesth 1962;34:576.
24. Bjork VO, Carlens E, Friberg O. Endobronchial anesthesia. Anesthesiology 1953;14:60.
25. Moody JD. Endobronchial occlusion during pulmonary resection. J Thorac Surg 1948;18:82.
26. Brodsky JB. Complications of double-lumen tracheal tubes. In: Bishop MJ, ed. Problems in anesthesia. Volume 2. Philadelphia: JB Lippincott, 1988; 292.
27. Maguire DP, Spiro AW. Bronchial obstruction and hypoxia during one-lung ventilation. Anesthesiology 1987;66:830.
28. Adkins MO, Chan JC, Brodsky JB. Unsuccessful unilateral bronchopulmonary lavage in a patient with cystic fibrosis. J Cardiothorac Anesth 1989;3: 481.
29. Shivaram U, Finch P, Nowak P. Plastic endobronchial tubes in the management of life-threatening hemoptysis. Chest 1987;92:1108.
30. Oakes DD, Sherck JP, Brodsky JB, et al. Therapeutic thoracoscopy. J Thor Cardiovasc Surg 1984;87:269.
31. Brodsky JB, Welti RS, Mark JBD. Thoracoscopy for

retrieval of intrathoracic foreign bodies. Anesthesiology 1981;54:91.
32. Carlon GC, Kahn R, Howland WS, et al. Acute life-threatening ventilation-perfusion inequality: an indication for independent lung ventilation. Crit Care Med 1978;6:380.
33. Benjaminsson E, Klain M. Intraoperative dual-mode independent lung ventilation of a patient with a bronchopleural fistula. Anesth Analg 1981; 60:118.
34. Hurst JM, DeHaven CB, Branson RD. Comparison of conventional mechanical ventilation and synchronous independent lung ventilation (SILV) in the treatment of unilateral lung injury. J Trauma 1985;25:766.
35. Frame SB, Marshall WJ, Clifford TG. Synchronized independent lung ventilation in the management of pediatric unilateral pulmonary contusion: case report. J Trauma 1989;29:395.
36. Carlon C, Teba L, Maloney B, et al. Recurrent unilateral lung disease. Intensive Care Med 1981;7: 313.
37. Van Renen RG, Schoonbee CG. Short-term asynchronous ventilation and differential positive end-expiratory pressure in the treatment of aspiration pneumonia. S Afr Med J 1985;67:96.
38. Siegel JH, Stoklosa JC, Borg U, et al. Quantification of symmetric lung pathophysiology as a guide to the use of simultaneous independent lung ventilation in posttraumatic and septic adult respiratory distress syndrome. Ann Surg 1985; 202:425.
39. Stow PJ, Grant I. Asynchronous independent lung ventilation: its use in the treatment of acute unilateral lung disease. Anaesthesia 1985;40:163.
40. Bochenek KJ, Brown M, Skupin A. Use of a double-lumen endotracheal tube with independent lung ventilation for treatment of refractory atelectasis. Anesth Analg 1987;66:1014.
41. Brodsky JB, Abramawitz MD, Mehrez MP. Endobronchial intubation for protection intraoperatively of a single functioning lung. Anesth Analg 1976;55:340.
42. Wood RE, Campbell D, Razzuk MA, et al. Surgical advantages of selective unilateral ventilation. Ann Thor Surg 1972;14:173.
43. Dalens B, Labbe A, Haberer JP. Selective endobronchial blocking vs selective intubation. Anesthesiology 1982;57:555.
44. Conacher ID. The urinary catheter as a bronchial blocker. Anaesthesia 1983;38:475.
45. Gottlieb LS, Hillberg R. Endobronchial tamponade therapy for intractable hemoptysis. Chest 1975; 67:482.
46. Gourin A, Garzon AA. Control of hemorrhage in emergency pulmonary resection for massive hemoptysis. Chest 1975;68:120.
47. MacGillivay RG. Evaluation of a new tracheal tube with a movable bronchus blocker. Anaesthesia 1988;43:687.
47a. Kelley JG, Gaba DM, Brodsky JB. Bronchial cuff pressures of two tubes used in thoracic surgery. J Cardiothorac Vasc Anesth 1992;6:190.
48. Latto IP, Rosen M, eds. Difficulties in tracheal intubation. In: Vaughan RS. Endobronchial intubation. London: Bailliere-Tindall, 1985:156.
49. White GMJ. A new double-lumen tube. Brit J Anaesth 1960;32:232.
50. Bryce-Smith R. A double-lumen endobronchial tube. Br J Anaesth 1959;31:274.
51. Bryce-Smith R, Salt R. A right-sided double-lumen endobronchial tube. Br J Anaesth 1960;32:230.
52. Hammond JE, Wright DJ. Comparison of the resistances of double-lumen endobronchial tubes. Br J Anaesth 1984;56:299.
53. Alfery DD. Increasing the margin of safety in positioning left-sided double-lumen endotracheal tubes. Anesthesiology 1988;69:149.
54. Sibai AN, Baraka A. A new double lumen tube adaptor. Anaesthesia 1986;41:628.
55. Viljoen JF. A new double-lumen endobronchial tube connector. Anesthesiology 1967;28:950.
56. White GMJ. A two-way union for double lumen tubes. Anaesthesia 1960;15:77.
57. Tanguturi S, Capan LM, Patel K, et al. A new double-lumen tube adaptor. Anesth Analg 1980;59: 507.
58. Andersen HW, Ozaki GT, Benumof JL. A new improved double-lumen tube adaptor. Anesthesiology 1982;56:54.
59. Salt RH. A modified two-way union for double-lumen tube. Anaesthesia 1970;25:418.
60. Welsh BE, Conn AW. A catheter mount for double-lumen endobronchial tubes. Can J Anaesth 1970;17:183.
61. Linter SP. Disposable double-lumen tubes. A cost-effectiveness survey. Anaesthesia 1985;40:191.
62. McKenna MJ, Wilson RS, Botelho RJ. Right upper lobe obstruction with right-sided double-lumen endobronchial tubes: a comparison of two tube types. J Cardiothorac Anesth 1988;2:734.
63. Shulman MS, Brebner J, Cain J, et al. Bronchopulmonary lung lavage. Anesthesiology 1983; 59:597.

64. Burton NA, Watson DC, Brodsky JB, et al. Advantages of a new polyvinyl chloride double-lumen tube in thoracic surgery. Ann Thorac Surg 1983; 36:78.
65. Clapham MC, Vaughan RS. Bronchial intubation. A comparison between polyvinyl chloride and red rubber double lumen tubes. Anaesthesia 1985; 40:1111.
66. Simpson PM. Tracheal intubation with a Robertshaw tube via a tracheostomy. Br J Anaesth 1976; 48:373.
67. Seed RF, Wedley JR. Tracheal intubation with a Robertshaw tube via a tracheostomy. Br J Anaesth 1977;49:639.
68. Coe VL, Brodsky JB, Mark JBD. Double-lumen endobronchial tubes for patients with tracheostomies. Anesth Analg 1984;63:882.
69. Taylor S, Walford A, McLellan I. A disposable double-lumen tracheostomy tube—a prototype. Anaesth Intensive Care 1984;12:57.
70. Jesseph JE, Merendino KA. The dimensional interrelationships of the major components of the human tracheobronchial tree. Surg Gynecol Obstet 1957;105:210.
71. Hannallah M, Gomes M. Bronchial rupture associated with the use of a double-lumen tube in a small adult. Anesthesiology 1989;71:457.
72. Smith GB, Hirsch NP, Ehrenwerth J. Placement of double-lumen endobronchial tubes. Correlation between clinical impressions and bronchoscopic findings. Br J Anaesth 1986;58:1317.
73. Brodsky JB, Shulman MS, Mark JBD. Malposition of left-sided double-lumen endobronchial tubes. Anesthesiology 1985;62:667.
74. Saito S, Dohi S, Tajima K. Failure of double-lumen endobronchial tube placement: congenital tracheal stenosis in an adult. Anesthesiology 1987; 66:83.
75. Brodsky JB, Mark JBD. A simple technique for accurate placement of double-lumen endobronchial tubes. Anesth Rev 1983;10:26.
76. Benumof JL, Partridge BL, Salvatierra C, et al. Margin of safety in positioning modern double-lumen endotracheal tubes. Anesthesiology 1987; 67:729.
77. Burke WJ III. Should a fiberoptic bronchoscope be routinely used to position a double-lumen tube? Anesthesiology 1988;68:826.
78. Greene ER Jr, Gutierrez FA. Tip of polyvinyl chloride double-lumen endotracheal tube inadvertently wedged in lower lobe bronchus. Anesthesiology 1986;64:406.
79. Gibbs N, Giles K. Malposition of left-sided PVC double-lumen endobronchial tubes. Anaesth Intensive Care 1986;14:92.
80. Cohen E, Kirschner PA, Goldofsky S. Intraoperative manipulation for positioning of double-lumen tubes. Anesthesiology 1988;68:170.
81. Cohen JA, Denisco RA, Richards TS, et al. Hazardous placement of a Robertshaw-type endobronchial tube. Anesth Analg 1986;65:100.
82. Nazari S, Trazzi R, Moncalvo F, et al. Selective bronchial intubation for one lung anaesthesia in thoracic surgery. A new method. Anaesthesia 1986; 41:519.
83. Nazari S, Trazzi R, Moncalvo F. A new method for separate lung ventilation. J Thorac Cardiovasc Surg 1988;95:133.
84. Trazzi R, Nazari S. Clinical experience with a new right-sided endobronchial tube in left main bronchus surgery. J Cardiothorac Anesth 1989;3:461.
85. Benumof JL. Improving the design and function of double-lumen tubes. J Cardiothoracic Anesth 1988;2:729.
86. Black AMS, Harrison GA. Difficulties with positioning Robertshaw double lumen tubes. Anaesth Intensive Care 1975;3:299.
87. Matthew EB, Hirschmann RA. Placing double-lumen tubes with a fiberoptic bronchoscope. Anesthesiology 1986;65:118.
87a. Gaeta RR, Brodsky JB. A new laryngoscopy blade to facilitate double-lumen tube placement. J Cardiothor Vasc Anesth 1991;5:418.
87b. Brodsky JB, Benumof JL, Ehrenwerth J, et al. Depth of placement of left double-lumen endobronchial tubes. Anesth Analg 1991;73:570.
88. Brodsky JB, Adkins MO, Gaba D. Bronchial cuff pressure measurements of double-lumen tubes. Anesth Analg 1989;69:608.
88a. Slinger PD, Chripko D. Clinical comparison of bronchial cuff pressure in three different designs of left double-lumen tubes. Anesth Analg 1993;77, 305.
88b. Neustein SM, Eisenkraft JB. Proper lateralization of left-sided double-lumen tubes. Anesthesiology 1989;71:996.
89. Ovassapian A. Fibreoptic bronchoscope and double-lumen tracheal tubes. Anaesthesia 1983; 38:1104.
90. Hirsch NP, Smith GB. Malposition of left-sided double-lumen endobronchial tubes. Anesthesiology 1985;63:563.
91. Slinger PD. Fiberoptic bronchoscopic positioning

of double-lumen tubes. J Cardiothorac Anesth 1989;3:486.

92. Grum DF, Porembka D. Misconceptions regarding double-lumen tubes and bronchoscopy. Anesthesiology 1988;68:826.
93. Shulman MS, Brodsky JB, Levesque PR. Fiberoptic bronchoscopy for tracheal and endobronchial intubation of double-lumen tubes. Can J Anasth 1987;34:172.
94. Benumof JL. Separation of the two lungs (double-lumen tube intubation). In: Benumof JL, ed. Anesthesia for thoracic surgery. Philadelphia: WB Saunders, 1987:223.
95. Shafieha MJ, Sit J, Kartha R, et al. End-tidal CO_2 analyzers in proper positioning of the double-lumen tubes. Anesthesiology 1986;64:844.
95a. Bardoczky GI, Levarlet M, Endelman E, et al. Continuous spirometry for detection of double-lumen endobronchial tube displacement. Brit J Anaesth 1993:70:499.
96. Saito S, Dohi S, Naito H. Alteration of double-lumen endobronchial tube position by flexion and extension of the neck. Anesthesiology 1985;62:696.
97. Brodsky JB, Shulman MS, Swan M, et al. Pulse oximetry during one-lung ventilation. Anesthesiology 1985;63:212.
98. Jenkins AV. An endobronchial cuff indicator for use in thoracic surgery. Br J Anaesth 1979;51:905.
99. Kay J, Fisher JA. Control of endotracheal tube cuff pressure using a simple device. Anesthesiology 1987;66:253.
99a. Brodsky JB, Mark JBD. Balloon method for detecting inadequate double-lumen tube cuff seal. Ann Thor Surg 1993:55:1584.
100. Diaz JH. Continuous monitoring of intracuff pressures in endotracheal tubes. Anesthesiology 1988;68:813.
101. Resnikoff E, Katz JA. A modified epidural syringe as an endotracheal tuve cuff pressure-controlling device. Anesth Analg 1990;70:208.
101a. Hannallah MS, Benumof JL, McCarthy PO, et al. Comparison of three techniques to inflate the bronchial cuff of left polyvinylchloride double-lumen tubes. Anesth Analg 1993;77:990.
102. Read RC, Friday CD, Eason CN. Prospective study of the Robertshaw endobronchial catheter in thoracic surgery. Ann Thor Surg 1977;24:156.
103. Newman RW, Finer GE, Downs JE. Routine use of the Carlens double-lumen endobronchial catheter. An experimental and clinical study. J Thorac Cardiovasc Surg 1961;42:327.
104. Guernelli N, Bragaglia RB, Briccoli A, et al. Tracheobronchial ruptures due to cuffed Carlens tubes. Ann Thorac Surg 1979;28:66.
105. Burton NA, Falls SM, Lyons T, et al. Rupture of the left main-stem bronchus with a polyvinyl chloride double-lumen tube. Chest 1983;83:928.
106. Wagner DL, Gammage GW, Wong ML. Tracheal rupture following the insertion of a disposable double-lumen endotracheal tube. Anesthesiology 1985;63:698.
107. Brodsky JB, Shulman MS, Mark JBD. Airway rupture with a disposable double-lumen tube. Anesthesiology 1986;64:415.
108. Heiser M, Steinberg JJ, MacVaugh H III, et al. Bronchial rupture, a complication of use of the Robertshaw double-lumen tube. Anesthesiology 1979;51:88.
109. Foster JM, Lau OJ, Alimo EB. Ruptured bronchus following endobronchial intubation. A case report. Br J Anaesth 1983;55:687.
110. Roxburgh JC. Rupture of the tracheobronchial tree. Thorax 1987;42:681.
111. Kumar SM, Sujit PK, Cohen PJ. Tracheal laceration associated with endotracheal tubes. Anesthesiology 1977;47:298.
112. MacGillivray RG, Rockne DA, Mahomedy AE. Endobronchial tube placement in repair of ruptured bronchus. Anaesth Intensive Care 1987;15:459.
113. Ruiz-Neto PP. Bronchial cuff pressure: comparison of Carlens and polyvinylchloride (PVC) double lumen tubes. Anesthesiology 1987;66:255.
114. Wells DG, Zelcer J, Podolakin W, et al. Cardiac arrest from pulmonary outflow tract obstruction due to a double-lumen tube. Anesthesiology 1987; 66:422.
115. Dryden GE. Circulatory collapse after pneumonectomy (an unusual complication from the use of a Carlens catheter): case report. Anesth Analg 1977; 56:451.

CHAPTER

13

Anesthetic Management of One-Lung Ventilation

Edmond Cohen

Currently, a variety of thoracic surgical procedures, such as lobectomy, pneumonectomy, esophagogastrectomy, pleural decortication, bullectomy, and bronchopulmonary lavage are commonly performed.[1] Present knowledge of the physiology of lung ventilation, the variety of currently available double-lumen tubes, fiberoptic bronchoscopy, and the development of new monitoring devices, render the management of thoracic anesthesia a challenge for the anesthesiologist. The hallmark of thoracic anesthesia is the use of double-lumen tubes (DLT) and the management of one-lung ventilation (OLV). This chapter will provide the essentials of OLV and addresses the issues of indications for OLV, the degree of shunt, choice of anesthetics, methods of lung separation and fiberoptic bronchoscopy, and the management of OLV.

Indications for One-Lung Ventilation

The indications for OLV are summarized in Table 13-1. Customarily, they are classified either as absolute or relative indications.

Absolute Indications

These should be considered life-saving maneuvers to protect individuals from life-threatening complications. An absolute lung separation is indicated when the nondiseased contralateral lung must be protected from a contamination source located in the diseased lung.

Massive bleeding (hemoptysis), and pus (empyema or lung abscess). Contamination from blood or pus may result initially in severe atelectasis and hypoxemia followed by pneumonia and sepsis.

Bronchopleural and bronchocutaneous fistulae are absolute indications because they offer a low resistance pathway for the delivered tidal volume during positive-pressure ventilation. In these circumstances, isolation from the ventilation is mandatory to avoid massive air leaks with wasted ventilation.

Giant unilateral bullae may rupture, increase in size during positive-pressure ventilation, and result in tension pneumothorax with hemodynamic instability.[2]

Bronchopulmonary lavage for alveolar proteinosis, cystic fibrosis, or prevention of contralateral lung drowning from the lavage fluid, is essential.[3]

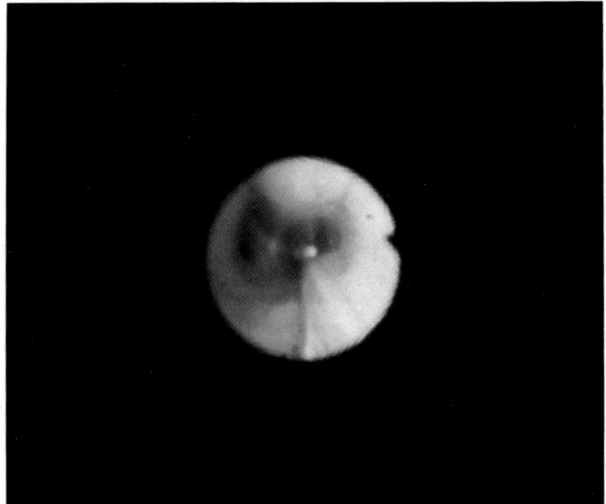

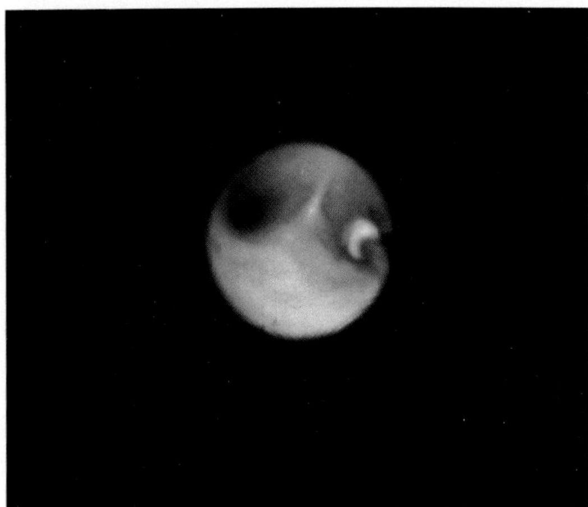

Color Plates 1 and 2. Fiberoptic bronchoscopy view of the bronchial blocker of the Univent tube inserted into the right mainstem bronchus. The bronchial cuff of the Univent tube is of a clear color.

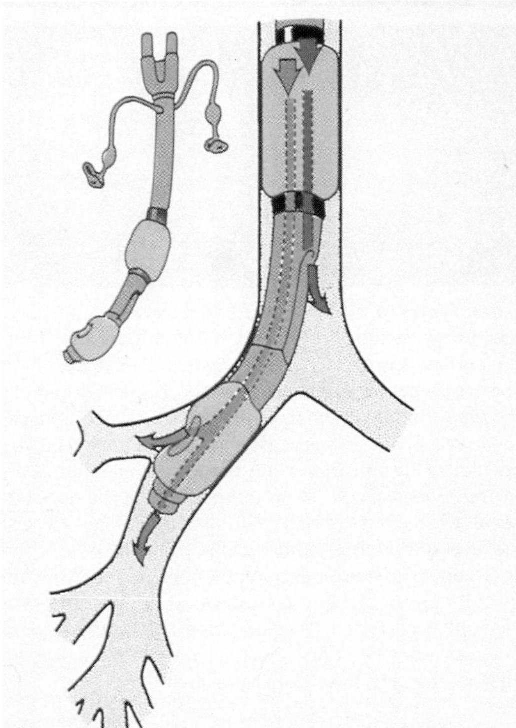

Color Plate 3. When right bronchial intubation is required, a rubber double-lumen tube may be the better choice.

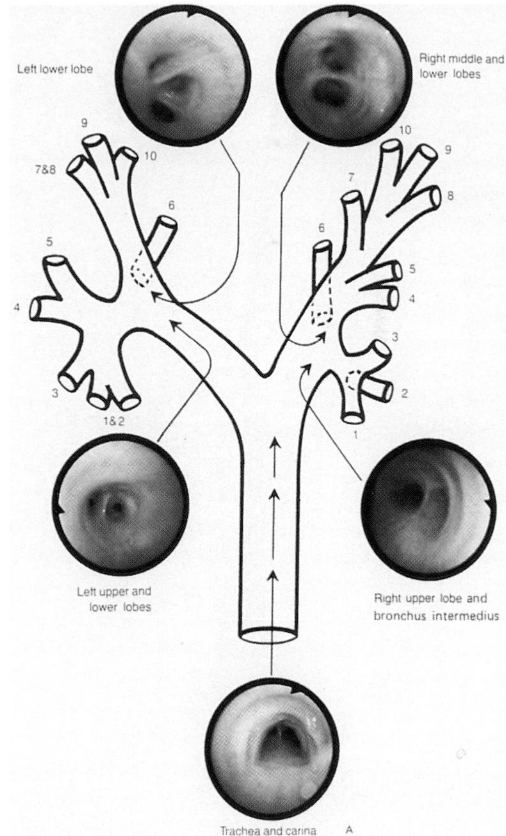

Color Plate 4. Fiberoptic presentation of the main carina and of the right and left bronchial carina.

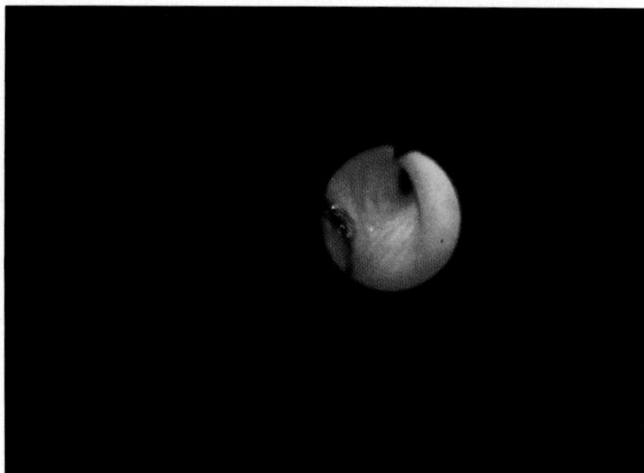

Color Plate 5. Endoscopic view of the left sided double-lumen tube positioning. The tip of the blue cuff of the bronchial lumen is visible at the carina. The right main stem bronchus orifice is fully open and is unobstructed by the bronchial cuff. This represents the proper position of the left sided tube.

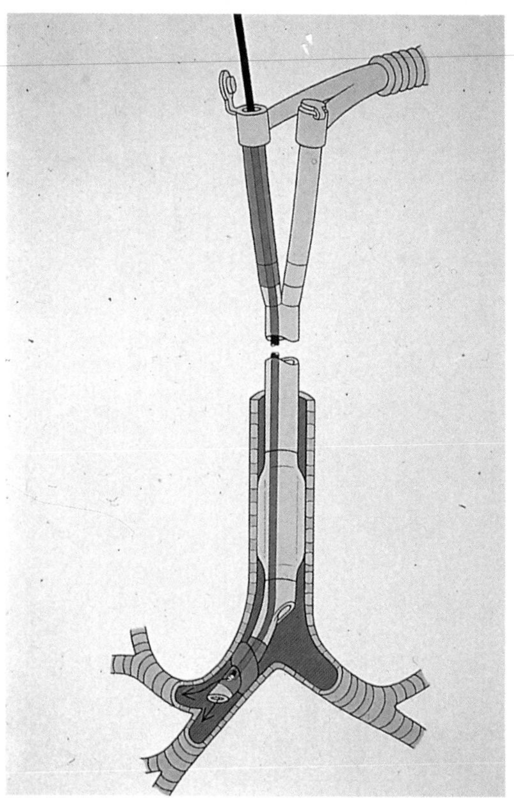

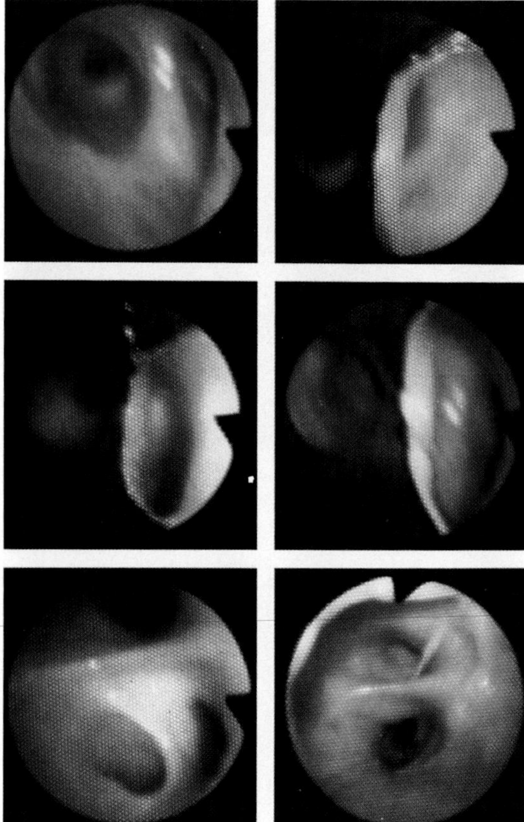

Color Plates 6 and 7. Endoscopic view of right-sided endobronchial tube positioning. A. Right upper lobe bronchus orifice and bronchus intermedius. B. The tip of the fiberscope at the upper level of the bronchial cuff slit showing the side opening of the bronchial tube and tracheal wall. C. As the fiberscope and tube are advanced, the opening of the right upper lobe bronchus comes into view. D. The bronchial cuff slit positioned against the right upper lobe bronchus orifice. The distal border of the orifice at the level of the distal border of the bronchial slit. E. The fiberscope is advanced through the bronchial cuff slit into the right upper lobe bronchus showing three segments of the right upper lobe. F. The fiberscope is advanced beyond the distal opening of the bronchial lumen to visualize the right middle and lower lobe bronchial orifices.

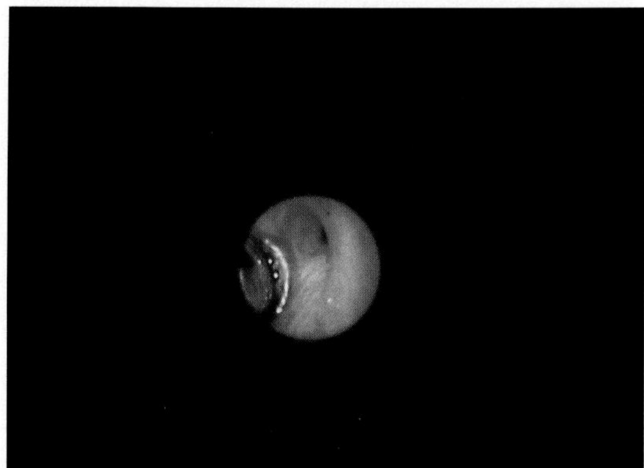

Color Plate 8. The carina is visualized; only the proximal edge of the endobronchial cuff should be identified just below the tracheal carina.

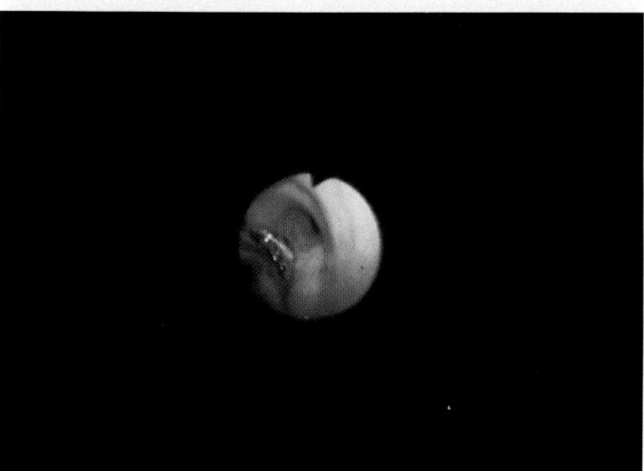

Color Plate 9. The blue bronchial cuff of the disposable PVC DLT is easily identified.

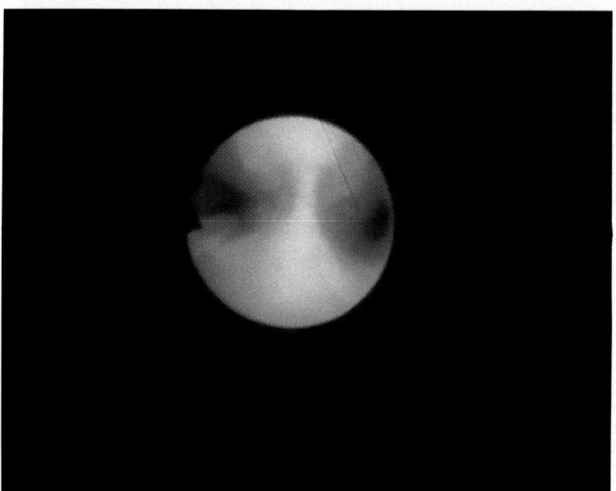

Color Plate 10. The bronchial carina and the patent left upper lobe orifice can be identified.

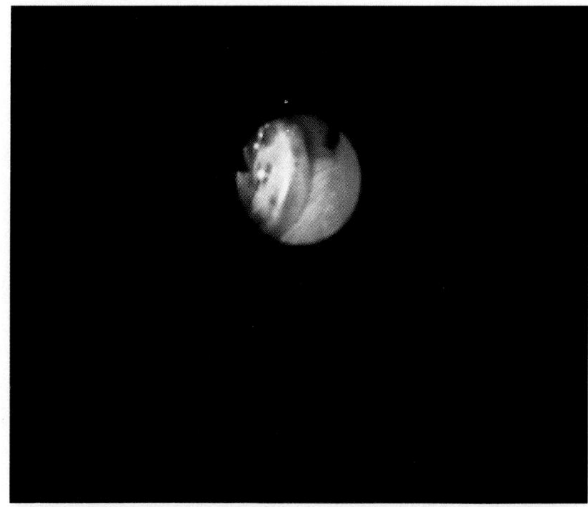

Color Plate 11. The tube is too far in and the tip of the bronchial lumen occluded the left upper lobe orifice.

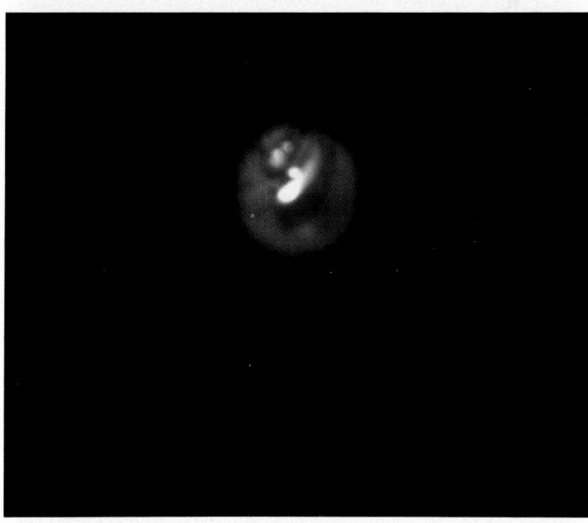

Color Plate 12. The bronchial cuff is herniated over the carina to occlude the ipsilateral main bronchus.

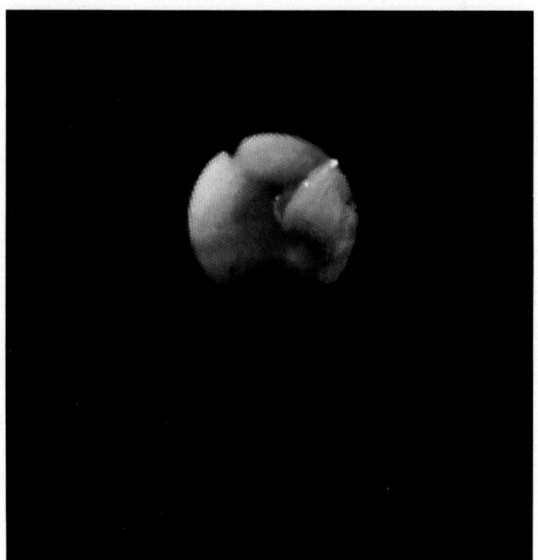

Color Plate 13. The bronchial blocker is directed into the main bronchus to be blocked.

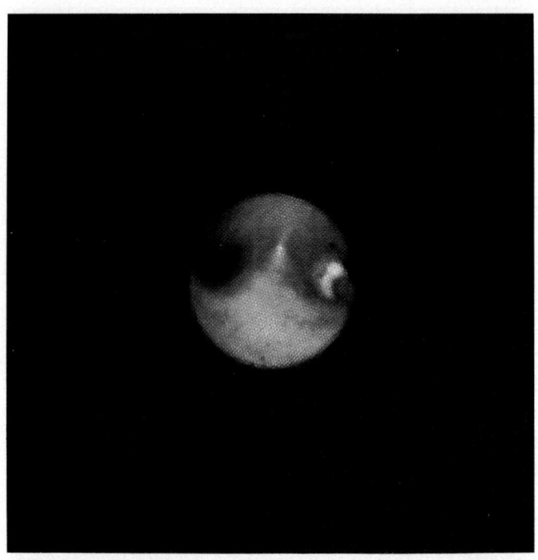

Color Plate 14. The bronchial blocker cuff is inflated to block the main bronchus lumen.

Table 13-1. Indications for One-Lung Ventilation

ABSOLUTE (to prevent life threatening complications)
1. Protection of the healthy lung from ipsilateral lung pathology
   A. Massive hemorrhage: to prevent spillage of blood
   B. Infection: to prevent spillage of pus.
   C. Unilateral lung lavage: to prevent spillage of water and lung drowning
2. Prevention of ventilation to one lung to protect from:
   A. Wasting ventilation: bronchopleural fistula, bronchopleural cutaneous fistula, or bronchial disruption or trauma
   B. Excessive pressure and rupture: unilateral cyst or unilateral bullae
3. Video-assisted thoracoscopy under general anesthesia

RELATIVE (for surgical exposure)
1. Pneumonectomy
2. Lobectomy (most commonly used)
3. Thoracic aortic aneurysm
4. Resection of the upper esophagus

Recently, the popularity of **video-assisted thoracoscopy (VAT)** has sharply increased. A considerable number of procedures, such as lung biopsy, pleural exploration and biopsy, random wedge resections, resection of a solitary lung lesion, talc insufflation, and pleuroabrasion, are all performed with VAT. In most circumstances general anesthesia is used. For an adequate resection, a well-collapsed lung is essential to allow proper visualization of the pleural space and the operative field. If the lung at the operative hemithorax is not adequately collapsed, the surgeon may have difficulty visualizing the operative field because this lung is pushing against the video camera. In addition, certain lung lesions that are not at the surface of the lung may be difficult to identify with a partially inflated lung. For these reasons, VAT should be included in the list of the absolute indication not for protection of the dependent lung but rather for the ability to perform the procedure.

Relative Indications

High-priority relative indications include **lobectomy**, particularly of the right upper lobe, which is considered technically the most difficult to perform. It is particularly important if the resection is performed via median sternotomy.[5] **Pneumonectomy** is greatly facilitated with good exposure of the lung hilum. **Thoracic aortic aneurysm repair** requires exposure of the entire length of the thoracic aorta.

Lower or middle lobectomy, esophageal resection and **thoracic spine procedures** are low priority.

In clinical practice, the vast majority of procedures using DLT's are in essence relative indication, and only a small fraction are absolute. The use of OLV for relative indications depends on the practice and preference of the surgeon-anesthesiologist. When the lung is well collapsed excessive lung retraction or compression is not needed; trauma to the lung and impairment of gas exchange is less.[6] Adequate surgical exposure facilitates the identification and separation of the dissection planes and lung fissures and reduces operative time.

Degree of Pulmonary Shunt

Nondependent Lung Factors

In estimating the degree of pulmonary shunt created during OLV, it should be kept in mind that, in the lateral position 40% of cardiac output perfuses the nondependent lung, and the remaining 60% perfuses through the dependent lung.[7–10] The degree of shunt depends on the hypoxic pulmonary vasoconstriction (HPV) response, which is a protective reflex whereby vasoconstriction diverts blood flow away from the nondependent hypoxic lung into the ventilated lung to reduce venous admixture. Typically, with an intact (noninhibited) HPV response, the transpulmonary shunt through the nondependent lung is approximately 23% of the cardiac output.[11–13]

Factors that Influence Degree of Shunt

- **Malposition of the DLT**, which is present in as many as 40–45% of patients. Such malposition may not be recognized by routine clinical evaluation such as inspection and auscultation. In most cases it is related to some degree of obstruction of the left upper lobe with left-sided double-lumen tubes or with inability to adequately ventilate the right upper lobe with right sided double-lumen tubes. In addition, migration and obstruction of a main bronchus or the trachea by a bulging or overinflated bronchial cuff may be present.[14–17]
- The nondependent lung has a ventilation-perfusion (V/Q) ratio of zero, which results in an obligatory transpulmonary shunt through that lung. **The degree of shunt depends on the degree of blood flow through the nondependent lung, the preoperative condition and the V/Q ratio of the dependent lung.**[18–19] The blood flow through the nondependent lung is gravity-dependent (passive mechanism) and depends on the degree of HPV (active mechanism). Hypoxemia is unlikely during OLV if less than 35% of the cardiac output is perfusing the nondependent lung. Hypoxemia is seen in 10–15% of patients if the perfusion of the nondependent lung is between 35–45% and in more than 30% of patients if the blow to that lung is over 45% of the cardiac output.[20–21]
- **The disease for which the procedure is performed.** In the past, thoracic procedures were performed for the treatment of tuberculosis, bronchiectasis, or extensive tumor occupying most of the hemithorax. These pulmonary diseases involved the lung extensively, and the blood flow through the nondependent lung was already markedly reduced. Thus the exclusion of that lung from the ventilation would have minimal impact on PaO_2.[22] In contrast, in patients who are admitted for resection of a coin-size lesion diagnosed on a routine chest x-ray, OLV would most likely have a major impact on arterial oxygenation because preoperatively, blood flow through that lung is high. Kerr et al[23–24] found that patients undergoing resection of pulmonary lesions had less of a decline in PaO_2 compared to those who had thoracotomies for nonpulmonary procedures.

Dependent Lung Factors

In addition to the reduction in functional residual capacity (FRC), poor ventilation of the dependent lung is a result of several factors. The dependent lung is generally compressed by the weight of the mediastinal structures from above and by the operative table and rolls from below. Transudate and interstitial edema from gravity lead to a further decrease in dependent lung FRC and compliance. Dependent lung atelectasis either from absorption (exposure to high oxygen concentration) or from cephalad compression of the abdominal content (a decrease in lung volume and an increase in airway closure) further increases the degree of shunt. Finally, difficulty in secretion removal may cause the development of poorly ventilated atelectatic area.

Choice of Anesthetic

The choice of anesthetic for thoracic surgery depends primarily on two factors: airway reactivity and HPV. A more detailed discussion on the choice of anesthetic and HPV can be found in Chapter 4.

Airway Reactivity and Resistance

General anesthesia reduces FRC, which usually produces an increase in airway resistance (Tables 13-2 and 13-3).[25–27] Most patients undergoing thoracic surgery have an increased airway reactivity and are susceptible to bronchoconstriction. The majority of these patients have chronic obstructive pulmonary disease (COPD) as a result of heavy smoking associated with increased mucous secretion. Indeed, there is a close association between the amount of secretions, the degree of coughing, bronchoconstriction, and mortality risk with the number of cigarettes smoked per day and the number of years of smoking.[28] In addition, airway reactivity increases in response to the insertion of double-lumen tube and surgical manipulation.[29]

Table 13-2. Effect of Volatile Agent and Narcotics on Cardiopulmonary Function and Airway Reactivity

Volatile	Narcotics
Desirable • Permits use of high FiO_2 • Bronchodilatation (all) • Diminished airway reflexes • Readily eliminated	**Desirable** • Stable hemodynamics (Fentanyl) • No inhibition of HPV • Postoperative analgesia
Undesirable • Myocardial depression Decrease BP Decrease CO Increase filling pressures Mild RV depression (Sevoflurane) • Arrhythmias (Halothane) • "Coronary steal" (Isoflurane) • Inhibits HPV 1 MAC Isoflurane increase Qs/Q_T by 4%	**Undesirable** • Respiratory depression Systemic narcotics in combination with epidural/intrathecal • Histamine release (Morphine, Meperidine) • Not readily eliminated • Not a general anesthetics

Table 13-3. Effect of Intraveneous Agents and Muscle Relaxants on Cardiopulmonary Function and Airway Reactivity

Ketamine
Desirable
Cardiovascular stability; the drug of choice for
Hypovolemia
Trauma
Cardiac tamponade
No inhibition of HPV
Reduce airway irritability
Undesirable
Myocardial ischemia: produced by
Increase contractibility
Tachycardia
Hypertension
↓
Increase myocardial oxygen demand
Emergence delirium
Thiopental
Short acting
Release histamine
May decrease BP, CO, Increase HR
Propofol
Desirable
Short acting, rapid and smooth recovery
Decrease post-op nausea and vomiting
Ideal for bronchoscopy, or HFV (infusion)
Undesirable
Hypotension, bradycardia
Venoirritaion
High cost
Etomidate
Desirable
No release of histamine
No cardiac depression
Useful in high risk patients
Undesirable
Venoirritation
Aderocortical suppression
Excitatory phenomena
High cost
Muscule relaxant
d-tubocurarine
Release histamine at clinical dosage
Pancuronium
Tachycardia
Atracurium
Release histamine at high doses
Short acting
Vecuronium
No cardiovascular effects
No release of histamine
Short acting
Mivacurium
Release histamine at high doses
Ultra short acting (bronchoscopy)
Doxacurium
Pipecuronium
No release of histamine
Long acting

Most of the potent **inhaled anesthetics** such as isoflurane, halothane, and enflurane have a beneficial effect; they all produce bronchodilatation. They are considered to be the anesthetics of choice for patients with reactive airways.[30–31] The more severe the degree of bronchoconstriction, the greater the predisposition for response to bronchodilators. Halothane may be preferred for inhalational induction because it is less pungent. Halothane produces relaxation of direct smooth muscle of the bronchial tree.[32] This effect may occur through alteration of the release of bronchoconstrictor mediators rather than via a centrally controlled reflex pathway.[33] The relationship between halothane and histamine release is more complex.[34–35] Halothane impairs the release of histamine induced by *d*-tubocurarine, and it attenuates the bronchoconstriction produced by administration of histamine.[36]

Isoflurane may be the preferred anesthetic agent because it increases the threshold of cardiac dysrhythmia and provides greater cardiac stability.[30–37] Patients who are receiving chronic treatment with aminophylline or beta-adrenergic agonist are susceptible to ventricular arrhythmias and may benefit from receiving isoflurane. Recent studies have suggested the relaxation of the smooth muscle by isoflurane is mediated through nitric oxide (NO). Isoflurane may cause increased production of NO from the vascular endothelium that activates guanylate cyclase in smooth muscle to cause relaxation.[38]

The **intravenous drugs** can potentially release histamine with the undesirable effect of bronchospasm. Fentanyl does not release histamine and provides relatively stable hemodynamics. It has no effect on the bronchomotor tone, does not cause an increase in plasma histamine level, and is the most popular agent used in N_2O narcotic-relaxant or inhaled narcotic-relaxant agents. In contrast, morphine releases histamine and increases central vagal tone.[39–43] Histamine release is undesirable, as it may precipitate bronchial constriction and hypotension. Ketamine and thiopental are the preferred drugs for induction of anesthesia in patients with reactive airways. Ketamine, which has a bronchodilating effect, is advantageous for hypovolemic patients because of its relative myocardial stability. Ketamine protects against antigen-induced bronchospasm, whereas thiopental does not. Thiopental has been associated with bronchospasm, probably not because of the degree of histamine release but as a result of the light level of anesthesia that leaves the airway reflexes relatively intact during the crucial time of endotracheal intubation and airway manipulation.[44]

Histamine release with propofol is uncommon. However, in a study where propofol was used for induction and maintenance during OLV, a significant decrease in systemic blood pressure occurs during induction.[45–46] This may be related to some degree of depression of left ventricular function by propofol. Etomidate has an excellent myocardial stability and does not release histamine, even in patients with asthma. This agent has been advocated for patients with severe bronchospasm.[47–48]

Of the **muscle relaxants**, curare is known to release histamine and to increase airway resistance; it should be avoided. Atracurium releases histamine in high doses (>0.6 mg/kg).[49] Pancuronium and vecuronium do not release histamine and both can be used for thoracic surgery.[50–51] Mivicurium, a new muscle relaxant, is a short-acting nondepolarizing agent which is rapidly metabolized by plasma cholinesterase at about 75% the rate of succinylcholine. It has a tendency to release histamine only at doses above 0.2 mg/kg, which is very similar to atracurium. Pipcuromium and doxacurium, which are potent, long-acting drugs, do not release histamine and have no cardiovascular side effects.[53] The patients' medical conditions, duration of the procedures, and cost-effectiveness should be considered when selecting the muscle relaxant.

Lidocaine, 1–2 mg/kg, can be given immediately prior to intubation to protect from reflex bronchoconstriction. Inhaled lidocaine given in an ultrasonic aerosol has been shown to prevent and to reverse increase in airways resistance.[54] It appears that administration of lidocaine either via the airway or intravenously protects against the development of bronchospasm in patients with reactive airways. Of the neuromuscular reversal agents, neostigmine and physostigmine are both cholinesterase-blocking agents that may increase airway resistance.[55] The simultaneous administration of atropine, a cholinergic blocker, reverses that effect, in addition to its direct bronchodilator action on the airways.

Effect on Hypoxic Pulmonary Vasoconstriction

One theme that has been a focus of extensive investigation is the effect of these drugs on hypoxic pulmonary vasoconstriction (HPV). An extensive review of the physiopathology of HPV can be found in Chapter 4.

Basically, HPV is a protective mechanism that diverts blood flow away from the hypoxic lung region into a functioning nonhypoxic lung region. It is a homeostatic mechanism for maintaining normal V/Q relationship to achieve efficient oxygenation.[56–59] It is important to stress that the blood flow diversion is not mechanical due to kinking of the vessels of the atelectatic area. The mechanism is active, as demonstrated by the fact that reexpansion of the atelectatic area by ventilation with nitrogen fails to restore blood flow. On the other hand, ventilation with oxygen does return blood flow to the lobe (Fig. 13-1).

Several studies have evaluated the effect of inhaled versus intravenous anesthetics on HPV in human and animal models. A fundamental property of inhalational anesthetic agents is decreased HPV. In a dog model, Buckley et al[60] found that N_2O increases HPV response but that 0.5% halothane, which had no significant effect on cardiac output, decreased HPV.

In vivo studies consistently show that intravenous agents have no effect on HPV. In con-

Figure 13-1. Flow to the left lower lobe test segment as a fraction of cardiac output is shown for 6 dogs. Left lower lobe atelectasis and left lower lobe hypoxic ventilation each produced similar reduction in test segment perfusion suggesting that HPV rather than mechanical factors is largely responsible for decreasing blood flow to an atelectatic lung. (Adapted with permission from Benumof JL. Mechanism of decreased blood flow to atelectatic lung. J App Physiol 1979;46:1047.)

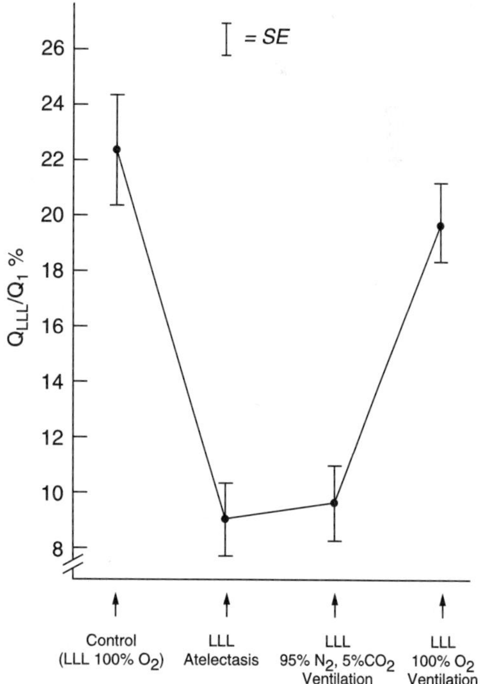

trast, a dose-related depression of HPV by halothane, enflurane, and isoflurane have been demonstrated. The results are somewhat conflicting, however, and the degree of influence on HPV varies from preparation to another. In rate, 0.5 minimal alveolar concentration (MAC) produce 50% inhibition of HPV, whereas in dogs, 1 MAC resulted in only 21% inhibition of HPV. The degree of HPV inhibition does not derive from a single factor of anesthetic concentration but is a result of a complex interaction of anesthetic concentration, cardiac output, oxygen consumption, shunt, surgical manipulations of the lung, the application of positive end-expiratory pressure (PEEP), and the mixed venous oxygen saturation (PvO_2).[61–65] For example, PvO_2 is very important determinant of HPV response. Therefore, anesthetics that depress cardiac output also reduce PvO_2 secondary to a decrease in oxygen delivery; such agents may produce a more potent stimulus to HPV.

Clinical studies are obviously more relevant to the clinician. Intravenous agents such as thiopental, ketamine, various narcotics, propofol, or etomidate have no direct influence on HPV.[66–67] The study by Weinreich et al[68] of ketamine infusion in 110 patients resulted in a mean PaO_2 of 130 mmHg using FiO_2 of 1.0. These researchers postulated that because ketamine has positive effects on the cardiovascular system and is an intravenous agent with no inhibitory effect on HPV, patients may have had a higher PaO_2 compared with other studies in which halothane was used. In another study by Rees et al,[68a] a comparison of ketamine and enflurane in 24 patients undergoing lung resection found no difference in shunt fraction or PaO_2 in both techniques. The authors concluded that ketamine has no advantage over enflurane in terms of PaO_2 or the degree of shunt during OLV. Left ventricular stroke index was greater in the ketamine group, however.

The effect of inhalational agents on HPV in clinical studies has been an issue of a long-standing debate. Rogers and Benumof[69] compared the effects of inhaled anesthetics (isoflurane and halothane) with intravenous anesthetics (methohexital and ketamine) during OLV in 20 patients. They concluded that inhaled anesthetics at 1 MAC concentrations do not significantly affect HPV in humans. In subsequent studies Benumof et al[70] explored the changes in PaO_2 and the percentage of shunt following conversion from halothane or isoflurane to intravenous anesthesia during OLV. They reported that "halothane and isoflurane only slightly impaired arterial oxygenation during one-lung ventilation in patients undergoing thoracotomy;" because discontinuing halothane and isoflurane causes some increase in PaO_2 and decrease in Q_S/Q_T. However, in their conclusion they stated that "because continuous positive airway pressure to the nondependent lung is usually effective in improving PaO_2 during OLV, the use of halogenated drugs in patients undergoing OLV is no longer a significant issue."

Perhaps the most significant clinical guide to the degree of influence of inhalational anesthetic on HPV was reported by Domino et al.[71] The authors reported that the administration of 1 MAC isoflurane anesthesia causes an increase of 4% in Q_S/Q_T. That increase may be significant during OLV if the shunt is already high, and an increase in FiO_2 has no beneficial effect on arterial oxygenation. More recently, the effect of sevoflurane anesthesia for OLV was evaluated in a sheep model. Sevoflurane had a slight depressant effect on right ventricular function in concentration of 2.0–4.0%. Arterial oxygenation remained unchanged, however.[72] Overall, inhaled anesthetics are the drugs of choice during thoracic surgery. One should keep in mind that at the doses used clinically, they slightly inhibit HPV. In contrast, intravenous anesthetics do not affect HPV. Selection of the anesthetic technique is dictated primarily by patient needs and the specific requirements of the procedure. Induction of anesthesia can be performed using any of the available induction agents such as thiopental, ketamine, propofol, or etomidate depending on the anesthesiologist's experience and the patient's age and condition. Following establishment of an airway, paralysis can be induced with vecuronium, atracurium, or pancuronium. This is preferable over succinylcholine to avoid the side effects such as bradycardia or fasciculation. Most important, it allows enough time for insertion and positioning of the double-lumen tube. Lidocaine administered intravenously or by laryngotracheal spray is important for blunting the airway response to tracheal manipulations.

Maintenance of anesthesia can be accomplished with moderate concentrations of isoflurane (0.5–1.0 MAC) and small doses of narcotics. Fentanyl or sufentanyl are preferable if early extubation is planned. Generally, 100% oxygen is used during OLV; N_2O can be safely used with close monitoring of oxygenation by pulse oximeter and arterial blood gases, however. Administration of adequate levels of anesthesia with lower concentration of potent inhalational agents may be sufficient.

Today thoracic epidural or intrathecal morphine prior to skin incision is popular for postoperative pain management. Parental administration of narcotic should be carefully monitored to avoid an additive effect with the drugs administered via the epidural route. This may result in respiratory depression. (See Chapter 16 on Postoperative Pain Management.)

Clinical Approach to Management of One-Lung Ventilation

Once the patient has been placed in the lateral decubitus position, proper positioning with axillary roll and protection of all pressure points should be assured (Table 13-4) as described extensively in Chapter 11 on Positioning and Complications of the Supine and Lateral Positions.

Checking of Proper Double-Lumen Tube Position

Since dislocation during position change is not uncommon, Chapter 12 on Separation of the Lungs describes the steps of insertion and correct positioning of double-lumen tubes by auscultation or by fiberoptic bronchoscopy in detail. This paragraph only briefly refers to the intraoperative management of the double-lumen tube or the Univent tube.

The double-lumen tube should be coated with a water soluble lubricating ointment (Surgilube, Atlanta, GA; Melville, NY) prior to insertion. A silicone spray ([silkospray] Rush AG, Waibligen, West Germany) provides excellent lubrication. The tracheal cuff should be tested to accommodate 20 mL of air; the bronchial

Table 13-4. Clinical Approach to Management of One-Lung Ventilation (OLV)

1. Use FiO_2 of 1.0
2. Ventilate with a tidal volume of 10–12 mL/kg
3. Respiratory rate to maintain $PaCO_2$ between 33–35 mmHg
4. Check the double-lumen tube position subsequent to the lateral decubitus positioning
5. If peak airway pressure exceed 40 mmHg during one-lung ventilation, double-lumen tube malposition should be excluded.
6. For hypoxemia, apply CPAP, 10 cm H_2O, to the nondependent lung.
7. If additional correction of hypoxemia is necessary, add PEEP, 5–10 cm H_2O, to the ventilated lung.
8. If hypoxemia persists and it is feasible, ask the surgeon to occlude the pulmonary artery of the nondependent lung or intermittently inflate and deflate the operated lung.
9. Keep in mind that arterial oxygenation can decrease up to 45 minutes following initiation of OLV.

cuff should be checked using a 3 mL air syringe. For intubation a Mackintosh 3 blade is preferred, since it provides the largest area through which to pass the tube. Insertion of the tube is performed with the distal concave curvature facing anteriorly. When the tip of the tube is passed the vocal cords, the stylet should be removed. This is important to prevent tracheal laceration from the rigid stylet. The polyvinyl chloride (PVC) tubes have a black ring at the level of the bronchial cuff, which serves as a landmark. Once the black ring is passed through the vocal cord, a left-sided tube is then rotated 90 degrees to the left, whereas a right-sided tube is turned to the right. Advancement of the tube ceases when moderate resistance to further passage is encountered.

First, the tracheal cuff should be inflated, then bilateral equal breath sounds should be confirmed. To avoid mucosal damage from excessive pressure applied by the bronchial cuff, the cuff is inflated with incremental volume to seal air leak around the bronchial cuff into the tracheal lumen. Inflation of the bronchial cuff seldom requires more than 2 mL of air. Bilateral breath sounds should be rechecked to confirm that the bronchial cuff is not herniating over to impede the ipsilateral lung ventilation. An important step is to verify that the tip of the bronchial lumen is located in the designated bronchus. One simple way to check is to first clamp the tracheal lumen (always at the level of the connector!), observe, and auscultate. Usually, inspection reveals unilateral ascent of the ventilated hemithorax. If both hemithorax are ventilating, the tip of the bronchial lumen is located above the carina. Following proper auscultation, the bronchial lumen is clamped to ventilate the tracheal lumen. Each time a right-sided double-lumen tube is used, appropriate ventilation of the right upper lobe should be ensured. This can be accomplished by careful auscultation over the right upper lung field or more accurately by fiberoptic bronchoscope. When a left-sided double-lumen tube is used, the risk of occluding the left upper lobe bronchus by the bronchial tip advanced far into the left main bronchus should be kept in mind. If peak airway pressure is of 20 cm H_2O during two-lung ventilation for the same tidal volume, that pressure should not exceed 40 cm H_2O on OLV.

Perhaps the most important advancement in confirming the proper positioning of double-lumen tubes is the introduction of **fiberoptic bronchoscopy** to clinical practice. Researchers recently used fiberoptic bronchoscopy to show that double-lumen tubes, thought to be correctly positioned by inspection and auscultation, were malpositioned in 20–48% of cases.

The simplest method to evaluate proper positioning of a left-sided double-lumen tube is **bronchoscopy via the tracheal lumen** (Fig. 13-2). The carina is then visualized; only the proximal edge of the endobronchial cuff should be identified just below the tracheal carina. Herniation of the bronchial cuff over the carina to occlude the ipsilateral main bronchus partially should be excluded (Fig. 13-3). The bronchial blue cuff of the clear disposable PVC double-lumen tube is easily visualized, whereas the nondisposable rubber double-lumen tube contains yellow bronchial cuffs somewhat more difficult to recognize. **Bronchoscopy should then be performed via the bronchial lumen** to identify the patent left upper lobe orifice (Fig. 13-2B). When using a right-sided double-lumen tube, the carina is visualized through the tracheal lumen. More importantly, the right upper lobe bronchial orifice must be identified while the bronchoscope is passed through the right upper lobe ventilating slot (Fig. 13-4). This is somewhat complex to accomplish and requires a relatively skilled endoscopist.

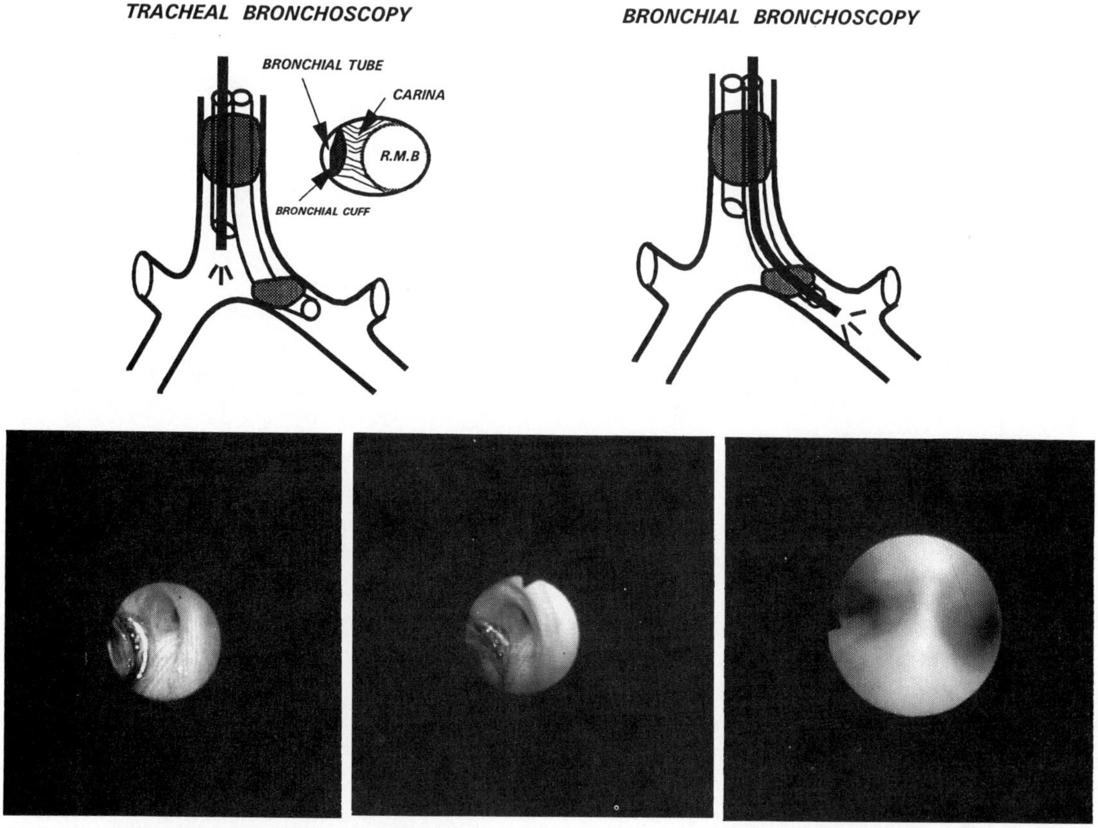

Figure 13-2. Left-sided DLT: Correct Position. A. The carina is visualized; only the proximal edge of the endobronchial cuff should be identified just below the tracheal carina. The blue bronchial cuff of the disposable PVC DLT is easily identified. B. The bronchial carina and the patent left upper lobe orifice can be identified. See Color Plates 8, 9, and 10.

Several sizes of bronchoscope are available for clinical use: 5.6, 4.9, and 3.9 mm of external diameter (Machida Co. or the LF-2 from the Olympus Co.). The 3.9-mm-diameter bronchoscope can easily be passed through a 37F or larger tube, whereas it is a tight fit through a 35F tube. It should be emphasized that fiberoptic confirmation for proper positioning is not indispensable for detection of gross malposition (ie, the bronchial tip is not located in the appropriate side) but for those fine ones easily missed by the clinical evaluation (ie, tube is too far in or not far enough). Fiberoptic confirmation is critical when absolute lung separation is indicated, since malposition can be life-threatening. The high incidence of undiagnosed malposition undoubtedly justifies that recommendation.

Problems Associated with Double-Lumen Tube Positioning

The use of double-lumen tubes is associated with a number of potential problems. First, due

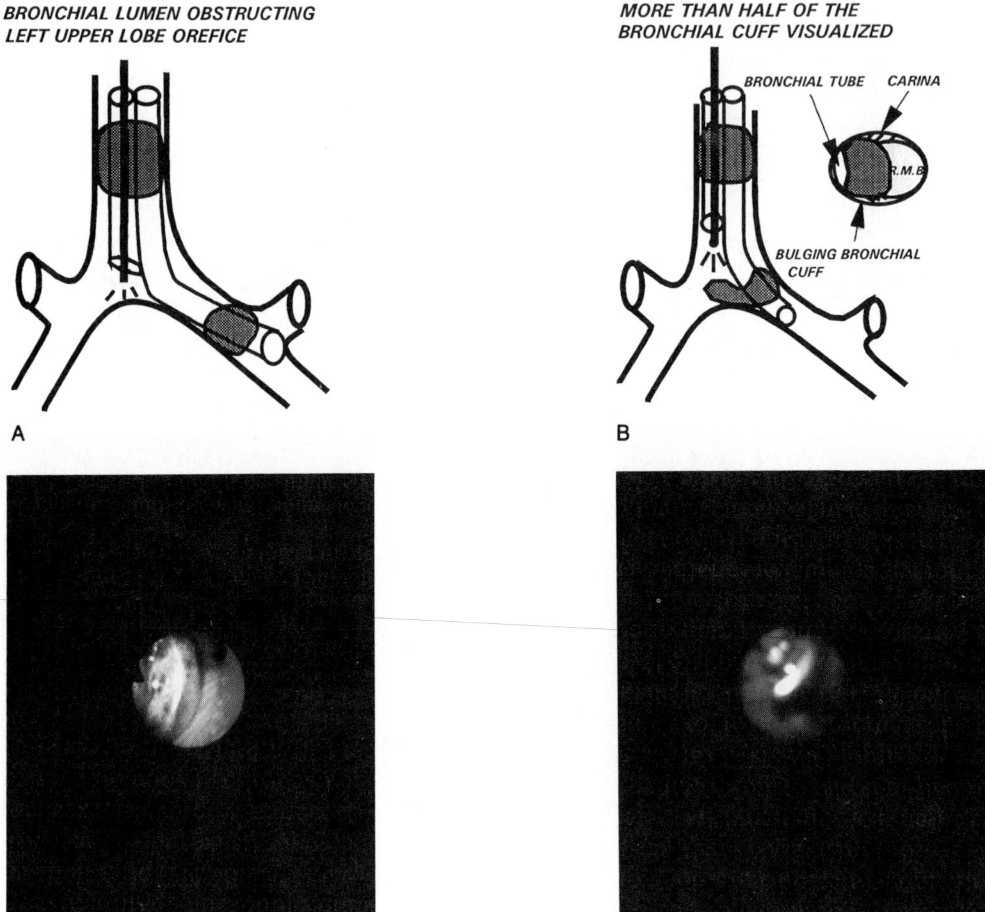

Figure 13-3. Left-sided DLT: Malposition. A. The tube is too far in and the tip of the bronchial lumen occluded the left upper lobe orifice. B. The bronchial cuff is herniated over the carina to occlude the ipsilateral main bronchus. See Color Plates 11 and 12.

to the morphology of the tube curvature, tracheal or bronchial lacerations may result during insertion. Second, if a left-sided tube is inserted into the right mainstem bronchus, ventilation to the right upper lobe is impaired. In this case fiberoptic bronchoscopy through the bronchial lumen can direct the tube to the left. This also can be accomplished by *turning the head to the right* while turning the DLT to the left and advancing it blindly. Third, the tube may not be introduced far enough into the mainstem bronchus, and the orifice of the bronchial lumen will be located above the carina. In this case, breath sounds are present bilaterally when ventilating through the bronchial lumen, whereas none are audible when ventilation is through the tracheal lumen. Fourth, a right-sided tube may occlude the right upper

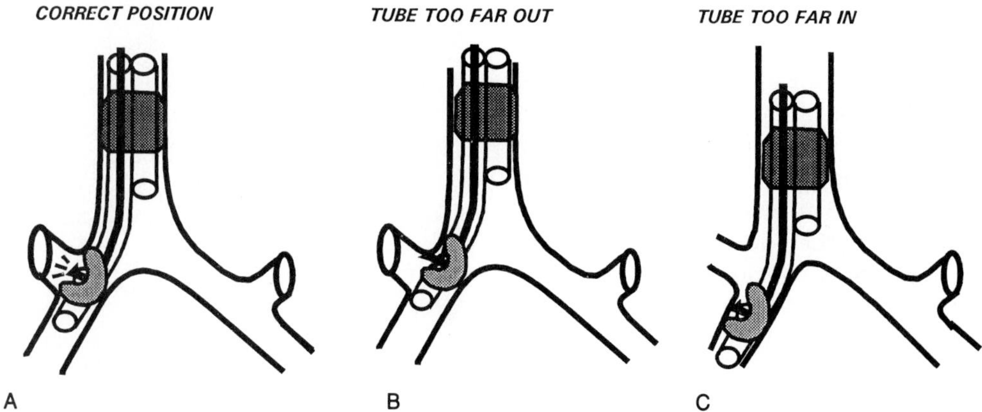

Figure 13-4. Right-sided DLT: Fiberoptic Bronchoscopy. A. Correct position. B. Tube is too far out. C. Tube is too far in. See Color Plates 6 and 7.

lobe orifice because of the short distance from the carina to the right upper lobe takeoff (2.3 ± 0.17 cm in males and 2.1 ± 0.7 cm in females). The right-sided double-lumen tube has a slot to allow ventilation of that lobe. Yet, the margin of safety is only between 1–8 mm, and it is hard to ensure appropriate ventilation to that right upper lobe. Fifth, a left-sided double-lumen tube may also obstruct the left upper lobe orifice.[73–78] Recently Benumof et al[79] reported that although the left upper lobe takeoff is between 5.0 and 5.5 cm from the carina, it is feasible to obstruct the left upper lobe by the bronchial tip and still have the tracheal orifice above the carina. Lastly, herniation of the bronchial cuff may obstruct the bronchial lumen when excessive volume is applied during its inflation. Tracheal rupture is rare but has been previously reported.[80,81] To reduce the risk of this serious complication during positioning of the double-lumen tube, it is important to remove the stylet before double-lumen tube rotation. Each time the patient's position is altered, or when OLV is no longer required, the bronchial cuff should be kept deflated. This minimizes bronchial mucosal damage due to prolonged excessive cuff pressure. Obviously, when OLV is an absolute indication, deflation of the bronchial cuff cannot be performed. There are two other practical points that are of clinical importance. First, tying the DLT, and second, how to change from single-lumen to DLT and vice versa.

First, an easy way to tie a double-lumen tube. After the correct placement of a double-lumen endotracheal tube (DLT), the positioning of the patient in the lateral decubitus position can result in substantial displacement of the DLT due to accidental pulling, flexion or extension of the neck, and traction exerted by the weight of the attached anesthesia circuit. In an attempt to prevent this, it is customary to firmly secure the DLT at the level of the lips using adhesive or umbilical tape. Often multiple knots are tied in this area, which, with time, become very slippery due to the continuous exposure to saliva and other secretions.

The traditional methods used to secure the DLT create additional difficulties if repositioning of the DLT is required. Frequently, following fiberoptic bronchoscopy or intraoperatively, adjustments requiring the untying or loosening of the DLT have to be made in the lateral decubitus position.

A simple and practical method for securing the DLT is to use a simple single tie around the tube at the level of the lips (Fig. 13-5), followed by a bow-tie at the bifurcation of the DLT connector (Fig. 13-6). Using this technique, stabilization of the tube is not dependent on tight knots around the tube itself, but is instead accomplished by the bow-tie around the connector bifurcation which prevents the tube from pulling out. If readjustments are needed, the DLT can be freed by simply pulling on either end of the bow-tie loops.

The second issue that frequently arises is how to change from single-lumen to DLT and vice versa. This is extremely important in the case of a difficult airway. Often, initial intubation may be performed with a single-lumen tube for mediastinoscopy or flexible bronchoscopy, and then it will be changed to a DLT for the lung resection. In addition, at the termination of the procedure, if the patient needs ventilatory assistance, the DLT is changed to a single-lumen tube for postoperative care. If the airways were somewhat difficult, or to avoid repeated laryngoscopies, a tube exchanger may be used. The tube exchanger used for single-lumen tube will pass through a 7.0 mm internal diameter but will not pass through the lumen of a DLT. Only a smaller size diameter stiff tube

Figure 13-5. A simple tie around the DLT. (Reproduced with permission from Cohen E, Koorn R. An easy way to safely tie a double-lumen tube. J Cardiothorac Anesth 1991;5:194.)

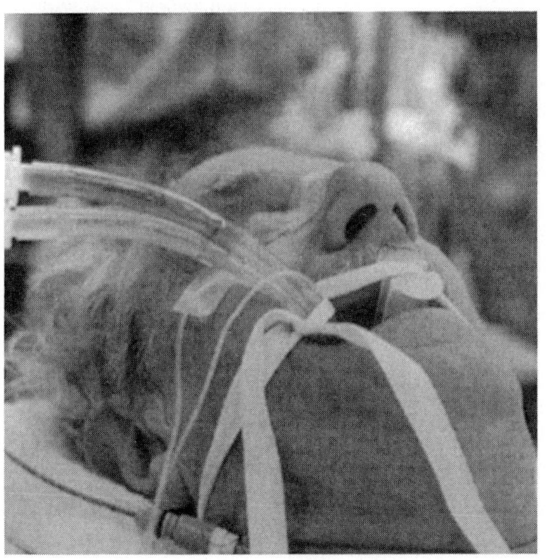

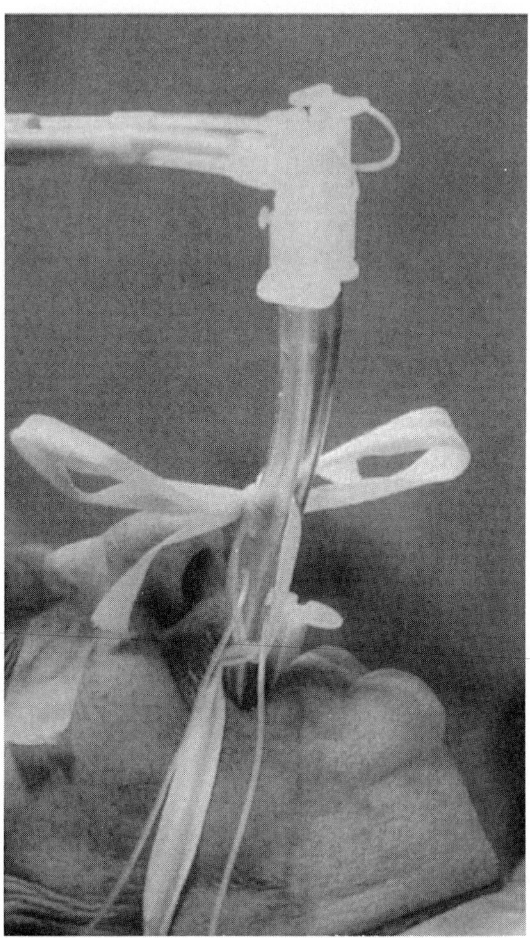

Figure 13-6. The DLT is stabilized with a bow-tie at the bifurcation of the DLT connector. (Reproduced with permission from Cohen E, Koorn R. An easy way to safely tie a double-lumen tube. J Cardiothorac Anesth 1991;5:195.)

exchanger will pass through a 4.0 mm ID.* Figure 13-7 A–E shows the sequence of events. Also, the tube exchanger should be longer than the bronchial lumen of the DLT and should be sprayed with Silkospray (Rusch, Waibligen, West Germany) for smooth manipulation. The exchanger is passed through the single-lumen tube, then it is removed and the exchanger is kept in the tracheal lumen. Finally, the DLT is passed over the exchanger through the bronchial lumen and is guided over the exchanger to be placed endobronchially. This method may be used for changing DLT into a single-lumen. Finally, if a rigid bronchoscopy is performed by the surgeon to establish an airway, this method can be used to place a DLT directly from a rigid bronchoscope (Fig. 13-8).

The Univent Tube

The Univent tube (Univent, Fuji Systems Corp.; Tokyo, Japan) is a novel new means of achieving bronchial blockade (Fig. 13-9).[82–84] The bronchial blocker technique has been modified so that the bronchial blocker is passed along a single-lumen endobronchial tube. The bronchial blocker is housed in a small anterior lumen containing a thin (2 mm internal diameter) tube with a distal balloon (blocker tube). The blocker tube can be advanced beyond the tip of the tracheal tube into a mainstem bronchus to serve as a blocker. Before intubation the blocker cuff is deflated, and the blocker is completely retracted into the small lumen. Intubation is routinely carried out as with single-lumen tube. The tracheal tube is then rotated to the side to be occluded under direct visualization with a fiberoptic bronchoscope, and the blocker is manipulated into the desired mainstem bronchus. To achieve lung separation the blocker cuff is inflated under direct vision to seal the bronchial lumen (6–7 mL of air). The Univent tube has the advantage of using a single-lumen tube instead of a double-lumen tube, and there is no need to change over at the end of the procedure if postoperative ventilatory support is required. It is also possible to suction through the blocker lumen or to apply CPAP to improve oxygenation in case of hypoxia.

The disadvantages of the tube are its relatively large, internal diameter, dislocation of the blocker during surgical manipulation, possible problems achieving a satisfactory bronchial seal and lung separation. In addition, the relative small diameter of the blocker lumen makes the removal of secretions more difficult, and prolongs the time required to achieve a complete deflation of the nondependent lung. A more detailed description of the Univent tube can be found in Chapter 12.

Inspired Oxygen Concentration

Two-lung ventilation should be maintained for as long as possible. OLV most likely results in a reduction of PaO_2, and depends on several factors, which are discussed extensively here and in Chapters 4 and 5. An FiO_2 of 1.0 provides a high margin of safety to protect against possible hypoxemia. With an FiO_2 of 1.0, assuming an intact HPV response, PaO_2 during OLV should be between 150–210 mmHg. Reduced oxygen concentrations, such as FiO_2 of 0.5, produce acceptable oxygenation in these patients (mean PaO_2: 68–84 mmHg).[85, 86] In a study by Cohen et al[87] the initiation of OLV using FiO_2 of 0.5 resulted in a significant decrease in PaO_2 to a mean of 80 mmHg. Theoretically, a high FiO_2 could cause lung injury from oxygen, although it is unlikely to occur in the time frame of the surgery. High FiO_2 can produce absorption at-

* Cook Critical Care (C-CAE–11.0–83), Bloomington, IN, USA presently is the only model of the tube exchanger available for DLT.

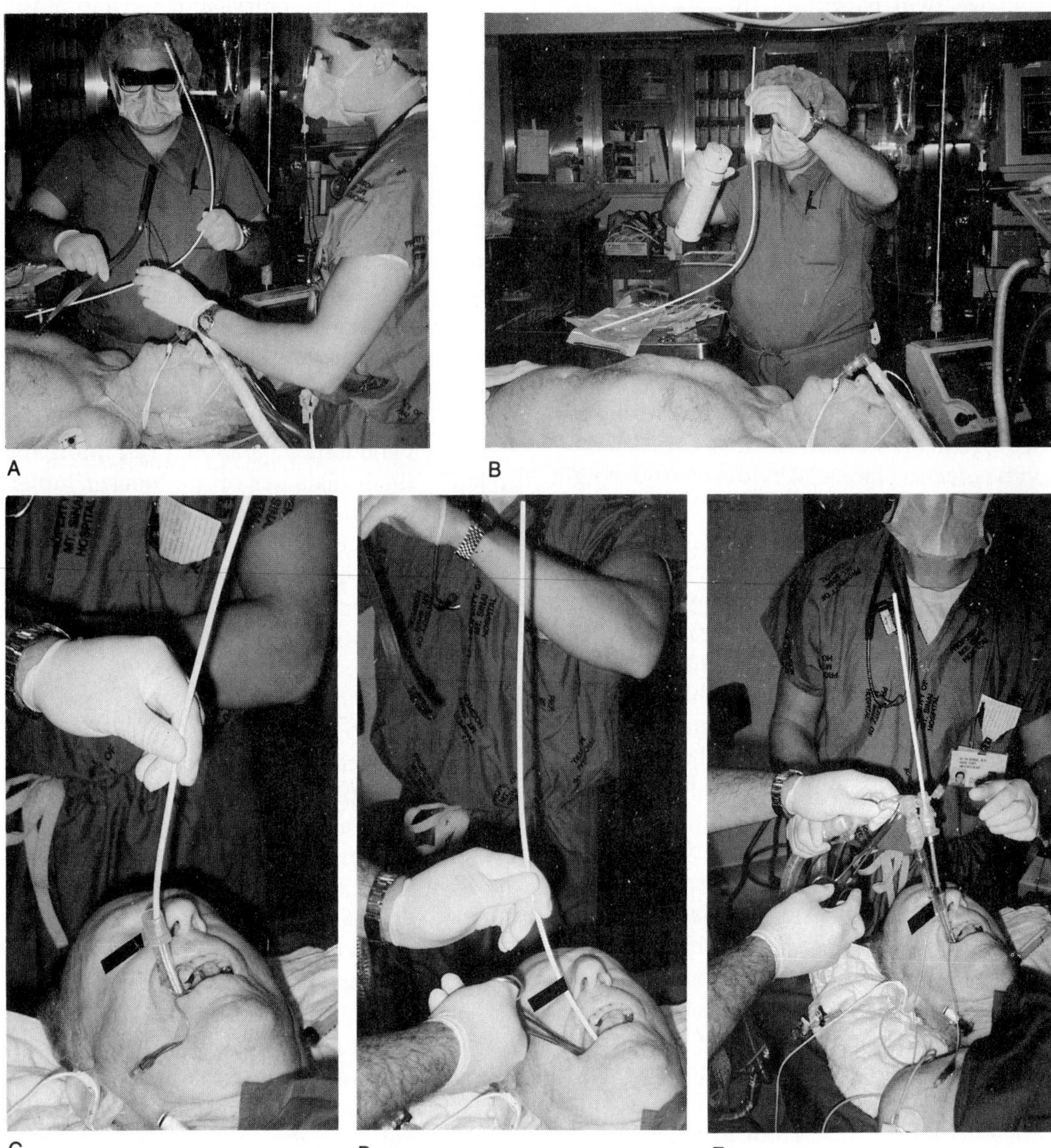

Figure 13-7. A. The tube exchanger should be longer than the DLT (The Cook exchanger is 83 cm). B. The exchanger should be well lubricated or sprayed with Silkospray. C. The exchanger is passed through a single-lumen tube. D. The single-lumen tube is then removed and the exchanger is kept in the tracheal lumen. E. Finally, the DLT is passed over the exchanger *through the bronchial lumen* and is guided over the exchanger to be placed endobronchially.

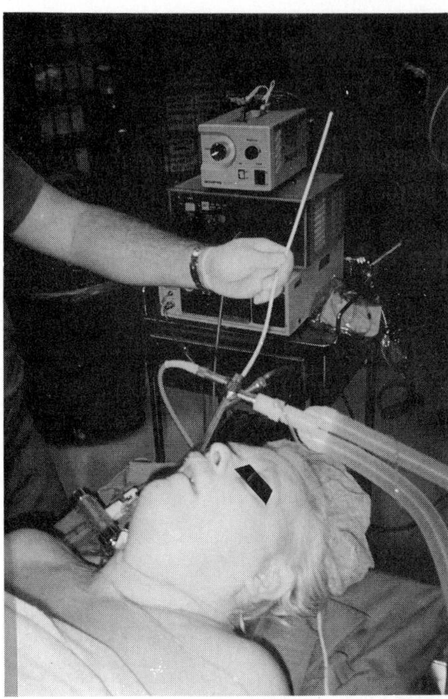

Figure 13-8. This method can be used to place a DLT directly from a rigid bronchoscope.

electasis and potentially further increase the shunt fraction. Despite the theoretical risk of oxygen toxicity, the beneficial effect of ventilating the lung with high oxygen concentration is by far more important. Nitrous oxide reduces the necessity for high concentrations of potent inhaled anesthetics with less myocardial depression, which may be beneficial in high-risk patients. It can be safely used during OLV with continuous monitoring of arterial saturation by pulse oximetry and arterial blood gases. It is important to keep in mind that those patients with a relatively well-preserved lung function, such as tumor found on a routine chest x-ray, are more prone to develop hypoxemia during OLV. On the other hand, patients who are scheduled for a thoracotomy for treatment of extensive tuberculosis or bronchiectasis already have compromised lung function in that collapsed lung and exhibit a less pronounced reduction in PaO_2. The risks and benefits for each patient should be considered for optimal management.

Tidal Volume and Respiratory Rate

Patients should be ventilated with a tidal volume of 10–12 mL/kg at a ventilatory rate to maintain a $PaCO_2$ of 35 ± 3 mmHg that can be estimated from the end-tidal CO_2 value. Individual response to an alteration of tidal volume is unpredictable, and that makes clinical studies inconclusive. Low tidal volume (8 mL/kg) may produce atelectasis in the ventilated lung (reduced FRC) and increases in the degree of shunt. High tidal volume (15 mL/kg) may shift blood flow into the nondependent lung (similar to the application of PEEP) to increase the transpulmonary shunt. A dependent lung tidal volume of 10 mL/kg affects arterial oxygenation least.[88]

In a study by Flacke et al[89] the dependent lung tidal volume was changed from 8 to 15 mL/kg during OLV. Changes in PaO_2 were unpredictable with considerable individual variation in both direction without change in the mean value (Fig. 13-10). Torda et al[95] found no difference in pulmonary shunt and PaO_2 between two groups of patients in which dependent lung ventilation was performed at 12 and 24 breaths/min with an unchanged tidal volume. On the other hand, Kerr et al[24] found that a decrease in tidal volume during OLV resulted in a progressive increase in shunt fraction from the beginning to the end of surgery. When the same tidal volume used for two-lung ventilation was continued during OLV, there was no decrease in the shunt fraction by the end of surgery, however. Katz et al[90] compared tidal

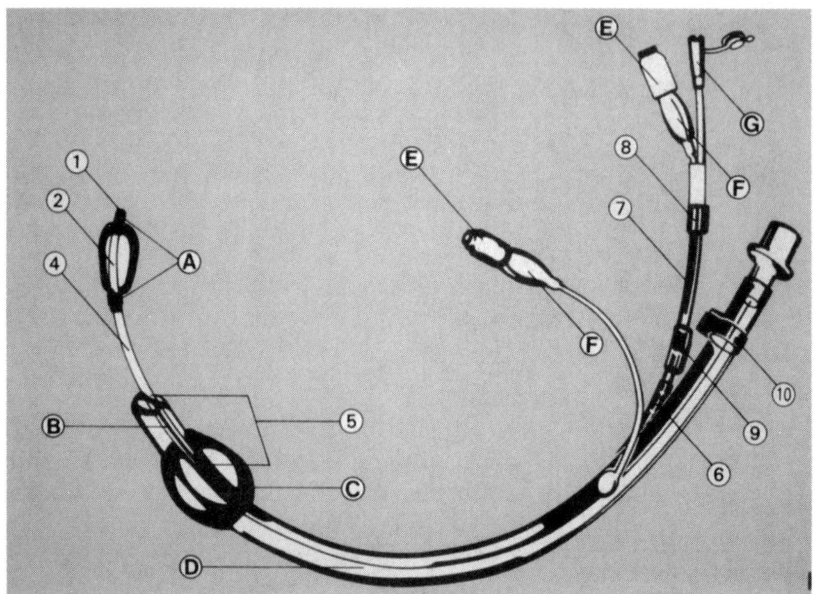

A

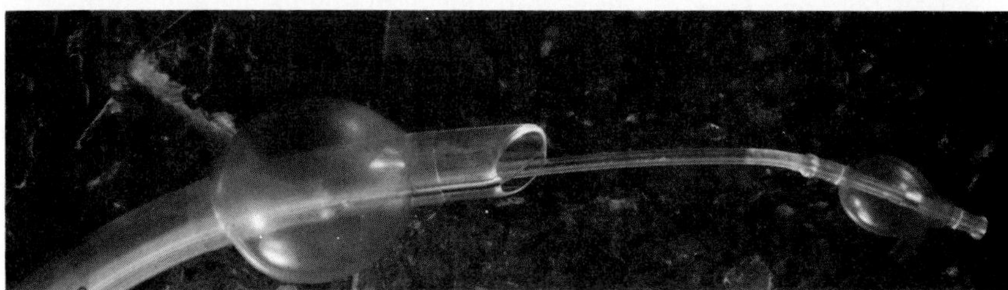

B

Figure 13-9. A. The Univent tube. 1. Open lumen tip (x-ray opaque). 2. Blocker cuff. 3. Setting end mark. 4. Blocker bend. 5. Pocket for blocker cuff. 6. Blocker mantle tube. 7. Blocker. 8. Blocker grip. 9. Cap stopper. 10. Band stopper. A. Blocker cuff band. B. X-ray opaque line. C. Endotracheal tube cuff. D. Endotracheal tube. E. One-way valve. F. Pilot balloon. G. Blocker cap connector.
B. Tip of the tracheal tube. The bronchial blocker is advanced beyond the top of the tracheal tube.

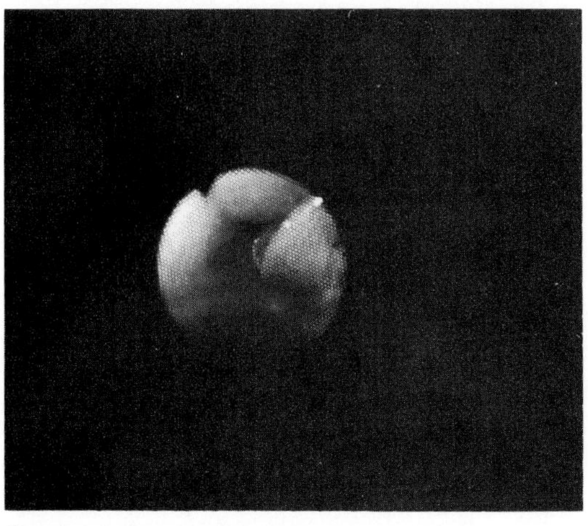

C

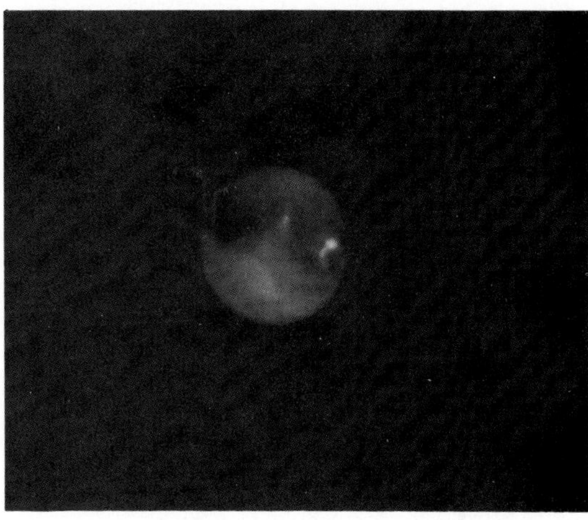

D

Figure 13-9. (Continued) C. The bronchial blocker is directed into the main bronchus to be blocked. See Color Plate 13. D. The bronchial blocker cuff is inflated to block the main bronchus lumen. See Color Plate 14.

volume of 8% versus 16% of total lung capacity. Minute ventilation was kept constant by adjusting the respiratory rate. They reported a higher PaO_2 with a larger tidal volume than with a smaller tidal volume (Fig. 13-11). They suggested that this increase in PaO_2 is secondary to improve lung compliance, probably because of a recruitment of atelectatic-dependent lung at end respiration. This type of atelectasis may be expected if the dependent lung has a low initial volume.

Although ventilation and perfusion are considerably mismatched during OLV, the elimination of carbon dioxide usually does not pose a problem even with an unchanged minute ventilation for three reasons. One, the $P(a\text{-}v)CO_2$ difference is normally about 6 mmHg, and the OLV shunt has a trivial influence on $PaCO_2$. Two, carbon dioxide is 20 times more diffusible than oxygen; thus, it is easily eliminated. Three, OLV decreases the dead space/tidal volume ratio, which enhances carbon dioxide elimination. The respiratory rate can be adjusted to maintain $PaCO_2$ at 40 mmHg. Overventilating the dependent lung produces excessive increase in dependent lung vascular resistance and may inhibit HPV in the nondependent lung.

Management of Hypoxemia

Following the initiation of OLV, PaO_2 can continue to decrease for up to 45 minutes (Fig. 13-12). Hence, close monitoring of arterial blood gases or the use of a pulse oximeter are indispensable. Should hypoxia occur patients should be ventilated with 100% oxygen if N_2O was used during OLV. Proper positioning of the double-lumen tube should be reconfirmed by fiberoptic bronchoscopy as described above. Once the double-lumen tube is properly positioned, other causes of hypoxemia such as bronchospasm or obstruction of main bronchi by secretion or mucous plugs should be excluded. Vigorous lung suctioning or the administration of bronchodilators should improve oxygenation.

In the vast majority of the cases, however, the hypoxemia is a direct result of the transpulmonary shunt through the nondependent

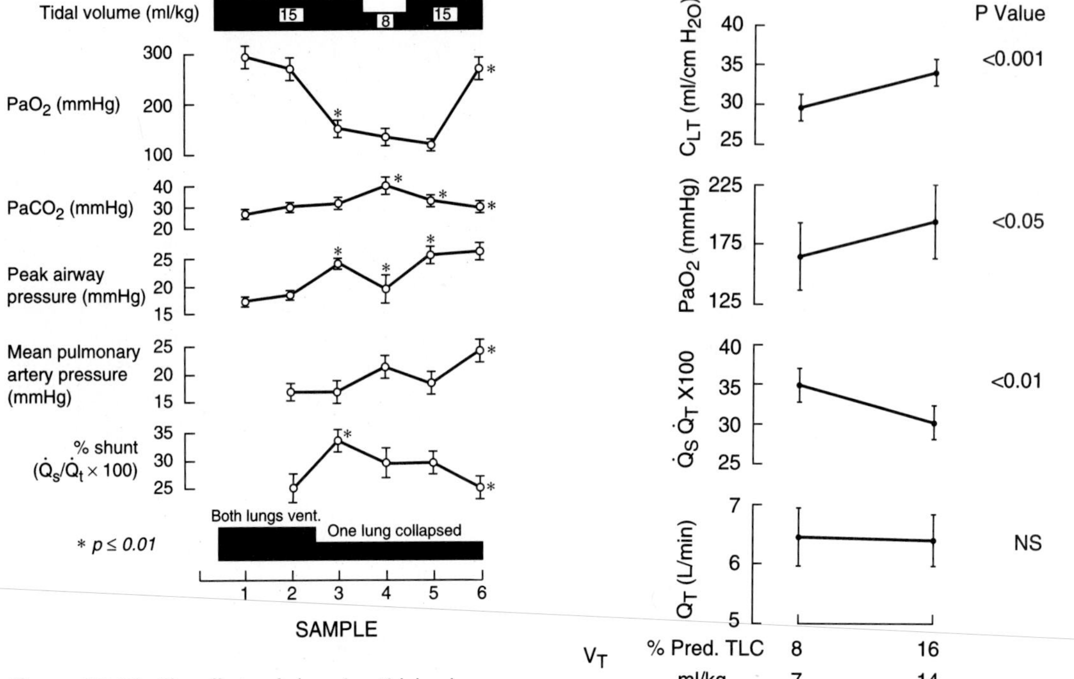

Figure 13-10. The effects of changing tidal volume on arterial blood gas values, peak airway pressure, pulmonary artery pressure, and shunt during one-lung ventilation. PaO_2 and percentage shunt are not significantly affected by changing the tidal volume from 15 to 8 mL/kg or vice versa. (Adapted with permission from Flacke JW, Thompson DS, Reed RC. Influence of tidal volume and pulmonary artery occlusion on arterial oxygenation during endobronchial anesthesia. South Med J 1976;69:619.)

Figure 13-11. Effect of tidal volume (VT) during one-lung ventilation (mean ± SE, n = 13). Data were analyzed using Student's *t* test for paired data. CLT = lung-thorax compliance; PaO_2 = arterial oxygen partial pressure; $\dot{Q}s/\dot{Q}T$ = physiologic shunt; and QT = cardiac output. (Adapted with permission from Katz JA, Laverne RG, Fairley HB. Pulmonary oxygen exchange during endobronchial anesthesia: Effects of tidal volume and PEEP. Anesthesiology 1982;56:164.)

lung. Therefore, further maneuvers such as the application of PEEP to restore the decreasing FRC of the dependent lung or the application of CPAP to the nondependent lung are effective for the treatment of hypoxemia.

Application of Positive End-Expiratory Pressure to the Dependent Lung

The application of PEEP to improve oxygenation during OLV is certainly appealing because of its simplicity and its immediate availability on most contemporary anesthesia delivery systems. This maneuver, however, has been displaced by CPAP to the nonventilated lung, which has so far proven to be more effective in improving PaO_2. With the recent increase in the number of VAT procedures, the role of PEEP needs to be reevaluated. During VAT for lung resection or bullectomy, the operated lung must be completely collapsed and immobile.

Data from previous studies show that the application of 5–10 cm H_2O of PEEP during OLV either did not change PaO_2 or actually de-

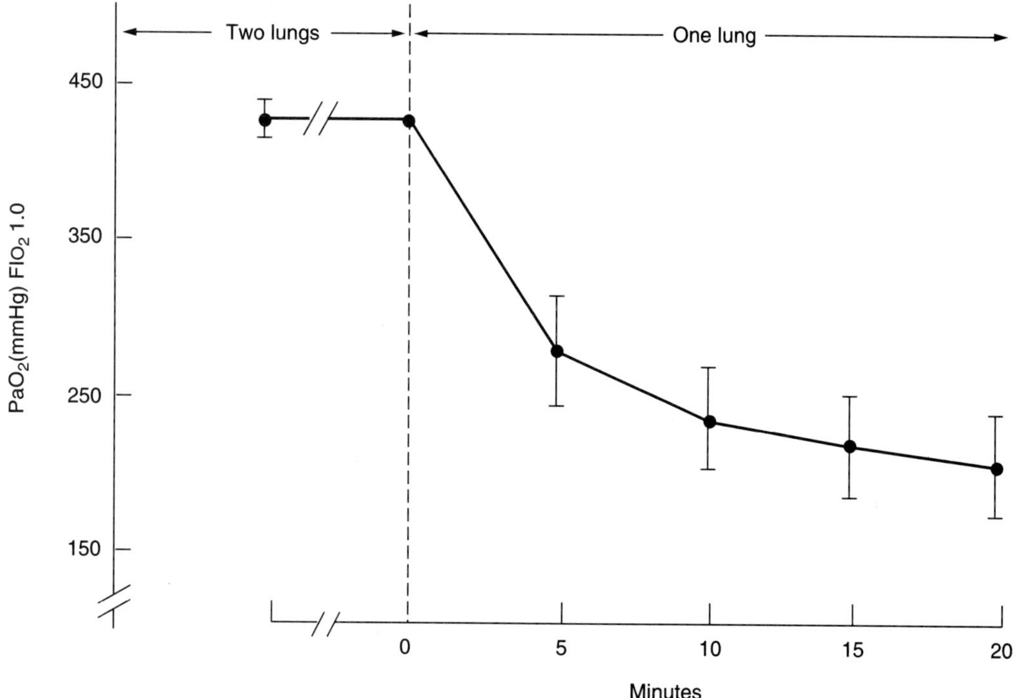

Figure 13-12. Arterial Oxygen Partial Pressure During One-Lung Ventilation. These are mean (±SE) PaO_2 values obtained in 17 patients in the lateral position. The broken vertical line indicates the start of one-lung ventilation. The mean PaO_2 value during two-lung ventilation was significantly different from all other measurements ($P<.001$). The means PaO_2 value at 5 minutes during one-lung ventilation was significantly different ($P<.05$) from all other measurements. Mean PaO_2 values at 10, 15, and 20 minutes demonstrated no statistically significant differences. (Adapted with permission from Katz JA et al. Pulmonary oxygen exchange during endobronchial anesthesia: Effect of tidal volume and PEEP. Anesthesiology 1982;56:164.)

creased it.[86,87,91–97] Dependent lung volume (Table 13-5) is often reduced during OLV, and the lateral position in a paralyzed ventilated patient causes an alteration in the distribution of pulmonary blood flow. Airway pressure generally falls to atmospheric during expiration, and the mediastinum tends to sink under its own weight into the lower hemithorax. This results in a decrease in the volume of the dependent lung and atelectasis. The blood flow to the non-dependent lung is gravity dependent, and with the addition of HPV, V/Q mismatch results from maldistribution in both lungs. Ventilation is greater than perfusion in the non-dependent lung, whereas perfusion is greater than ventilation in the dependent lung.[98–99]

The beneficial effect of PEEP, if any, is via an increase in lung volume at end-expiration. This augmentation in FRC prevents airway and alveolar closure, and recruits airways and alveoli during inspiration. PEEP increases the expansion of already open alveoli, prevents the collapse of unstable alveoli at end-expiration, and counteracts physical forces such as surface

Table 13-5. Application of PEEP to the Dependent Lung, Insufflation of Oxygen to the Nondependent Lung, Effect on Arterial Oxygenation During OLV

Authors	Total Volume (mL/kg)	PEEP (cm H_2O)	CPAP (cm H_2O)	Changes in PaO_2
Increasing Dependent Lung Tidal Volume				
Khanam et al.[102]	7 vs 10	—	—	NS
Flacke et al.[89]	7 vs 15	—	—	NS
Katz et al.[88]	7 vs 14	—	—	↑
Application of Dependent Lung PEEP				
Tarhan et al.[1]	Manual Ventilation	10		↓
Khanam et al.[102]	7	10		NS
Capan et al.[96]	—	10		↓
Katz et al.[90]	7	10		NS
	14	10		↓
Cohen et al.[87]	12	10		NS
Aalto-Setala et al.[86]	—	5		NS
Insufflation of Oxygen to the Nondependent Lung				
Capan et al.[96]	—		10	↑
O'Shea et al.[104]	10		5, 10	↑
Rees et al.[103]	10		Insufflation	↑
Cohen et al.[87]	12		10	↑
Benumof et al.[111]	12		10 (Univent)	↑
Slinger et al.[108]	10		10	↑
Gunnar et al.[105]	12		Intermittent Insufflation	↑
Hogue et al.[109]	12		2-5(Broncocath)	↑

tension changes that keep alveoli collapsed at end-inspiration, thus improving gas exchange. The latter mechanism is mediated by a long alveolar inflation time that renders PEEP more effective than ventilation using large tidal volumes (Fig. 13-13).[100–102]

The risk of the application of PEEP is that it may cause compression of small intra-alveolar vessels with a rise in vascular resistance, which may cause diversion of blood flow into the nondependent lung. The shunt fraction is ultimately determined by the balance between recruitment of atelectatic-dependent lung and increase vascular resistance that occurs following an increase in intra-alveolar pressure.

The effect of tidal volume on oxygenation seems to depend on the initial PaO_2 value during OLV. Specifically, the effect of high or low TV depends on the resulting modification of FRC and pulmonary vascular resistance in the dependent lung. Application of PEEP appears to have no beneficial effect on PaO_2 during OLV, and in most cases causes a further decrease in PaO_2. PEEP has been applied in patients who had a relatively high PaO_2 (155–210 mmHg) during OLV.[96]

Using FiO_2 of 0.5, Cohen et al[87] found that 10 cm of H_2O of PEEP delivered to the dependent lung increased PaO_2 in those patients with a PaO_2 less than 80 mmHg, while the PaO_2 decreased or remained unchanged in patients with a higher PaO_2. One possible explanation is that an increase in FRC above normal may alter the vascular resistance to that lung during the application of PEEP. The direction of that change depends on the initial lung volume.

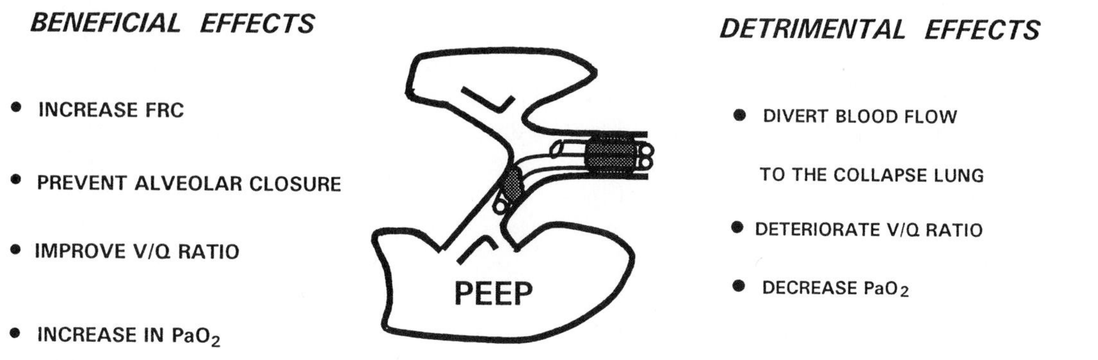

BENEFICIAL EFFECTS

- INCREASE FRC
- PREVENT ALVEOLAR CLOSURE
- IMPROVE V/Q RATIO
- INCREASE IN PaO_2

PEEP

DETRIMENTAL EFFECTS

- DIVERT BLOOD FLOW TO THE COLLAPSE LUNG
- DETERIORATE V/Q RATIO
- DECREASE PaO_2

Figure 13-13. Dependent Lung PEEP. The beneficial and detrimental effects of the application of PEEP to the dependent lung during OLV.

Pulmonary vascular resistance (PVR), which is a composite of the resistance of large and small vessels, is least at lung volumes near the ideal FRC and increases rapidly once lung volume varies from this ideal value. If the FRC is restored to normal from an initially low volume, the PVR should fall, resulting in increased blood flow through the ventilated lung, decreased Qs/QT, and an increase in PaO_2 (Fig. 13-14). If however, PEEP increased the FRC from an initially normal value, PVR increases and a larger proportion of the blood flow would

Figure 13-14. If the application of PEEP restores FRC to normal from an initially low volume, then the PVR falls resulting in increased blood flow through the ventilated lung, decreased $\dot{Q}s/\dot{Q}T$, and an increase in PaO_2.

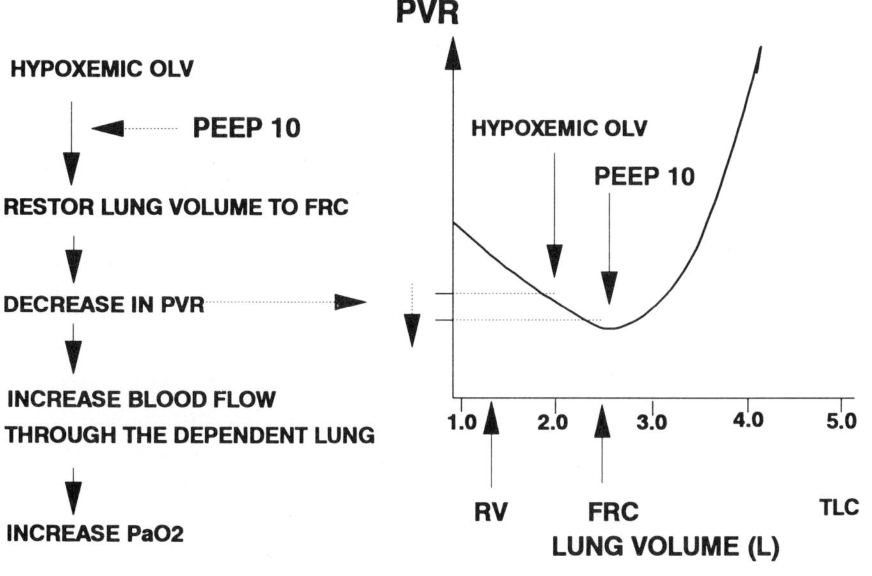

be shunted through the nondependent lung, resulting in a decrease in PaO_2.

The argument that PEEP decreases oxygenation by increasing PVR and diverting blood flow to the nonventilated lung merits some reconsideration. It is generally accepted that the best way to improve oxygenation is to apply 10 cm H_2O of CPAP ($CPAP_{10}$) to the nonventilated lung. $CPAP_{10}$ has been shown to be effective because of its apneic oxygenation effect in the nonventilated lung and not because it diverts blood flow to the dependent ventilated lung. Benumof et al[100] showed that the application of $CPAP_{10}$ using nitrogen to the nondependent lung failed to improve oxygenation. This clearly demonstrated the minimal role of positive pressure in diverting blood flow.

Nevertheless, PEEP to the ventilated lung is commonly considered to be responsible for diverting blood flow against gravity and HPV into the nonventilated lung and therefore deteriorates oxygenation. One can argue, however, that $CPAP_{10}$ is applied to an open hemithorax, while $PEEP_{10}$ is applied to the closed one.

Maneuvers Applied to the Nondependent Lung

As previously stated, the most effective maneuver for improving PaO_2 is the application of a CPAP of 10 cm H_2O ($CPAP_{10}$) to the nondependent lung. This finding is not surprising, because the primary cause of decreased arterial oxygenation during OLV is the deflation of the nondependent lung. Manipulation of this lung either by insufflation of oxygen or by decreasing the perfusion is most likely to improve oxygenation.

Clamping of the Pulmonary Artery

Reduction of blood flow to the nondependent lung by clamping the pulmonary artery to that lung and eliminating the shunt increases PaO_2. This approach may be useful in cases where pneumonectomy was planned; dissection of the pulmonary artery is not surgically appropriate otherwise. In addition, this procedure is time-consuming and the surgeon needs a collapsed lung to achieve control of the vessels.

Insufflation of Oxygen

Rees et al[103] found that continuous insufflation of oxygen to the nondependent lung during OLV, essentially an apneic oxygenation, effectively minimized the degree of shunt and attenuated the decrease in arterial oxygenation over the first 45 minutes of OLV in 24 patients (Fig. 13-15). This method can be applied where inflation of the operative lung by positive pressure may interfere with the surgical procedure (eg, with VAT). Insufflation alone without positive pressure may have a limited benefit during the first 45 minutes, however, and is certainly effective for a longer period of time. It should be mentioned that in both animal and human studies, oxygen insufflation at zero airway pressures did not significantly improve PaO_2. This is probably the result of the inability of such transtracheal pressures to maintain airway patency and overcome the critical opening pressure.[104]

Intermittent Reinflation of the Collapsed Lung with Oxygen

The clinical usefulness of and the effect of intermittent oxygen reinflation (Fig. 13-16) of the collapsed lung was studied by Gunnar.[105] During O_2/N_2O-balanced anesthesia, the nondependent lung was intermittently inflated and deflated with oxygen at five-minute intervals in a group of patients. The PaO_2 values in the intermittent insufflation group were higher compared to a control group. In addition, intermittent inflation every five minutes consistently

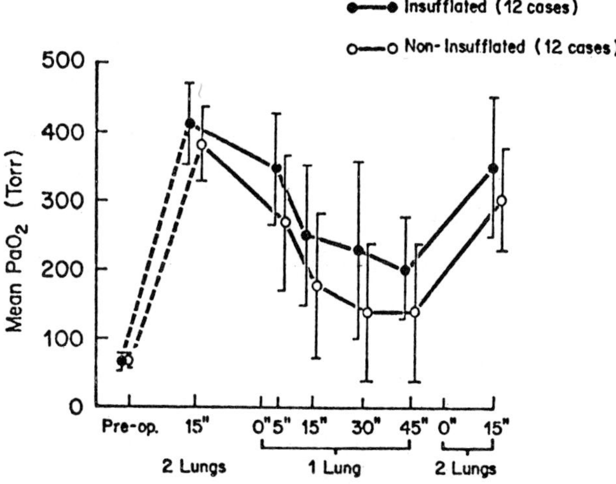

Figure 13-15. Plot of mean ($\pm$SD) arterial oxygen tension against time for insufflated and non-insufflated patients. Preoperative data plotted merely to illustrate similarity of both groups in prestudy period. Statistically significant group differences ($p<0.05$) ooccurred during period of one-lung ventilation. (Reproduced with permission from Rees DI, Wansbrough SR. One-lung anesthesia and arterial oxygen tension during continuous insufflation of oxygen to the non-ventilated lung. Anesth Analg 1982;61:501.)

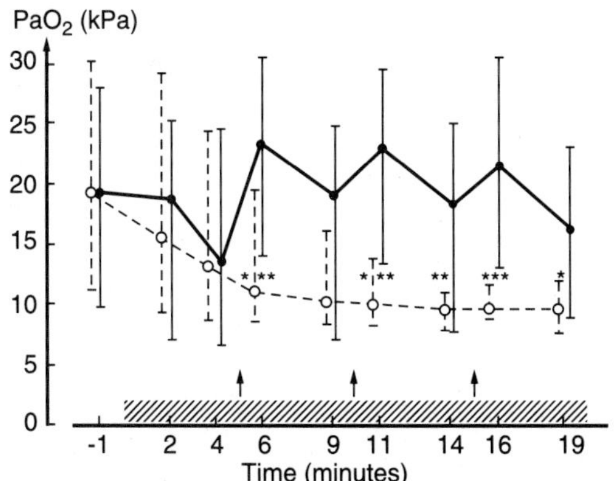

Figure 13-16. Arterial oxygen tension (PaO_2, median and range) in the control group (o---o) and inflation group (•—•). Arrows indicate inflation.s *P* values for differences between groups denoted by *$P<0.05$; **$P<0.02$, and ***$P<0.01$. (Adapted with permission from Gunnar M. Maintenance of oxygenation during one-lung ventilation: Effects of intermittent reinflation of the collapsed lung with oxygen. Anesth Analg 1989;68:763.)

increases oxygenation in all patients. The drawback of this technique is that it may interfere with the surgeon's work. Therefore it is recommended only as a last resort or when a CPAP device is not readily available.

Continuous Positive Airway Pressure to the Nondependent Lung

In all clinical studies to date, the single most effective maneuver to improve oxygenation is the application of CPAP to the nondependent lung. This technique consists of insufflation of oxygen under positive pressure to keep a lung "quiet" while preventing it from collapsing completely. The beneficial effect of CPAP is not secondary to the positive pressure effect, which potentially causes blood flow diversion to the dependent perfused lung, but from distending the alveoli with oxygen to allow gas exchange. The ability of CPAP to improve oxygenation substantially is highly reliable, as has been demonstrated in numerous studies in humans and dogs. Most studies in humans have showed that CPAP, 5–10 cm H_2O, to the nondependent lung significantly increases PaO_2 during OLV (Fig. 13-17). Capan et al[96] reported that the application of PEEP to the dependent lung decreased a mean PaO_2 of 155 ± 25 mmHg to 85 ± 11 but the application of CPAP to only the nonventilated lung resulted in an increase of 248 ± 41. This procedure was superior to the combination of both maneuvers. Cohen et al[87] using N_2O/O_2 (50%/50%) evaluated the effect of these maneuvers during OLV. The collapse of the nondependent lung resulted in a mean PaO_2 of 80 ± 6 mmHg. The application of CPAP 10 cm H_2O alone or in combination with PEEP 10 cm H_2O significantly increased PaO_2 to a mean of 125 ± 11 (Fig. 13-18). In a dog study Alfery et al[100] have shown during OLV that the application of CPAP, 10 cm H_2O, by the insufflation of 100% oxygen improve PaO_2, whereas the insufflation of nitrogen to the nonventilating lung failed to do so. This suggested that mechanical flow diversion alone is not the sole mechanism whereby CPAP, 10 cm H_2O, improves oxygenation. Rather the main mechanism of action is apneic oxygenation with alveolar recruitment of the nonventilated lung that reduces the degree of shunt. In fact, increasing the CPAP application to 15 cm H_2O leads to blood flow directed to the dependent lung however with no improvement in PaO_2. The application of CPAP should follow a delivery of a tidal volume to keep the patency of the alveoli distended and allow apneic oxygenation.[106–108] In general, low doses of CPAP, 5–10 cm H_2O, do not interfere with the surgeon from over-expurition of the lung. Sometimes keeping the lung quiet but in a constant state of inflation facilitates intralobar dissection and helps pleural decortication.

Recently, the ability of the application of

Figure 13-17. PaO_2, (A-a) DO_2, and $\dot{Q}s/\dot{Q}_T$ during two-lung ventilation and ventilation of the dependent lung with and without up-lung CPAP. (Abbreviations: ZEP, zero end-expiratory pressure; DEFL, deflation). Up-lung CPAP improves PaO_2, (A-a) DO_2 and $\dot{Q}s/\dot{Q}_T$ significantly. (Modified with permission from Capan LM, Turndorf J, Chandrakant P, et al. Optimization of arterial oxygenation during one-lung anesthesia. Anesth Analg 1980;59:847.)

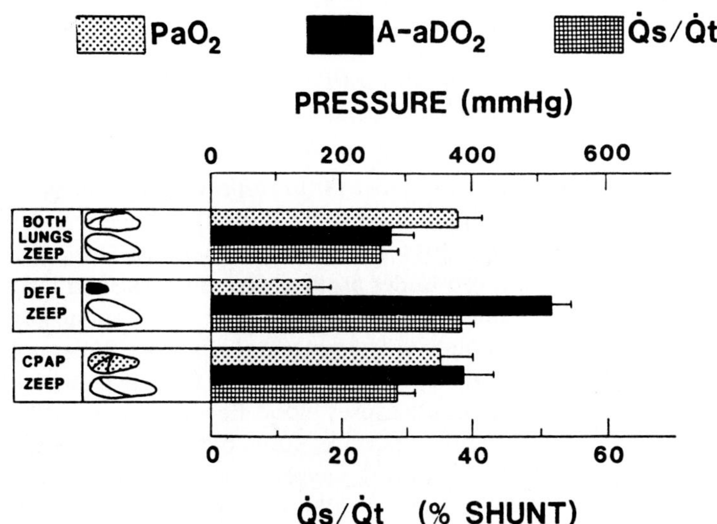

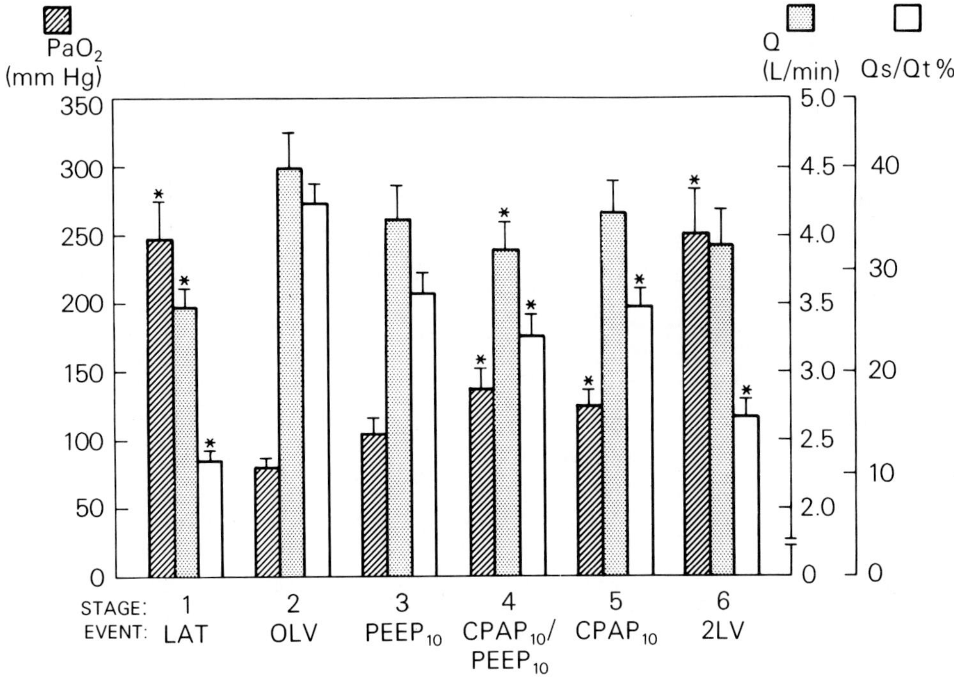

Figure 13-18. Changes in PaO_2, Q, and Q_S/Q_T% during the six stages of the study. All comparisons made with values obtained during stage 2 (OLV). (Reproduced with permission from Cohen E, Eisenkraft JB, Thys DM, et al. Oxygenation and hemodynamic changes during one-lung ventilation: effects of $CPAP_{10}$, $PEEP_{10}$, and $CPAP_{10}/PEEP_{10}$. J Cardiothorac Anesth 1988;1:34.)

low levels of CPAP, 2 and 5 cm H_2O, have been evaluated. Using a Bronchcath CPAP system (see below in CPAP devices) Hogne reported improved PaO_2 using 2 cm H_2O from 126 ± 75 to 270 ± 112 and CPAP, 5 cm of H_2O from 173 ± 79 to 386 ± 66.[109] This showed that low levels of CPAP may be therapeutic and have the advantage of avoiding hyperinflation of the operative lung. Hyperinflation of nitrogen under positive pressure into the nondependent lung failed to improve PaO_2. Most studies confirmed the occurrence of dramatic improvement in PaO_2 values with the application of $CPAP_{10}$.

Several systems used to apply CPAP to the nondependent lung all have essentially identical features:[86, 96] an oxygen source, tubing that connects the oxygen source to the nonventilated lung, a pressure-relief valve that allows the magnitude of the delivered CPAP to be adjusted, and a pressure gauge (Fig. 13-19). The arrangement of the oxygen source, pop-off valve, and the pressure manometer is not crucial. Two important points should be kept in mind. One, the system that has the capability to adjust the CPAP level by the built-in bleed valve, may be more prone to barotrauma from increase in oxygen flow or from inadvertent closure of the valve. Two, some systems can deliver fixed, predetermined levels by changing the PEEP valve. The chance of lung trauma is less with this

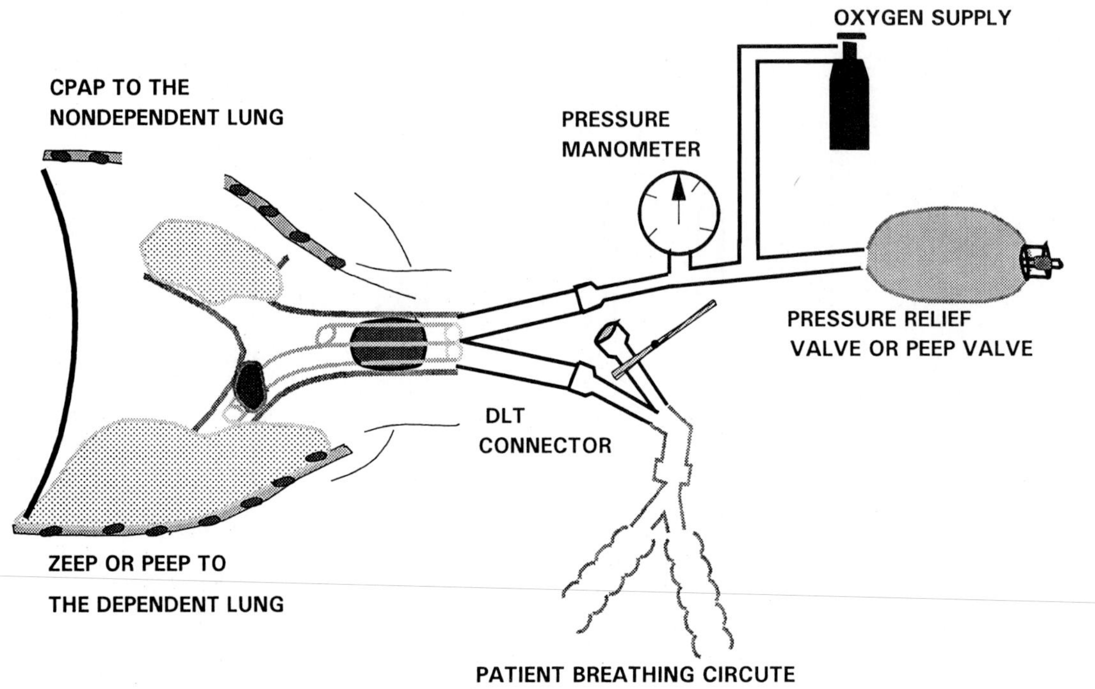

Figure 13-19. Non-dependent lung CPAP system.

system. Using a modified Ayre's T piece circuit, the nondependent lung is commonly insufflated with 5 L/min of oxygen, and the valve on the expiratory limb is adjusted to the desired $CPAP_{10}$ as read on an attached pressure gauge. One manufacturer currently encloses a disposable CPAP circuit with a double-lumen tube (Fig. 13-20) (Mallinckrodt, Argyle, NY).[109–110] The advantage of this system is that the therapeutic levels of CPAP can be titrated and low levels of CPAP can be given. If the level of the given CPAP is not sufficient to expand an atelectatic lung, the improvement in oxygenation is limited. The level of CPAP should be adjusted to balance between the degree of lung expansion and the negative effect of impeding surgery from overdistension. However, it is important to remember that the application of CPAP should be initiated *following* a delivery of a tidal volume to the nondependent lung. A level exceeding 5 cm of H_2O is seldom needed to improve oxygenation. Recently Benumof et al[111] reported the possibility of improved PaO_2 during OLV with the application of CPAP via the bronchial blocker of the Univent tube (Fig. 13-21).

High-Frequency Ventilation

High-frequency ventilation (HFV) uses a high-pressure gas source that delivers a pulse of gas through a small catheter at a frequency that ranges between 100 and 150 per minute.[112] The delivered small tidal volume is less than the anatomic dead space. In thoracic surgery HFV is mostly recommended in cases of a large air leak such as bronchopleural or cutaneous fistula, where conventional ventilation results in a

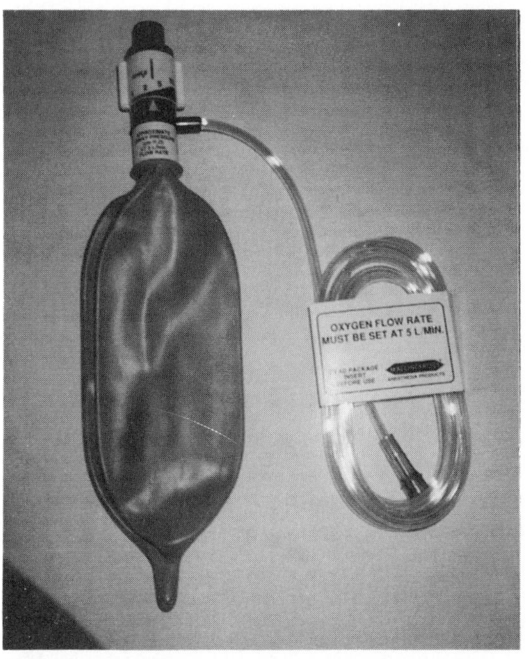

A

larger leak and inability to eliminate CO_2. Another example of the use of HFV is during sleeve pneumonectomy, where ventilation can be maintained while the open airways are being repaired. During OLV, HFV may be used in the deflated lung instead of CPAP. Malina et al[113] evaluated gas exchange during thoracotomy using HFV to both lungs. Using FiO_2 of 0.5, the authors reported PaO_2 above 75 mmHg in all patients. Despite the low tidal volume delivered, however, the nondependent lung was expanded and interfered with the surgeon's work. In clinical practice the use of HFV instead of CPAP to the nonventilated lung adds significant complexity and does not offer any advantage over CPAP. In addition, it may produce continued lung movement and overexpansion of the operative lung.

In summary, the preferred method for management of hypoxemia during OLV is by

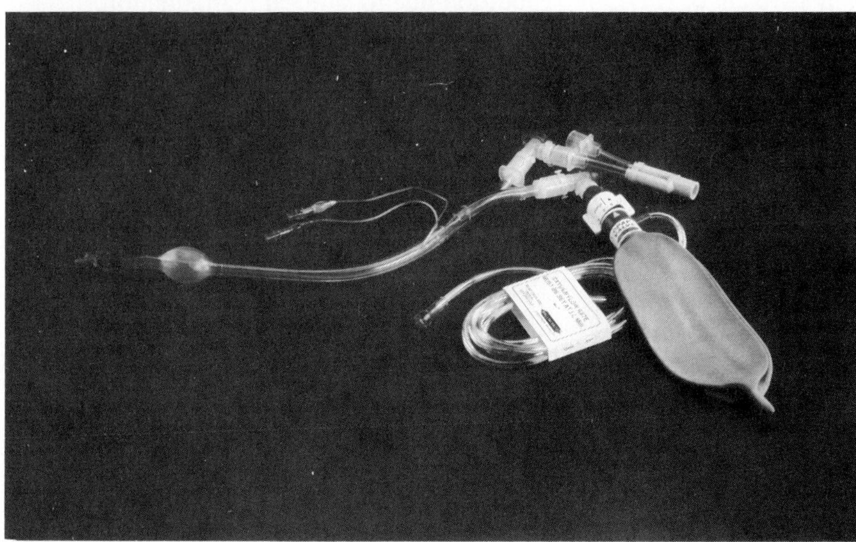

B

Figure 13-20. A. Disposable CPAP device (Mallinckrodt, Argyle, NY). The level of PEEP can be achieved by dialing the desired number at the CPAP valve. B. The CPAP device is attached to the connector of the DLT.

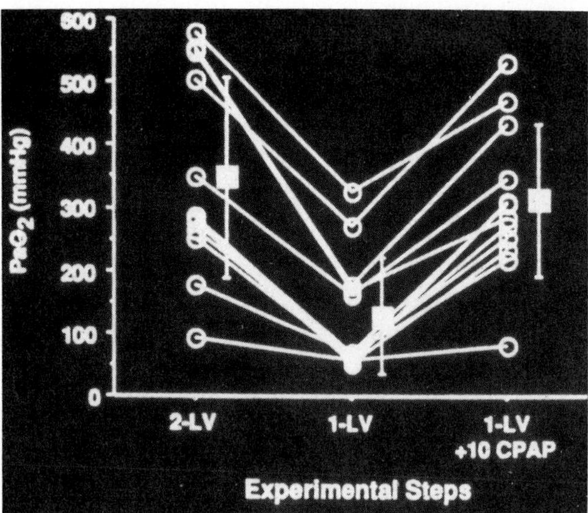

Figure 13-21. The PaO_2 values during two-lung ventilation, OLV, and OLVT 10 of CPAP which was applied through the bronchial blocker lumen of the Univent tube. The improvement in PaO_2 is evident.

application of CPAP to the nondependent lung with a search for an optimal combination of PEEP and CPAP (between 5–10 cm of H_2O). In exceptional cases, despite all of these maneuvers, PaO_2 fails to improve and intermittent ventilation of the nondependent lung should be reinstituted with the surgeon's collaboration. Depending on the stage of the surgery, if a pneumonectomy is planned, ligation of the pulmonary artery eliminates the shunt through that lung. Should doubt arise as to the stability of the patient (eg, the patient becomes hypotensive, dusky, or tachycardic), two-lung ventilation should be resumed until the problem is resolved. It should be appreciated that the majority of the thoracic cases represent only relative indications for OLV.

Finally, several important issues should be kept in mind during management of OLV. First, when using a right-sided double-lumen tube, adequate ventilation to the right upper lobe should always be confirmed with the help of fiberoptic bronchoscopy. Second, when using a left-sided tube for right thoracotomy where the patient is dependent on the left lung, the tip of the left-sided tube may obstruct the left upper lobe orifice. Thus, should hypoxemia result during right thoracotomy with left-sided tube, correct position of the tube should be reconfirmed with fiberoptic bronchoscopy. Withdrawal of the tube by 1 cm and reexpansion of the left upper lobe typically resolve the hypoxemia. Manipulation of the double-lumen tube can involve the surgeon as well. Palpation and manual occlusion of the main bronchial lumens can guide the tip of the tube to the correct position. Finally, peak airway pressure, delivered tidal volume (as measured by spirometer), and the capnogram shape, should be inspected continuously to identify an obstructive or a low end-tidal value from inadequate gas exchange subsequent to double-lumen tube malposition. A peak airway pressure of up to 40 cm of H_2O on OLV is acceptable. A sudden increase in the peak airway pressure may result from tube dislocation due to surgical manipulation.

Termination of the Surgery

At the completion of the procedure, the lung should be appropriately expanded in collaboration with the surgeon using a sustained positive pressure to reopen previously collapsed alveoli. This maneuver permits testing of the integrity of the resected bronchus suture line. An airway pressure of 40 cm H_2O with an open chest cavity filled with saline detects a gross air leak from a bronchial stump or the lung parenchyma. At the completion of a lobectomy, a chest tube is placed and connected with underwater seal suction to allow proper lung expansion. Following pneumonectomy, no chest tube is placed, since no lung tissue needs expansion. While in the supine position, an aspirating needle is used to equalize the cavity pressure to atmospheric levels. This maneuver allows the mediastinum to reposition in midline and avoid hypotension from mediastinal shift. The decision whether to extubate the patient at the conclusion of the procedure depends on the preoperative condition and the extent of lung resection. In addition, adequate temperature, complete reversal of muscle relaxant, and recovery from the presence of inhaled anesthetic or residual narcotic, should be ascertained. Except for high-risk patients with limited cardiopulmonary reserve, the majority of patients tolerate extubation in the operating room once the extubation criteria are met. Following extubation, respiratory rate, adequate air exchange, chest symmetry, and the presence of cyanosis should be closely observed in the operating room for a few minutes with an oxygen face mask in place to ensure proper gas exchange and oxygen saturation. Prompt reintubation of the postthoracotomy patient in the operating room, under most control circumstances could be life-saving.

References

1. Rutkow IM. Thoracic and cardiovascular operations in the United States, 1979 to 1984. J Thoracic Cardiovasc Surg 1986;92:181.
2. Cohen E, Kirschner PA, Benumof J. Simultaneous bilateral bullectomy for bullous emphysema with severe pulmonary insufficiency. J Cardiothorac Vasc Anesth 1990;4:119.
3. Cohen E, Eisenkraft JB, Thys DM, et al. Unilateral lung lavage: a case report with continuous monitoring of arterial and mixed venous oxygen saturation. J Cardioth Vasc Anesth 1990;4:609.
4. Barker SJ, Clarke C, Trivedi N, et al. Anesthesia for thoracoscopic laser ablation of bullous emphysema. Anesthesiology 1993;78:44.
5. Urschel HJ Jr, Razzuk MA. Median sternotomy as a standard approach for pulmonary resection. Ann Thorac Surg 1986;41:130.
6. Thompson DF, Campbell D. Changes in arterial oxygen tension during one-lung anesthesia. Br J Anaesth 1973;45:611.
7. West JB, Dollery CT, Naimark A. Distribution of blood flow in isolated lung: relation to vascular and alveolar pressures. J Appl Physiol 1964;19:713.
8. Wulff KE, Aulin I. The regional lung function in the lateral decubitus position during anesthesia and operation. Acta Anesthesiol Scand 1972;16:195.
9. Rehdar K, Wenthe FM, Sessler AD. Function of each lung during mechanical ventilation with ZEEP and with PEEP in man anesthetized with thiopental-meperidine. Anesthesiology 1973;39:597.
10. Benumof JL. Anesthesia for Thoracic Surgery. Philadelphia: WB Saunders. 1987;211.
11. Marshall BE, Marshall C, Benumof JL, et al. Hypoxic pulmonary vasoconstriction in dogs: effects of lung segment size and oxygen tension. J Appl Physiol 1981;51:1543.
12. Benumof JL. One lung ventilation and hypoxic pulmonary vasoconstriction: implications for anesthetic management. Anesth Analg 1985;64:821.
13. Domino KB, Borowee L, Alexander CM, et al. Influence of isoflurane on hypoxic pulmonary vasoconstriction in dogs. Anesthesiology 1986;64:423.
14. Brodsky JB, Shulman MS, Mark JBD. Malposition of left-sided endobronchial tubes. Anesthesiology 1985;62:667.
15. Smith GB, Hirsch NP, Ehrenwerth J. Placement of double-lumen endobronchial tubes. Br J Anaesth 1986;58:1317.
16. McKenna MJ, Wilson RS, Botelho RJ. Right upper lobe obstruction with right-sided double-lumen endobronchial tubes: a comparison of two tubes types. J Cardiothorac Anes 1988;2:734.
17. Alliaume B, Coddens J, Deloof T. Reliability of auscultation in positioning of double-lumen endobronchial tubes. Can J Anaesth 1992;39:687.
18. Benumof JL. Mechanism of decreased blood flow to atelectatic lung. J App Physiol 1979;46:1047.
19. Benumof JL. One-lung ventilation and hypoxic pulmonary vasoconstriction: implications for anesthetic management. Anesth Analg 1985;64:821.
20. Nomoto Y. Perioperative pulmonary blood flow and one-lung anesthesia. Can J Anaesth 1987;34:447.
21. Hurford WE, Kolker AC, Strauss W. The use of ventilation/perfusion lung scans to predict oxygenation during one-lung anesthesia. Anesthesiology 1987;67:841.
22. Virtue RW, Permutt S, Tanaka R, et al. Ventilation-perfusion changes during thoracotomy. Anesthesiology 1966;27:132.

23. Kerr JH. Physiological aspects of one-lung (endobronchial) anesthesia. Int Anesth Clin 1972;10:61.
24. Kerr JH, Smith AC, Prys-Roberts C, et al. Observations during endobronchial anaesthesia II. Oxygenation. Br J Anaesth 1974;46:84.
25. Rehdar K, Sessler AD. Function of each lung in spontaneously breathing man anesthetized with thiopental-meperidine. Anesthesiology 1973;38:320.
26. Froese AB, Bryan AC. Effects of anesthesia and paralysis on diaphragmatic mechanics in man. Anesthesiology 1974;42:242.
27. Don HF, Wahba M, Cuadrado L, et al. The effects of anesthesia and 100 percent oxygen on the functional residual capacity of the lungs. Anesthesiology 1970;32:521.
28. Fielding JE. Smoking: health effects and control. N Engl J Med 1985;313:491.
29. Bennett DJ, Torda TA, Horton DA, et al. Severe bronchospasm complicating thoracotomy. Arch Surg 1970;101:555.
30. Hirshman CA, Edelstein G, Peetz S, et al. Mechanism of action of inhalational anesthesia on airways. Anesthesiology 1982;56:107.
31. Hirshman CA. Airway reactivity in humans. Anesthesiology 1983;58:170.
32. Patterson RW, Sullivan SF, Malm JR, et al. The effects of halothane on human airway mechanics. Anesthesiology 1969;29:900.
33. Waltemath CL, Bergman NA. Effect of ketamine and halothane on increased respiratory resistance provoked by ultrasonic aerosols. Anesthesiology 1974;41:473.
34. Hermens JM, Edelstein G, Hanifin JM, et al. Inhalational anesthesia and histamine release during bronchospasm. Anesthesiology 1984;61:69.
35. Shah MV, Hirshman CA. Mode of action of halothane on histamine-induced airway obstruction in dogs with reactive airways. Anesthesiology 1986; 65:170.
36. Kettlekamp NS, Austine DR, Downes H, et al. Inhibition of d-tubocurarine-induced histamine release by halothane. Anesthesiology 1987;66:666.
37. Johnston RR, Eger EI, Wilson C. A comparative interaction of epinephrine with enflurane, isoflurane, and halothane in man. Anesth Anal 1976; 55:709.
38. Moore PG, Kien ND, Reitan J. Inhibition of nitric oxide synthesis causes systemic and pulmonary vasoconstriction in isoflurane-anesthetized dogs. J Cardioth Vasc Anesth 1994;8:310.
39. Hermens JM, Ebertz JM, Hanifin JM, et al. Comparison of histamine release in human skin mast cells induced by morphine, fentanyl, and oxymorphine. Anesthesiology 1985;62:124.
40. Shemano I, Wendel H. Effects of meperidine hydrochloride on morphine sulphate on the lung capacity of intact dogs. J Phrmacol Exp Ther 1965;149: 379.
41. Hirshman CA, Downes H, Farbood A, et al. Ketamine block of bronchospasm in experimental canine asthma. Br J Anaesth 1979;51:713.
42. Vitkun SA, Foster WM, Chang H, et al. Bronchodilating effects of the anesthetic ketamine in an in vitro guinea pig preparation. Ling 1987;165:101.
43. Corssen G, Gutierrez J, Reeves JG, et al. Ketamine in the anesthetic management of asthmatic patients. Anesth Analg 1972;51:588.
44. Hirshman CA, Edelstein G, Ebertz JM, et al. Thiobarbiturate-induced histamine release in human skin mastcells. Anesthesiology 1985;63:353.
45. Doenick A, Lorenz W, Stamwerth D, et al. Effects of propofol ("Diprivan") on histamine release, immunoglobulin levels and activation of complement in healthy volunteers. Postgrad Med J 1986;61S:15.
46. Withington DE. Basophil histamine release studies in the evaluation of a new anesthetic agent. Agents Actions 1988;23:337.
47. Guldager H, Sondergaard I, Jensen FM, et al. Basophil histamine release in asthma patients after in vitro provocation with althesin and etomodate. Acta Anaesthesiol Scand 1985;29:352.
48. Walkins J. Etomidate: an "immunologically" anesthetic agent. Anaesthesia 1983;38S:34.
49. Moss J, Roscow CE, Savarese JJ, et al. Role of histamine in the hypotensive action of d-tubocurarine in humans. Anesthesiology 1981;55:19.
50. Basta SJ, Ali HH, Savarese JJ, et al. Clinical pharmacology of atracurium besylate: a new nondepolarizing muscle relaxant. Anesth Analg 1982;61:723.
51. Scott RPF, Savarese JJ, Basta SJ, et al. Atracurium: Clinical strategies for preventing histamine release and attenuating the hemodynamic response. Br J Anaesth 1985;57:550.
52. Stoops CM, Curtis CA, Kovach DA, et al. Hemodynamic effects of mivacurium chloride administered to patients during oxygen-sufentanil anaesthesia for coronary artery bypass grafting or valve replacement. Anesth Analg 1989;68:333.
53. Tassonyi E, Neidhart P, Pittet J, et al. Cardiovascular effects of pipecuronium in patients undergoing

coronary artery bypass grafting. Anesthesiology 1988;69:793.
54. Brandus V, Joffe S, Benoit CV, et al. Bronchial spasm during general anesthesia. Canad Anaesth Soc J 1970;17:269.
55. Gal TJ. Airway responses in normal subjects following topical anesthesia with ultrasonic aerosols with 4 percent lidocaine. Anesth Analg 1980;59:123.
56. Marshall BE, Marshall C. Continuity of response to hypoxic pulmonary vasoconstriction. J Appl Physiol 1980;59:189.
57. Benumof JL. One-lung ventilation and hypoxic pulmonary vasoconstriction: implications for anesthetic management. Anesth Analg 1985;64:821.
58. Benumof JL. Mechanism of decreased blood flow to atelectatic lung. J App Physiol 1979;46:1047.
59. Carlsson AJ, Bindslev L, Hedenstierna G. Hypoxia pulmonary vasoconstriction in the lung. Anesthesiology 1987;66:312.
60. Buckley MJ, McLaughlin JS, Fort L, et al. Effects of anesthetic agents on pulmonary vascular resistance during hypoxemia. Surgical Forum 1964;15:183.
61. Pirlo AF, Benumof JL, Trousdale FR. Atelectatic lung lobe blood flow: open vs. closed chest, positive pressure vs. spontaneous ventilation. J Appl Physiol 1981;50:1022.
62. Glasser SA, Domino KB, Lindgren L, et al. Pulmonary pressure and flow during atelectasis. Anesthesiology 1982;57:A504.
63. Carlsson AJ, Bindslev L, Santesson J, et al. Hypoxic pulmonary vasoconstriction in the human lung: the effect of prolonged unilateral hypoxic challenge during anesthesia. Acta Anesthesiol Scand 1985;29:346.
64. Domino KB, Wetstein L, Glosser SA, et al. Influence of mixed venous oxygen tension (PvO_2) on blood flow to atelectatic lung. Anesthesiology 1983;59:428.
65. Benumof JL, Pirlo AF, Trousdale FR. Inhibition of hypoxic pulmonary vasoconstriction by decreased PvO_2: a new indirect mechanism. J Appl Physiol 1981;51:871.
66. Benumof JL, Wahrenbrock EA. Local effect of anesthetic on regional hypoxic pulmonary vasoconstriction. Anesthesiology 1975;43:525.
67. Bjertnaes LJ. Intravenous versus inhalational anesthesia-pulmonary effects. Acta Anaesthesiol Scand 1982;75:18.
68. Weinteich AI, Silvay G, Lumb PD. Continuous ketamine infusion for one lung anaesthesia. Can Anaesth So J 1980;27:485.
68a. Rees DI, Gaines GY. One-lung anesthesia: A comparison of pulmonary gas exchange during anesthesia with ketamine and enflurane. Anesthes Analg 1984;63:521.
69. Rogers SM, Benumof JL. Halothane and isoflurane do not decrease PaO_2 during one-lung ventilation in intravenously anesthetized patients. Anesth Analg 1985;64:946.
70. Benumof JL, Augustine SD, Gibbins J. Halothane and isoflurane only slightly impair arterial oxygenation during one-lung ventilation in patients undergoing thoracotomy. Anesthesiology 1987; 67:910.
71. Domino KB, Borowec L, Alexander CM, et al. Influence of isoflurane on hypoxic pulmonary vasoconstriction in dogs. Anesthesiology 1986;65:423.
72. Fujita Y, Yamasaki T, Masuhiko T, et al. Sevoflurane anaesthesia for one-lung ventilation with PEEP to the dependent lung in sheep: effects on right ventricular function and oxygenation. Can J Anaesth 1993;40:1195.
73. Smith GB, Hirsch NP, Ehrenwerth J. Placement of double-lumen endobronchial tubes. Br J Anaesth 1986;1317.
74. McKenna MJ, Wilson RS, Botelho RJ. Right upper lobe obstruction with right-sided double-lumen endobronchial tubes: a comparison of two tubes types. J Cardiothorac Anes 1988;2:734.
75. Alliaume B, Coddens J, Deloof T. Reliability of auscultation in positioning of double-lumen endobronchial tubes. Can J Anaesth 1992;39:687.
76. Lewis JW, Serwin JP, Gabriel FS, et al. The utility of a double-lumen tube for one-lung ventilation in a variety of noncardiac thoracic surgical procedures. J Cardiothorac Vasc Anes 1992;5:705.
77. Hurford WE, Alfille PH. A quality improvement study of the placement and complications of double-lumen endobronchial tubes. J Cardiothorac Vasc Anes 1993;7:517.
78. Read RC, Friday CO, Eason CN. Prospective study of the Robertshaw endobronchial catheter in thoracic surgery. Ann Thorac Surg 1977;24:156.
79. Benumof JL, Partridge BL, Salvatierra C, et al. Margin of safety in positioning modern double-lumen endotracheal tubes. Anesthesiology 1987;67:729.
80. Burton NA, Falls SM, Lyons T, et al. Rupture of the left mainstem bronchus with a polyvinyl chloride double lumen tube. Chest 1983;83:928.
81. Wagner DL, Gammage GW, Wong ML. Tracheal rupture following insertion of disposable double-lumen endotracheal tube. Anesthesiology 1986;63:698.
82. Kamaya H, Krishna PR. New endotracheal tube (Univent tube) for selective blockade of one lung. Anesthesiology 1985;63:342.

83. Karande SV. A new tube for single lung ventilation. Chest 1987;92:761.
84. Gayes JM. One-lung ventilation is best accomplished with the Univent tube. J Cardiothorac Vasc Anesth 1993;7:103.
85. Lunding M, Fernandes A. Arterial oxygen tension and acid-base status during endobronchial anesthesia. Acta Anasthesiol Scand 1967;11:43.
86. Aalto-Setala M, Heinonen J, Salorinne Y. Cardiorespiratory function during thoracic anaesthesia: comparison of two-lung ventilation and one-lung ventilation with and without PEEP. Acta Anaesthesiol Scand 1975;19:287.
87. Cohen E, Eisenkraft JB, Thys DM, et al. Oxygenation and hemodynamic changes during one lung ventilation: effects of $CPAP_{10}$, $PEEP_{10}$, and $CPAP_{10}/PEEP_{10}$. J. Cardiothorac Anesth 1988;2:34.
88. Katz JA, Ozanne G, Zinn Se, et al. Time course and mechanisms of lung-volume increase with PEEP in acute pulmonary failure. Anesthesiology 1981;54:9.
89. Flacke JW, Thompson DS, Read RC. Influence of tidal volume and pulmonary artery occlusion on arterial oxygenation during endobronchial anesthesia. South Med J 1976;69:619.
90. Katz JA, Laverne RG, Fairley HB. Pulmonary oxygen exchange during endobronchial anesthesia. Effects of tidal volume and PEEP. Anesthesiology 1982; 56:164.
91. Tarhan S, Lundborg RO. Effects of increased respiratory pressure on blood gas tensions and pulmonary shunting during thoracotomy with use of the Carlens catheter. Can Anaesth Soc J 1970;17:4.
92. Brown RD, Caer RED, Roberson OV, et al. Improved oxygenation during thoracotomy with selective PEEP to the dependent lung. Anesth Analg 1977; 56:26.
93. Tarhan S, Lundborg RO. Carlens endotracheal catheter versus regular endotracheal tube during thoracic surgery: a comparison of blood tensions and pulmonary shunting. Can Anaesth Soc J 1971;18:594.
94. Hatch D. Ventilation and arterial oxygenation during thoracic surgery. Thorax 1966;21:310.
95. Torda TA, McCullogh CH, O'Brien HD, et al. Pulmonary venous admixture during one-lung anesthesia, effect of inhaled oxygen tension and respiration rate. Anaesthesia 1974;29:274.
96. Capan LM, Turndorf H, Chandrakant P, et al. Optimization of arterial oxygenation during one-lung anesthesia. Anesth Analg 1980;59:847.
97. Slinger PD, Hickey D, Gottfried S. Intrinsic PEEP during one-lung ventilation. Anasth Analg 1989; 68:S269.
98. Benumof JL. One-lung ventilation: which lung should be PEEPed? Anesthesiology 1982;56:161.
99. Benumof JL. Mechanism of decreased blood flow to atelectatic lung. J App Physiol 1979;46:1047.
100. Alfery DD, Benumof JL, Trousdale FR. Improving oxygenation during one-lung ventilation in dogs: the effects of positive end-expiratory pressure and blood flow restriction to the nonventilated lung. Anesthesiology 1981;55:381.
101. Khanam T, Branthwaite MA. Arterial oxygenation during one-lung anaesthesia (1). A study in man. Anaesthesia 1973;28:132.
102. Khanam T, Branthwaite MA. Arterial oxygenation during one-lung anaesthesia (2). Anaesthesia 1973; 28:280.
103. Rees DI, Wansbrough SR. One-lung anesthesia and arterial oxygen tension during continuous insufflation of oxygen to the non-ventilated lung. Anesth Analg 1982;61:501.
104. O'Shea PJ, Savagw TM, Walton B. Effect of oxygen insufflation during one-lung anaesthesia. Proc R Soc Med 1975;68:772.
105. Gunnar M. Maintenance of oxygenation during one-lung ventilation: effects of intermittent reinflation of the collapsed lung with oxygen. Anesth Analg 1989;68:763.
106. Eisenkraft JB, Cohen E, Neustein SM. Anesthesia for thoracic surgery. In: Barash PG, Cullen BF, Stoelting RK, eds. Clinical anesthesia, second edition. Philadelphia: JB Lippincott 1992, 961.
107. Benumof JL. Anesthesia for thoracic surgery. Philadelphia: WB Saunders, 1987, 275.
108. Slinger P, Triolet W, Wilson J. Improving arterial oxygenation during one-lung ventilation. Anesthesiology 1988;68:291.
109. Hogue C Jr. Effectiveness of low levels of nonventilated lung continuous positive airway pressure in improving arterial oxygenation during one-lung ventilation. Anesth Analg 1994;79:364.
110. Body SC, Casieri T, DeMur C, Topulos GP. Flow sensitivity of the Mallinckrodt continuous continuous positive airway pressure device (letter). J Cardiothrac Vasc Anesth 1992;6:771.
111. Benumof JL, Gaughan S, Ozaki GT, et al. Operative lung CPAP with bronchial blocker. Anesth Analg 1992;74:406.
112. Wilkins D, Schmamunn T, Riley R, et al. Selective high frequency jet ventilation of the operative lung improves oxygenation during thoracic surgery. Anesthesiology 1985;63:A568.
113. Malina JF, Nordstrom FG, Skostrand UH, et al. Clinical evaluation of high-frequency positive-pressure ventilation (HFPPV) in patients scheduled for open-chest surgeries. Respir Care 1981;27:1380.

SECTION

IV

Postoperative Care of the Thoracic Surgery Patient

CHAPTER

14

Postoperative Care

Michael M. Hansen
John W. Hoyt

Care of the patient who has just undergone a major surgical procedure involving the thorax can be a challenging, especially if the patient has a history of preoperative cardiopulmonary disease, as is the case in the majority of adult patients. Ensuring that the patient with severe emphysema has adequate oxygenation and ventilation both during and after surgery or that the patient with a severe cardiomyopathy retains adequate cardiac function and oxygen delivery can be a tremendous test of clinical acumen. Many of the greatest challenges in treating the thoracic surgical patient occur in the postoperative period, which begins in the operating suite.

Extubation Versus Continued Mechanical Ventilation

Extubation

Many relatively healthy patients who have not undergone extensive surgical procedures can be extubated either in the operating room or the recovery room after their ability to maintain adequate oxygenation and ventilation on minimal support is ensured. In spite of sometimes severe alterations in pulmonary function, only a minority of patients require continued mechanical ventilation to support gas exchange in the postoperative period.[1] Several simple tests and observations can be made in the immediate postoperative period to determine which patients can be extubated. Minimum criteria have been established to identify those patients who may be candidates for early extubation and those who should remain intubated until minimum criteria are met (Table 14-1).[2]

Vital Capacity

Initial assessment of respiratory muscle strength is undertaken before extubation to ensure that patients are able to generate adequate tidal volumes, and often more importantly, are able to mount an adequate cough to clear retained secretions and blood that may be present in the tracheobronchial tree. Vital capacity (VC), a simple indicator of the single-breath exhalation capacity of the patient, is used to measure respiratory muscle strength. VC is measured by attaching a spirometer to the end of the endotracheal tube and can be easily performed in the operating room or the recovery room. The patient takes a maximal inspiration, and when end-inspiration is reached, the pa-

Table 14-1. Weaning Criteria*

Gas exchange variables
$PAO_2 \geq 60$ mmHg on $FIO_2 \leq 0.35$
Alveolar-arterial PO_2 gradient of < 350 mmHg
PaO_2/FIO_2 ratio of > 200
$PaCO_2$ > 45 mmHg
Ventilatory pump
Vital capacity of > 10–15 mL/kg body weight
Maximum negative inspiratory pressure < −30 cm H_2O
Minute ventilation (VE) < 10 L/min
Maximum voluntary ventilation more than twice resting VE

* Data from Tobin, MJ. Weaning from mechanical ventilation. Crit Care Clin 1990;6:725.

tient forcefully exhales through the endotracheal tube with the attached spirometer down to end expiration (residual volume [RV]). The VC is read from the spirometer. The procedure is repeated three times to check for consistency.

VC is measured most commonly with a turbine spirometer such as the Wright spirometer. This hand-held unit, which is attached to the end of the endotracheal tube, measures the volume of air that passes through the unit, setting a series of turbines in motion. The speed of the turbines and duration of spin is translated into exhaled volume and is read off a dial display. Both VC and VT can be measured with this technique.

The minimum VC needed to consider extubation is 10–15 mL/kg.[3–5] Below this value, there is concern that the patient will not have the muscle strength or ability to generate sufficient expulsive force to clear retained material from the airways. Minimum VC is approximately two times the predicted tidal volume (VT).[6] In preoperative evaluations of patients with pulmonary function tests, it has been shown that a VC less than 50% of the predicted value is an indicator of those patients who are at high risk for pulmonary complications and postoperative ventilator dependence.[1]

It must be remembered that VC is measured on a single breath and is an adequate test to evaluate for strength of cough and ability to clear secretions, but it does not relate to the ability of the patient to sustain spontaneous ventilation. Therefore VC is not a good predictor of endurance or ability to eliminate carbon dioxide or regulate pH. It must also be remembered that measurement of the forced vital capacity (FVC) is an effort-dependent test. Patient cooperation is required; otherwise the test yields a falsely low result and may prolong intubation unnecessarily. The patient must be awake and alert enough to understand and follow instruction on how to perform the test.

VC is a commonly used weaning criteria, but recent studies have questioned its reliability in predicting successful extubation. Milbern[7] found that a FVC of 15 mL/kg in 33 postoperative patients was falsely positive in 15% of study patients and falsely negative in 63%. Using a lower VC threshold of 10 mL/kg, Tahvanainen[8] found that 18% of patients failed extubation when they were predicted to tolerate weaning, though these were not in postoperative patients.

Maximum Inspiratory Pressure

Another easily performed test to assess weanability is the maximum inspiratory force or pressure (MIP). MIP is considered to be a valuable predictor of neuromuscular performance.[9–11] This procedure is performed by attaching an aneroid manometer to the end of the endotracheal tube. The open end of the tube is then occluded with a thumb or finger and the patient is asked to forcefully inspire against the closed endotracheal tube. The maximum negative pressure measured at the tube is called the MIP. This maneuver can be effort-dependent, but if the endotracheal tube is left occluded for 30–45 seconds, the test becomes less dependent on the cooperation of the patient as the drive to inhale becomes involuntary. In this way, MIP is a more reliable predictor of neuromuscular performance than is measuring the FVC. But like FVC, MIP is only a predictor of neuromuscular strength on a single-breath basis and is not a good predictor of respiratory endurance and ability to sustain adequate minute ventilation to eliminate carbon dioxide.

A minimum value for MIP prior to extubation is 30 cm H_2O. In a study by Sahn,[12] patients who were able to generate a MIP of more than 30 cm H_2O were all successfully extubated, whereas those that were only able to generate a MIP of less than 20 cm H_2O were not successfully weaned. One important point concerning the measurement of MIP is that the results are very dependent on lung volume. The compliance or pressure-volume curve of the lung is not linear (Fig. 14-1).[13,14] When the lung is at very high or very low volumes, the compliance of the lung is decreased. Greater effort must be exerted by the patient to bring on the pressure change needed for a given volume change. The measured pressure change may not accurately reflect the patient's effort, and the patient will fail weaning criteria and remain intubated. For this reason, MIP is usually measured when the patient is at the end of a normal, unforced exhalation (ie, functional residual capacity [FRC]). At FRC, the lungs usually are on the steep intermediate slope of the pressure-volume curve where volume change for a given change in pressure is maximal. Intraoperative changes in lung volumes include a decrease in FRC that my place the patient on the lower, noncompliant, section of the curve. Lung compliance is decreased, and even with a strong inspiratory effort, the MIP can be unacceptably low, which should prompt continued intubation and subsequent reevaluation.[9]

Figure 14-1. Pressure-volume curve for the lungs. Note that at a normal functional residual capacity (FRC), large volume changes are associated with small changes in transmural pressure. As lung volumes become high or low, large changes in pressure are needed to move volume into the lungs, leading to increases in the work of breathing.

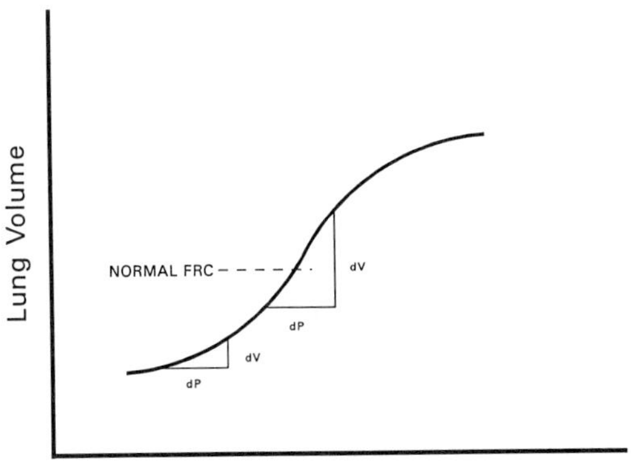

Minute Ventilation

Minute ventilation, also referred to as expired minute volume, VE is the measure of the volume of gas expired by the patient in 1 minute. Its predictive value lies in its ability to determine whether the patient will have adequate ventilatory endurance to allow adequate carbon dioxide removal after extubation. The predictive value is increased when coupled with the measurement of the maximum voluntary ventilation in 1 minute (MVV).[12] VE which is equal to the respiratory rate times the VT, is usually measured in two ways. One, an in-line spirometer that measures the volume exhaled over two or three breaths and converts that into volume exhaled in 1 minute can be used. Two, a Wright hand-held spirometer that measures breath-to-breath volume and also displays a cumulative exhaled volume that can be measured for 1 minute is also effective.

Minute volume is related to the amount of work the patient needs to perform to maintain a given P_{CO_2} level. In a spontaneously breathing patient, a minute volume of less than 10 L/min is desired before extubation.[12] Minute volume is determined both by the carbon dioxide production and the amount of dead space ventilation (VD). VD is the amount of tidal volume that is inspired but does not participate in gas exchange and thus does not contribute to carbon dioxide removal. A patient with a normal dead space to tidal volume ratio (VD/VT) of 0.3 to 0.4 requires a minute ventilation of less than 10 L/min to maintain a normal arterial PCO_2 as long as the carbon dioxide production is within normal limits. A VD/VT ratio of greater than 0.6 usually precludes successful extubation.[15] Spontaneous VT for a healthy adult at rest is in the range of 5–7 mL/kg.[16] When compared to MIP and VE, VT is not a sensitive indicator of extubation potential, although very low VTs can indicate that the patient does not have an adequate ventilatory drive (eg, when the patient is still under the effects of anesthesia or sedation). VT can also be low when the lungs are very noncompliant, and the patient is not strong enough to overcome the lung stiffness. In this case, the patient often meets the minute volume requirements by taking rapid shallow breaths, which are much less efficient at removing carbon dioxide because of the increase in the VD/VT ratio.

Work of Breathing and Compliance

The minute ventilation and actual work of breathing must be strongly considered. Work of breathing relates to the amount of energy that needs to be exerted by the patient to achieve movement of adequate volume in and out of the lungs to eliminate carbon dioxide. Work of breathing can be defined by the following formula:[11]

$$\text{(14-1)} \quad \text{Work} = \overline{P} \times \Delta V$$

where $\overline{P}$ = mean airway pressure and ΔV = volume change.

The volume of gas moved into the lungs depends on the pressure change in the airways during inspiration also relates to the airway resistance. If airway resistance is high, less gas is moved per unit time with the same change in pressure. Compliance of the lungs also plays a role in the amount of work necessary to generate the needed pressure differential to move adequate gas into the lungs.

Compliance is the volume of gas moved for a given change in pressure; it can be graphically represented by a pressure-volume curve (Fig. 14-1). The normal lung lies on the mid portion of the curve such that at FRC, small changes in pressure result in large changes in lung volume. In noncompliant lungs, such as in pulmonary fibrosis, adult respiratory distress syndrome, or pulmonary edema, the patient is often breathing at a lower lung volume and FRC. This is reflected by a downward shift in the pressure-volume curve. The patient must exert additional energy to bring about the change in pressure needed to allow adequate volume ventilation In severe cases, the curve is shifted downward and to the right.[17]

Compliance can be assessed in the operating room.[18,19] Peak inspiratory airway pressure is directly related to lung compliance. As the lungs become more stiff, as is seen with increased lung water, the peak airway pressure will rise. Dynamic compliance (C_{dyn}) can be measured while the patient is on positive-pressure ventilation by dividing the inflation volume by the peak airway pressure. Normal values exceed 50 mL/cm H_2O. The most common cause of decreased compliance in the operating room is pulmonary edema. If excessive lung water is suspected, diuresis is indicated, which should improve compliance as lung water is moved out of the interstitial spaces. Low compliance ($C_{dyn} < 35$ mL/cm H_2O) means that the patient is not likely to be able to maintain a high spontaneous minute ventilation if required because of the higher work of breathing involved.

Airway resistance also contributes to the work of breathing and needs to be considered before extubation. Bronchoconstriction, which is evident as increased wheezing on auscultation of the lungs, causes marked increases in airway resistance. To overcome this resistance to air flow, the patient is required to perform additional mechanical work.[20] This can contribute to extubation failure if not treated. On positive-pressure ventilation, bronchoconstriction also causes an elevation in the measured airway pressures due to the obstruction to air flow through the bronchial tree. Bronchoconstriction is treated initially with nebulized β_2-agonist drugs administered into the endotracheal tube (eg, albuterol, metaproteronol).[21,22] If needed, intravenous methylxanthine drugs are administered in a continuous drip fashion (eg, aminophylline).

Arterial Blood Gases

Measurement and interpretation of arterial blood gases have to be considered in light of the entire clinical picture. Actually no minimum arterial PO_2 value reliably predicts ability to be weaned and tolerate extubation, but some guidelines may be followed. Arterial PO_2 should be at least 60 mmHg while being administered at an inspired oxygen concentration (F_{IO_2}) of less than 35%.[5] Some clinicians use the PaO_2/F_{IO_2} ratio that should be greater than 200.[5] Since arterial oxygenation depends on the diffusion of oxygen from the alveoli across the respiratory epithelium, following the gradient of oxygen partial pressure from the alveoli to the systemic arterial blood can also be helpful assessing the overall ability of the lung to take up oxygen at the time of measurement. The alveolar-arterial (A-a) oxygen gradient can be calculated by first determining the alveolar concentration of oxygen P_{AO_2} using the alveolar air equation:

$$(14\text{-}2)\quad P_{AO_2} = P_{IO_2} - PaCO_2/R$$

where P_{AO_2} is the alveolar oxygen tension, P_{IO_2} is the oxygen tension of inspired air, $PaCO_2$ is the arterial carbon dioxide tension, and R is the respiratory quotient.

$$(14\text{-}3)\quad P_{IO_2} = (P_B - P_{H_2O}) \times F_{IO_2}$$

where P_B is the barometric pressure, P_{H_2O} or PH_2O is the partial pressure of water in the airways (equals 47 mmHg at 100% saturation), and F_{IO_2} = fraction of inspired oxygen. Therefore:

$$(14\text{-}4)\quad P_{AO_2} = ([P_B - PH_2O] \times F_{IO_2}) - PaCO_2/R$$

The alveolar-arterial oxygen gradient can then be calculated by subtracting the arterial oxygen tension from the calculated alveolar oxygen tension:

$$(14\text{-}5)\quad \text{A-a gradient} = P_{AO_2} - PaO_2$$

The concentration of oxygen in the alveoli depends on several factors. Within a gas mixture, the sum of the individual partial pressures of the different gases equals total barometric pressure (P_B). The component gases present in the alveoli are chiefly nitrogen, oxygen, carbon dioxide, and water. Alveolar gas is assumed to be 100% saturated with water vapor at body temperature. Alveolar carbon dioxide concentration, which is difficult to measure accurately, is usually close to arterial PCO_2, and so PCO_2 is substituted in the equation. The respiratory quotient (R) is equal to the carbon dioxide production divided by the oxygen consumption and cannot be measured in the operating room. It is assumed to be close to the average value of 0.8. To calculate the alveolar-arterial gradient, the measured arterial PO_2 is subtracted from the calculated alveolar PO_2. The value should be less than 350 mmHg before extubation is considered,[15] but when the FIO_2 is less than 0.35 in the normal adult, the A-a gradient is less than 15–20 mmHg.[23] The gradient increases as the FIO_2 rises due to small intrapulmonary shunts, and when the normal patient is breathing an FIO_2 of 1.0, it is close to 100 mmHg.[23]

Optimal oxygen uptake in the lung depends on blood flow passing through pulmonary capillaries adjacent to well-ventilated alveolar units. Gas exchange depends on the distribution of ventilation in relation to blood flow.[24,25] Ideally, the ventilation-perfusion ratio (V/Q) would be perfectly matched and equal (V/Q = 1). As different segments of the lung drift further in either direction from this optimum value, hypoxemia occurs because of the mismatch of ventilation and perfusion.

In the extreme case of perfusion in the absence of ventilation, a shunt is produced because the deoxygenated pulmonary artery blood is shunted through the lungs without picking up oxygen. In the normal person, a small amount of such unoxygenated blood returns to the left-sided circulation. Less than 2% of the right ventricular output is shunted through physiologic shunts made up of the bronchial circulation, thebesian veins, and pulmonary arteriovenous anastomoses.[24] As a result of V/Q mismatches in the normal person, an intrapulmonary shunt that usually involves less than 5% of the cardiac output delivered to the lungs.[24] An intrapulmonary shunt of greater than 15% usually contributes to significant arterial hypoxemia.

As V/Q mismatching worsens, arterial oxygenation falls as the pulmonary venous blood receives a higher and higher component of poorly oxygenated blood. In the absolute sense, a true shunt (V/Q = 0), cannot be overcome by increasing the FIO_2 as the inspired air never comes in contact with the pulmonary blood flow, so no diffusion of oxygen can take place. Conversely, hypoxemia that occurs as a result of V/Q ratios greater than zero can usually be overcome by increasing the FIO_2.[9]

Calculating the shunt requires being able to measure the oxygen content in mixed venous blood.[26]

$$\text{(14-6)} \quad \frac{\dot{Q}_{SP}}{\dot{Q}_T} = \frac{(CcO_2 - CaO_2)}{(CcO_2 - C\bar{v}O_2)}$$

where $\dot{Q}_{SP}$ = shunt blood flow, $\dot{Q}_T$ = total blood flow from right heart, CcO_2 is the ideal end-capillary blood oxygen content, CaO_2 is the arterial oxygen content, and $C\bar{v}O_2$ is the mixed venous oxygen content.

Peripheral venous blood is not an accurate substitute when measuring the mixed venous oxygen content. Accurate sampling of the mixed venous blood requires placement of a pulmonary artery catheter. If the patient is hypoxic and the shunt is found to be high ($Q_{SP}/Q_T > 0.15$), attempts are made to treat the shunt.[27] Because the V/Q abnormalities are often due to atelectatic areas of the lung, better expansion is tried. The application of positive end-expiratory pressure (PEEP) is most commonly attempted. Adding PEEP reexpands atelectatic segments of the lung and makes areas with low V/Q ratios more effective by increasing the ventilation. The application of PEEP also raises the FRC and places the lung on a more optimal portion of the compliance curve, thus allowing better alveolar expansion.[28] It must always be kept in mind that poor oxygenation is usually the result of V/Q mismatching and has little relationship to minute volume.[25] As can be seen by the alveolar air equation, the alveolar PO_2 only decreases significantly if the PCO_2 markedly increases.

PEEP is usually started at 5 cm H_2O. The optimum PEEP is that level which allows the best V/Q ratio to be established, thus resulting in the best oxygenation and lowest shunt fraction.[29] But as PEEP levels increase, more pressure is transmitted into the thoracic cavity and ultimately begins to impede venous return; therefore cardiac output drops.[30] Perfusion starts to fall, and the V/Q ratio begins to worsen. The best PEEP is often determined by measuring the oxygen saturation of the mixed venous blood (SvO_2) that is maximal at the PEEP level allowing optimal alveolar expansion with the least impedance of venous return. This brings the V/Q ratio closer to one.

Overall, the optimal PEEP is considered to be that amount of PEEP at which Q_S/Q_T is lowest with no drop in the cardiac output. Sometimes optimal PEEP is defined as that level which provides maximum oxygen delivery with the lowest dead space to tidal volume ratio (V_D/V_T).[31] It is thought that a "physiologic" PEEP is exerted by the nose and upper airway structures in the nonintubated individual.[29] This PEEP, which is estimated to be 3–5 cm H_2O, keeps the lungs at a more ideal FRC to optimize compliance and minimize atelectasis. For this reason, having an intubated patient on zero PEEP is believed not to be physiologic and contributes to V/Q mismatching and hypoxia. Most clinicians routinely add low level PEEP in almost all intubated patients. There is still considerable controversy on the benefits, optimum level, and exact mechanism of action of PEEP.[28,32]

Arterial PCO_2 and pH are related to the minute volume (V_E). Given that a normal V_T is approximately 5–7 mL/kg and a normal respiratory rate is 10–12 breaths/min, then a normal resting minute ventilation for a 70-kg adult is about 5–6 L/min. Adequate minute ventilation is that which is needed to maintain a normal $PaCO_2$ and pH. If carbon dioxide production rises or V_D increases then minute ventilation must increase to normalize $PaCO_2$. V_D is usually expressed as a ratio of dead space to tidal volume (V_D/V_T). The normal value is 0.3–0.4. As V_D rises, minute ventilation must increase to eliminate carbon dioxide. If the V_D/V_T ratio is greater than 0.6, then the patient is considered not weanable and should be left on mechanical ventilation because minute volume demands probably cannot be met by spontaneous ventilation.[15] Monitoring V_D/V_T is based on the Enghoff modification of the Bohr equation:

$$(14\text{-}7) \quad V_D/V_T = (PaCO_2 - P_ECO_2)/PaCO_2$$

where: V_D is dead space, V_T is tidal volume, $PaCO_2$ is arterial carbon dioxide tension, and P_ECO_2 = mixed expired gas carbon dioxide tension. Inspired PCO_2 is considered insignificant. Arterial PCO_2 is available from a routine arterial blood gas measurement.

Monitoring the V_D/V_T ratio was not common in the past because of the difficulty in measuring mixed expired PCO_2. The expired gases had to be collected in a large Douglas bag and analyzed, which was time-consuming and inconvenient. Today, more sophisticated expired gas analysis can be performed using a metabolic cart. This cart can be measure both oxygen consumption and carbon dioxide production as well as mixed P_ECO_2. This allows direct calculation of the V_D. Such measurements are best left for the recovery room or the intensive care unit, because this procedure is time-consuming and requires bulky equipment at the bedside.

From a practical standpoint, in the immediate postoperative period, ventilatory capability has to be assessed by pH, PCO_2, and minute ventilation using a spirometer. Studies have shown that an arterial PCO_2 greater than 45 mmHg, a pH less than 7.35,[33] and a V_E of more than 10 L/min[12] are strong predictors of failure to tolerate extubation. In addition, the respiratory rate should be reasonable (in the range of 8–35 breaths/min).[34] A lower value may indicate hypoventilation and respiratory depression from the residual effects of anesthesia or sedation. A respiratory rate much higher than

35 breaths/min indicates that the patient is having to work excessively hard at breathing and has a good chance at failing extubation secondary to progressive respiratory muscle fatigue. If the patient fails to meet any of these criteria, extubation should be withheld until reevaluation can be performed in the recovery room or intensive care unit. Obviously, many patients with chronic pulmonary disease do not meet minimum criteria at baseline but still lead productive lives.

Other Factors

Other factors to consider prior to early extubation relate to the need for continued airway protection and secretion removal. If patients have a high volume of secretions or a weak ability to cough, the endotracheal tube should be left in place for frequent suctioning. Voluminous secretions are often seen in patients with a lung abscess, pneumonia, bronchiectasis, and chronic obstructive pulmonary disease (COPD), as well as in patients with hemoptysis from tumor or operative resection. Thick, tenacious secretions as in patients with cystic fibrosis can also indicate the need for continued intubation. Treatment of such secretions involves good pulmonary toilet prior to extubation and includes humidified air to loosen secretions and frequent suctioning. In addition, it is important to make sure the patient is adequately hydrated to aid in thinning of the secretions. Nebulized 2%-N-acetyl-cysteine (Mucomyst) has been used as a mucolytic agent to try and loosen tenacious secretions,[35] but its propensity to cause significant bronchospasm[36] and its unproven efficacy has made this treatment less popular. We believe that it is useful only when direct application of the agent onto inspissated secretions through a fiberoptic bronchoscope can be performed.

Ability to protect the airway is an important consideration before extubation. The physician must ensure that the patient's level of consciousness is high enough to be able to sustain an adequate respiratory rate and to cough effectively enough to clear retained secretions. One simple method of ascertaining the level of consciousness is to see whether the eyes open on verbal stimulation. Eye-opening returns rather late as the patient emerges from general anesthesia and is an indicator of depth of anesthesia. It is believed that if a patient can open his or her eyes on command, the risk of developing laryngospasm following extubation is low. Airway protection may be limited, however, if significant airway edema occurs following extubation. Ability to cooperate with the FVC and MIP maneuvers are also good indicators of adequate level of consciousness.

Most patients without significant preexisting cardiopulmonary disease who have not undergone an extensive procedure are able to be weaned quickly and extubated within a very short time after surgery. Using the previously mentioned weaning criteria allows the majority of patients to be on minimal supplemental oxygen via mask or nasal cannula within the first few hours after their procedure. If minimal weaning criteria are not met in the operating room; the patient has had an extensive or prolonged procedure; known, preexisting severe cardiac or pulmonary disease; or intraoperative instability; then the patient should remain intubated and be transported to the recovery room or directly to the intensive care unit (ICU) for further monitoring. In the recovery room and the ICU, newer techniques of monitoring respiratory status can help in later reassessment for possible extubation. These techniques include the evaluation of arterial oxygen saturation via pulse oximetry, transcutaneous and transconjunctival oxygen monitoring, and real-time expired gas carbon dioxide analysis via capnographic end-tidal carbon dioxide measurement. More studies still need to be performed to confirm the applicability of these techniques in weaning intubated patients before they can be considered standard weaning criteria.

Monitoring Oxygenation

Because the thoracic surgery patient is at high risk for developing postoperative hypoxemia, monitoring oxygenation is of paramount importance in the early period following surgery. Much of the risk is secondary to the changes in lung function and pulmonary physiology that are related to the operative procedure and general anesthesia. Decreases in FRC, RV, and VC all occur as a result of patient positioning and the effects of anesthesia.[37–39] During the surgery, the diaphragm usually lies much further within the thorax, leading to diminished lung volume and a tendency towards atelectasis.[40–42] The open thorax also causes the lung to collapse as the negative intrapleural pressure is lost; this allows the lung to recoil into an atelectatic state. Since blood flow can usually continue through the collapsed segments, a large increase in the intrapulmonary shunt occurs as the V/Q ratio in these areas approaches zero.[43] Some of this atelectasis is carried into the postoperative period and contributes to postoperative hypoxemia. Intraoperative manipulation of the lung can also lead to lung edema that contributes to the hypoxia.

Limiting the monitoring of oxygenation to intermittent arterial blood gas analysis carries the risk of the development of significant hypoxia that can remain unrecognized. Checking the patient for the development of cyanosis is also insensitive, since approximately five grams of desaturated hemoglobin per deciliter must be present before cyanosis is apparent. If the patient has had a significant intraoperative blood loss or has postoperative anemia for any reason, the arterial PO_2 may be very low before five grams of hemoglobin become desaturated. Cyanosis can also be seen in patients with poor peripheral perfusion, although the central arterial blood is adequately oxygenated.

Pulse Oximetry

Continuous monitoring of arterial oxygen saturation with a pulse oximeter has become standard practice in the operating room, the recovery room, and the ICU.[44–46] This instrument can be used to aid in the extubation process and with further monitoring of oxygenation. Newer transcutaneous pulse oximeters use the technology of transmission spectrometry, with high-intensity, light-emitting diodes that are designed to eliminate variability resulting from skin thickness or pigmentation. Minimum saturation criteria from values obtained from the pulse oximeter, however, have not yet been established. Since an arterial PO_2 of 60 mmHg is considered the minimum required to prevent tissue hypoxia, a corresponding arterial oxygen saturation of 90% is usually accepted as adequate, as predicted by the adult hemoglobin-oxygen saturation curve.[46–50] However, Jubran and Tobin[51] have found that the pulse oximeter is much less reliable in predicting accurate and adequate arterial oxygen concentrations in critically ill patients. In their study, the variation in the minimum pulse oximeter reading that corresponded to a PO_2 greater than 60 mmHg was large. The variation was greatest in black patients; significant arterial hypoxemia was often present even when pulse oximetry readings exceeded 90%. The minimum pulse oximeter reading to assure an adequate arterial PO_2 (a $>$ 60 mmHg in black patients) was 95%. Less variation was noted in white patients, but still a minimum pulse oximeter reading of 92% was needed to guarantee adequate arterial oxygenation.

Carbon Dioxide Analysis

Improved technology in expired gas analysis has allowed the emergence of bedside capnography as a helpful adjunct in both intraoperative as well as postoperative respiratory monitoring. By means of either an in-line sensor placed in the expiratory circuit or a sidestream gas sampling port, carbon dioxide concentration in the exhaled gas can be measured. Infrared spectrophotometry is used.[50] Because carbon dioxide is measured on a continuous real-time basis, a graphical representation of the concentration can be displayed as a continuous waveform on a bedside monitor. In addition, the end-tidal carbon dioxide concentration, as determined by the maximum concentration measured at the end of a breath, is usually displayed as well.

In the normal lung, the end-tidal PCO_2 is usually very close to the alveolar PCO_2 level because the last expired air usually originates from the alveoli.[52] The accuracy of the correlation of end-tidal PCO_2 to the alveolar PCO_2 and to the arterial PCO_2 depends on equal and homogeneous expansion and emptying of the alveoli throughout the lung. This is, of course, not the case. Because V/Q abnormalities occur throughout the lung, a gradient usually develops between the end-tidal PCO_2 and the arterial PCO_2.[53] This gradient is usually less than 10 mmHg but can vary in patients with pulmonary disease.[54] Abnormal V/Q ratios, increasing shunt, and dead space lead to an increase in the end-tidal PCO_2 arterial PCO_2 gradient as carbon dioxide elimination becomes less efficient.[55] If the patient's gradient has been stable during surgery, however, the capnogram can be very helpful in warning the clinician of carbon dioxide retention secondary to ventilatory failure. Following the end-tidal PCO_2 to alveolar PCO_2 gradient can also alert the clinician to severe alterations in the V/Q ratio. If the gradient is high, extubation may need to be deferred until further improvement in the patient is seen. Although no extubation criteria for capnography have been established, it is reasonable to make 10 mmHg the upper limit of the end-tidal PCO_2 to arterial PCO_2 gradient that precludes early extubation.

Capnography also gives additional information on airway resistance that can be helpful in assessing the overall work of breathing in the intubated patient.[56,57] Normally, during passive exhalation air flows easily and in a laminar fashion from the alveoli to the upper airways. This gives a characteristic shape to the expired carbon dioxide curve (Fig. 14-2). During inspiration, the carbon dioxide level is zero unless rebreathing occurs. Shortly after the start of expiration, this level rises rapidly and is close to the maximum level that is measured at the end of expiration (ie, the end-tidal PCO_2). As inspiration begins, the level rapidly returns to zero as fresh gas, devoid of carbon dioxide, is inhaled. If emptying of the alveoli is impaired in any way, as in severe bronchospasm or emphysema, then the shape of the capnogram assumes a ramp pattern due to the slow rise of expired

Figure 14-2. Capnogram tracings. A: normal capnogram; B: capnogram reflecting severe airway obstruction.

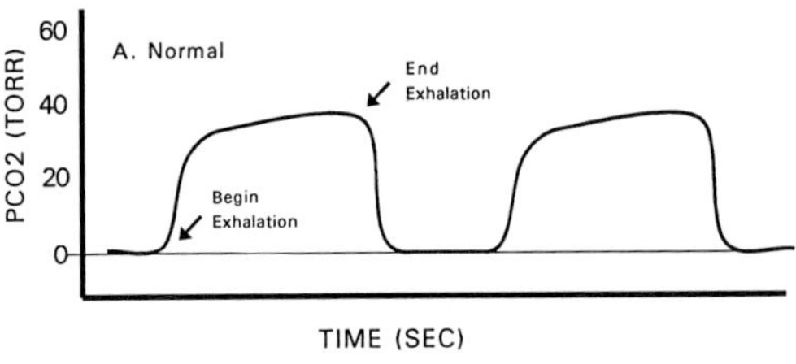

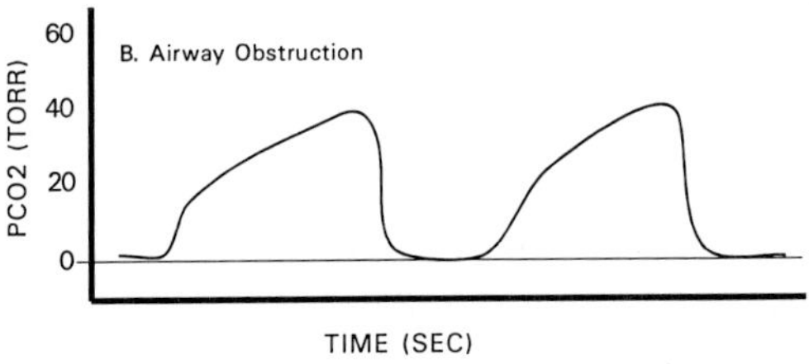

carbon dioxide towards the maximum level. Even without auscultatory findings of bronchospasm, the shape of the curve can be a very sensitive indicator of impaired carbon dioxide elimination due to bronchoconstriction or air trapping. More aggressive therapy with bronchodilators may be necessary before extubation can be contemplated.[58]

Other Considerations

Additional factors must be taken into consideration before early extubation of the postoperative patient. In the patient who has an indwelling pulmonary artery catheter, assessment of the hemodynamic status can provide useful information about potential problems that may occur following removal of the endotracheal tube and the application of positive pressure ventilation. Pulmonary capillary wedge pressure (PCWP) can be a valuable indicator of the likelihood of developing pulmonary edema with concurrent hypoxia. If the PCWP exceeds 20 mmHg, significant lung water is likely to be present. This water also contributes to low lung compliance and increases the work of breathing to a level that may exceed the patient's capabilities.[59] High pulmonary vascular resistance can indicate significant lung disease. The potential of cardiovascular decompensation exists as well should the patient deteriorate from the oxygenation standpoint; hypoxia further worsens pulmonary hypertension resulting in increased strain on the right ventricle.[60]

Direct Admission to the Intensive Care Unit

Certain patients should be considered as candidates for direct admission to the intensive care unit (ICU) following surgery without planning for extubation in the operating room or recovery room. Such patients usually have severe underlying medical problems that predispose them to early postoperative complications or difficult weaning. They may have had an extensive procedure that puts them at an increased postoperative risk. Patients that have also exhibited marked intraoperative instability or have suffered a severe intraoperative complication should also be considered for direct ICU admission.

Patients who have undergone cardiac or thoracic vascular surgery, (including major pulmonary resections), especially lengthy operations, are often taken automatically to the ICU for postoperative monitoring while still intubated. In addition to still being under the effects of anesthesia, these patients are at an increased risk for developing severe pulmonary dysfunction as well as early postoperative complications such as bleeding and hemodynamic instability. They are usually left intubated at least overnight until the risk of early complication is less and the patients are more fully awake. This allows for better assessment of pulmonary function and measurement of weaning parameters.

Preoperative Assessment

The universal deterioration of pulmonary function seen in the perioperative period makes pulmonary risk assessment a very important part of the preoperative evaluation of thoracic surgery patients. Many patients who need additional postoperative ventilatory support can be identified preoperatively. Many concerns are associated with the identification of such patients. Many of the same factors used to assess medical resectability can be applied to define a group of patients at high risk for postoperative respiratory failure.[1] Early indications that pulmonary complications were the most common cause of morbidity and mortality in the postoperative setting led to interest in identifying patients at risk for such complications.[61] It is also important to remember that coexistent medical conditions can also contribute to postoperative instability. Such conditions themselves may put the patient at high risk for possible continued mechanical ventilatory support even when the operative procedure would otherwise not have placed them at risk.

Pulmonary Function Testing

The most common way to evaluate a patient preoperatively to determine if they are at increased risk for postoperative respiratory complications involves the use of pulmonary function testing (PFT) and preoperative baseline arterial blood gas analysis. PFTs are a group of physiologic studies that are used as tools for the evaluation and diagnosis of underlying lung disease.[62] The spirometric tracing, which is obtained by measuring exhaled volume over time as the patient performs a forced expiratory maneuver from end-inspiration (total lung capacity) to end-expiration (RV), is the most commonly used procedure.

As early as the 1950s, investigators noted that abnormalities in the timed segments of a spirometric tracing coupled with the forced vital capacity (FVC) identified patients at risk for major postoperative complications or death following thoracic surgery.[63,64] In 1955, Gaensler[63] looked at the value of spirometric testing in patients who were undergoing surgery for pulmonary tuberculosis. His work showed that the most specific test in predicting mortality from postoperative pulmonary complications was the maximum breathing capacity (MBC), which is also known as the maximum minute ventilation (MMV) or maximum volume ventilation (MVV). The MBC is the maximum volume of air a patient is able to move in and out of the lungs in 1 minute. In this study all deaths except for one, occurred in patients with an MBC less than or equal to 50% of its predicted value. However, many of the surviving patients had MBCs that were less than 50% of the predicted value; thus the correlation with postoperative mortality was not very strong.

Several other measurements can be made from a simple spirometric tracing when looking at the volumes exhaled over specific time intervals. The forced expiratory volume over the first second of a forced exhalation (FEV_1) is often expressed as a percentage of the FVC (FEV_1/FVC). The average flow rate from 25% to 75% of the forced vital capacity, $FEF_{25\%-75\%}$ is thought to correlate with the resistance to air flow in the smaller airways. Both the FEV_1/FVC ratio and the $FEF_{25\%-75\%}$, are reduced in severe COPD.[65] Increased surgical risk has been traditionally thought to occur when any of these values are less than 50% of their predicted norm.[66] Patients with such values are also at a much higher risk for more prolonged postoperative ventilatory support.

Overall PFTs appear to correlate well with the incidence of severe postoperative pulmonary complications in patients undergoing lung surgery. This is especially true when PFTs are combined with arterial blood gases and split-perfusion radionuclide lung scanning. Olsen, et al also used preoperative right heart catheterization in addition to PFTs and lung scanning to evaluate high-risk pulmonary resection candidates.[67] The risk of postoperative pulmonary failure in those patients having high pulmonary vascular resistance and abnormal PFTs was increased. Fee[60] noted that a pulmonary vascular resistance higher than 190 $dyn \cdot s^{-1} \cdot cm^{-5}$ during exercise was a better predictor of death in patients undergoing resection for lung cancer than a FEV_1 of less than 50% of the predicted value.

Other Methods of Assessment

Arterial blood gases alone are not sufficient to predict postoperative complications. When compared to arterial PCO_2, baseline arterial PO_2 is not as good a correlate to postoperative pulmonary problems. Although preoperative arterial hypoxemia ($PO_2 < 50$ mmHg) with a severe widening of the alveolar-arterial PO_2 gradient has been reported to be a contraindication to thoracic surgery,[66] this is not a very reliable indicator. In some patients the lung zone to be resected may have significant atelectasis with lack of ventilation but still retain its perfusion. Such an area of lung contributes to the hypoxia due to the pulmonary shunt. Removal of this lung section can actually improve the arterial PO_2 dramatically.

Arterial PCO_2 is a much better indicator and predictor of postoperative pulmonary problems.[68] In most patients, an increase in the resting baseline arterial PCO_2 above 45 mmHg signifies a marked loss of lung function.[69] This is usually associated with advanced pulmonary disease and minimal pulmonary reserve. In addition, patients are also likely to have very low spirometric flow values such as FEV_1 and $FEF_{25\%-75\%}$. An arterial PCO_2 of more than 45 mmHg coupled with an FEV_1 of less than 800 mL is a direct contraindication for further lung resection. The patient will probably not be able to achieve an adequate minute volume to eliminate carbon dioxide and regulate pH.[70,71]

It is standard practice to perform PFTs on any patient before pneumonectomy or major thoracic surgery that is not emergent. Resection of lung tissue results in more impairment of pulmonary function in the postoperative period than does other types of surgery. If the PFTs are markedly abnormal, further testing is performed to try to determine if the patient will tolerate removal of lung tissue without suffering debilitating pulmonary insufficiency. Otherwise, the patient will be destined to live on mechanical ventilation. Radionuclide ventilation-perfusion scanning can determine as well as the predicted postoperative PFTs and the relative contribution of each lung to either total ventilation or perfusion.[72] Tisi has proposed four categories of predicted change in postoperative pulmonary function based on quantitative radionuclide ventilation-perfusion scanning (Table 14-2).[66] A predicted postoperative FEV^1 of at least 800 mL is required for pneumonectomy. Otherwise significant retention of carbon dioxide occurs as a result of inadequate minute ventilation and gas exchange.[73] In certain situations, surgery still needs to be considered even when the predicted FEV_1 is less than 800 mL. In these cases an invasive study is performed using a balloon-tipped pulmonary artery catheter. After the catheter is directed into the lung or segment being evaluated for resection, the balloon is inflated and the resultant arterial blood gases are measured along with the pulmonary artery pressure and cardiac output. If the pulmonary artery pressure rises above a mean of 35 mmHg or the PaO_2 falls to less than 45 mmHg, the patient is believed not to be a candidate for resection.[71]

Mechanical Ventilation

Mechanical ventilation is required when the patient is unable to sustain adequate ventila-

Table 14-2. Preoperative Evaluation of Lung Function as a Predictor of Postoperative Performance*

If baseline PFTs and ABGs markedly abnormal then:
Quantitative ventilation-perfusion scan:

Function of Resected Segment	Predicted Result
1. V/Q (resection) equals V/Q of remaining lung	Decline in function proportional to extent of resection
2. V/Q (resection) = O/O	No loss of function
3. V/Q (resection) >>> V/Q of remaining lung	Decline in function >>> extent of resection
4. V/Q (resection) much worse than V/Q of remaining lung	May improve function

* Data from Tisi, GM. State of the art: preoperative evaluation of lung function. Am Rev Respir Dis 1979;119:293.

atory capacity while breathing spontaneously. It is also used to gain control of a marginally functioning respiratory system. In addition, mechanical ventilation may be effective when total rest of the respiratory system may benefit the patient because of the decrease in oxygen consumption produced with total ventilatory support. Such is the case in a patient with a failing cardiovascular system, which results in an inability to match oxygen delivery to the oxygen consumption of the muscles involved in ventilation. Taking away the work of breathing by fully supporting ventilation by mechanical means may provide the life-saving benefit of lowering oxygen consumption in a decompensated patient.

Types of Ventilators

Three basic classes of ventilators are available: negative-pressure ventilators; positive-pressure ventilators; and most recently developed, high-frequency ventilators.[9]

Negative-pressure ventilators generate a negative pressure around the thorax and abdomen leading to distension and deformation of the thorax. A pressure gradient from the ambient air to the alveoli is created, causing air to flow into the lungs. Exhalation is by passive flow of the air from the lungs once the negative pressure is released or by active application of positive pressure in the chamber. These ventilators were popular in the 1940s and 1950s when the poliomyelitis epidemic left patients unable to use their respiratory muscles and dependent on external devices to move air into and out of their lungs.[74,75,76]

Positive-pressure ventilators cause inspiratory gas flow by raising the airway pressure above atmospheric pressure. All such ventilators require that the patient be attached to the ventilator by means of a tight-fitting face mask, endotracheal tube, or tracheostomy tube. The volume of gas delivered to the patient depends on the amount of pressure that is applied to the airways, the length of time that the pressure is applied, and the mechanical characteristics of the patient's lungs and thorax. Positive-pressure ventilators commonly in use fall into three categories: pressure-cycled, volume-cycled, and time-cycled. They are classified according to the mechanism used to terminate inspiration.[9]

Pressure-cycled ventilators terminate inspiration when a present airway pressure is reached. Examples of this type of ventilator are the Bird Mark-7 and Bennett PR-2 ventilators. Tidal volume is determined by the inspiratory flow rate, compliance of the respiratory system, and resistance to airflow in the bronchial tree. Tidal volume varies and is difficult to predict for the following reasons. In poorly compliant lungs, the terminating airway pressure may be reached at inadequately low lung volumes. If airway resistance is high, the preset pressure limit is also reached with a potentially inadequate tidal volume. With a pressure-cycled ventilator, a consistent tidal volume cannot be guaranteed.

To obtain a desired tidal volume, a spirometer can be connected to the expiratory limb of the circuit and pressure can be adjusted. This needs to be done on almost a breath-to-breath basis, however, because of changing thoracic mechanics, which limits the utility of this mode of ventilation. Pressure-cycled ventilators can be used to apply intermittent positive-pressure ventilation (IPPB) in nonintubated patients with atelectasis that has not responded to deep breathing exercises, incentive spirometry, or other modes of lung expansion (see Intermittent Positive-Pressure Ventilation.)

Volume-cycled ventilators are the most popular class of ventilators in use today.[9] These ventilators deliver a preset volume of gas to the ventilator circuit even if high airway pressure are generated. To minimize the risk of barotrauma, a high-pressure alarm system automatically terminates the breath or vents remaining delivered air to the surrounding environment when the preset pressure limit is exceeded. Exhaled volumes are monitored to confirm adequate minute ventilation. Measurement of these volumes also confirms that the patient is receiving the set tidal volume. In addition, such measurements indicate potential air leaks in the system if the exhaled volume is significantly less than the preset tidal volume.

In volume-cycled generators tidal volume is created by a variety of mechanisms, which include bellows compression, a flow generator interfaced with a flow sensor, or by gas compression in a piston chamber.[77] Bellows compression is used in the Bennett MA-2 ventilator. This ventilator is classified as an electronically controlled and powered, volume-cycled, constant-flow generator. Flow begins at the start of inspiration, remains constant throughout the inspiratory phase, and then abruptly ends, allowing exhalation. A square waveflow pattern is produced because the flow rate varies little throughout inspiration. The MA-2 ventilator also allows control over the mode of ventilation, as well as inspiratory flow rate, mandated respiratory rate, tidal volume, FIO_2, and PEEP.

The Puritan-Bennett 7200 ventilator is a microprocessor-controlled, volume-cycled, generator that uses a flow generator interfaced with a flow sensor. Microprocessing control of the flow generator via solenoids allows different inspiratory flow patterns to be used in delivering a tidal volume. The types of flow patterns available on the 7200 ventilator are square wave, sine wave, and decelerating or ramp configuration. All of these flow patterns can be affected to a degree by changes in the patient's airway pressure, resulting in some variation in the flow pattern (Fig. 14-3).

A nonconstant flow generator, which usually uses a rotary-driven piston with compressed gas, produces gas flow rates that vary throughout inspiration. The variation in flow rate is constant from breath to breath, unlike the variable flow patterns in the microprocessor-controlled flow generator used in the Puritan-Bennett 7200. A constant-cycling, rotary-driven piston produces an inspiratory flow pattern that resembles a true, positive, sinusoidal wave. The Emerson 3-PV and 3-MV and the Engstrom 150 ventilators use this type of nonconstant flow generation.

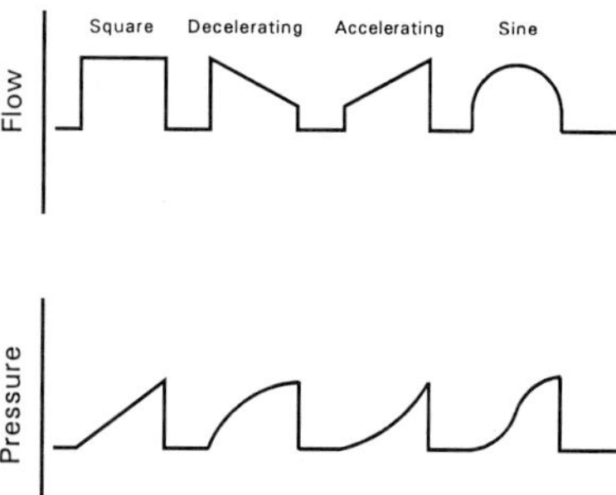

Figure 14-3. Inspiratory flow patterns and the corresponding airway pressure tracings. (Modified from Segal B, et al. Mechanical ventilation. In: Macdonnel K, Fahey P, Segal B, eds. Respiratory intensive care. Boston: Little Brown, 1987:134.)

Time-cycled ventilators terminate the inspiratory flow after a predetermined time interval. Tidal volume is determined by manipulation of the flow rate and the inspiratory time interval. The ventilatory cycle is often set by adjusting the inspiratory and expiratory time, manipulating the inspiratory time and total ventilatory cycle time, or setting the inspiratory time as a percentage of the total expiratory time. Examples of time-cycled ventilators in use today are the Siemens 900B and 900C models. Although the Emerson-IMV ventilator is considered a time-cycled ventilator, tidal volume is not determined by inspiratory and expiratory time intervals. Tidal volume depends on the excursion of a piston, which is not altered by changing the inspiratory or expiratory times.

Modes of Ventilation

Ventilator modes differ in the amount of spontaneous ventilation the patient is allowed. Positive pressure can also be applied to the airway at different times during the ventilatory cycle. Some modes can be combined to allow both mandated machine-delivered preset tidal volumes as well as inspiratory, pressure-supported, spontaneous ventilations.

CONTROLLED MANDATORY VENTILATION. During controlled mandatory ventilation (CMV), the ventilator delivers a set number of breaths per minute at a preset tidal volume. The patient is unable to trigger additional supported breaths. The patient is only allowed to inspire additional volume between breaths by activating a valve in the circuit. This is not considered a mode of spontaneous ventilation, since the negative inspiratory pressure needed to activate the inspiratory valve is prohibitively high. Because of the air hunger that develops in an alert patient who is trying to regulate ventilation with spontaneous breaths, this method is usually reserved for patients who have severe neurologic dysfunction and depression of level of consciousness to the point of depression of respiratory drive. CMV can also be used for patients who are heavily sedated or under the influence of neuromuscular blocking agents.[9]

Since CMV mode is insensitive to the patient's inspiratory efforts and delivers a preset minute volume as determined by the clinician, the risk of hypo- or hyperventilation exists if the metabolic status of the patient changes. The patient who is sufficiently conscious to respond to these changes often breathes "out of sync" with the ventilator, and the work of breathing increases tremendously to an unacceptable level. For this reason CMV is reserved for patients with depressed levels of consciousness.[79]

ASSISTED VENTILATION. Modes of assisted ventilation were developed to provide inspiratory support for patient-initiated breaths. Originally, the idea that assisted ventilation removed much of the patient's work of breathing by allowing the machine to do the majority of the work during the inspiratory cycle was thought to be correct. This is only true if the inspiratory flow rate provided by the ventilator exceeds patient demand or if the patient ceases to breathe. Studies by Marini and others have shown that the patient is often required to perform significant work while breathing on an assisted mode of mechanical ventilation.[80–82] Supplying the negative pressure necessary to activate the inspiratory valve during spontaneously initiated breaths and to overcome an insufficient inspiratory flow rate to meet demand requires effort.

To try and reduce the work involved in opening the inspiratory valve, some newer ventilators are equipped with inspiratory valves that have a lower threshold pressure requirement to open the valve. In addition, many ventilators allow adjustment of the sensitivity of the inspiratory valve. Research has also shown that a patient does not cease inspiratory efforts once a mechanical breath has been initiated. Instead, respiratory muscle contraction continues until the end of inspiration. At low inspiratory flow rates that do not match or exceed the patient's demand, the patient must perform the majority of the work of respiration, even in an assisted mode. It is important to realize that if the patient is doing excessive work while on assisted ventilation, then the respiratory rate of the ventilator should be increased to match the patient's demand rate. Alternatively, the inspiratory flow rate should be increased to exceed the patient's demand. If this results in hyperventilation, a different mode of ventilation should be attempted or the patient should be sedated in an attempt to decrease the excessive respiratory drive.

ASSIST-CONTROL MODE. The assist-control (AC) mode combines features of both CMV and assisted ventilation. Although the ventilatory rate can be set by the patient's inspiratory effort in AC mode, a back-up rate is set, as in CMV, to ensure at least a minimally acceptable minute ventilation. All breaths are delivered via positive pressure, but unlike CMV, the patient's triggering effort can exceed the preset rate, providing additional breaths at the preset tidal volume. If the patient's rate exceeds the set rate, the patient receives a full tidal volume breath from the machine each time. The patient can raise the minute volume by increasing the respiratory rate but take advantage of full ventilator support on the breaths that exceed the set minimum respiratory rate.

One of the common drawbacks of the AC mode is that the machine is triggered by each respiratory effort, however small. This can easily lead to hyperventilation, since each breath is supported to the full tidal volume. Agitated patients or other patients with a high respiratory rate can easily receive excessive minute volumes and develop significant respiratory alkalosis. Fine-tuning of the sensitivity of the patient triggering mechanism is required. If the sensitivity is too high, the ventilator may "autocycle," as it is set to provide a breath at the least little movement of the patient or change in the airway pressure. If the trigger is not sufficiently sensitive, a large negative pressure is required to activate the ventilator. The generation of high negative pressures adds to the work of breathing and can contribute to ventilation failure even in those patients who are assumed to be on full support because they have been placed on the AC mode.[80] If adjusting the sensitivity does not successfully control any resultant hyperventilation, then the patient needs to be evaluated for sedation or another mode of ventilation, such as intermittent mandatory ventilation (see below).

INTERMITTENT MANDATORY VENTILATION. In the intermittent mandatory ventilation (IMV) mode, the patient is able to breathe at spontaneous rates and tidal volumes. In addition to the spontaneous breaths, the patient receives periodic pressure-supported breaths at a preset rate and tidal volume. In this way, a minimum respiratory rate and minute volume are guaranteed.

IMV ventilation is probably the most common mode of ventilation used today, especially in critical care units. Proponents of this mode of ventilation have suggested that IMV has several advantages over other modes, but little factual evidence support this claim.[83–85] IMV supposedly prevents the patient from "fighting" the ventilator better than AC or CMV modes. In addition, IMV decreases the need for sedation and neuromuscular paralysis. Because spontaneous breaths above the preset rate are not supported with a full tidal volume, the chance of developing respiratory alkalosis is less. IMV is also thought to improve alveolar ventilation and ventilation-perfusion matching,[83] reduce oxygen consumption[85] and respiratory muscle fatigue, improve cardiac output, and achieve more rapid weaning from the ventilator. Evidence to support these claims is often comes from trials comparing IMV with CMV. Since CMV is rarely used, these studies can be misleading when comparing the advantages of IMV over AC or inspiratory pressure-support ventilation. New trials comparing IMV to other newer modes of ventilation are needed to document the distinct advantages of this method.

Allowing the patient to breathe both spontaneously and mechanically, with positive pressure-supported breaths, should theoretically lead to diminished negative effects on hemodynamic performance. Positive-pressure ventilation results in increases in intrathoracic pressures and can lead to a decrease in the venous return to the heart and a fall in cardiac output. Administering fewer positive-pressure breaths and allowing the patient to make more spontaneous efforts decreases the effect on intrathoracic pressure and results in less potential deterioration of cardiac output. This is balanced, however, by the increased work of breathing involved in spontaneous ventilation.

IMV circuits, which are usually set up in parallel with a conventional breathing circuit, either provide a continuous flow of gas through the circuit or include a demand-valve that must be activated to open the circuit and allow air flow during a spontaneous ventilation. It has been repeatedly demonstrated that some ventilators with IMV circuits with demand-valves require excessive reductions in airway pressure to open the valves; this delay causes a lag in the start of air flow. Both of these facts contribute to the marked increase in the work of breathing involved with some present-day mechanical ventilators when placed in the IMV mode.[86] Some studies have demonstrated a twofold increase in the work of breathing using IMV ventilation provided through a demand-valve system.[86]

Synchronized intermittent mandatory ventilation (SIMV) refers to the fact that the demand valve "senses" when the patient is initiating a spontaneous breath. The machine can then synchronize mandated positive-pressure supported breaths to coincide with the patient's effort. In this way, excessive tidal volumes are not administered because a machine breath is "stacked" on top of a spontaneous breath.

INSPIRATORY PRESSURE-SUPPORT VENTILATION. Inspiratory pressure-support ventilation (IPSV) has reemerged as a form of positive-pressure ventilation that allows application of positive pressure to the airways only during the inspiratory phase of spontaneous breaths.[87] It differs from other forms of positive-pressure ventilation in that a preset airway pressure is chosen; during inspiration, this pressure is kept at the preselected level by microprocessor-controlled servo valves that open or close in response to measured airway pressure. The flow rate is determined by the applied pressure, the resistance to airflow in the airways, and the lung and thoracic compliance. Termination of the applied pressure support is determined either by the initial flow rate generated by the patient at the beginning of the spontaneous breath or by the peak flow achieved. Inspiratory pressure support is terminated when the inspiratory flow drops below a percentage of either the initial flow rate or the peak flow rate. The value used to end pressure support is often 25% of the of the peak flow.[88]

IPSV can be used in two ways.[88] Using low-level IPSV (2–10 cm H_2O), the work of breathing required to overcome the resistance of the endotracheal tube and respiratory circuit can be decreased. This allows partial unloading of the respiratory muscles and yet lets the patient do the majority of the work needed during spontaneous ventilations. High-level IPSV (15–50 cm H_2O) can be used to support ventilation totally and still allows the patient to determine the respiratory rate. The level of inspiratory pressure support is adjusted to provide a tidal volume of 10–12 mL/kg. In this way IPSV can be used as a stand-alone mode of ventilation as long as the patient is alert and cooperative enough to set an appropriate respiratory rate. IPSV can also be used in combination with IMV ventilation to augment the spontaneous breaths.

The advantages of IPSV revolve around patient interaction with the ventilator and control over respiratory rate and minute ventilation. Unquestionably the work of breathing can be reduced with IPSV, but whether this mode of ventilation has a distinct advantage over other more conventional modes is unclear. Many physicians feel that IPSV has a weaning advantage in that the patient can be slowly required to do more of the ventilatory work by decreasing the amount of inspiratory pressure support applied. Before using IPSV as the sole mode for weaning, it must be assumed that the patient has a stable and reliable ventilatory drive and that ventilatory requirements are not changing significantly. Before using IPSV alone, conditions must be stable, since the achieved tidal volume depends on the lung and thoracic compliance along with the airway resistance.

Care of the Intubated Patient

Treatment of Agitation

Continued mechanical ventilation often results in agitation secondary to inability to speak, feelings of air hunger, and feelings of loss of control over one's environment. Postoperative pain also contributes to the agitation commonly seen in postsurgical patients. Agitation can lead to increased oxygen consumption, difficulty in providing mechanical ventilation secondary to the patient's efforts to fight the ventilator, and potential for other postoperative complications such as angina and hypertension from high endogenous catecholamine levels. Sedation is often used to try and control agitation that does not result from hypoxia, severe pain, or other identifiable sources such as poor cerebral perfusion. Short-acting benzodiazepines such as midazolam in doses of 1–5 mg, administered intravenously, can be used on an intermittent basis as needed. The longer acting benzodiazepines such as diazapam or lorazepam may also be used.[89] Neuroleptics can also be helpful in controlling excessive agitation especially with associated delirium. Haloperidol given in doses of 1–5 mg per nasogastric tube or intramuscular or intravenous injection is often successful in calming the agitated patient.[90,91] High-dose haloperidol, at doses exceeding 100 mg per day, has also been used safely in agitated cardiac patients.[92]

When agitation is sufficiently severe to compromise the hemodynamic or respiratory status to the point of being a threat to the patient, neuromuscular paralysis may be effective. Muscle relaxants can also be helpful in the unstable patient who requires a maximum decrease in oxygen consumption as in the case of inadequate oxygen delivery due to severe cardiogenic shock. Vecuronium, a nondepolarizing, neuromuscular blocking agent, has proved very effective for induction of paralysis in unstable, critically ill patients.[93] Because this drug has no appreciable effects on the cardiovascular system, it is an ideal agent for use in patients with unstable hemodynamics who require muscle paralysis.[94]

Prevention and Treatment of Postoperative Atelectasis

If the patient is extubated in the operating room or early in the recovery period after thoracic surgery, the usual postoperative care involves the addition of supplemental oxygen by face mask at an FIO_2 of at least 50% until an adequate PO_2 is reached. Arterial blood gases should document a value of more than 60 mmHg. At most institutions, standard pulse oximetry is used to assure the physician that the oxygen saturation is at least 92%. If the validity of the pulse oximetry reading is in question, as is often seen when patients experience peripheral vasoconstriction due to hypothermia, hypovolemia, medications, or high catecholamine levels, a formal arterial blood gas should be sent to document adequate oxygenation or to dictate further support of the respiratory system.[47]

When the positive pressure of the ventilator is removed, the patient is at increased risk of developing worsened atelectasis as a result of an inability to reexpand the lungs fully and decreased airway pressures.[95] This inability may have several causes, including severe pain at the surgical site, residual effects of inadequately reversed anesthetics, neuromuscular blocking agents or sedatives, pulmonary edema and alveolar fluid sequestration from intraoperative compression or overload fluid administration, phrenic nerve dysfunction from the cooling effects of the iced cardioplegic solutions used in cardiac surgery, or simply poor positioning of the patient in the postoperative period. In addition, ventilation-perfusion abnormalities are exacerbated, which can lead to severe hypoxemia.[96]

Postoperative Pain Control

Pain can be severe after an open thorax procedure, and adequate pain relief in the postoperative thoracic surgery patient is of high importance (See also Chapter 16, Postoperative Pain Management.) Traumatic wide separation of the sternum or ribs with transection and disruption of muscle and connective tissue and direct trauma to the intercostal nerves contribute to overall discomfort. Patients with posterolateral incisions have increased pain as compared to those patients who have undergone median sternotomy. This pain is likely a result of intercostal nerve injury and postoperative movement of the surgical site during respiratory excursions or coughing.[97] Inadequate analgesia leads to shallow breathing and poor lung expansion with splinting of the involved areas of the thorax, as well as a loss of sighing, causing underventilation, which further contributes to the poor expansion of the alveoli.[95,96] In addition this leads to segmental atelectasis in both the dependent portions of the lung and the areas underneath the splinted chest wall. Pain also results in an increase in sympathetic nervous system activity, which is manifested by tachycardia, hypertension, and increased oxygen consumption; this latter condition predisposes the patient to myocardial ischemia.[98]

Too often, the clinician is overly concerned with suppressing respirations if narcotics are administered. As a result, the patient is left undermedicated and without adequate ventilatory efforts due to the increased discomfort caused by deep breathing or coughing. Coughing is important to clear excessive secretions and blood from the airways but can lead to significant pain at the surgical site. Using a firm "cough pillow" held tightly against the chest wall over the incision during a cough often helps to decrease the associated pain, as it splints the chest wall under the pillow and minimizes excessive movement. When pain seems to be the limiting factor to deep breathing, intravenous morphine in 3–5-mg increments is used until adequate analgesia is obtained and the patient's respiratory efforts are adequate. We also use the lipophilic narcotic fentanyl intravenously in doses of 0.5–2 μg/kg as needed for pain control. The benefits of adequate analgesia must be balanced against possible oversedation, cough suppression, and respiratory depression.[99]

If the patient requires frequent doses of analgesia that often cause periods of oversedation interspersed with periods of painful undersedation, a continuous intravenous drip of narcotics can be used. Continuous infusion allows a higher steady-state concentration to be maintained, which results in adequate analgesia without the more severe side effects seen when intermittent boluses produce high blood levels of narcotic just after being administered.[100,101] Fentanyl given in doses of 0.5–3 μg/kg/hour after an adequate loading dose has been administered is quite useful. Morphine can also be used in this fashion, although the effects are slightly more difficult to titrate because of the drug's longer half-life.

We have also found that after the first 12–24 hours, an intravenous pump can be activated by the cooperative patient to administer a preset dose of analgesic. Patient-controlled analgesia (PCA) can be very useful in both titrating pain relief according to the patient's needs as well as allowing the patient to have some control over their postoperative care.[102] To reduce the possibility of a drug overdose, the dose per activation as well as the total dose over a specified time (lockout time) is preset by the physician. Once the PCA system is set up, it also relieves the nurse of the time-consuming job of measuring and administering frequent doses of medication.

In the past 20 years, research concerning the administration of narcotics directly into the central nervous system by way of either an epidural or intrathecal route has been tremendous.[103,104] If the fact that the patient is to undergo an extensive procedure or one that is often associated with significant postoperative pain (eg, thoracic aneurysm repair, major pulmonary resection, etc) is known before surgery, placement of an epidural infusion catheter for either intermittent bolus or continuous infusion of analgesics and local anesthetics can be very beneficial. Both vital capacity (VC) and functional residual capacity (FRC) increase with analgesia,[105,106] and research has shown that VC is 15–20% greater with epidural anesthesia than with systemic analgesia.[107] Many anesthesiologists choose to place the epidural catheter at the beginning of the procedure and use it throughout the case to administer local anesthetics; this reduces or eliminates the need for muscle relaxants.[105] Epidural narcotics started before the end of the procedure allow patients to be extubated uneventfully after they have awakened free of pain in the operating room. Although the catheter has traditionally been placed in the lumbar position, thoracic placement is becoming more accepted as the practice and management and monitoring of this very effective mode of patient analgesia become increasingly widespread.

However, at least two studies indicate that thoracic placement has no real advantage over lumbar administration in either the dose or frequency of administration of narcotics in upper abdominal or thoracic procedures.[108,109,110] If a continuous epidural infusion is not possible, intermittent boluses of preservative-free morphine can be given, starting with 2–5-mg doses that can last up to 12 hours or more. It is important to remember that the intrathecal dose is usually one-tenth of the epidural dose. Continuous infusion via the intrathecal route is usually not used because of the increase in the number and intensity of side effects, which may include severe headache secondary to the dural puncture.[111] Side effects, usually manifested as nausea, vomiting, pruritus, especially in the involved dermatomes, bladder retention, hypotension, or respiratory depression, are less common with epidural administration, but they can be severe in some cases. In addition, sympathetic outflow from the spinal cord can be inhibited, leading to a type a "spinal shock" state that causes hypotension if the analgesic or anesthetic migrates rostrally. This is much more common when local anesthetics are used, however, and is almost never seen after administration of epidural narcotics alone. Treatment usually consists of fluid administration but occasionally requires blood pressure support with alpha-agonist pressor agents such as dopamine or phenylephrine.

Intramuscular or intravenous antiemetics such as prochlorperazine are often effective in treating gastrointestinal intolerance. Either diphenhydramine or hydroxyzine may combat pruritus. Although bladder retention occurs in

30%–50% of patients who receive epidural analgesics, it is rarely a problem initially as most patients have an indwelling bladder catheter that is usually left in place until the epidural or intrathecal analgesia is discontinued.[112,113] Clinically significant respiratory depression caused by the cephalad migration of the instilled analgesic or anesthetic is reported to occur in 0.2%–1.0% of patients and is more common when agents with a low lipophilic nature are used.[114] Severe side effects from any of the opiates can be effectively treated with the narcotic antagonist naloxone. The dose is either administered intermittently, 5–10 μg/kg intramuscularly or intravenously, or continuously, as a 5–10 μg/kg/h infusion. It must be remembered that the half-life of naloxone is only about 15 minutes, which is much shorter than the half-life of most opioids; repeat doses may be necessary for continued reversal of unwanted side effects. Some clinicians believe that the analgesic properties of epidural narcotics persist even during treatment with low-dose naloxone.[115]

Angle intercostal nerve blocks for pain relief have been used with fairly successfully to treat chest wall pain following thoracic procedures. Analgesia can be initiated in the operating room by the surgeon after placement of catheters at the posterior rib angles at the incision line and two intercostal spaces above and below the incision. Alternatively, transcutaneous injection can be carried out with a small-gauge needle along the inferior borders of the involved ribs. Intercostal nerve blockade has been shown to provide effective postoperative pain relief and probably reduces the need for systemic narcotics.[116] In addition, it appears to improve FEV and VC.[116,117]

Endotracheal Suctioning

Suctioning of secretions from the endotracheal tube as well as from the upper airways is necessary in all intubated patients. The frequency and level of aggressiveness should be individualized. Often the need for repeated suctioning is evidenced by the production of either voluminous or tenacious secretions. Auscultating the lungs reveals coarse, moist, rhonchal breath sounds as secretions increase. Many times localized wheezing can be heard as the inspired and expired air flows past inspissated fluids and other material contaminating the airways. Before beginning suctioning, adequate oxygenation must be ensured. Before the aspiration catheter is passed into the endotracheal tube, the borderline patient is hyperoxygenated by administering increased F_{IO_2} either via the ventilator or by manually hyperinflating the lungs with a hand-held, self-expanding ventilation bag connected to 100% oxygen. For patients receiving PEEP, an increased risk of alveolar collapse due to loss of the airway pressure exists.[118] A right-angled connector with a self-sealing orifice can be used to minimize the loss of airway pressure during suctioning.

Self-contained suction catheters that remain attached to the endotracheal tube connector are becoming more common. They are encased in a protective plastic sleeve that serves to reduce the amount of contamination and colonization. Since the catheters are never exposed to the hands of the caregiver, they are not easily contaminated with bacteria from the hands. Because the incidence of significant bacterial colonization markedly increases after 24–48 hours, these catheters are replaced after this time. Higher numbers of bacteria increase the risk of developing nosocomial pneumonia secondary to the contamination of the tracheobronchial tree.

Patients often cough due to the noxious stimulation of the endotracheal and endobronchial mucosa, but this can aid in mobilizing distal secretions. Endotrachial suctioning can be repeated several times, but between each attempt the patient should be hyperventilated and reoxygenated. Each pass of the suction catheter should be limited to 10 seconds or less to reduce the risk of hypoxia and airway collapse.[118]

Attempts to direct the suction catheter into one bronchus as opposed to another is usually unsuccessful.[119] Statistically, the catheter will pass down the right mainstem bronchus more than 60% of the time owing to the more acute angulation of the left mainstem bronchus. Attempts to catheterize the left mainstem bronchus by turning the patient's head to the right, lowering the shoulder, or positioning the body in other ways usually increases the chances of success to no more than 40% when a common, straight-tipped catheter is used. Using a catheter with an angulated tip can increase the success rate to approximately 50%.[119]

Preinstillation of various fluids into the tracheobronchial tree have been used to try to loosen and mobilize tenacious secretions before suction is attempted. Evidence showing any advantages to this practice is sparse, but the procedure is still quite common. Often 2–10 mL of sterile 0.9% normal saline is injected into the endotracheal tube, and the patient is hyperinflated with a hand-bag for several breaths. This is followed by the introduction of the suction catheter. 2% N-acetylcysteine has been used to try to thin highly viscous and tenacious secretions, but its tendency to provoke intense bronchospasm due to mucosal irritation in patients with or without reactive airway disease limits its usefulness.[120] Sodium bicarbonate ($NaHCO_3$), 1.5%–2.5%, has also been used to aid in the evacuation and mobilization of secretions. The mechanism is unknown but is thought to involve several factors, which include hypertonicity, decreased adhesiveness of secretions, and improved local environmental conditions for endogenous enzyme activity.[120]

Several risks and complications are associated with endotracheal suctioning. The most common is the development of arterial hypoxemia. As suction is applied to the catheter, supplemental oxygen is removed from the endobronchial tree, thus causing the inspired oxygen concentration to fall. This lead to a decrease in the alveolar oxygen concentration with potential hypoxemia in borderline oxygenated patients. In addition, airway pressure falls during the application of suction. The resting lung volume decreases when some patients especially those who require PEEP, are removed from the ventilator. With the application of suction, the resting lung volume falls further. Preoxygenating and hyperventilating the patient and keeping the suctioning time short can minimize this problem.[118]

Cardiac arrhythmias can occur during suctioning.[121] Hypoxia caused by the procedure coupled with the discomfort of the suction catheter can easily lead to a sinus tachycardia. When patients are less stable and when catecholamine levels are high due to pain and agitation, ventricular arrhythmias can occur but rarely need treatment. Some patients may have profound bradycardia,[122] which is not usually due to severe hypoxia but appears to be secondary to a strong vagally mediated reflex. It can be prevented by the preadministration of atropine. Monitoring the arterial oxygen saturation with a pulse oximeter is standard practice, as in all postoperative thoracic surgery patients. Pulse oximetry can identify patients who are becoming severely hypoxic during the suctioning procedure.

Further Treatment and Prevention of Atelectasis

The majority of cases of pulmonary atelectasis, the most common postoperative respiratory complication,[123] are self-limited and clinically insignificant. Comparison of the various modalities used to prevent or treat this disorder has led to more confusion than answers.[123, 124] Evidence has suggested that patients with an inspiratory capacity of more than 1 liter needs no additional lung reexpansion as long as they are able to breathe deeply.[123] O'Donohue[125] found that in a national survey, physicians in only 21% of hospitals were measuring actual lung volumes where lung expansion maneuvers were being ordered for the treatment of postoperative atelectasis. Keys to optimizing postoperative respiratory function appear to revolve around early mobilization and adequate pain control. Several techniques that may be used in attempts to prevent the development of postoperative atelectasis or to treat this condition are discussed below.

Postoperative thoracic surgery patients, especially those who have undergone median sternotomy and cardiopulmonary bypass, develop severe alterations in pulmonary function and gas exchange leading to significant drops in VC and $PA{O_2}$ (Table 14-3).[126–128] Restrictive defects in pulmonary function persist for more than two weeks, and both FRC and $PA{O_2}$ remain well below preoperative values.[129] Instructing patients to expand the lungs by deep breathing, often with a prolonged end-inspiratory hold maneuver, is one way to overcome these problems. Forceful coughing; vigorous chest physiotherapy using either a cupped-hand technique of slapping the chest wall or a mechanical, vibrating diaphragm applied to the chest wall; and postural drainage loosen and mobilizes secretions. Intermittent positive-pressure breathing (IPPB) or continuous positive airway pressure (CPAP) are also used in an attempt to treat or prevent further reductions in lung volumes with increased atelectasis.

Table 14-3. Postoperative Changes in Lung Function Following Coronary Bypass Surgery*

Parameter	% Change
Vital capacity	−34
Total lung capacity	−28
Inspiratory capacity	−34
Functional residual capacity	−20
Diffusion capacity	−03
Arterial PO_2	−12

* Data from Braun SR. Pre- and postoperative pulmonary function abnormalities in coronary revascularization surgery. Chest 1978;73:316.

Incentive Spirometry

Incentive spirometry is the most commonly used method for treating postoperative atelectasis in the United States.[125] Usually a hand-held cannister with either a piston or light-weight plastic balls enclosed in air chambers is used. The piston or the balls travel upward in relation to the amount of negative pressure generated during a forced inspiration through an attached mouthpiece. The estimated volume of the inspired breath is indicated by the distance the piston travels or the number of balls that can be sustained in air by the inspiratory flow. It is important that the patient be watched very closely to make sure the technique is adequate; the full inspiration should be held as long as possible to encourage expansion of atelectatic areas of the lung.

Incentive spirometry is not always effective, however. In one small, uncontrolled study postoperative coronary bypass patients incentive spirometry was no more beneficial than early patient mobilization or maximum breathing exercises.[130] Another study that looked at 110 males undergoing myocardial revascularization confirmed these results. There were no differences in arterial blood gases or bedside pulmonary function tests whether the patients were treated postoperatively with incentive spirometry or deep breathing exercises and early mobilization.[131]

Intermittent Positive-Pressure Breathing

Intermittent positive-pressure breathing (IPPB) is another modality that has been used with variable success in the treatment or prevention of postoperative atelectasis.[124,132,133] Positive airway pressure is applied either with a tight-fitting face mask or a mouthpiece. Pressure is set (usually 15–40 cm H_2O) to deliver a desired inspiratory volume. The desired target volume is 1.5–2.5 times the tidal volume and usually exceeds 1 liter in the average-sized adult. Cooperation of the patient is necessary to allow maximum lung expansion at the preset pressure. Air swallowing, which can potentially lead to gastric distension and aspiration, is common, but these serious complications occur infrequently.

Continuous Positive Airway Pressure

Continuous positive airway pressure (CPAP) is used to maintain a continuous increased airway pressure at the mouth and nose with a soft, tight-fitting, self-sealing mask (Fig. 14-4). Usually a gas-powered Venturi device that delivers a continuous gas flow of greater than 90 L/min through a threshold resistor valve is used. This is adjusted to keep the upper airway pressure at a desired level,[134] usually in the range of 5–15 cm H_2O. As the patient initiates a spontaneous breath, the drop in airway pressure is sensed, and the pressure is immediately increased to the preset level. Conversely, when the patient begins expiration, the slight increase in the airway pressure is sensed, and the pressure is reduced. Airway pressure is kept relatively constant using this mechanism. A large decrease in pressure would allow alveolar collapse to occur. In addition, the stenting open of the small airways and alveoli keep the alveoli on a more optimal portion of the pressure-volume curve, thus allowing easier expansion during inspiration. This is one of the reasons believed responsible for the decreased pulmonary shunt often seen with CPAP administration.[135,136]

Figure 14-4. CPAP mask.

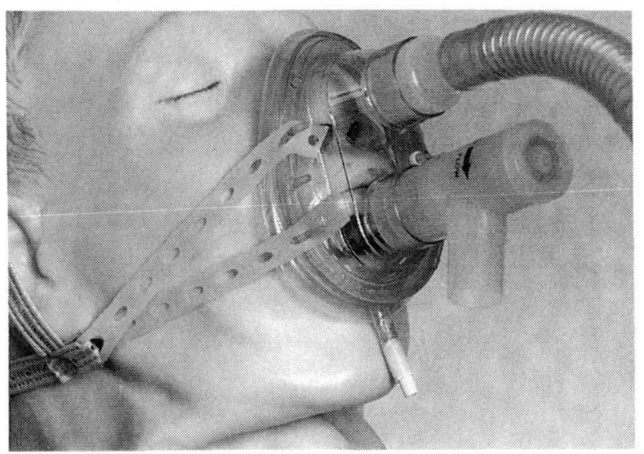

One of the major drawbacks in using mask CPAP is lack of patient comfort. The tight-fitting mask can be very claustrophobic, and the constant pressure on the facial tissues, especially over the bridge of the nose, can lead to pressure necrosis and sloughing. In addition, the constant positive pressure in the posterior pharynx predisposes the patient to air-swallowing with resultant gastric distension and possible vomiting and aspiration. Since the mask is tightly strapped to the face, quick removal (as is necessary in case of vomiting) is difficult. Some clinicians place a nasogastric tube to combat gastric distension, but the tube often interferes with the tight fit of the mask, causing a loss of pressure and effectiveness.

CPAP has been compared to incentive spirometry and conservative therapy in postoperative cardiac patients, but has not been shown to be more effective in the prevention or treatment of postoperative pulmonary changes than either of the other modalities.[134] CPAP can still be an effective means of temporizing respiratory failure resulting from a quickly treatable cause such as bronchospasm, mild-to-moderate atelectasis, or fluid overload that is responsive to diuretics.[137,138]

Oxygenation Techniques

During the transfer of the patient from the operating room to the recovery room, supplemental oxygen is always applied. If the patient is still intubated, a hand-held ventilation bag attached to a 100% oxygen supply is usually used until the patient is either connected to a mechanical ventilator or to a T-tube apparatus that is connected to supplemental oxygen. If the patient is extubated, a simple face mask is used to deliver an FIO_2 of at least 0.50. Ideally, a pulse oximeter is left attached to the patient to alert the medical staff to any deterioration of the arterial oxygen saturation (SaO_2). An (SaO_2) of less than 92% should prompt further investigation into the possible causes of hypoxemia. Depending on the patient's level of consciousness, ability to protect the airway, pulmonary secretions, and ability to effect adequate gas exchange, a decision concerning extubation or intubation is made. Frequent reassessment is performed to determine when a patient is a good candidates for extubation.

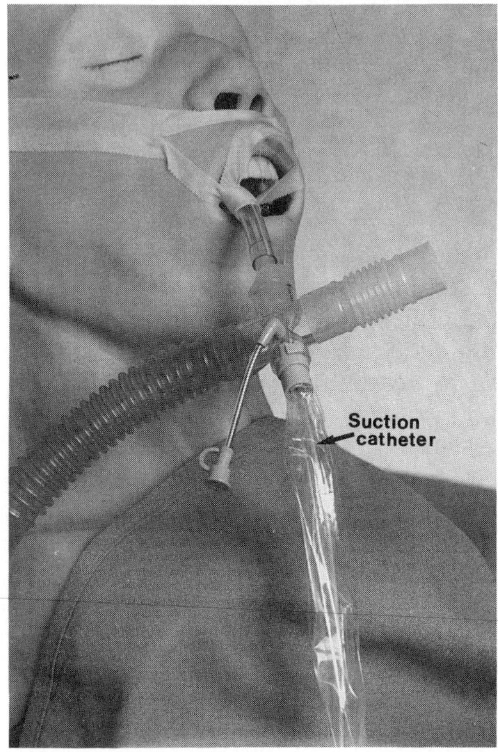

Figure 14-5. T-tube system.

T-tube

For an intubated patient who is breathing spontaneously but is still awakening from anesthesia or is otherwise unable to protect the airway, a T-tube circuit can be used to deliver humidified air with an enriched oxygen concentration (Fig. 14-5). This system has several disadvantages. Because of lack of adequate monitoring, a patient can develop respiratory and ventilatory insufficiency that may go unnoticed by the caregivers until the situation is potentially life-threatening. Checks for cardiac arrhythmias and monitoring of blood pressure, pulse, and arterial oxygen saturation occur, but the medical staff receives little warning of a hypoventilating patient. Carbon dioxide retention and progressive respiratory acidosis may result. By the time the pulse rate, blood pressure, or arterial oxygen saturation change, the patient can be dangerously acidotic. This can further provoke cardiac irritability, leading to arrhythmias as well as increased pulmonary vascular resistance, which place an excessive burden on the often already stressed myocardium. If the ability of the patient to exhale adequate carbon dioxide is in question, mechanical ventilation with a mandated respiratory rate should be maintained to ensure adequate ventilation. Attaching the patient to a formal capnograph to measure end-tidal carbon dioxide solves the problem of not being able to monitor carbon dioxide removal. Many recovery rooms and most ICUs are not equipped with this technology at this time, however.

Another problem with using a T-tube circuit on spontaneously breathing patients who are still under the influence of sedatives, analgesics, or other respiratory depressants involves the lack of increased airway pressure during the ventilatory cycle. The resulting propensity to develop micro- and macroatelectasis can be significant. This is especially true if the patient is taking shallow, suboptimal breaths, which worsens arterial oxygenation as the V/Q mismatch deteriorates from progressive alveolar collapse. As previously discussed, the postoperative patient has already suffered a decline in most of the spirometric parameters, including TV, VC, and FRC, and is predisposed to developing significant lung collapse.

Face Mask

After the patient is extubated, a face mask is applied to deliver oxygen-enriched, humidified air at a high flow rate. FiO_2 is usually started at least 0.50. The patient is monitored for any signs of increasing respiratory distress or arterial oxygen desaturation. The pulse oximeter should exceed 92% arterial saturation, and the actual partial pressure of oxygen in the arterial blood should be confirmed by arterial blood gas analysis as soon as possible.

Four general types of face masks that provide supplemental oxygen and humidification are available:[139] simple, partial rebreathing non rebreathing, and air entrainment or high-flow.

The simple face mask consists of a molded, flexible, plastic mask that fits rather loosely over the nose and mouth and contains no valves or a reservoir (Fig. 14-6). The mask is connected to an oxygen source that delivers oxygen at a flow of 6–10 L/min. The achievable FiO_2 is approximately 0.35 to 0.50. Determinants of the actual FiO_2 attained depend primarily on the oxygen flow rate and even more importantly on the patient's respiratory rate and effort. Oxygen flow must exceed the patient's minute ventilation to prevent rebreathing of exhaled gas. In addition, the oxygen flow rate must be greater than the patient's inspiratory flow rate. If the inspiratory flow rate does not match or exceed the patient's inspiratory flow because the patient is taking rapid or forceful inhalations, then ambient room air is entrained through the side vents or around the edges of the mask. As a result of dilution, the oxygen concentration falls. A study showed that a simple oxygen mask delivery of 2–4 L/min offered no advantage over either a nasal cannula or catheter in providing a higher or more consistent FiO_2 (Table 14-4).[140]

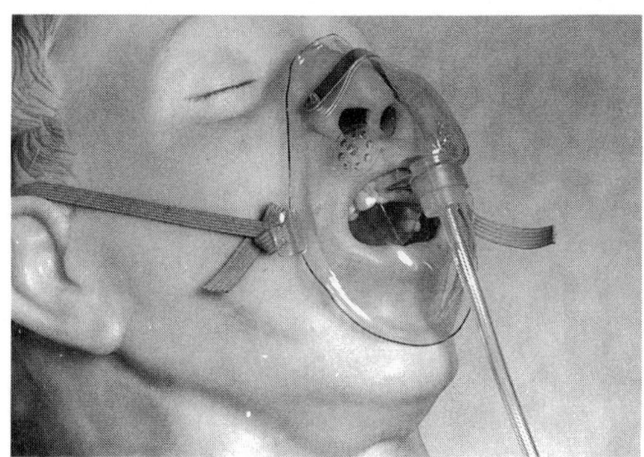

Figure 14-6. Simple face mask.

For delivery of oxygen via mask at concentrations higher than 0.50, either a partial rebreathing or nonrebreathing mask can be used. Both of these masks make use of a reservoir bag to store some of the oxygen-enriched gas mixture to be inhaled by the patient (Fig. 14-7). In a partial rebreathing mask, the oxygen reservoir is about 200 mL. The mask has no valves but does have side ports open to the room air. When the patient exhales, the initial 200 mL of expired gas (ie, principally the high-oxygen content gas retained in the upper airways) re-

Table 14-4. Estimation of FiO_2 for Low-Flow Systems

Flow Rate (L/m-100% O_2)	FiO_2
Nasal Cannula	
1	0.24
2	0.28
3	0.32
4	0.36
5	0.40
6	0.44
Oxygen (simple) mask	
5–6	0.40
6–7	0.50
7–8	0.60
Mask with reservoir	
6	0.60
7	0.70
8	0.80
>10	0.80+

turns to the bag. When the bag is inflated, the remainder of the exhaled gas passes out of the side ports of the mask into the room. This allows the exhaled gases that are rich in carbon dioxide (ie, gas from the distal airways and alveoli) to be liberated into the room and not be rebreathed by the patient. Since the oxygen requirements for the partial rebreathing mask are much less than for high-flow masks, this mask is ideal in situations where the oxygen supply may be limited (eg, during patient transport). When the oxygen flow into the mask is 10 L/min, the FiO_2 ranges from 0.6 to 0.8 in the majority of patients.[139, 141]

A nonrebreathing mask contains a reservoir with a volume that exceeds that of the patient's tidal volume. In addition, one-way valves on the side of the mask allow air only to pass out of the mask, and a one-way valve located at the opening to the reservoir prevents exhaled gases from entering the reservoir. Oxygen is supplied to the reservoir at a rate required to keep the reservoir inflated. In this way, when the patient inhales, air is pulled in from the reservoir and not from the surrounding ambient air. As with the other masks, the delivery rate has to provide sufficient oxygen to exceed the patient's overall minute inspiratory volume. More than 15 L/min is usually required. Routine single humidification systems cannot provide a higher flow rate. If a patient has an extremely high minute volume, a second humidifier is added to the system to produce the necessary flow. The nonbreathing mask must be secured tightly to the patient's face to prevent air entrainment around the sides of the mask, which would dilute the inspired oxygen.

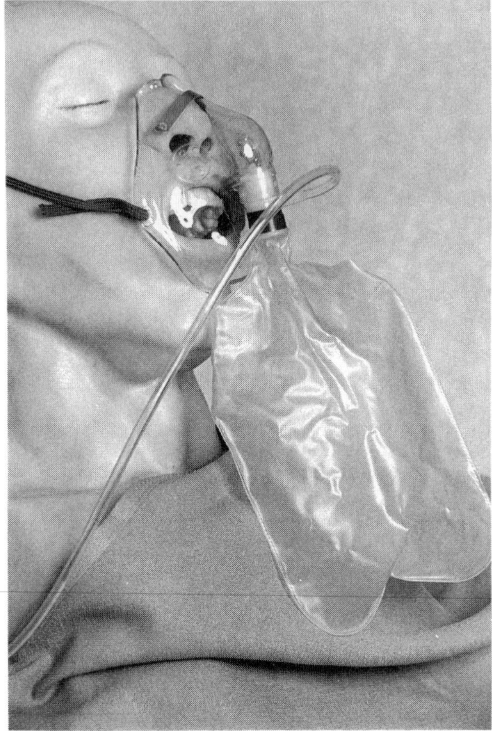

Figure 14-7. Reservoir mask.

Fixed oxygen concentration masks, also known as oxygen-powered air entrainment masks or Venturi masks, are used when a constant concentration of delivered oxygen is desired (Fig. 14-8). With these devices, 100% oxygen is mixed with ambient air to attain the

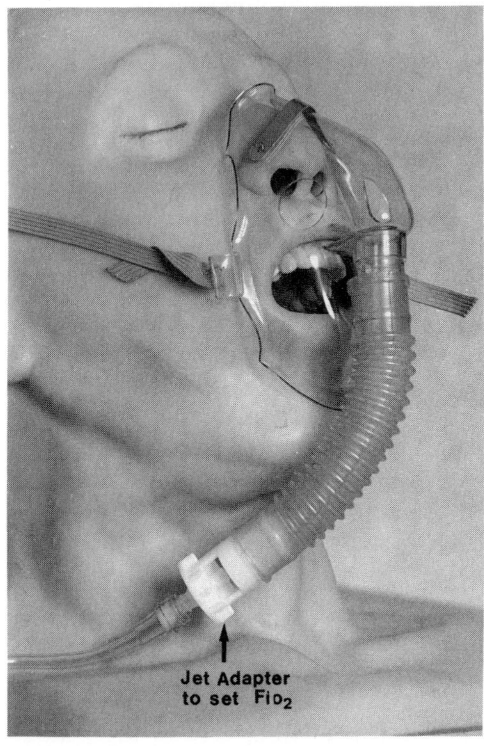

Figure 14-8. Venti-mask. The F_{IO_2} is determined by the size of the jet in the attached adapter.

desired F_{IO_2}; the oxygen is supplied to a small tube or jet-mixing device that increases the gas velocity. As the high-velocity jet of 100% oxygen exits the device, room air at an F_{IO_2} of 0.21 is entrained into the gas stream and dilutes the pure oxygen. Depending on the size of the central jet and side ports on the jet-mixing assembly, the F_{IO_2} of the gas mixture reaching the mask varies, but it is relatively precise and constant. Since the flow rate of gas delivery to the mask far exceeds the patient's minute volume, the air-entrainment system is not affected by changes in the patient's respiratory pattern. In addition, because of the high flow rates, no valve system or reservoir is needed to prevent rebreathing.

Although this air-entrainment system is often referred to as the 'venti-mask' system, implying the use of a true Venturi tube, the air dilution is actually accomplished by jet-mixing. The F_{IO_2} that can be attained with available air-entrainment masks is determined by the inflow rate of oxygen and the adaptor attached to the mask. The available adapters usually allow the F_{IO_2} to be set in the range of 0.24 to 0.50 and are often color coded to indicate the delivered F_{IO_2} at a given oxygen inflow delivery rate. Venti-masks can be very useful in providing accurate oxygen administration to patients who may be at risk for suppression of respiratory drive if excessive or uncontrolled oxygen is given (eg, patients with severe COPD with a hypoxic respiratory drive).

Nasal Cannula

When a high F_{IO_2} is not needed and the patient does not require administration of nebulized or aerosolized gas, oxygen delivery via a nasal cannula can be used. Administration of 1–8 L/min of oxygen provides for an increased F_{IO_2} and is second only to the oxygen face tent for patient comfort and tolerance. The major drawback is the variability in the received F_{IO_2}. F_{IO_2} is primarily determined by the patient's ventilatory pattern, and the actual value depends not only on the oxygen flow rate, but also on the patient's minute volume, respiratory rate, and anatomical reservoir (naso- and oropharynx). The actual increase in the F_{IO_2} is usually assumed to be between 0.03 and 0.04 for each liter per minute of oxygen flow. Since the maximum tracheal F_{IO_2} is usually no greater than 0.45 to 0.50, regardless of the oxygen inflow rate, there is little reason to place the patient on higher flow rates than 8 L/min. Higher rates increase patient discomfort, especially if the gas is not humidified; this leads to substantial drying of the nasal mucosa and possible epistaxis. When the flow rate exceeds 2 L/min, the oxygen should be passed through a humidifier to improve patient comfort.

Face Tent

When a patient needs supplemental oxygen but cannot tolerate a nasal cannula or face mask, an oxygen face tent can be tried. This tent consists of a molded plastic apparatus in the shape of the blade of a shovel, hence the term 'face-shovel' (Fig. 14-9). The face tent is held flush with the chin or neck and then loosely flares outward and upward. Oxygen is connected to the face tent, and the face is bathed in an oxygen-rich mixture of air. Moisture can also be added by means of a humidifier or nebulizer. Although the oxygen concentration feeding the face tent can be fairly accurate, the exact FIO_2 of the inspired air cannot be predicted accurately, as mixing with the room air is variable. FIO_2 probably does not exceed 0.50 to 0.75, even with 100% oxygen supplying the apparatus.

Providing Moisture

Airway humidity is absolutely crucial to the integrity, function, and maintenance of a normal respiratory epithelium. Allowing the airways to dry out predisposes to irritation, bleeding, infection, and inspissated secretions that may lead to small airway occlusion. Under normal conditions room air, which has a relative humidity of approximately 50%, is warmed to 34°C and its relative humidity is raised to 80%–90% as it passes through the nose.[142] By the time the air reaches the carina it is 100% humidified and its temperature is the same as body temperature (usually 37°C). Even when the patient is breathing by mouth, the air is fully warmed and humidified by the time it reaches the major bronchi. If the mouth and upper airways are bypassed by placement of an endotracheal tube or tracheostomy, the normal heating and humidification system is lost. If anhydrous medical gases are administered to the patient, the respiratory mucosa becomes dried and damaged. Ciliary function is impaired, hampering the clearance of secretions and bacteria and interfering with the normal protective mucin layer. Dry gas must be humidified before it is administered to the patient. This is accomplished with the use of a humidifier, which delivers water vapor, or a nebulizer, which generates an aerosol of water droplets (Fig. 14-10).

Figure 14-9. Face tent. Patient tolerance improves when exact oxygen concentrations not needed.

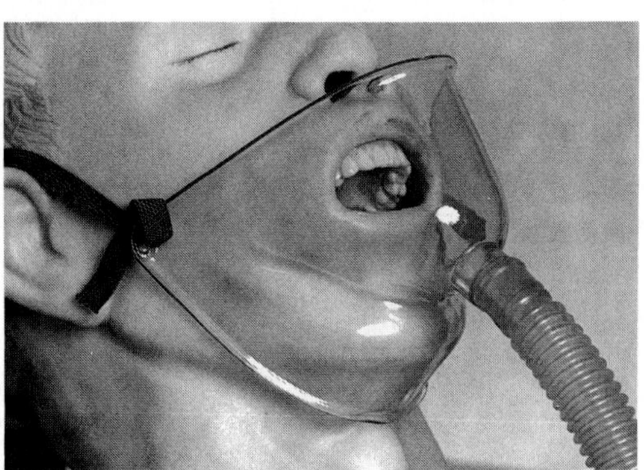

Humidifiers

Humidity refers to the moisture or water vapor in a gas. As previously stated, room air has a relative humidity of approximately 50%. In a normal individual inspired air is 100% saturated with water by the time it reaches the carina and is warmed to body temperature. If upper airway mechanisms for humidification are bypassed or insufficient, external humidification must be provided to try to prevent mucosal dehydration and drying of secretions. The humidification system used when administering oxygen via nasal cannula, partial or non-

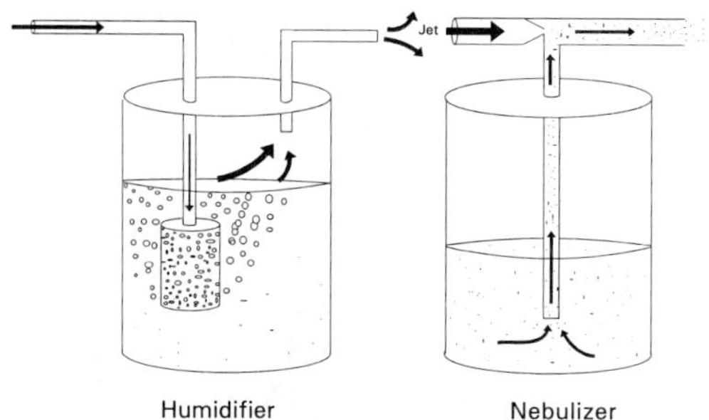

Figure 14-10. Humidifier and nebulizer. The humidifier produces water vapor, and the nebulizer produces an aerosol and is subject to the "rain-out" effect. (Modified from Tobin, MJ. Mechanical ventilation and weaning. In: Dantzker, DR, ed. Cardiopulmonary critical care. Orlando: Grune & Stratton, 1986:238.)

rebreathing mask, or air-entrainment mask consists of passing the gas through a water bath at ambient temperature. Usually the gas is passed through a grid that produces many tiny bubbles, which increases the surface area of the gas-water interface. This type of system results in the relative humidity at room temperature that approaches 80%–90%.[143]

When both humidification and heating are required, such as in the case of the intubated patient or the patient with a tracheostomy, then a heated humidifier or aerosol generator is used. This is often accomplished by heating the water bath that the air bubbles pass through (eg, in the Puritan-Bennett Cascade humidifier). The temperature can either be set manually or controlled by a servo mechanism in response to proximal airway temperature measured with a thermistor probe. Other models, such as the Bird humidifier, use a water-saturated wick system that allows dry gas to pass by the saturated wick in a heated chamber; moisture is transferred from the wick to the passing air, which is eventually heated as well as 100% humidified by the time it reaches the patient. The temperature is closely monitored to prevent tracheal mucosa burn.[144]

Nebulizers

In respiratory therapy aerosols, suspensions of particulate fluid droplets in the gaseous phase, are generated by nebulizers. Humidification of inspired gases through aerosolization is believed to be more beneficial in improving clearance of secretions over vaporized humidification systems.[142, 145] Aerosolized gases, which are rich in water droplets, are thought to loosen and break up desiccated secretions, thus allowing them to be more easily mobilized and either coughed or suctioned from the respiratory tree.[142]

Nebulizers are often wall-mounted and used to supply moisture-rich, oxygenated air to the patient via a face mask, face tent, or T-adaptor connection to an endotracheal tube. Oxygen-enriched air is fed through a restricted orifice creating a high-velocity jet stream. The jet stream passes over the end of a small tube immersed in sterile water. Subatmospheric pressure is generated over the end of the tube from the high-velocity jet and water is drawn up the tube. At the water-jet interface, the water is fractionated into small droplets (aerosolized) and carried to the inspiratory circuit along with the jet stream of oxygen-rich gas. The gas can also be heated to provide warmed, humidified gas to the respiratory tree.

Nebulizers powered by oxygen usually have an adjustable air-entrainment system that provides an FIO_2 of 0.35–1.0. Certain factors can alter the FIO_2 that the patient receives, however. Oxygen supply to most nebulizers is limited by the jet orifice restrictions and the pressure of the oxygen gas source. The most common oxygen-outlet pressure for wall-mounted units is 50 pounds per square inch gauge, and the resultant flow of humidified oxygen from the nebulizer is usually limited to 14–16 L/min.[146] If the patient's inspiratory minute volume (VI) exceeds this capacity, then room air is entrained either from around the edges or through the vents of the face-mask or from the open end of the T-connector. This lowers the FiO_2 according to the amount of dilution with ambient air. In the case of either a face mask or tracheostomy collar, an additional nebulizer unit can be interfaced in parallel to provide the necessary flow. For additional reservoir space, short segments of reservoir tubing can be attached to the open side vents of the face mask, thus making available humidified, oxygen-enriched gas that otherwise would be lost to the room. In the case of a patient with a T-tube, reservoir tubing can be added to the distal end of the tube adaptor to provide the additional space.

Nonconventional Support of the Respiratory System

High-Frequency Ventilation

High-frequency ventilation (HFV) refers to several forms of mechanical ventilation that use small tidal volumes delivered at rapid respiratory rates to ventilate the patient. This technique was developed in 1967 by Sjostrand,[147,148] who thought that ventilation accomplished with a lower tidal volume (VT) at higher respiratory rates would have less deleterious effects on the cardiovascular system and less chance of barotrauma than conventional ventilatory techniques that generated higher airway pressures. Sanders also described the use of HFV to augment ventilation during rigid bronchoscopy.[149] Smith has categorized HFV into three types: high-frequency positive-pressure ventilation (HFPPV), high-frequency jet ventilation (HFJV), and high-frequency oscillation (HFO).[150]

HFPPV, the system described initially by Sjostrand,[147] uses a time-cycled, volume-controlled ventilator that delivers VT at 60–110 breaths/min. The VT is usually close to the calculated dead space (VD) volume. The gas is delivered via a low-compliance ventilator and circuit equipped with a pneumatic valve that closes during inspiration, and no external air entrainment is involved. The Siemens-Elema Servo Ventilator was once used for this mode. Newer ventilators now permit cycling frequencies of up to 150 breaths/min.

HFJV uses a system that delivers gas through a small (14- or 16-gauge) catheter at rapid flow rates. The tip of the catheter is located in the trachea or is incorporated into the side wall of a specially-constructed endotracheal tube. Gas is delivered under high pressure and accelerates through the orifice of the injector catheter. Frequencies are usually 60–200 cycles per minute. Due to the Bernoulli principle, the pressure at the tip of the injector-catheter is lower than the pressure in the surrounding environment, and humidified air is entrained into the trachea and augments inspiratory flow and tidal volume.[151,152] Both HFPPV and HFJV are "open" systems that allow egress of gas at high volumes from the lungs. In essence, exhalation is a passive process. In HFJV, atmospheric gas or gas from an oxygen source is drawn in by bias flow or air entrainment. It is difficult to determine the true FiO_2 in a HFJV system, as varying degrees of mixing of the jet stream and biased gas occur. Humidification of the biased gas is difficult and inadequate moisture can lead to significant drying of the airways. Currently, one of the most popular ways to humidify the jet stream is to nebulize sterile water at 5–30 mL/h and deliver it to the jet cannula by means of a Y-connector feeding into the jet catheter.[153]

Applications of HFJV are not yet fully defined.[154,155] The peak airway pressure is definitely lower in HFJV than with other conventional modes of mechanical ventilation.[156,157] The attractive potential benefits of this form of ventilation are that the reduced airway pressure is less likely to cause barotrauma and interfere with cardiovascular function through its reduced influence on venous return. Considerable controversy still exists regarding the applications of HFJV. Some of the strongest indications are in the treatment of bronchopleural fistula (BPF),[158,159] where large portions of the tidal volume can be lost through the fistula. With conventional mechanical ventilation, increasing the delivered VT or increasing the peak airway pressure usually worsens the leak. With HFJV, lower peak airway pressures and decreased tidal volume produced can potentially reduce the magnitude of the leak. Other applications where HFJV has been beneficial include ventilatory support during bronchoscopy, laryngoscopy, and microlaryngeal and tracheal surgery.[160] HFJV has been used in many other applications requiring mechanical ventilation, but it has yet to show consistent advantage over conventional modes of ventilation.

HFO delivers small volumes of gas at rates of 600–3000 cycles per minute. This type of HFV differs from HFPPV and HFJV in that it moves gas in an oscillatory manner without depending on bulk flow of air.[161] The actual mechanism for gas exchange is unclear. The use of HFO has been limited to the pediatric population, mainly in patients with respiratory distress syndrome.[162]

Extracorporeal Membrane Oxygenation

Since the 1970s extracorporeal membrane oxygenation (ECMO) has been successfully used to treat newborn infants with severe respiratory failure.[163] The basis of ECMO is the transport of oxygen across a semipermeable membrane into the blood. ECMO involves prolonged extracorporeal cardiopulmonary bypass using extrathoracic vascular cannulation. The ECMO system is designed from cardiopulmonary bypass equipment; there is no standard ECMO machine. The basic components include vascular catheters, polyvinyl chloride tubing, a roller pump, a reservoir bag, an alarm system to warn of a drop in blood flow, a membrane oxygenator, oxygen and carbon dioxide flow meters, an oxygen blender to regulate the oxygen fraction going to the membrane, and a heat exchanger with a heating unit that also acts as a bubble trap (Fig. 14-11).[164]

Although there has been great enthusiasm for using ECMO in adults with severe cardiorespiratory failure, studies have not suggested that it has advantages over conventional hemodynamic and pulmonary support. In a multicenter study of patients with severe acute respiratory failure, ECMO conferred no survival advantage compared to continued mechanical ventilation.[165] The study did find that ECMO was a safe, effective method of treatment in these patients. ECMO is touted as being beneficial in those patients who are at risk of pulmonary toxicity from mechanical ventilation and oxygen therapy because it gives the lungs a chance to be 'put at rest' and allows a period of healing. Gattinoni has developed a modified ECMO technique using low-frequency positive-pressure ventilation with extracorporeal carbon dioxide removal.[166] In a study of adults suffering from acute respiratory failure he found a 49% survival rate in those treated with ECMO. Pennington,[167] who has used ECMO in patients with refractory cardiogenic shock, has shown that some patients benefit from this therapy and ultimately can be weaned off ECMO after they recover some cardiac function. Others studies of the use of ECMO to treat cardiopulmonary failure have not shown promising results.[168,169] Nawa[170] has compared ECMO against and in combination with intra-aortic

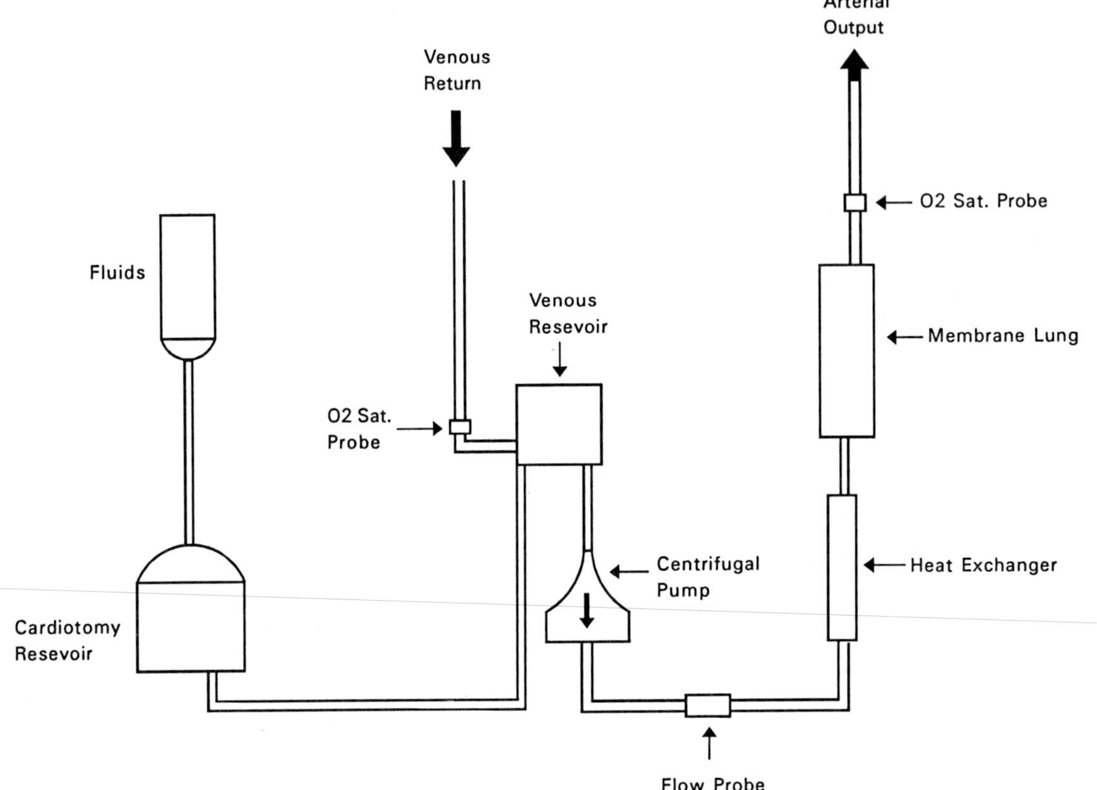

Figure 14-11. Extracorporeal membrane oxygenation (ECMO) perfusion circuit. This system utilizes a membrane lung and a standard centrifugal pump.

balloon pumping and venoarterial bypass in postcardiac surgery patients with cardiac failure. Although the small group of patients did not do well overall, the researchers believed that ECMO can provide temporary support of the cardiopulmonary system and serve as a bridge until further definitive therapy, such as cardiac transplant, is available.

Care of the Chest Tube

The majority of thoracic surgery patients have an indwelling chest tube placed in the pleural space following the operative procedure. The exact placement of the tube depends on the type of procedure performed and the preference of the surgeon. The unique physiology of the pleural space imparts a negative pressure in the pleural cavity, and all patients who undergo a thoracotomy have some residual pneumothorax due to the inability to completely evacuate all the air at the time of chest closure. The decision concerning whether to place a thoracostomy tube and the size and number of chest tubes depends on the propensity for either continued air leakage into the pleural space or the need for continued drainage of blood or fluids.

In the case of a pneumonectomy, the pleural space is not drained unless there is continued bleeding, a high suspicion that a major air leak will occur, or a high risk of infection with necessary drainage of purulent material.[98] Obliteration of the pleural space is accomplished by reexpansion of the remaining lung, shift of the mediastinum into the operative hemithorax, narrowing of the ipsilateral intercostal spaces, and elevation of the ipsilateral hemidiaphragm. Attempts to close the chest cavity are usually made to create a slightly negative pressure in the operated hemithorax and to place the mediastinum in a midline or more neutral position.

Once a chest tube is placed, it is either left to water seal or is attached to a vacuum source to aid in the evacuation of air and fluids in the pleural space. The negative pressure also serves to reexpand the collapsed lung segments. In some medical centers, a conventional two- or three-bottle evacuation system is used (Fig. 14-12): a drainage bottle to collect evacuated fluids, a water-seal cannister, and a suction-control bottle. Although this system is effective, it is cumbersome; the greater number of bottles and necessary connections increases the chances for system breaks, leading to air leakage back into the pleural space with a resultant pneumothorax. In addition, if the collection bottle is elevated above patient level, fluids can be drawn back into the pleural cavity via a siphon action. Alternative devices that package the two- or three-cannister system into a single apparatus have been developed; these require only two connections to be made to complete the system (see Fig. 14-12).

Clamping of the chest tube is discouraged. This is especially true for patients maintained on positive pressure ventilation. If air leakage from the lung or bronchial tree is appreciable, a life-threatening tension pneumothorax can quickly occur if the chest tube has been clamped or blocked in any way. Kinking of the tube during transfer or repositioning of the patient may also lead to life-threatening hemo- or pneumothorax. If tension pneumothorax is suspected, an emergent chest radiograph is ordered and the surgeon is notified immediately. All connections in the chest tube drainage and suction system are verified and any kinks in the tubing removed. In some cases, chest tube function is impaired because of blood clots or tissue

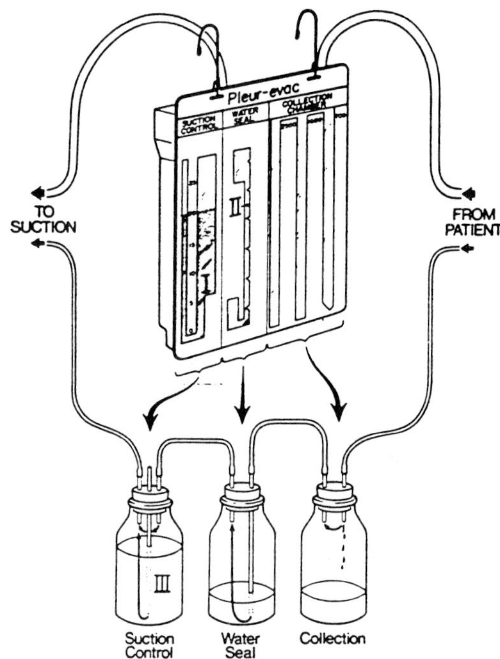

Figure 14-12. Chest tube system. The Pleur-evac is one of the many kinds of compartmentalized, three-bottle suction apparatus. It can be used without suction as a water-seal system. The height of the column in the suction control chamber determines the amount of negative pressure applied to the pleural space (I). An additional feature of the Pleur-evac is the ability to measure the amount of negative pressure developed by the patient (II and III). (Reproduced, with permission, from Hartz, RS. General principles of postoperative care. In: Shields, T, ed. General thoracic surgery. Philadelphia: Lea and Febiger, 1989: 322).

occluding both the end and side ports of the chest tube or the drainage tubing. Occasionally these obstructions can be evacuated by "milking" or "stripping" the connecting tubing,[171,172] Routine stripping may not be needed, however.[173]

Suction is applied to the chest tube if a large air leak or voluminous drainage is anticipated. The chest tube is initially left to suction at 15–25 cm H_2O for at least 12–24 hours. If air leakage is significant, suction is maintained until the leak subsides. After no significant air leakage is apparent, the chest tube system is put to water seal. Water seal drainage is maintained for another 12–24 hours. If the lung remains expanded and the amount of drainage is not significantly high, the chest tube is then removed. A follow-up chest radiograph is obtained to document that the lung is still expanded and a pneumothorax has not been created during the removal process as a result of the inadvertent entry of air into the pleural cavity.

References

1. Todd T, Keenan R. Ventilatory support of the postoperative patient. In: Shields T, ed. General thoracic surgery. 3rd ed. Philadelphia: Lea & Febiger, 1989: 325.
2. Irwin R. Mechanical ventilation. Part II: Weaning. In: Rippe J, Irwin RS, Alpert JS, et al, eds. Intensive care medicine. 2nd ed. Boston:Little, Brown, 1991: 575.
3. Bendixen HH, Egbert LD, Hedley-White J. Respiratory care. St. Louis:CV Mosby, 1965:149.
4. Feeley TW, Hedley-White J. Weaning from controlled ventilation and supplemental oxygen. N Engl J Med 1975:292:903.
5. Pierson DJ. Weaning from mechanical ventilation in acute respiratory failure: concepts, indications, and techniques. Respir Care 1983;28:646.
6. Sahn SA, Lahshminarayan S, Petty TL. Weaning from mechanical ventilation. JAMA 1976;235:2208.
7. Milbern SM, Downs JB, Jumper LC. Evaluation criteria for discontinuing mechanical ventilatory support. Arch Surg 1978;113:1441.
8. Tahvanainen J, Salmenpera M, Nikki P. Extubation criteria after weaning from intermittent mandatory ventilation and continuous positive airway pressure. Crit Care Med 1983;11:707.
9. Tobin MJ, Dantzker DR. Mechanical ventilation and weaning. In: Dantzker DR, ed. Cardiopulmonary critical care. Orlando: Grune and Stratton, 1986:203.
10. Black, LF, Hyatt RE. Maximal respiratory pressures: normal values and relationship to age and sex. Am Rev Respir Dis 1969;99:696.
11. Tobin MJ, Yang K, Weaning from mechanical ventilation. Crit Care Clin 1990;6:733.
12. Sahn SA, Lakshminarayan S. Bedside criteria for discontinuation of mechanical ventilation. Chest 1973;63:1002.
13. Rochester DF, Arora NS. Respiratory muscle failure. Med Clin North Am 1983;67:573.
14. Mecca RS. Pulmonary physiology. In: Kirby RR, Taylor RV, eds. Respiratory failure. Chicago:Yearbook Medical, 1986:310.
15. Pontoppidan H, Laver MB, Geffen B. Acute respiratory failure in the surgical patient. In: Welch CE, ed. Advances in surgery. Chicago:Yearbook Medical, 1970:163.
16. Tobin MJ, Chadha TS, Jenouri G, Breathing patterns. 1. Normal subjects. Chest 1983;84:202.
17. Boysen PG. Respiratory muscle function and weaning from mechanical ventilation. Respir Care 1987;32:572.
18. Hubmayr RD, Gay PC, Tayyab M. Respiratory system mechanics in ventilated patients: techniques and indications. Mayo Clin Proc 1987;62:358.
19. Marini J. Monitoring during mechanical ventilation. Clin Chest Med 1988;9:73.
20. Mecca RS. Respiratory: Essential physiologic concerns. In: Civetta JM, Taylor RW, Kirby RR, eds. Critical care. Philadelphia:JB Lippincott, 1988: 1023.
21. Patterson JW, Woolcock AJ, Shenfield GM. State of the art: bronchodilator drugs. Am Rev Resp Dis 1979;120:149.
22. Vozeh S, Kewitz G, Perruchoud A. Theophylline serum concentrations and therapeutic effect in severe acute bronchial obstruction. The optimal use of intravenously administered aminophylline. Am Rev Resp Dis 1982;125:181.
23. Mellemgard K. The alveolar-arterial oxygen difference. Its size and components in normal man. Acta Physiol Scand 1966;67:10.

24. West JB. Ventilation-perfusion relationships. Am Rev Resp Dis 1977;116:119.
25. West JB. Ventilation-perfusion inequality and overall gas exchange. In: West JB, ed. Ventilation/blood flow and gas exchange. London:Blackwell Scientific Publications, 1977:33.
26. Cane RD, Shapiro BA, Harrison RA. Minimizing errors in intrapulmonary shunt calculations. Crit Care Med 1980;8:294.
27. Gallagher TJ, Civetta JM, Kirby RR. Terminology update: optimal PEEP. Crit Care Med 1978;6:323.
28. Shapiro BA, Cane RD, Harrison RA. Positive end-expiratory pressure in adults with special reference to acute lung injury. A review of the literature and suggested clinical correlations. Crit Care Med 1984; 12:127.
29. Shapiro BA. General principles of airway pressure therapy. In: Shoemaker WC, Ayres S, Grenvik A, et al, eds. Textbook of critical care. Philadelphia:WB Saunders, 1989:505.
30. Dorinsky DM, Whitcomb ME. The effect of PEEP on cardiac output. Chest 1983;2:210.
31. Suter DM, Fairley HG, Isenberg MD. Optimum end-expiratory pressure in patients with acute pulmonary failure. N Engl J Med 1975;292:284.
32. Tyler D. Positive end-expiratory pressure: a review. Crit Care Med 1983;11:300.
33. Milbern SM, Downs JB, Jumper LC. Evaluation of criteria for discontinuing mechanical ventilatory support. Arch Surg 1978;113:1441.
34. Morganroth ML, Grum CM. Weaning from mechanical ventilation. Intensive Care Med 1988;3: 109.
35. Irwin RS, Thomas HM III. Mucoid impaction of the bronchus: diagnosis and treatment. Am Rev Resp Dis 1973;108:955.
36. Bernstein IL, Ausdenmoore RW. Iatrogenic bronchospasm occurring during clinical trials of a new mucolytic agent, acetylcysteine. Dis Chest 1964; 46:469.
37. Nunn JF, Bergman NA, Coleman AJ. Factors influencing the arterial oxygen tension during anaesthesia with artificial ventilation. Br J Anaesth 1965;37:898.
38. Rehder K, Sessler AD, Marsh HM. General anesthesia and the lung. Am Rev Resp Dis 1975;112:541.
39. Matthay MA, Weiner-Kronish JP. Respiratory management after cardiac surgery. Chest 1989;95:425.
40. Westbrook PR, Stubbs SE, Sessler AD, et al. Effects of anesthesia and muscle paralysis on respiratory mechanics in normal man. J Appl Physiol 1973;34:81.
41. Tusiewicz K, Bryan AC, Froese AB. Contributions of changing rib cage-diaphragm interactions to the ventilatory depression of halothane anesthesia. Anesthesiology 1977;47:327.
42. Schmid ER, Rehder K. General anesthesia and the chest wall. Anesthesiology 1981;55:668.
43. Tokics L, Hedenstierna G, Strandberg A, et al. Lung collapse and gas exchange during anesthesia: effects of spontaneous breathing, muscle paralysis, and positive end-expiratory pressure. Anesthesiology 1975;42:160.
44. Cote CJ, Goldstein EA, Cote MA, et al. A single-blind study of pulse oximetry in children. Anesthesiology 1988;68:184.
45. Smith DC, Canning JJ, Crul JF. Pulse oximetry in the recovery room. Anaesthesia 1989;44:345.
46. Curley FJ, Smyrnios NA. Routine monitoring of critically ill patients. In: Rippe JM, Irwin RS, Alpert JS, et al, eds. Intensive care medicine. 2nd ed. Boston: Little, Brown, 1991:199.
47. Tobin MJ. State of the art: respiratory monitoring in the intensive care unit. Am Rev Resp Dis 1988; 138:1625.
48. Eichorn JH, Cooper JB, Cullen DJ. Standards for patient monitoring during anesthesia at Harvard Medical School. JAMA 1986;256:2017.
49. American Society of Anesthesiologists. Standards for basic intraoperative monitoring. ASA Directory of Members, 1991:670.
50. Clark JS, Votteri B, Ariagno RL, et al Park Ridge, IL: State of the art: noninvasive monitoring of blood gases. Am Rev Respir Dis 1992;145:220.
51. Jubran A, Tobin M. Reliability of pulse oximetry in titrating supplemental oxygen therapy in ventilator-dependent patients. Chest 1990;97:1421.
52. Scheid P, Teichman J, Adaro F, et al. Gas-blood CO_2 equilibration in dog lungs during rebreathing. J Appl Physiol 1972;33:582.
53. Clark JS, Cutillo AG, Criddle M, et al. Gas-blood PCO_2 and PO_2 equilibration in a steady-state rebreathing dog preparation. J Appl Physiol 1984; 56:1229.
54. Nye RE. Influence of the cycle pattern on pulmonary gas exchange. Respir Physiol 1970;10:321.
55. Hatle L, Rokseth R. The arterial to end-expiratory carbon dioxide gradient in acute pulmonary embolism and other cardiopulmonary disease. Chest 1974;66:352.
56. Carlon GC, Cole R, Miodownik S, et al. Capnography in mechanically ventilated patients. Crit Care Med 1988;16:550.

57. Kalenda Z. Capnography during anesthesia and intensive care. Acta Anaesthesiol Belg 1978;29:201.
58. Watson R, Benumof J, Clausen J, et al. Expiratory CO_2 plateau predicts airway resistance. Anesthesiology 1989;71:A1072. Abstract.
59. O'Quinn R, Marini J. Pulmonary artery occlusion pressure: clinical physiology, measurement, and interpretation. Am Rev Respir Dis 1983;128:319.
60. Fee HJ. Role of pulmonary vascular resistance measurements in preoperative candidates for pulmonary resection. J Thorac Cardiovasc Surg 1978; 75:519.
61. King DS. Postoperative pulmonary complications: a statistical study based on two years' personal observation. Surg Gynecol Obstet 1932;56:43.
62. Zibrak, JD, O'Donnell CR, Marton K. Indications for pulmonary function testing. Ann Intern Med 1990; 112:763.
63. Gaensler EA, Cugell DW, Lindgren I, et al. The role of pulmonary insufficiency in mortality and invalidism following surgery for pulmonary tuberculosis. J Thorac Cardiovasc Surg 1955;29:163.
64. Woodruff W, Merkel CG, Wright GW. Decision in thoracic surgery as influenced by the knowledge of the pulmonary physiology. J Thorac Cardiovasc Surg 1953;26:156.
65. Becklake MR, Permutt S. Evaluation of tests of lung function for screening for early detection of chronic obstructive lung disease. In: Macklemm PT, Permutt S, eds. The lung in the transition between health and disease. New York: Marcel Dekker, 1979:345.
66. Tisi GM. State of the art: preoperative evaluation of lung function. Am Rev Respir Dis 1979;119:293.
67. Olsen GN, Block AJ, Tobias JA. Prediction of post-pneumonectomy pulmonary function using quantitative macroaggregate lung scanning. Chest 1974;66:13.
68. Burrows B, Earle RH. Prediction of survival in patients with chronic airway obstruction. Am Rev Respir Dis 1969;99:865.
69. Segall JJ, Butterworth BA. Ventilation capacity in chronic bronchitis in relation to carbon dioxide retention. Scand J Respir Dis 1966;47:215.
70. Kristersson S, Lindell SE, Svanberg L. Prediction of pulmonary function loss due to pneumonectomy using ^{133}Xe-radiospirometry. Chest 1972;62:694.
71. Olsen GN. Pulmonary function evaluation of the lung resection candidate: a prospective study. Am Rev Respir Dis 1975;111:379.
72. Juhl B, Frost N. A comparison between measured and calculated changes in the lung function after operation for pulmonary cancer. Acta Anesthesiol Scand Suppl 1975;57:39.
73. Cherniack NS. The clinical assessment of the chemical regulation of ventilation. Chest 1976;70(Suppl): 274.
74. Grenvik A, Eross B, Powner D. Historical survey of mechanical ventilation. Int Anesthesiol Clin 1980; 18:1.
75. Ibsen B. The anesthetist's viewpoint on treatment of respiratory complications in poliomyelitis during the epidemic in Copenhagen. Proc R Soc Med 1954;47:72.
76. Lassen HC. Preliminary report in the 1952 epidemic of poliomyelitis in Copenhagen. Lancet 1953;1:37.
77. Smith RA. Respiratory Care: mechanical. In: Miller R, ed. Anesthesia. 2nd ed. New York: Churchill Livingstone, 1986:2177.
78. Kacmarek RM, Meklaus GJ. The new generation of mechanical ventilators. Crit Care Clin 1990;6:551.
79. Segal BJ, Johnston RP, Donovan DJ, et al. Mechanical ventilation. In: MacDonnell KF, Fahey PJ, Segal BJ, eds. Respiratory intensive care. Boston: Little, Brown, 1987:131.
80. Marini JJ, Capps JS, Culver BH. Mechanical ventilatory support. JAMA 1985;24:90.
81. Rodriguez RM, Marini JJ, Lamb V. Inspiratory work requirement of assisted ventilation. Am Rev Respir Dis 1985;131:A131.
82. Ward ME. Role of initiating inspiratory effort in determining work of breathing during mechanically assisted ventilation. Am Rev Respir Dis 1985; 131:A131.
83. Downs JB, Block AJ, Vennum KB. Intermittent mandatory ventilation in the treatment of patients with chronic obstructive pulmonary disease. Anesth Analg 1974;53:437.
84. Downs JB, Douglas ME. Intermittent mandatory ventilation: why the controversy? Crit Care Med 1981;9:622.
85. Downs JB, Perkins HM, Modell JH. Intermittent mandatory ventilation: an evaluation. Arch Surg 1974;109:519.
86. Marini JJ. Strategies to minimize breathing effort during mechanical ventilation. Crit Care Clin 1990;6:635.
87. MacIntyre NR. Respiratory function during pressure support ventilation. Chest 1986;89:677.
88. MacIntyre NM. Pressure support ventilation. In: Banner MJ, ed. Problems in critical care. Philadelphia: JB Lippincott, 1990:225.

89. White PF. What's new in intravenous anesthetics? Anesthesiol Clin North Am 1988;6:2.
90. Cameron OG. Safe use of haloperidol in a patient with cardiac dysrhythmia. Am J Psychiatry 1978; 135:1244.
91. Sos J, Casssem NH. Managing postoperative agitation. Drug Ther 1980;10:103.
92. Tesar GE, Murray GB, Cassem NH. Use of high-dose intravenous haloperidol in agitated cardiac patients. J Clin Psychopharmacol 1985;5:344.
93. Darrah WC, Johnston JR, Mirakhur RK. Vecuronium infusions for prolonged muscle relaxation in the intensive care unit. Crit Care Med 1989;17:1297.
94. Morris RB, Cahalan MK, Miller RD, et al. The cardiovascular effect of vecuronium (OrgNC45) and pancuronium in patients undergoing coronary artery bypass grafting. Anesthesiology 1983;58:438.
95. Bendixen HH, Bullwinkel B, Hedley-White J, et al. Atelectasis and shunting during spontaneous ventilation in anesthetized patients. Anesthesiology 1964;25:297.
96. Hamilton WK, McDonald JS, Fischer HW, et al. Postoperative respiratory complications. Anesthesiology 1964;25:607.
97. Gorty S. Recovery room care after thoracic surgery. Int Anesthesiol Clin 1983;21:173.
98. Hartz RS. General principles of postoperative care. In: Shields T, ed. General thoracic surgery. 3rd ed. Philadelphia: Lea & Febiger, 1989:319.
99. Egbert LD, Bendixen HH. Effect of morphine on breathing pattern: A possible factor in atelectasis. JAMA 1964;188:485.
100. Ready LB. Acute postoperative pain. In: Miller RD, ed. Anesthesia. New York: Churchill Livingstone, 1990:2137.
101. Sun X, Quinn T, Weissman C. Patterns of sedation and analgesia in the postoperative ICU patient. Chest 1992;101:1625.
102. Tamsen A, Hartvig P, Fagerlund C, et al. Patient-controlled analgesic therapy: Clinical experience. Acta Anesthesiol Scand 1982(Suppl 74)26:157.
103. Wang JK, Nauss LA, Thomas JE. Pain relief by intrathecally applied morphine in man. Anesthesiology 1979;50:149.
104. Behar M, Olshwang D, Magora F, et al. Epidural morphine in the treatment of pain. Lancet 1979; 1:527.
105. Brodsky JB, Shulman MS, Mark BD. Management of postoperative thoracotomy pain: lumbar epidural narcotics. In: Kittle CF, ed. Controversies in thoracic surgery. Philadelphia: WB Saunders, 1986: 228.
106. El-Baz N. Continuous epidural morphine analgesia for pain relief after thoracic surgery. Anesthesiology 1982;57:A205.
107. Miller L, Gertel M, Fox GS, et al. A comparison of narcotic and epidural analgesia on postoperative respiratory function. Am J Surg 1976;131:291.
108. Steidl LJ, Fromme GA, Danielson DR. Lumbar versus thoracic epidural morphine for postthoracotomy pain. Anesth Analg 1984;63:277.
109. Fromme GA, Steidl LJ, Danielson DR. Comparison of lumbar and thoracic epidural morphine for the relief of postthoracotomy pain. Anesth Analg 1985;64:454.
110. Larsen VH, Iversen AD, Christensen P, et al. Postoperative pain treatment after upper abdominal surgery with epidural morphine at the thoracic or lumbar level. Acta Anaesthesiol Scand 1985;29:566.
111. Gregg R. Spinal analgesia. Anesthesiol Clin North Am 1989;7:79.
112. Bromage PR, Camporesi EM, Durant PAC, et al. Nonrespiratory side effects of epidural morphine. Anesth Analg 1982;61:490.
113. Durant PAC, Yaksh TL. Drug effects on urinary bladder tone during spinal morphine-induced inhibition of micturition reflex in unanesthetized rats. Anesthesiology 1988;68:325.
114. Lilley JP, Fromme GA, Wang JK. Management of acute pain. Adv Anesthesiol 1987;4:347.
115. Scott DB. Acute pain management. In: Cousins MJ, Bridenbaugh PO, eds. Neural blockade in clinical anesthesia and management of pain. Philadelphia: JB Lippincott, 1988:861.
116. Crawford ED, Skinner DG. Intercostal nerve block with thoracoabdominal and flank incisions. Urology 1982;19:25.
117. Galway JE, Caves PK, Dundee JW. Effect of intercostal nerve blockade during operation on lung function and relief of pain following thoracotomy. Br J Anaesth 1975;47:730.
118. Shapiro BA, Harrison RA, Kacmerek RM, et al. Maintenance of artificial airways and extubation. In: Shapiro BA, Harrison RA, Kacmerek RM, et al, eds. Clinical applications of respiratory care. 3rd ed. Chicago: Yearbook Medical, 1985:251.
119. Haberman PB, Green JP, Archibald C, et al. Determinants of successful selective tracheobronchial suctioning. N Engl J Med 1973;289:1060.
120. Hirsch SR. In vitro evaluation of expectorant and mucolytic agents. Bull Physiopathol Respir 1973; 9:435.
121. Shim C. Cardiac arrhythmias resulting from tracheal suctioning. Ann Intern Med 1969;71:1149.

122. Sloan HE. Vagus nerve in cardiac arrest. Surg Gynecol Obstet 1950;91:257.
123. O'Donohue WJ. Prevention and treatment of postoperative atelectasis: can it and will it be adequately studied? Chest 1985;87:1. Editorial.
124. Pontoppidan H. Mechanical aids to lung expansion in nonintubated surgical patients. Am Rev Respir Dis 1980 (Part 2);122:109.
125. O'Donohue WJ. National survey of the usage of lung expansion modalities for the prevention and treatment of postoperative atelectasis following abdominal and thoracic surgery. Chest 1985;87:76.
126. Gale GD, Sanders DE. The Bartlett-Edwards incentive spirometer: a preliminary assessment of its use in the prevention of atelectasis after cardiopulmonary bypass. Can J Anaesth 1977;24:408.
127. Turnbull KW, Miyagishima RT, Gerein AN. Pulmonary complications and cardiopulmonary bypass. Can J Anaesth 1974;21:181.
128. Gale GD, Teasdale SJ, Sanders DE, et al. Pulmonary atelectasis and other complications after cardiopulmonary bypass and investigation of aetiologic factors. Can J Anaesth 1979;26:15.
129. Braun SR, Birnbaum ML, Chopra PS. Pre- and postoperative pulmonary function abnormalities in coronary artery revascularization surgery. Chest 1978;73:316.
130. Dull JL, Dull WL. Are maximal inspiratory breathing exercises or incentive spirometry better than early mobilization after cardiopulmonary bypass? Phys Ther 1983;63:655.
131. Jenkins LC, Moxham J. Physiotherapy after coronary artery surgery: are breathing exercises necessary? Thorax 1989;44:634.
132. Bartlett RH. Respiratory therapy to prevent pulmonary complications of surgery. Respir Care 1984; 29:667.
133. Baker JP. Magnitude of usage of intermittent positive-pressure breathing. Am Rev Respir Dis 1974; 11(Suppl):170.
134. Stock MC, Downs JB, Cooper RB, et al. Comparison of continuous positive airway pressure, incentive spirometry, and conservative therapy after cardiac operations. Crit Care Med 1984;12:969.
135. Civetta JM, Brons R, Gabel JC. A simple and effective method of employing spontaneous positive-pressure ventilation. J Thorac Cardiovasc Surg 1972; 63:312.
136. Shah DM, Newell JC, Dutton RE, et al. Continuous positive airway pressure versus positive end-expiratory pressure in respiratory distress syndrome. J Thorac Cardiovasc Surg 1977;74:557.
137. Branson RD, Hurst JM, DeHaven CB. Mask CPAP: state of the art. Respir Care 1985;30:846.
138. DeHaven CB, Hurst JM, Branson RD. Postextubation hypoxemia treated with a continuous positive airway mask. Crit Care Med 1985;13:46.
139. Smith RA. Oxygen therapy. In: Civetta JM, Taylor RW, Kirby RR, eds. Critical care. Philadelphia: JB Lippincott, 1988:137.
140. Sellers WFS, Huggs CMB. Comparison of tracheal oxygen concentrations using Hudson mask, nasal cannula, and nasal catheter. Anesth Analg 1987; 66:S153.
141. Johanson WG, Peters JI. Critical care. In: Murray JF, Nadel JA, eds. Textbook of respiratory medicine. Philadelphia: WB Saunders 1988:1976.
142. Shapiro BA, Harrison RA, Kacmerek RM, et al. Clinical applications of respiratory care. 3rd ed. Chicago: Yearbook Medical, 1985:91.
143. Klein EF, Shah DA, Modell JH, et al. Performance characteristics of conventional and prototype humidifiers and nebulizers. Chest 1973;64:690.
144. Klein EF, Graves SA. "Hot pot" tracheitis. Chest 1974;65:225.
145. Gammage GW. Airway management. In: Civetta JM, Taylor RW, Kirby RR, eds. Critical care. Philadelphia: JB Lippincott 1988:197.
146. Farney RJ, Morris AH, Berlin SL, et al. Oxygen therapy: appropriate use of nebulizers. Am Rev Respir Dis 1977;115:567.
147. Sjostrand U. Review of the physiologic rationale for and development of high frequency, positive-pressure ventilation HFPPV. Acta Anaesth Scand Suppl 1977;644:7.
148. Sjostrand U. High-frequency positive-pressure ventilation (HFPPV): a review. Crit Care Med 1980; 8:345.
149. Sanders RD. Two ventilating attachments for bronchoscopes. Del Med J 1967;39:172.
150. Smith RB. Ventilation at high respiratory frequencies. Anaesthesia 1962;37:1011.
151. Froese AB. High-frequency ventilation. A critical assessment. In Shoemaker WC, ed. Critical care: state of the art. Fullerton CA: Society of Critical Care Med, 1984;5:1.
152. Banner MJ. Technical aspects of high-frequency ventilation. Curr Rev Respir Ther 1985;7:91.
153. Smith RB. Humidification during high-frequency ventilation. Respir Care 1982;27:1371.
154. Gallagher TJ, Klain MM, Carlon GC. Present status of high-frequency ventilation. Crit Care Med 1982; 10:613.

155. Schuster DP, Klain MM, Snyder JV. Comparison of high-frequency jet ventilation to conventional ventilation during acute respiratory failure in humans. Crit Care Med 1982;10:625.
156. Klain MM, Keszler H. High-frequency jet ventilation. Surg Clin North Am 1985;65:917.
157. Carlon GC, Griffin J, Miodownik S, et al. Tidal volume and airway pressure on high-frequency jet ventilation. Crit Care Med 1983;11:83.
158. Carlon GC, Ray C, Klain M, et al. High-frequency positive-pressure ventilation in management of patient with bronchopleural fistula. Anesthesiology 1980;52:160.
159. Derderian SS, Rajagopal KR, Abbrecht PH, et al. High-frequency positive-pressure jet ventilation in bilateral bronchopleural fistulae. Crit Care Med 1982;10:119.
160. Borg U, Eriksson I, Sjostrand U. High-frequency positive-pressure ventilation (HFPPV): a review based upon its use during bronchoscopy and for laryngoscopy and microlaryngeal surgery under general anesthesia. Anesth Analg 1980;59:594.
161. Butler WJ, Bohn DJ, Bryan AC, et al. Ventilation by high-frequency oscillation in humans. Anesth Analg 1980;59:577.
162. Kolton M. A review of high-frequency oscillation. Can J Anaesth 1984;31:416.
163. Bartlett RH, Gazzaniga AB, Jeffries MR, et al. Extracorporeal membrane oxygenation (ECMO) cardiopulmonary support in infancy. Trans Am Soc Artif Intern Organs 1976;22:80.
164. Short BL, Anderson KD. Extracorporeal membrane oxygenation in neonates. In: Shoemaker WC, Ayres S, Grenvik A, et al, eds. Textbook of critical care. 2nd ed. Philadelphia: WB Saunders, 1989:661.
165. Zapal WM. Extracorporeal membrane oxygenation in severe acute respiratory failure: a randomized prospective study. JAMA 1979;242:2193.
166. Gattinoni L, Presenti A, Mascheroni D, et al. Low-frequency positive-pressure ventilation with extracorporeal CO_2 removal in severe acute respiratory failure. JAMA 1986;256:881.
167. Pennington DG, Merjavy JP, Codd JE, et al. Extracorporeal membrane oxygenation for patients with cardiogenic shock. Circulation 1984;70:I130.
168. Bartlett RH, Gazzaniga AB, Fong SW, et al. Extracorporeal membrane oxygenation for cardiopulmonary failure: experience in 28 cases. J Thorac Cardiovasc Surg 1977;73:375.
169. Hill JD. Discussion of the paper by Bartlett RH, et al: Extracorporeal membrane oxygenation support for cardiopulmonary failure. J Thorac Cardiovasc Surg 1975;73;375.
170. Nawa S, Yamada M, Teramato S. Evaluation of conventional circulatory assist devices. Chest 1989; 95:261.
171. Sabiston DC, Spencer F, Gibbons C, eds. Surgery of the chest. 2nd ed. Philadelphia: WB Saunders, 1976:183.
172. Beal JM, ed. Critical care for surgical patients. New York: Macmillan, 1982:124.
173. Lim-Levy F, Babler SA, De Groot-Kosolcharoen J, et al. Is milking and stripping the chest tubes really necessary? Ann Thorac Surg 1986;42:77.

CHAPTER

15

Postoperative Complications

Michael M. Hansen
John W. Hoyt

Postoperative Respiratory Failure

The postoperative thoracic surgery patient has several risk factors for the development of respiratory failure following surgery. Perioperative factors include independent effects of anesthesia, the surgical procedure, and cardiopulmonary bypass effects on pulmonary function.[1] Following thoracic surgery a universal rise in the alveolar-arterial oxygen gradient occurs. The most significant factor in the development of a widened alveolar-arterial gradient is an increase in right-to-left intrapulmonary shunting.[2,3] Arterial hypoxemia is not uncommon. Worsening of the ventilation-perfusion mismatch may also be seen as a result of a variety of factors. Residual effects of anesthetics or other medications that may block hypoxic pulmonary vasoconstriction allow perfusion into poorly ventilated areas of the lung.[4,5] Pulmonary edema from a cardiogenic or noncardiogenic source may also cause worsening oxygenation.

The most common reason for the deterioration of oxygenation is atelectasis, however. Intraoperative changes in lung volume caused by positioning and the effects of anesthesia are well known and contribute to the development of atelectasis.[6–8] Atelectasis promotes entrapment of secretions and worsens the ventilation-perfusion ratio, especially if regional hypoxic-pulmonary vasoconstriction is inadequate and diverts blood flow away from hypoxic areas of the lung toward better ventilated segments.

Delayed respiratory failure that occurs after the immediate postoperative period is a dreaded complication in thoracic surgery. It is the most common serious complication after pulmonary resection. In a recent paper that studied patients undergoing pulmonary resection for bronchial carcinoma, the overall incidence of respiratory failure in the postoperative period was 4.4%. In those patients who developed respiratory failure, the mortality was 50%.[9] In addition, mortality following right-sided pneumonectomy was greater than that following left-sided pneumonectomy; researchers believed that this finding was due to the smaller size of the remaining right lung.

Respiratory failure in postoperative cardiac surgery patients is uncommon. The vast majority of such patients are extubated within the first 12–18 hours after surgery. Although atelectasis, especially in the left lower lobe, is common, few patients require continued mechanical ventilation.[10,11] In addition, the defects in pulmonary function following surgery improve rapidly after mobilization, although they usually do not return to normal for several months.[12] Preexisting lung disease predisposes the patient to postoperative lung complications and respiratory failure. Chronic obstructive pulmonary disease is the most common preoperative lung disorder. Pulmonary function tests performed before surgery may help to identify the patient at high risk for respiratory failure and ventilator dependence in the postoperative period. A patient with a forced expiratory volume in 1 second (FEV_1) of less than 50% of forced vital capacity or less than 50% predicted or an FEV_1 less than 1–1.5 L has an increased risk of postoperative respiratory failure.[13,14] Although the predictive value of preoperative pulmonary function tests for postoperative respiratory failure is not absolute, there is a strong tendency to avoid major thoracic procedures in patients with markedly subnormal pulmonary function tests for fear of resultant ventilator dependence.

Pulmonary Edema

Pulmonary edema may be due to a cardiogenic or noncardiogenic etiology, and postoperative pulmonary edema may cause postoperative respiratory failure. Several factors determine the shift of fluid out of the intravascular space into the surrounding interstitium and ultimately into the alveolar air spaces, where alveolar flooding leads to hypoxemia (Fig. 15-1). Excessive capillary hydrostatic pressure due to volume overload or heart failure results in fluid leakage from the capillaries. Cardiogenic causes of pulmonary edema most commonly involve left ventricular dysfunction with poor systolic or diastolic performance that allow end-diastolic pressures to rise. As left ventricular end-diastolic pressure rises, the back pressure is

$$F = K([P_{mv} - P_i] - S[O_{mv} - O_i])$$

where:
- F = transvascular fluid flux
- K = hydraulic fluid conductance
- P = hydrostatic pressure
- mv = microvascular
- i = interstitial
- S = protein reflection coefficient
- O = protein oncotic pressure

Figure 15-1. The Starling equation. Fluid moves across microvascular endothelium in response to several forces. Increased microvascular hydrostatic pressure (P_{mv}), decreased microvascular oncotic pressure (O_{mv}), and decreased protein reflection coefficient (S) leading to increased permeability and elevated interstitial oncotic pressure (O_i) all promote movement of fluid out of the intravascular space.

transmitted up through the left atrium and into the pulmonary veins and ultimately into the pulmonary capillaries. Pulmonary artery wedge pressure is elevated, reflecting the increased pressure in the left side of the heart. Although an increased wedge pressure often signifies left ventricular failure with a corresponding increase in left ventricular failure and a rise in the left ventricular end-diastolic volume, the wedge pressure may also be elevated in the case of a poorly compliant left ventricle where a relatively normal end-diastolic volume leads to a marked increase in the intraventricular pressures.[15] The patient is not truly volume overloaded but suffers from a stiff ventricular wall that does not allow for normal diastolic relaxation (Fig. 15-2). Diastolic dysfunction is seen in a variety of disorders including hypertrophy,[16] stunned myocardium from postbypass cooling, and ischemia.[17,18] The high diastolic pressures result in pulmonary edema secondary to excessive pulmonary capillary hydrostatic pressure, even though the patient may not be volume overloaded. Some investigators advocate use of a left atrial catheter to measure left-sided pressure.[19] In the first 12 hours after surgery, the pulmonary capillary wedge pressure

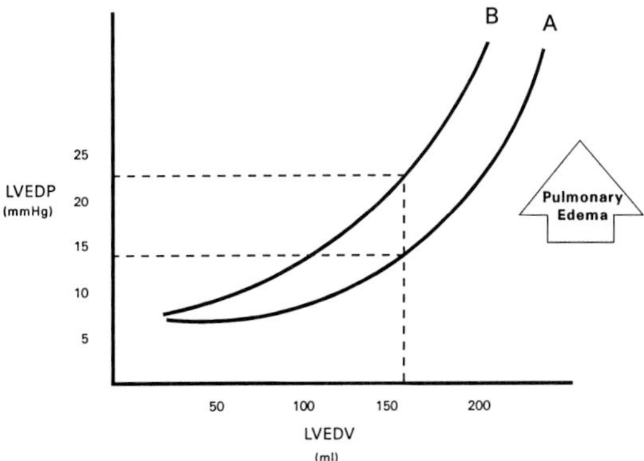

Figure 15-2. Left ventricular compliance curves. The compliance of the ventricle depends on a number of factors. [A] represents a normal compliance curve, and [B] represents a more noncompliant ventricle. With normal left ventricular end-diastolic volumes (LVEDVs), the end-diastolic pressures (LVEDPs) are not elevated to a range that leads to cardiogenic pulmonary edema in a normally compliant heart. In a stiff, noncompliant heart, normal end-diastolic volumes lead to elevated end-diastolic pressures and promote pulmonary edema.

(PCWP) usually exceeds the left atrial pressure, probably because of increased interstitial pulmonary fluid.

The treatment of pulmonary edema may include not only diuretics, but also the addition of agents that increase the compliance of the left ventricle, thus allowing it to accommodate higher filling volumes without leading to excessively high pressures. Nitroglycerine, angiotensin-converting agents, and calcium-channel antagonists have the ability to increase ventricular compliance.[20] Nitroglycerine is also used to treat ischemia that may be contributing to the poor compliance.

Valvular heart disease, including severe mitral stenosis, mitral regurgitation, aortic stenosis with left ventricular decompensation and dilatation may all lead to pulmonary edema secondary to increased pulmonary capillary hydrostatic pressure. Typical murmurs may help suggest the diagnosis. Large V waves in the pulmonary capillary wedge tracing suggests mitral regurgitation. In the postmyocardial infarction patient who develops a new systolic murmur with rapidly progressing pulmonary edema, the diagnosis of ruptured papillary muscle must be entertained.

Noncardiogenic pulmonary edema results from leakage of fluid into the interstitial and alveolar space from causes other than heart failure, poor myocardial compliance, or valvular disease. In this situation, fluid leaks from the intravascular compartment into the interstitium secondary to an increase in capillary permeability or a decrease in the intravascular colloid oncotic pressure.[21] Increases in capillary permeability can be seen in a variety of conditions. Coronary bypass patients tend to develop increased permeability believed to be secondary to the activation of white blood cells and the complement cascade with release of circulating mediators.[22–24] Inflammatory processes such as sepsis syndrome or pneumonia are common causes of capillary leak. Leukoagglutinin reaction from blood transfusions can also increase pulmonary capillary permeability secondary to the release of mediators from the trapped white blood cells in the transfused blood.[25] Anaphylaxis increases capillary permeability partly because of the local effects of histamine; a variety of other mediators are also responsible.[26]

Adult Respiratory Distress Syndrome

Adult respiratory distress syndrome (ARDS) is a severe form of respiratory failure that is secondary to both infectious and noninfectious causes. The syndrome can develop relatively quickly, in less than 24 hours, or can take several days or more to become established. The cardinal appearance on chest radiograph in the absence of cardiogenic pulmonary edema is one of diffuse, bilateral infiltrates.[27–29] Many definitions stipulate that the PCWP be less than

18 mmHg for diagnosis to exclude fluid overload or congestive heart failure as the cause (Table 15-1).[30] (Other characteristics of ARDS include hypoxemia with a widened alveolar-arterial oxygen gradient; stiff, noncompliant lungs; and increased pulmonary capillary permeability resulting in noncardiogenic pulmonary edema. Severe hypoxemia is one of diagnostic criteria for ARDS. The exact etiology of the hypoxemia is unknown. Initial attempts to demonstrate excessive extravascular lung water as the cause of the hypoxemia have failed.[31,32] Ventilation-perfusion mismatching with the loss of pulmonary hypoxic vasoconstriction appears to be one of the major sources of the significant hypoxemia that is often seen.[33,34]

ARDS therapy revolves around initial treatment of the suspected underlying cause. In severe cases, mechanical ventilation is required to establish adequate oxygenation and ventilation. Oxygenation is provided with the application of increased FIO_2 and the addition of positive end-expiratory pressure (PEEP). Oxygen is thought to be toxic at levels of FIO_2 greater than 0.50.[35,36] Therefore PEEP is often added up to 20 cm H_2O or more in an attempt to minimize FIO_2 requirements. Lung compliance is often very poor, and the risk of barotrauma increases as the airway pressures rise. Thus attempts at minimizing high peak airway pressures are made by lowering the tidal volume, increasing the inspiratory time, or by using less conventional modes of ventilation such as pressure-control ventilation, inverse-ratio ventilation, or high-frequency ventilation.[37] These latter modes are used with neuromuscular blocking agents to allow for better tolerance of the ventilator, to decrease the chest wall resistance to lung expansion, and to prevent coughing episodes that would increase airway pressures to dangerous levels.

Table 15-1. Criteria for the Diagnosis of Adult Respiratory Distress Syndrome from the Multicenter Trial for Corticosteroid Therapy*

1. Hypoxemia
   a. $PAO_2 < 70$ mmHg on $FIO_2 = 0.40$, or
   b. $PAO_2/PAO_2 < 0.3$
2. Diffuse bilateral infiltrates on chest x-ray
3. Pulmonary artery occlusion pressure < 18 mmHg

* From: Bernard GR, Luce JM, Sprung CL, et al. High-dose corticosteroids in patients with the adult respiratory distress syndrome. N Engl J Med 1987;317:1565.

Other approaches to ventilation that are being evaluated in the ARDS patient include airway pressure-release ventilation (APRV) where the patient is maintained in inspiration for prolonged cycles interspersed with brief intermittent exhalations[38] and permissive hypercapnia where the patient is allowed to become hypercapneic with or without permissive acidemia.[39,40] Extracorporeal membrane oxygenation (ECMO)[41] and extracorporeal carbon dioxide removal (ECCOR)[42] systems have also been used in the treatment of the severe ARDS. Despite a variety of treatment options, the mortality of patients who develop full-blown ARDS still exceeds 60%.[43] Recent studies have indicated that there may be subsets of patients who have a lower mortality depending on the severity of the syndrome.[44,45]

Postoperative Bleeding

Significant postoperative bleeding requiring transfusion occurs in a minority of thoracic surgery patients. Many such patients have come from the operating room with pleural or mediastinal tubes in place, and excessive bleeding is usually manifested by steady or increasing drainage from one or more of these tubes. Although there is no absolute value for excessive postoperative blood loss, reexploration is usually undertaken if a chest tube is in place and if persistent blood loss is greater than 100 to 200 mL per hour.[46] Some clinicians also measure the hematocrit of the chest drainage; the usual hematocrit is less than 20%. The usual hematocrit will exceed 20% if significant postoperative bleeding occurs into the pleural space or into a mediastinum with a drainage tube in place. The lack of significant drainage does not rule out the possibility of significant postoperative bleeding. Drainage tubes may become clogged with coagulated blood or may not be draining the space where significant bleeding is occurring. Significant amounts of bleeding are usually, but not always, accompanied by overt signs of hypovolemia such as hypotension, tachycardia, and oliguria. If there signs of hypovolemia and bleeding continue to persist, a chest radiograph is obtained to rule out the possibility of a tension hemothorax or pneumothorax. Postoperative bleeding necessitating surgical intervention occurs in approximately 3% of all thoracotomy patients.[47] In cases of major postoperative bleeding requiring a return to the operating room, mortality is quite high and approaches 25%.[47]

In cases of rapid blood loss due to a major vessel leak, life-saving treatment must be instituted in the recovery room or intensive care unit before exsanguination occurs. Measures may include reopening the chest at the bedside, trying to maintain as sterile environment as possible. If the bleeding source is identified, a vascular clamp is placed, if possible, or a ligature is applied while the operating room is being prepared. Of course, blood products are administered as soon as available if indicated by the situation, coagulation profile, or platelet count.

In open-heart patients, approximately 5% of patients require a trip back to the operating room for reexploration within the initial 24 hours to try to control significant postoperative hemorrhage.[48] In most cases, the bleeding source can be identified as a single vessel. Despite meticulous attention to hemostasis and ligation of open vessels prior to chest closure, some vessels may not exhibit significant bleeding until the postoperative period. In some instances, when the patient is reexplored, only diffuse oozing is found. In these circumstances, the bleeding may be attributable to a number of factors including thrombocytopenia, poor platelet function, decreased clotting factors, inadequate heparin reversal, primary fibrinogenolysis, or disseminated intravascular coagulation (DIC).[49]

Platelet function and numbers may be affected by a variety of factors. Preoperative treatment with antiplatelet drugs is one of the most common causes of perioperative platelet dysfunction. Aspirin irreversibly acetylates platelets and may affect bleeding time for up to seven days.[50] In addition, an acquired platelet defect from cardiopulmonary bypass itself appears to be directly related to time spent on the bypass machine.[51] Preoperative medical conditions such as renal failure or liver dysfunction may also adversely affect platelet function. Platelet dysfunction is often suspected when the platelet count is normal, but clot formation is inadequate and can be documented by a prolonged bleeding time. Desmopressin acetate (DDAVP) has been proposed as a treatment for platelet dysfunction based on its ability to raise von Willebrand factor levels, thus enhancing platelet performance.[52,53] Unfortunately, controlled trials have not shown clinical efficacy. The treatment of platelet dysfunction continues to be platelet transfusion.[54]

Thrombocytopenia

A low number of circulating platelets may be responsible for postoperative bleeding. Generally, significant bleeding does not occur until the platelet count falls below 50,000 platelets/dL.[55] Causes of a low platelet count are usually related to one or more etiologies. Excessive fluid administration or transfusion of significant amounts of packed red blood cells, which are low in platelets, may lead to a dilutional thrombocytopenia. In the cardiopulmonary bypass patient, platelets are destroyed while on the bypass circuit but rarely fall below 75,000/dL (assuming the patient's preoperative platelet count was normal).[56] Thrombocytopenia may also be induced by the presence of heparin-dependent antibodies.[57] In the most severe cases, patients with heparin-induced thrombocytopenia may develop intra-arterial thromboses. Heparin-dependent antibodies can be measured by in vitro testing.[58, 59] Treatment requires discontinuation of all heparin, including that present in flush solutions used to maintain patency of indwelling intravascular catheters. In addition, thrombocytopenia may result from a consumption phenomenon that can be seen with significant bleeding and attempted clot formation, or from DIC.[60]

Clotting Factor Abnormalities

Clotting factors or their function may be depressed during or following cardiopulmonary bypass.[61–63] The decrease in clotting factors during bypass appears to be on a dilutional basis. The magnitude of the drop is approximately equal to the fall in the hematocrit. More importantly, the drop in factor levels usually does not approach the level at which spontaneous bleeding occurs, which is at levels less than 30% of normal.[64] Some researchers have suggested that activation of the coagulation cascade occurs during cardiopulmonary bypass, resulting in coagulation factor consumption[65]; however, Wolk and his colleagues have disputed this.[48] DIC resulting in a consumption coagulopathy can occur, but fortunately this is rare. Significant factor deficiencies are manifest by elevation of the protime (PT) or partial thromboplastin time (PTT). The basis of treatment is replacement of the coagulation factors in the form of fresh-frozen plasma or cryoprecipitate. Fresh-frozen plasma, which is administered as a type-specific product, contains all of the clotting factors, including factor V and factor VIII. These two factors are labile factors and are present in stored blood in low concentrations. Cryoprecipitate is the cold-insoluble protein fraction of plasma and contains high levels of factor VIII, von Willebrand's factor, and fibrinogen. It is administered as a pooled product of eight to ten bags for the adult patient.[66]

Excess heparin effect may be implicated as a cause of postoperative bleeding in the postcardiopulmonary bypass patient. The influence of heparin on coagulation is measured by the degree of prolongation of either the PTT or the activated clotting time (ACT). The continuation of the heparin effect into the postoperative period may be secondary to excessive heparin dosing, heparin rebound, or improper protamine neutralization. Excessive protamine sulfate may also be a cause of significant bleeding.[67] Interestingly, Wolk and his colleagues and Umlas[67] have shown that in most cases of cardiopulmonary bypass, the protamine doses are too high for the amount of heparin administered and metabolized. They have suggested that a quantitative heparin assay be used before protamine is given. Although protamine is commonly infused in slight excess, a clinically apparent anticoagulant effect is usually not seen.

Excessive Fibrinolysis

Excessive fibrinolysis occurs in patients who have been treated with thrombolytic therapy as well as in patients who have been supported with extracorporeal circulation. In both instances the plasminogen activator that converts plasminogen to plasmin increases. Plasmin degrades the fibrin meshwork of any exposed clot surface. The result is a breakdown of fibrin with resultant clot weakening and potential bleeding.[68–70] Epsilon-aminocaproic acid (EACA) inhibits the proteolytic activity of plasmin and the conversion of plasminogen to plasmin by plasminogen activator. Several investigators have advocated the use of EACA either on a prophylactic basis[71] or when spontaneous bleeding occurs in the postoperative setting.[72–74] Fibrinogen is often consumed in a fibrinolytic state and may be replaced by administering pooled cryoprecipitate.[66]

Additional methods and treatments to attempt to decrease postoperative bleeding in the cardiac surgical population are numerous. The application of positive end-expiratory pressure (PEEP) has been advocated to decrease the amount of bleeding and to avert reexploration in patients with significant postoperative blood loss.[75,76] The mechanism is thought to involve increased mediastinal pressure resulting from augmented lung inflation and compression of small blood vessels. The routine application of PEEP in the postoperative period does not appear to affect the amount of blood loss, the need for reexploration for bleeding, or the blood requirements.[77,78] High-dose aprotinin, a plasmin and kallikrein inhibitor, has been used in a small number of patients; this agent may prove useful in decreasing the amount of postoperative blood loss in open-heart patients.[79]

Following pulmonary resection, the causes of significant postoperative bleeding are usually due to either slippage of a pulmonary vessel suture or ligature, diffuse bleeding from raw surfaces, or systemic arterial bleeding.[80] Slippage of a ligature off a major pulmonary vessel is often a postoperative catastrophe. Although the pulmonary vessels are part of a low pressure system, hemorrhage from these vessels is often massive because they usually bleed into a high volume space. Factors used to decrease the risk of postoperative bleeding from major pulmonary vessels include meticulous surgical technique, taking care to perform careful dissection; scrupulous detail to assure hemostasis prior to closure; single-lung ventilation; and occasionally an intrapericardial approach to lung resection.

Hemorrhage from the raw surfaces created during surgery is more common with pneumonectomy than lobectomy. Following lobectomy, the remaining lobes of the lung expand and directly appose the chest wall and mediastinum, allowing a tamponade effect to decrease the tendency to bleed. Raw pleural surfaces are especially prone to bleed when vascular connections between the visceral and parietal pleura have been divided. These connections are often seen when adhesions are present between the lung and the inner chest wall, such as in an organized loculated pleural effusion or a tumor extension from the lung.

Systemic arterial bleeding after pulmonary surgery occurs when one of the bronchial vessels has been cut or torn during surgery and has not been adequately ligated or coagulated before closure. Bronchial vessels are usually ligated during bronchial stump closure following resection, but they may retract into the connective tissue from spasm prior to ligation. Bleeding may occur postoperatively from these vessels when the spasm is spontaneously relieved. Other sources of systemic arterial bleeding include intercostal vessels that may be damaged from periosteal closure at the end of the case or during thoracostomy tube placement and mediastinal vessels that are damaged during dissection.[81]

Cardiac Tamponade

Cardiac tamponade results from blood or fluid accumulation in the pericardial space or mediastinum that restricts the diastolic filling of the ventricles. The resultant decrease in the end-diastolic volume leads to a progressive decline in cardiac output that may lead to frank shock. Cardiac tamponade after noncardiac surgery, which is an unusual occurrence, is rarely reported. The underlying cause of such a situation is often an inadvertent needle injury during the course of the surgical procedure.[82] In postoperative cardiac patients, the incidence is reported to be 3.4%–5.8% of patients.[83,84]

Classical signs of tamponade include tachycardia and hypotension coupled with an increase in the pulsus paradoxus and an associated rise in the central venous pressure (Table 15-2). If a pulmonary artery catheter is in place, there is a rise and equalization of the pulmonary artery wedge pressure, right ventricular end-diastolic pressure, central venous pressure, and the pulmonary diastolic pressure.[85] These indices presumably reflect the global increase in the pericardial pressure. Hypotension ensues because of poor ventricular filling due to external compression and deformation. In the postoperative patient, tamponade is frequently not uniform, and compression of one or more of the chambers may be asymmetric. This may lead to very atypical presentations or hemodynamics. Thus the diagnosis of pericardial tamponade must be entertained in any postoperative patient who is hemodynamically unstable and at risk.[86,87]

Table 15-2. Signs of Cardiac Tamponade

Increased pulsus paradoxus
Equalization and elevation of central venous pressure, pulmonary artery diastolic pressure, pulmonary capillary wedge pressure
Electrical alternans on ECG
Hypotension
Depressed cardiac output
Tachycardia
Mediastinal widening on chest x-ray
Echocardiographic findings
Fluid collection in pericardial space
Diastolic compression of right ventricle
Inadequate ventricular filling secondary to compression
Findings may be atypical in postoperative patient

Unfortunately, no single finding or constellation of findings is sufficient to diagnose pericardial tamponade. The differentiation between tamponade and a low output state due to myocardial insufficiency can be difficult. Elevation of the central venous pressure can be seen with fluid overload, right heart and biventricular failure, as well as with tamponade. Distant heart tones, enlarged cardiac silhouette on chest radiograph, and low voltage on the surface electrocardiogram (ECG), which are all very nonspecific, can be seen frequently in the postoperative cardiac patient without tamponade.

Echocardiogram has been the diagnostic test of choice in pericardial tamponade. The appearance of pericardial fluid with diastolic compression of the right ventricle is suggestive of the diagnosis. Although echocardiogram can help support the diagnosis, it does not establish tamponade physiology.[88,89] Transesophageal echocardiography has been more helpful in the diagnosis, especially when the presentation is atypical, as in tamponade from a posteriorly located clot that does not cause enlargement of the cardiac silhouette.

Tamponade may be present with any amount of fluid or clot in the pericardial space. Loculation of material may affect cardiac function leading to tamponade physiology.[90,91] Preexisting cardiac dysfunction can predispose a patient to tamponade and lower the requirements of intrapericardial fluid required to produce decompensation.[92]

Postoperative pericardial tamponade is usually evident within the first 24 hours after surgery. Most of the cases occur in patients who have had significant postoperative bleeding or who have a bleeding diathesis secondary to anticoagulation, DIC, thrombocytopenia, etc. Late presentation has been reported, and diagnosis may easily be missed by an atypical presentation.[93,94]

Treatment of cardiac tamponade requires urgent drainage of the pericardial space. Postoperative patients who manifest tamponade physiology early are usually taken back to the operating room for open drainage and evacuation of the pericardial cavity. Attention is directed at finding a possible source of pericardial bleeding. Temporizing measures that can be utilized prior to surgical drainage are volume loading, reduction of airway pressures by decreasing the PEEP and tidal volume in the intubated patient, and using inotropic and pressor agents to support blood pressure. Late tamponade may be treated by placing a drainage catheter into the pericardial space via a percutaneous approach. Even small amounts of fluid removal from the pericardial space may result in dramatic improvements in the patient's hemodynamic status.

Cardiac Herniation

Cardiac herniation is one of the major life-threatening complications of thoracic surgery in the immediate postoperative period. It is a relatively rare complication of intrapericardial pneumonectomy for lung cancer. The intrapericardial approach, which allows easier access to major vessels and a wider hilar dissection, may result in a large pericardial defect that is unable to be closed once pneumonectomy is accomplished. The heart then slips through the pericardial defect into the empty hemithorax and develops a volvulus that leads to obstruction of blood flow into and out of the heart. Hypotension and ultimately death may result if this condition is not corrected.[95–98] Overall mortality is 50%.[99,100]

The herniation, which can be either into the right or left hemithorax, is associated with profound cardiovascular compromise. In right-sided herniation, the entire heart protrudes through the pericardial defect and lies in the right hemithorax. Right-sided herniation usually causes cardiac torsion, resulting in obstruction at the atriocaval junction and ventricular outflow tracts.[101–103] Twisting of the superior vena cava causes acute superior vena cava syndrome, and twisting of the inferior vena cava leads to cardiac collapse due to the lack of venous return. The chest radiograph reveals the cardiac silhouette in the right chest; the apex of the heart is pointing to the right and at times even touches the chest wall. Other radiographic signs that may help with diagnosis are the presence of a notch between the right heart border and the great vessels, displaced thoracostomy tubes, clockwise rotation of the pulmonary artery catheter, and kinking of the central venous catheter at the brachiocephalic junction.[104,105]

In left-sided herniation, the ventricular apex protrudes through the pericardial defect into the left hemithorax. The ventricles become incarcerated as the heart is trapped at the level of the atrioventricular groove.[95] Myocardial ischemia with infarction or fibrillation ensues as the herniated segment of ventricle becomes more edematous. Ventricular outflow obstruction may occur, leading to hypotension. Electrocardiographic changes consistent with ischemia are common. The chest radiograph usually reveals that the heart has assumed a hemispherical shape and has been displaced laterally at a right angle to the mediastinum. A notch is seen between the great vessels and the more lateral herniating cardiac margin.[95,103]

Most cases of cardiac herniation occur within a few hours of surgery, and in the majority of these cases the condition develops immediately after the patient is turned from the lateral decubitus to the supine position. Other factors that can initiate cardiac herniation are (1) rolling the patient onto the side of the pericardial defect, allowing gravity to pull the heart into the empty hemithorax; (2) hyperinflation of the remaining lung that pushes the heart into the empty hemithorax; (3) application of suction to thoracostomy drainage tubes left in the operative hemithorax; and (4) coughing attacks that lead to an increase in pleural pressure in the remaining lung, promoting displacement of the heart into the contralateral hemithorax.[101]

The differential diagnosis includes myocardial ischemia and infarction, cardiac tamponade, massive pulmonary embolus, acute airway obstruction, and rapidly developing hypovolemia from acute hemorrhage. Treatment almost always involves immediate reexploration. Temporizing measures may be tried while the operating room is being readied for surgery. These more conservative measures may improve cardiovascular function before and during transfer to operating suite. Initially the patient should be placed in a lateral decubitus position with the operative hemithorax in the superior position. This encourages the return of the heart towards the midline and possibly back into the pericardial sac. Even if the heart does not reenter the pericardium, the torsion on the heart may be sufficiently relieved to allow restoration of adequate blood flow through the cardiac chambers. In addition, decreasing the level of positive-pressure ventilation in the remaining lung may allow the heart to return to a more normal position. This is accomplished by lowering the tidal volume and removing PEEP. The respiratory rate may need to be increased to maintain an adequate minute ventilation. Suction to the evacuated hemithorax should be discontinued to decrease any tendency of the negative intrahemithoracic pressure to draw the heart into the empty space. Some investigators have proposed injecting one to two liters of air into the operative hemithorax to push the heart and mediastinum towards the midline.[99,106,107]

Postoperative Arrhythmias

Arrhythmias following thoracic surgery are common, and both ventricular and supraventricular arrhythmias may be evident. Since the emergence of cardiac surgery in the 1950s, postoperative arrhythmias have been recognized as a common occurrence. Interestingly, the incidence and types of arrhythmias in the postthoracic surgery patient have not changed dramatically since the advent of the myocardial revascularization and the era of valve replacement. Several factors appear to contribute to the development of postoperative arrhythmias, including advanced age, hypoxia, preexisting coronary artery disease, and electrolyte problems.[108]

Supraventricular Arrhythmias

Sinus tachycardia is a common rhythm seen in the postoperative setting. The causes are myriad, but the clinician must consider possible serious etiologies. In the immediate postoperative period, pain and anxiety are frequent contributors to the development of sinus tachycardia. Catecholamine levels also tend to be elevated following surgery, predisposing patients to this arrhythmia.[109] Other important causes that must be excluded are hypovolemia, anemia, and hypoxia. Fever is usually accompanied by sinus tachycardia. Patients who require postoperative therapy with beta-adrenergic agents to support the cardiovascular system often become tachycardic. In addition, patients treated with systemic bronchodilators such as aminophylline may become tachycardic even when their serum concentrations are in the normal range.[110]

The incidence of supraventricular tachyarrhythmias is close to 30% following coronary artery bypass surgery,[111] and the number of occurrences is even higher following valve surgery and in the elderly. Supraventricular arrhythmias are seen in almost 60% of older patients undergoing aortic valve replacement.[112] Although sinus tachycardia is by far the most common arrhythmia seen, atrial fibrillation and flutter are also frequently observed. Paroxysmal atrial tachycardia and junctional rhythms are less common. All of these arrhythmias are also frequently seen following pulmonary surgery, especially pulmonary resection.[113, 114] Proposed causes of atrial arrhythmias following pulmonary resection include trauma to the heart, especially the right ventricle, during surgery; right atrial distension due to pulmonary hypertension; and hypoxia. The high incidence of preexisting cardiac disease in elderly patients appears to predispose them to postoperative arrhythmias.

Causes for supraventricular arrhythmias following cardiac surgery have been attributed to a number of factors, including unprotected ischemia,[115, 116] cardioplegic solution containing high levels of potassium,[117] pericarditis induced by the operation,[118] and the presence of pericardial fluid following surgery.[119] High catecholamine levels in the postoperative period also may play a role.[109] Interestingly, age, sex, severity of symptoms, cardiomegaly, heart failure, previous myocardial infarction, and number of bypass grafts do not appear to be independent risk factors for the development of atrial fibrillation following non-valve replacement cardiac surgery.[120]

Although supraventricular arrhythmias can occur at any time following surgery, they are most commonly seen between the third and fifth postoperative day.[121] Usually the occurrence of a supraventricular arrhythmia does not lead to hemodynamic deterioration. Most patients remain asymptomatic or experience a light feeling of palpitations. Blood pressure and cardiac output may fall but are usually maintained at an acceptable level. Certain marginal patients, who depend on atrial contraction for adequate ventricular filling, can experience an appreciable and sometimes destabilizing drop in the cardiac output. This is especially true for the patient with preexisting cardiac disease and marginal ventricular function. Blood pressure may also drop significantly if the rate of the arrhythmia is very fast, usually in excess of 180 beats/min. Inadequate time for diastolic filling of the ventricle may also result in a decreased cardiac output. Patients with partial or incomplete myocardial revascularization are unlikely to tolerate a rapid atrial tachyarrhythmia. The increase in myocardial oxygen consumption coupled with the low diastolic filling time leads to an imbalance in the oxygen supply and demand. This produces an ischemic state that can be manifest by anginal pain and ventricular dysfunction.[122]

Prophylaxis of Supraventricular Arrhythmias

Much controversy exists in the area of chemical prophylaxis of supraventricular tachyarrhythmias in patients undergoing cardiac surgery. Preoperative treatment with 1–1.5 mg of oral digoxin started two to three days before surgery has been advocated by some clinicians. Johnson[123] found that using this regimen resulted in a much lower incidence of postoperative supraventricular arrhythmias (5.5%) than in the control group (26%). Csicsko[124] also demonstrated that giving digoxin in the immediate postoperative period lowered the incidence of postoperative atrial tachyarrhythmias from 15% to 2%. Other studies have not been able to demonstrate a benefit of prophylactic digitalis, and some have shown that it may even favor the development of postoperative arrhythmias.[125]

Prophylactic use of digoxin has been recommended by some investigators for patients undergoing pulmonary resection, especially pneumonectomy.[114] Much of the data is based on retrospective analysis of these patients. Reports have also shown an actual increase in the number of more serious arrhythmias in those patients pretreated with digoxin prior to pulmonary resection.[126,127]

Beta-blocking agents have also been used in an attempt to prevent postoperative supraventricular arrhythmias. Numerous studies have shown that postoperative administration of propranolol can reduce the incidence of postoperative atrial tachyarrhythmias after cardiac surgery.[128–131] Some clinicians prefer to use both a beta-blocking agent along with digoxin to try to minimize the incidence of such arrhythmias.[132,133] Not all studies are conclusive concerning the use of beta-blocking agents or digitalis glycosides in the prevention of postoperative arrhythmias; many physicians begin medical therapy only after an arrhythmia has occurred.

Treatment of Specific Arrhythmias

Sinus Tachycardia

Sinus tachycardia is often not treated unless the physician believes that the patient may be compromised from the arrhythmia. Treatment, if undertaken, is directed toward the underlying cause. Hematocrit level, arterial blood gases, and electrolytes are checked to see if they can provide an explanation for the tachycardia. Fever is treated with antipyretics. Pain and anxiety are controlled with analgesics and sedative medications as needed. Fluid status is assessed for signs of hypovolemia; often a fluid challenge is given if the patient may possibly be intravascularly depleted.

If no obvious or easily correctable cause for the sinus tachycardia is apparent, and the patient is at risk for compromise because of the rapid rate, then pharmacologic therapy can be used. Beta-blocking drugs have been used the most for this purpose. Propranolol, 10–40 mg orally or 0.5–2 mg intravenously will controls the heart rate. Esmolol, a short-acting intravenous beta-blocker, can be used as a continuous infusion for rate control.[134] Since beta-blocking agents can exert a negative inotropic effect and provoke bronchospasm in patients at risk, administration of these drugs must be carefully monitored.

Atrial Tachyarrhythmia

Treatment of atrial arrhythmias should be aimed initially at correcting potential underlying etiologies such as hypoxia or electrolyte disturbances. Therapy is then directed at adequate rate control of the tachyarrhythmia and finally conversion back to sinus rhythm. Digoxin is the mainstay for the initial treatment of atrial arrhythmias with a non-life-threatening, rapid, ventricular response. Digoxin increases vagal tone and leads to a slowing in the heart rate. Orthograde conduction through the A-V node is delayed. Unfortunately, digoxin is not very effective in converting atrial tachyarrhythmias back to sinus rhythm.[135] In addition, the maximum effect of digoxin is not seen for a several hours after a loading dose is administered.[136]

For more immediate control of the ventricular response rate in atrial tachyarrhythmias, calcium-blocking agents are employed. Verapamil can be given intravenously in 2–5 mg-increments at 5–10-minute intervals. A maintenance infusion of verapamil at 5–15 mg/h can be used to sustain rate control if needed. Hypotension, which is not uncommon with bolus therapy, can be reduced by pretreatment with intravenous calcium.[137] Diltiazem is also available for intravenous treatment of atrial tachyarrhythmias.[138,139] A 10-mg loading dose is administered intravenously followed by an infusion of 10 mg/h. Additional doses are given as needed, and the drip can be increased up to 20 mg/h. Diltiazem may be associated with less hypotension and negative inotropic effect than verapamil.

Esmolol, an ultrashort-acting, intravenous beta-blocking agent, has recently been shown to be quite effective in controlling the ventricular response rate in postoperative atrial tachyarrhythmias.[134,140] Administration of a continuous infusion of the drug allows for smoother rate control. The short half-life also allows for efficient titration and rapid disappearance of the drug once the infusion is stopped should undesirable side effects occur. The incidence of conversion back to sinus rhythm may be superior to other agents such as verapamil and diltiazem.[141]

If the patient remains in a new atrial arrhythmia and the above measures do not result in conversion back to sinus rhythm, attempts are made to convert the patient with a type IA antiarrhythmic agent. The prototype drug is quinidine. Quinidine is usually administered orally with a loading dose of up to 1000 mg over 12 hours; a maintenance dose of 200–300 mg every six to eight hours is then continued. Most patients convert to sinus rhythm within the first two to three days if they are going to respond to the drug.[142] Intravenous procainamide can also be used. A loading dose of 10–20 mg/kg is given, which is followed by a continuous infusion of 2–3 mg/min.[143] Hypotension may be seen during loading and can be treated with fluid administration and by slowing the infusion rate. Type IA antiarrhythmic agents can accelerate conduction through the A-V node, and adequate pretreatment with digoxin or another rate-controlling medication should be used before administering the type IA drug for atrial fibrillation to protect against an accelerated ventricular response rate.

Intravenous adenosine triphosphate is a new agent for the rapid diagnosis and control of atrial tachyarrhythmias.[144] Intravenous adenosine works within seconds following a rapid initial bolus of 6–12 mg by blocking the antegrade slow pathway through the A-V node. This agent is usually reserved for patients with paroxysmal atrial tachycardia and is often ineffective in patients with atrial fibrillation. The drug is metabolized rapidly in the serum; its half-life is approximately 10 seconds.[144–146] Postbolus rhythms of bradycardia, transient asystole, and high-grade heart block may occur but are usually very short-lived. Many patients convert back to sinus rhythm as the reentrant circuit is blocked. The differentiation of a wide-complex tachycardia is another potential use for intravenous adenosine. If the occurrence of a ventricular tachycardia or a supraventricular tachycardia with aberrant conduction is in question, adenosine may very well terminate the supraventricular rhythm and convert the patient back to sinus rhythm.[147] With ventricular tachycardia, there is usually no response in the rhythm, and the short half-life of the drug and minimal side effects do not pose an ongoing risk to the patient. Side effects of a calcium-blocking agent can be significant.[148]

Electrical Cardioversion

Electrical cardioversion is attempted in patients who continue to have persistent, sustained supraventricular tachyarrhythmias despite drug therapy or who become hemodynamically unstable from the tachyarrhythmia. Cardioversion is more commonly required for patients who have undergone valve surgery, especially at the mitral location, since they appear to be more refractory to medical therapy.[149] Chronic sustained atrial fibrillation of more than one year's duration is usually resistant to attempts at conversion to sinus rhythm by either the pharmacologic or electrical route. Attempts at conversion in these patients with these conditions are not made. Even if sinus rhythm is established in this group of patients, almost all revert back to atrial fibrillation after a short time.

The major risk of cardioversion in patients with atrial fibrillation is thromboembolism. The overall risk appears to be around 0.5%.[150] Guidelines suggest that if patients have been in atrial fibrillation for longer than a few days, formal anticoagulation should be undertaken for a period of at least one week before cardioversion is attempted.[151–153] If the patient has been receiving digoxin to control the arrhythmia, cardioversion is avoided unless absolutely necessary as the postcardioversion arrhythmias increase. In patients on chronic digoxin therapy, the daily dose is withheld on the day of planned cardioversion.

Cardioversion is performed only in a monitored setting with resuscitation equipment close at hand. The patient is sedated with a drug that allows amnesia for the procedure. We use a short-acting benzodiazepine such as midazolam, 2–5 mg intravenously, and assess for adequate sedation before performing the cardioversion. Oxygen is given by nasal cannula or mask. Synchronized direct current shocks are administered in a stepwise fashion starting at a low energy level (20–50 J).

Overdrive Pacing

This technique involves pacing the atria at a rate exceeding the spontaneous rate and abruptly terminating pacemaker discharges. Electrocardiographic monitoring of several leads must document atrial capture at the overdrive rate. Normal sinus rhythm is frequently restored by this maneuver. Rapid stimulation of the atrium using surgically implanted epicardial pacemaker wires can frequently control and terminate atrial flutter and paroxysmal supraventricular tachycardia.[154] Atrial fibrillation is usually not responsive to atrial overdrive pacing. Patients who experience refractory or recurrent bouts of atrial flutter or supraventricular tachycardia should be treated with the addition of pharmacologic agents such as digoxin and a type IA antiarrhythmic, such as quinidine or procainamide, or a beta-blocking drug.

Ventricular Arrhythmia

Ventricular ectopy is common in the postoperative thoracic surgery patient. Ventricular ectopy is evident following pulmonary resection but is seen much less often than atrial arrhythmias.[155] Ventricular arrhythmias, including nonsustained ventricular tachycardia, that necessitate at least a short course of antiarrhythmic therapy are found in up to 50% of patients who have undergone open-heart surgery.[156, 157] In all cases the highest incidence occurs within the first week of surgery; it increases markedly on the third and fourth postoperative days.[156] Possible causal mechanisms include elevated circulating catecholamines, myocardial ischemia, hypoxia, electrolyte abnormalities, and side effects of medication.

The decision to treat postoperative ventricular arrhythmias is controversial. Clinicians generally agree that if the ventricular ectopy is sustained or leads to hemodynamic deterioration, it must be treated aggressively. Ectopy associated with myocardial infarction is treated as well. Once ventricular ectopy is noted, arterial blood gases, electrolytes, and a hematocrit are obtained. The ECG is checked for evidence of ischemia. Historically, occasional premature beats have not been treated unless they exceed six per minute. Other indications for treatment have included R-on-T phenomenon, frequent couplets, or multifocal beats.[157]

Intravenous lidocaine is used to treat ventricular ectopy initially.[158] A loading dose of 1 mg/kg is given, followed by a constant infusion of 2 mg/min. For persistent ectopy, lidocaine can be rebolused and the infusion increased to

4 mg/min if needed. Side effects include disorientation and agitation, especially in elderly patients with compromised hepatic function. If lidocaine fails to suppress the arrhythmia, intravenous procainamide is the second drug of choice. A loading dose of 5 to 10 mg/kg is given at a rate not exceeding 20–30 mg/min, followed by a constant infusion of 2 mg/min. Hypotension is not uncommon and is often effectively treated with fluids, a reduction in the administration rate of the loading dose, and occasionally, pressor agents.

Sustained ventricular tachycardia is always treated aggressively. If the patient is conscious and is not hemodynamically compromised, then a trial of intravenous lidocaine or a type I antiarrhythmic agent may be tried. Attention should also being given to the addition of oxygen and correction of any electrolyte abnormalities (Table 15-3). An empiric dose of 1–2 grams of intravenous magnesium is administered by many physicians. Close attention must be continually given to the patient because of the risk of hemodynamic destabilization or degeneration into ventricular fibrillation. Resuscitation equipment must be nearby. Sustained ventricular tachycardia with hemodynamic deterioration or ventricular fibrillation is most effectively treated with electrical direct-current countershock.[158]

Pulmonary Hypertension and Cor Pulmonale

Following pulmonary resection and especially pneumonectomy, the total cross section of the pulmonary vasculature markedly decreases. Significant increases in pulmonary vascular resistance may occur, and pulmonary hypertension usually ensues. The right ventricle may be unable to keep up with the higher workload imposed by the increased afterload. Right ventricular dilation and the poor filling of the left heart occur due to decreased pulmonary blood flow. Blood pressure may fall secondary to inadequate preload of the left ventricle. A shift in the ventricular septum to the left due to the contin-

Table 15-3. Antiarrhythmic Drugs*

Drug Class	Elimination Half-life (h)	Renal Clearance (%)	Protein Binding (%)	Daily Dose (mg)	Therapeutic Serum Level (μg/mL)
IA					
Quinidine	8	20	70	600–2400	2–6
Procainamide	3	65	15	1000–9000	4–10
Disopyramide	8	55	30	400–1600	2–5
IB					
Lidocaine	1–8	2	50	1–4mg/min	1–5
Mexiletene	10	10	70	600–1200	0.75–2
Tocainide	12	40	10	1200–2400	3–10
IC					
Flecainide	16	40	40	200–600	0.2–1.0
Propafenone	2–10	1	97	450–900	Not known
III					
Amiodarone	19–56 days	min	90	200–600	1.0–2.5

* Modified from: Dunbar DN, Pentel PR. Antiarrhythmic drug toxicity. In: Rippe JM, Irwin RS, Alpert JS, et al, eds. Intensive care medicine. 2nd ed. Boston: Little, Brown, 1991:1174.

ued enlargement of the right ventricle may also hamper left ventricular performance.[159]

Pulmonary venous hypertension of long duration, especially in patients with mitral valve disease, often leads to a marked increase in pulmonary vascular resistance. Pulmonary arterial hypertension results. Following normalization of the left atrial pressure, as in mitral valve replacement, the pulmonary vascular resistance returns toward normal, and the pulmonary arterial hypertension usually resolves. Some patients have persistent pulmonary hypertension despite adequate surgical correction.[160] In postoperative cardiac patients with persistent pulmonary hypertension, right ventricular failure can easily ensue secondary to the increased afterload effects. Poor preservation of the right ventricle during surgery promotes postoperative right ventricular dysfunction, and predisposes patients to ventricular decompensation in the face of pulmonary hypertension.

Treatment of pulmonary hypotension involves supporting right ventricular function with inotropic agents such as dobutamine or isoproterenol, which tend to have a favorable effect on pulmonary vascular resistance. Amrinone, a phosphodiesterase inhibitor, may also provide inotropic support and possesses pulmonary vasodilating properties.[161] Inotropic drugs are usually combined with vasodilating agents in an attempt to decrease right ventricular preload and afterload. Such agents as nitroprusside, nitroglycerine, and phentolamine are agents that have been used.[162] Prostaglandin E_1, a potent systemic and pulmonary vasodilator, may be used in refractory cases of severe pulmonary hypertension.[163] Intra-aortic balloon pumping may have a beneficial effect in decompensated right heart failure, especially if right ventricular ischemia has occurred as a result of coronary artery disease.[164] A pulmonary artery counterpulsation balloon has also been developed and has shown some promise in the treatment of right ventricular failure.[165] Correction of hypoxemia and acidosis is essential, as these conditions lead to further pulmonary vasoconstriction.

Pulmonary Embolism

The actual incidence of pulmonary embolism after thoracic surgery is unknown. Pulmonary embolism after cardiac surgery is thought to be rare. Systemic heparinization during cardiopulmonary bypass likely prevents the development of deep venous thrombosis, at least intraoperatively. Retrospective analysis has suggested that the incidence of pulmonary embolism after cardiac operations is less than 1%.[166] Risk factors in this study were prolonged preoperative or postoperative bed rest, prolonged hospitalization before surgery, recent cardiac catheterization through the groin, postoperative congestive heart failure, and deep venous thrombosis. In patients developing a postoperative pulmonary embolus, mortality was 34%.

The origin of pulmonary emboli are venous thromboses in over 90% of cases.[167] Virchow defined three factors that must be present in order for venous thrombosis to occur[168]: stasis of blood flow, hypercoaguable state, and endothelial injury. Research has shown that the intrinsic fibrinolytic system is markedly impaired following surgery or trauma when the risk for venous thrombosis is high.[169] The diagnosis of pulmonary embolism is often missed.[170] If the condition is left untreated, the recurrence rate is 30%. The acute mortality rate, which increases with each recurrent episode, is approximately 11%.

Signs and Symptoms

The most common symptom experienced in patients with acute pulmonary embolism is dyspnea (Table 15-4). The common ventilatory response is hyperventilation; the partial pressure of carbon dioxide measured by arterial blood gas is decreased, reflecting respiratory alkalosis.[171] Because of the low perfusion, the ventilation-perfusion ratio is elevated due to the increase in the dead space ventilation. Local bronchoconstriction may occur leading to localized wheezing,[172] and inadequate surfactant production in the area may result in alveolar collapse.[173]

Hypoxemia is almost universal in patients with pulmonary embolism.[174,175] Although the exact cause is not known, ventilation-perfusion abnormalities that accompany pulmonary embolism are the most likely cause of the hypoxemia. Other factors that may contribute to the fall in oxygen are anatomic right-to-left shunts, decreased cardiac output with lower mixed venous blood oxygen saturation, and impaired oxygen uptake in the lungs due to pulmonary edema.[176] If the pulmonary artery pressure becomes high enough, right ventricular and right atrial pressures rise and may allow opening of a probe-patent foramen ovale, which further contributing to arterial hypoxemia.

Table 15-4. Clinical Presentation of Pulmonary Embolism*

1. Worsening arterial hypoxemia and respiratory alkalosis in the spontaneously ventilating patient.
2. Worsening dyspnea and arterial hypoxemia unresponsive to bronchodilators despite a reduction in arterial PCO_2 in the patient with chronic lung disease and known CO_2 retention.
3. Worsening hypoxemia, hypercapnea, and respiratory acidosis in the sedated patient on controlled mechanical ventilation.
4. Unexplained fever or development of atelectasis or a pleural-based infiltrate.
5. Spontaneous development of pulmonary hypertension in a hemodynamically monitored patient.
6. Sudden elevation of central venous pressure in conjunction with evidence of impaired organ perfusion.
7. Development of unexplained tachycardia and tachypnea.

* From Benotti JR, Dalen JE, Alpert JS. Pulmonary embolism. In: Rippe JM, Irwin RS, Alpert JS, et al, eds. Intensive care medicine. 2nd ed. Boston: Little, Brown, 1991:308.

Hemodynamically, the most common response to pulmonary embolism is sinus tachycardia. The spectrum of presentation is wide, however, it ranges from tachycardia to overt cardiovascular collapse. In general, clinical manifestations reflect the extent of embolization and the pulmonary reserve.[177] Pulmonary hypertension is common, and it reflects not only the mechanical obstruction but also the effect of local mediators released from the clot.[178] With a large pulmonary embolism, the right ventricle may quickly progress into right heart failure as a result of the increased pulmonary artery pressure.[179,180] Right ventricular cardiac output falls, leading to a decrease in return of blood to the left heart. Overdistension of the right ventricle may result in a shift of the ventricular septum to the left, thus encroaching on the left ventricular cavity. This encroachment leads to a decrease in left ventricular filling as well as ventricular outflow. The overall result may be a life-threatening fall in cardiac output.

Other signs and symptoms of a pulmonary embolism in the postoperative patient are myriad. Chest pain, especially pleuritic in nature, may be experienced.[181] Hemoptysis is uncommon and usually is associated with a pulmonary infarct.[182,183] Supraventricular arrhythmias other than sinus tachycardia may be seen and likely represent increased atrial pressures and distension.[171] Although classic teaching emphasizes an $S_1Q_3T_3$ pattern on the EKG, the most common alterations are nonspecific ST-T wave changes.[177]

Diagnosis

The diagnosis of pulmonary embolism in the postoperative patient can be extremely challenging. The chest radiograph is commonly abnormal in the postoperative setting due to atelectasis, pulmonary edema, preexistent lung disease, or pneumonia. Classic signs such as oligemia in the affected segment (Westermark's sign) may be seen but are difficult to identify in this population. A pleural-based density may be seen in the case of pulmonary infarct (Fig. 15-3). The chest x-ray may be normal even in the face of a hemodynamically significant pulmonary embolus.

Initial screening of stable patients suspected of having a pulmonary embolism involves performing a radionuclide perfusion scan.[184, 185] Isotope-labeled macroaggregates of albumin are injected into the patient, which are then distributed to areas of perfused lung tissue. Scanning the patient with a gamma camera identifies lung tissue. Scanning the patient with a gamma camera also identifies areas of abnormally low or absent perfusion consistent with a pulmonary embolism. Sensitivity of the test may be increased by performing a ventilation scan at the same time, although this is not possible if the patient is on a ventilator. The scan is then ranked as either normal, or high, intermediate, or low probability for pulmonary embolism (Table 15-5). Unfortunately, many factors may alter the sensitivity of the examination. Atelectasis, bronchoconstriction, and bronchial obstruction due to tumor or secretions alter the ventilation component. In addition, patients with chronic lung disease usually have regional alterations in the ventilation-perfusion relationship, which make the scan difficult to interpret.[186]

Figure 15-3. Pulmonary infarct in the left lower lung field. The patient, who was confined to bed after cardiac surgery, developed chest pain and hemoptysis on postoperative day six. Deep vein thrombosis in the left leg is documented by venography.

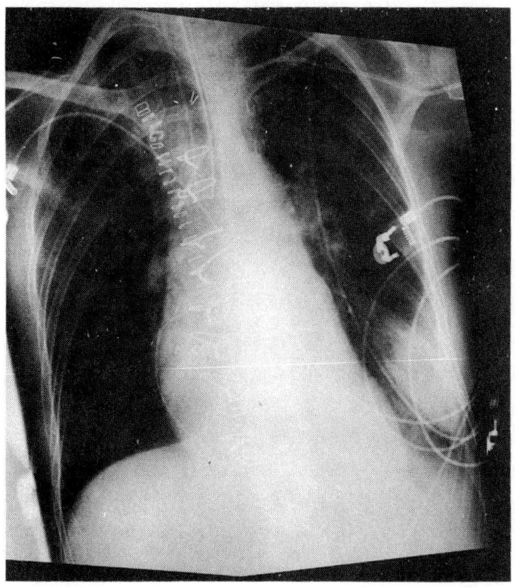

The definitive diagnosis of a pulmonary embolus is made by pulmonary angiogram. High-probability ventilation-perfusion scans in the appropriate setting are usually adequate to prove the diagnosis and to warrant treatment.[187] A pulmonary angiogram should be performed in (1) patients who have an indeterminate perfusion scan or who have a low-probability scan but a clinical picture consistent with pulmonary embolism or (2) in patients with a high-probability scan but major contraindications to anticoagulation. Some investigators advocate the use of venography or impedance plethysmography of the lower extremities in patients who have a low- or intermediate-probability scan but still are clinically suspect. A negative venogram or noninvasive studies allows these patients to be followed closely without specific treatment, since the probability of their having serious sequelae or recurrent pulmonary emboli is low.[188, 189]

Treatment

The standard treatment for deep venous thromboses and pulmonary embolism is anticoagulation. Heparin, the drug of choice, should be

Table 15-5. Ventilation/Perfusion Scanning*

Findings	Classification	Clinical Implication
Normal perfusion/ventilation	Normal	Rules out a pulmonary embolism. No further workup for embolism needed
No perfusion defects larger than a segment	Low probability	Need pulmonary angiogram if clinical suspicion high. May follow closely if venogram or noninvasive studies of the legs are negative
All segmental or larger perfusion defects are matched with ventilation defects	Intermediate/ Indeterminant	Need pulmonary angiogram or positive lower extremity venogram to confirm diagnosis or justify treatment
Segmental or larger perfusion defects with normal ventilation	High probability	Justifies treatment for pulmonary embolism. May need pulmonary angiogram to document if major contraindication to anticoagulation

* Data from Hull RD, Raskob GE. The diagnosis of clinically suspected pulmonary embolism: practical approaches. Chest 1986;89:4175.

administered as soon as a major pulmonary embolism is suspected. This agent alters both the intrinsic and extrinsic clotting cascade through its binding with antithrombin-III; its major effect is to prevent additional clot from forming at both the site of origin of the embolus and the site of entrapment in the pulmonary circulation. The heparin is initially administered as an initial intravenous bolus of 75–150 units/kg and then as a continuous infusion. The dose is adjusted to keep the activated partial thromboplastin time at 1.5–2 times control. Over the next five to seven days, the patient is transitioned to oral coumadin therapy. Although the risk of bleeding with heparin in the postoperative patient is increased, beginning heparin therapy if needed is generally safe after the third or fourth postoperative day if the patient has not had continued bleeding problems.[190]

For patients who are at high risk for bleeding or have recurrent emboli while on adequate anticoagulation, the treatment usually involves placement of a filter in the inferior vena cava.[191] The cone-shaped Greenfield filter results in a long-term patency rate of 97% and a recurrent embolism rate of 5%. Similar results have been achieved with other types of vena caval filter devices.[192] Potential side effects include chronic venous insufficiency and edema of the lower extremities. Case reports have also described migration of the filter devices, which may have devastating consequences.[193]

Massive Pulmonary Embolism

For the patient who has a suspected massive pulmonary embolism, the diagnosis must be made quickly and aggressive therapy instituted early. Pulmonary angiography is usually the diagnostic test of choice. Once massive pulmonary embolism is diagnosed, several options are available. Since thrombolytic agents are contraindicated in the postoperative patient, pulmonary embolectomy must be entertained. Results of open pulmonary embolectomy differ widely and reflect differences in patient population, timing of surgery, and experience with the technique. Mortality varies between 25 and 50%.[194,195] In cases of massive pulmonary embolism, catheter embolectomy using a steerable esuction-cup catheter inserted percutaneously from the femoral vein has been used under fluoroscopic guidance with some success.[196]

Pneumonia

Nosocomial pneumonia is the second most common hospital-acquired infection in the United States after urinary tract infections.[197] In the intensive care unit, it is the most common infection encountered.[198] The consequences of morbidity, mortality, and increased length of stay in the hospital are enormous.

In postoperative thoracic surgery patients several factors increase the risk of postoperative pneumonia. Many patients have a history of preexisting lung disease. Chronic obstructive pulmonary disease, history of tobacco smoking, pneumoconiosis, bronchial obstruction secondary to tumor, and impaired ciliary motility from a variety of conditions are associated with increased colonization of bacteria in the lower respiratory tree. Colonization with pathogenic organisms predisposes patients to the development of respiratory infections.[199] Once patients are intubated, the normal cough reflex and ability to eliminate secretions are markedly impaired and often lead to retention of contaminated secretions. Once patients are extubated, postoperative weakness may make it difficult to expel secretions. Chest wall pain also limits effective coughing and results in pooled secretions in the airways.

Pneumonia leads to an increase in secretions as well as a decrease in the arterial oxygenation. Alveolar flooding with secretions results in an increase in the ventilation-perfusion mismatch and worsens oxygenation of the pulmonary capillary blood. In severe cases, impairment of carbon dioxide elimination leads to hypercapnia with resultant acidosis. In an effort to eliminate the carbon dioxide, minute ventilation requirements rise, resulting in an increase in the work of breathing in spontaneously ventilating patients. The increase in the work of breathing, which causes a rise in carbon dioxide production, further exacerbates the need to increase minute ventilation. A downhill spiral may ensue, leading to reintubation and institution of mechanical ventilatory support.

Pneumonia is usually acquired via the aspiration of oropharyngeal organisms.[200,201] Once bacteria from the back of the throat are aspirated into the tracheobronchial tree, they may become colonized and, in the worst cases, progress into a pneumonia. Risk factors for aspiration of oropharyngeal contents are listed in Table 15-6. Of note is that the presence of an endotracheal tube does not prevent aspiration of oropharyngeal contents.[202] The incidence of aspiration around the cuff has markedly increased as the shift from high-pressure, low-volume endotracheal cuffs to high-volume low-pressure cuffs has occurred in the last two decades in an attempt prevent tracheal erosions and stenosis.

The organisms responsible for the development of postoperative pneumonia reflect the oropharyngeal flora. Gram-negative organisms predominate in patients admitted to the intensive care unit or in those with preexisting lung disease and gram-negative colonization.[203,204] Once admitted to the intensive care unit most patients exhibit a shift in their oropharyngeal flora from a predominance of anaerobic organisms to gram-negative bacteria. The incidence of pneumonia due to *Staphylococcus aureus* also

Table 15-6. Risk Factors for Bacterial Aspiration

Vomiting
Depressed level of consciousness
Depressed gag reflex
Presence of endotracheal tube
Presence of nasogastric tube
High gastric volume
Ileus or intestinal obstruction
Gastroesophageal reflux
Esophageal dysmotility
Supine position

increases in the postoperative patient. If gram-negative pneumonia occurs, mortality increases to at least to 50%, as opposed to 5–10% for a gram-positive organism. If the organism is *Pseudomonas aeruginosa*, the overall mortality is 70%.[205]

One area of considerable controversy is the potential of the gastric lumen as a source of organisms that may ultimately colonize the oropharynx, which therefore leads to the development of a nosocomial pneumonia if the organisms are aspirated. Concern has been especially high in those patients treated with acid-neutralizing regimens in an effort to prevent stress ulcer formation. The normal acidic environment of the stomach is very hostile to bacteria and does not allow significant growth of organisms in the lumen. Once the pH rises above 4, significant numbers of gram-negative bacteria may be found in the gastric contents of many patients.[206] Conditions that promote gastroesophageal reflux such as high gastric volume, decreased tone of the lower esophageal sphincter due to drugs or disease, high intra-abdominal pressures, or the presence of a nasogastric tube that may promote movement of bacterial laden secretions from the stomach to the oropharyngeal area further increase the chance of retrograde colonization.[207] Numerous studies[208–211] and editorial opinions both support and refute the concept of the stomach as a reservoir of bacteria responsible for nosocomial pneumonia and possible neutralization of the gastric pH increases the risk for pneumonia. The issue is still very much unresolved, however.[212]

The diagnosis of pneumonia is usually based on clinical findings (Fig. 15-4, Table 15-7). Although sputum samples are usually derived from an expectorated specimen or from a specimen obtained from the blind insertion of a suction catheter into the endotracheal tube, the clinician must be aware that the yield of these techniques may be relatively poor concerning identification of the causative organism.[213] If the patient is not responding to appropriate antibiotic therapy as dictated by bacteriologic cultures, bronchoscopic examination with bronchoalveolar lavage or protected specimen brush catheter culture should be considered. Successful treatment of a nosocomial pneumonia requires appropriate antibiotics as well as aggressive pulmonary toilet.

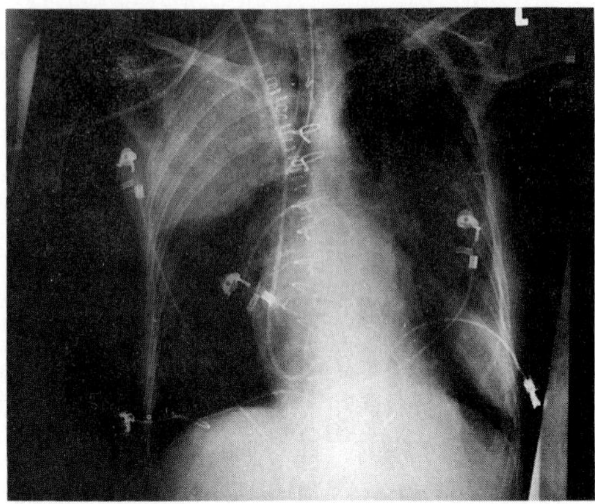

Figure 15-4. Right upper lobe pneumonia, which developed two weeks after aortic valve surgery. The patient has a history of emphysema with numerous bouts of pneumonia. Note a pulmonary infarct in the left lower lung field. The source of the infarct was thought to be a pulmonary artery catheter that had initially been positioned in the left lower lobe pulmonary artery for several days. Venous studies of the legs were normal.

Atelectasis

Postoperative atelectasis is an extremely common finding in thoracic surgery patients. Atelectasis has been reported in up to 100% of patients undergoing thoracotomy for pulmonary resection.[214] The great majority of patients undergoing cardiopulmonary bypass also have varying degrees of atelectasis in their early post-

Table 15-7. Clinical Diagnosis of Pneumonia

1. New infiltrate on chest x-ray
2. Increased white blood cell count
3. Fever
4. Purulent sputum (predominance of polymorphonucleocytes with few epithelial cells)
5. Pathogenic organism on sputum culture

operative course (Fig. 15-5).[215] Significant atelectasis leads to an increase in the ventilation-perfusion mismatch with resultant hypoxia and inability to clear trapped secretions from the area. This places patients at a high risk for development of postoperative pneumonia.

Studies suggest that atelectasis occurs in the operating room immediately after the induction of anesthesia.[216,217] It is well known that general anesthesia results in at least a 20%–30% decrease in the functional residual capacity (FRC).[218–220] Upon induction of general anesthesia, the diaphragm moves cephalad into the chest, promoting pulmonary collapse of the basal segments. The decrease in alveolar volume promotes closure of the alveoli secondary to the lack of distending pressure. Loss of the negative intrapleural pressure upon opening the chest further decreases the transalveolar pressure gradient. This pressure loss contributes to the development of significant atelectasis. As ventilation to the collapsed units is diminished, there is little concomitant decrease in pulmonary blood flow to those areas and a significant ventilation-perfusion inequality occurs, resulting in hypoxemia. Both lung collapse for surgical exposure and direct manipulation of the lung during surgery exacerbate postoperative atelectasis.

Figure 15-5. Atelectasis in a patient on the third postoperative day after coronary bypass surgery. Note the bilateral atelectasis of the lower lobes as well as the postoperative left pleural effusion. Most of the density seen on the lower left is secondary to volume loss of the left lower lobe.

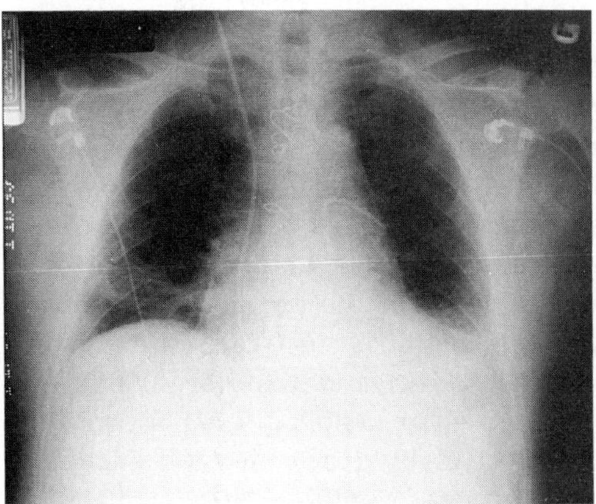

Conditions that may promote continued postoperative atelectasis are numerous. Intravenous narcotics used in the maintenance of general anesthesia may have residual effects in the early postoperative period. Narcotics may substantially reduce the hypoxic and hypercapneic respiratory drive, leading to inadequate ventilation and a poor spontaneous tidal volume with a reduction in the postoperative FRC. Continued treatment of postoperative pain with high doses of narcotic analgesics delay the resolution of the atelectasis due to poor respiratory effort. In contrast, inadequate pain relief leads to splinting of the chest wall with resultant lung collapse and continued atelectasis. Titration and proper monitoring of pain relief is essential for this reason.

Postoperative atelectasis is common after cardiac surgery, but the precise mechanism is unknown (Fig. 15-5). Atelectasis occurs much more commonly in the left lower lobe than the right. For this reason, investigators have speculated that the cause may be related to the retraction of the left lower lobe during surgery, postoperative gastric distension, or transient paresis of the left hemidiaphragm due to phrenic nerve injury from direct intraoperative trauma or from the application of the topical hypothermia solution used for myocardial preservation. (Fig. 15-6).[221–224] Although phrenic nerve dysfunction can lead to significant postoperative atelectasis, studies demonstrate that the majority of patients with significant atelectasis have normal phrenic nerve conduction studies.[222, 225] Several other factors seem to contribute including length of cardiopulmonary bypass time, violation of the pleural space, increased number of coronary artery bypass grafts, failure to use a right atrial drain or a cardiac insulating pad, and lower body temperature. Decreased surfactant activity contributing to a decrease in the FRC and early airway closure has also been proposed as a mechanism.[219, 226] The cause of postoperative atelectasis is most likely multifactorial.

Treatment

Considerable time and effort is spent in prevention and treatment of this atelectasis, which is the most common postoperative respiratory complication.[227] There is no absolute consensus on how to prevent or treat this condition. In general, a variety of techniques are used to try and prevent as well as resolve established atelectasis. None is clearly superior to all others.

Treatment of atelectasis usually begins in the operating room. The goal is to try and raise the FRC while on positive pressure ventilation. This is done by placing the patient on at least 5–10 cm H_2O of positive end-expiratory pressure (PEEP). In addition, the tidal volume is adjusted to provide 8–10 mL/kg of body weight. Periodic sighs of 1.5–2.5 times the tidal volume have been used as well.[228]

Once the patient is in the recovery room, PEEP is maintained if the patient is on mechanical ventilation. If atelectasis is noted on the chest radiograph or the patient has an increased alveolar-arterial oxygen gradient with no other obvious cause, active hyperinflation of the lung with a hand-held respiratory bag may be attempted if there is no contraindication to transient increased airway pressures. More formal recruitment of an atelectatic segment may be performed by placing the collapsed portion in a superior position and increasing the airway pressures through hyperinflation with a hold on exhalation.[229] Airway pressures of 30–40 cm H_2O are held by occluding the exhalation valve for a period of 30 seconds or more. Oxygen saturation is monitored by a pulse oximeter, and the patient is maintained on 100% oxygen before and during the maneuver. Airway pressure is released if changes in the oxygen saturation or the hemodynamic status are significant. It is often necessary to sedate patients prior to active recruitment for two reasons: (1) to allow better tolerance of the procedure and (2) to discourage coughing, which can result in significant transient increases in the airway pressure. A follow-up chest radiograph is performed to assess any changes in the atelectasis and to rule out barotrauma.

Figure 15-6. Phrenic nerve paralysis. Postoperative coronary bypass patient who has the typical elevation of the left hemidiaphragm with volume loss of the left lung. Ultrasound documented lack of descent of left hemidiaphragm on spontaneous inhalation.

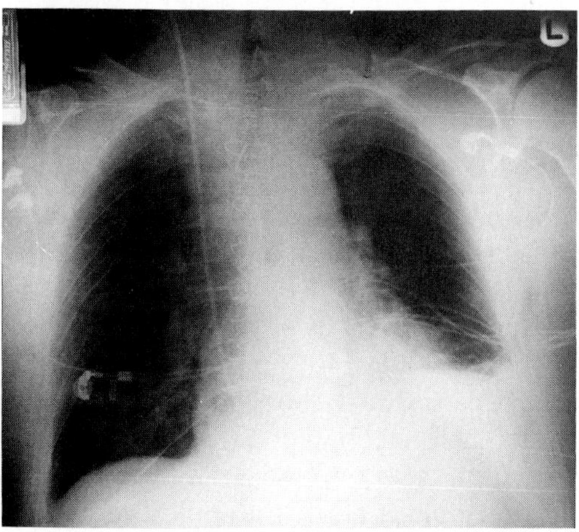

Once the patient is extubated, several treatment modalities are commonly used to treat postoperative atelectasis. Methods used include voluntary deep breathing, incentive spirometry, intermittent positive-pressure breathing (IPPB), chest physiotherapy, bronchoscopy, aerosol therapy, and continuous positive airway pressure (CPAP). A national survey published in 1985 revealed that more than 95% of hospitals in the United States use several of the above methods in the prevention and treatment of postoperative atelectasis.[230] In most instances, a combination of therapies are used. Incentive spirometry is used in over 95% of hospitals for established atelectasis closely followed by chest physiotherapy and intermittent positive-pressure ventilation. Intermittent CPAP by mask has become much more popular in larger hospitals over the last decade.[230–233]

Despite considerable numbers of studies comparing routine modalities, no mode or combination of modes has a proven clear advantage over any other. The work of Jenkins and colleagues showed no difference with the addition of breathing exercises or incentive spirometry to a regimen of early mobilization and coughing in 110 postcoronary bypass patients.[234] Dull also showed no benefit in either maximal inspiratory breathing exercises or incentive spirometry over early mobilization in 49 postcardiac bypass patients.[235] Stock demonstrated no clinical benefit in using mask CPAP over incentive spirometry or routine cough and deep breathing exercises in post cardiac patients.[233] However, her studies found the CPAP mask to be a less painful modality than the others.

Because the natural history of postoperative atelectasis is one of usual resolution, it is difficult to show true benefit of any one therapy. Most postoperative atelectasis is not clinically significant and does not need specific therapy. Up to 90% of postoperative cardiac patients develop radiographic evidence of atelectasis, especially on the left side. Only a small number of these patients experience clinically significant problems due to the volume loss. Most of the patients who experience significant clinical deterioration due to atelectasis are those who cannot perform adequate conservative voluntary treatment regimens such as deep breathing and coughing or for whom early mobilization is not possible. It has been suggested that lung volumes be measured to separate out patients at high risk for clinically significant atelectasis and apply more aggressive regimens only in those cases.[236] In the future, it will be important to compare treatment regimens in high risk groups alone to look for benefits of one therapy or another. In the majority of patients, it is clear that early mobilization with encouragement to breathe deeply and cough is likely as effective as the more labor-intensive and sometimes painful modalities used in the treatment and prevention of significant postoperative atelectasis. Patients who are unable to mobilize early following surgery because of weakness or ongoing medical problems are at increased risk for postoperative atelectasis and its consequences; in these patients more aggressive forms of treatment and prevention appear to be warranted.

Air Leak and Bronchopleural Fistula

Small air leaks, as evidenced by bubbling in the water-seal chamber of the thoracostomy drainage system, are common after thoracic surgery. Air leaks are more common after pulmonary resection, especially if the lung parenchyma and visceral pleura have been violated. Partial lobectomy, lung biopsy, or parenchymal damage from intraoperative trauma usually result in a postoperative air leak. Decortication procedures routinely lead to a significant postoperative air leak when the pleura has been removed. Oozing of air from the raw lung surfaces is the usual source of the leak.

Initially, the patient is treated with the application of negative pressure to the thoracostomy tube to ensure continued lung expansion. If the patient is on mechanical ventilation, airway pressures are kept to a minimum by decreasing tidal volume, removing PEEP, and allowing the patient to breathe spontaneously, which minimizes positive airway pressure. Suction is usually removed from the chest tube system within the first 24–48 hours to decrease the transalveolar gradient and discourage air leak. Most minor air leaks clear spontaneously within the first few days of surgery. Once the leak has stopped and the lung remains fully expanded on x-ray, the chest tube is removed.

A bronchopleural fistula (BPF), which represents an abnormal communication between the bronchial tree and the pleural space, is one of the most serious and dreaded complications of pulmonary surgery. The majority of BPFs occur after pneumonectomy and less commonly after partial lung resections.[237] The incidence has markedly decreased over the last three decades. In the 1950s, the incidence of BPF following pneumonectomy was 20%–30%,[238–240] and currently it is less than 5%[241] and decreasing. The mortality associated with this condition is still high, however. The mortality in the 1950s was greater than 60%,[242] and since 1975, the mortality has tended to level off at between 15% and 30%.[243–245]

The major pathophysiologic basis for the development of a BPF is the blood supply to the bronchus and the anatomic structure of the bronchus.[246–248] Although there are vascular variations, the majority of right bronchial arteries arise as a single artery and lack extensive collaterals. This means that the bronchial stump following a right-sided pneumonectomy is more likely to break down from lack of adequate blood flow than the left-sided bronchial stump, because the left side is often supplied by more than one bronchial artery. Either side may break down if close attention is not paid to preserving blood supply to the area of stump closure during resection. In addition, it appears that the natural tendency to recoil back to an open position due to the tubular cartilaginous skeleton promotes rupture of a sutured or stapled bronchial stump. Bronchial stumps appear to heal by secondary intention.[246] Covering the stump with, omentum, pleural tissue, pericardial fat, or muscle at the time of surgery has been reported to reduce the incidence of BPF following resection.[243,244,249–251]

BPF can occur at any time after pulmonary resection but most commonly in the first two weeks.[252] The patient usually presents with fever and cough. Associated signs and symptoms may include pain, dyspnea, subcutaneous emphysema, or hemoptysis. If a thoracostomy tube is already in place, air bubbles are evident in the water-seal chamber as the escaping air is drained from the pleural space. Depending on the amount of air being evacuated, a spectrum of bubbles ranging from only a few per breath during a positive pressure cycle to vigorous air bubbling in all phases of the respiratory cycle may be noted. If the patient is on positive pressure ventilation and no thoracostomy tube exists, the mean and peak airway pressures usually increase as the compliance of the lungs decreases due to the impending tension pneumothorax. Sometimes a notable shift in the trachea to the side opposite the pneumothorax is apparent. Late development of BPF occurring months or years after pneumonectomy is always associated with empyema,[253,254] but may not be related to a significant shift in the intrathoracic contents due to established adhesions to the inner chest wall.

Chest radiographs may demonstrate early signs of BPF. A falling air fluid level in a postpneumonectomy space is the classic sign.[255] Radiographic features also associated with a BPF include the development of a new air space, an increase in the size of an existing air space, or the failure of a remaining lung to expand.[256]

Documentation of a BPF can be attempted via several modalities. Fiberoptic bronchoscopy has been used try to locate and document a BPF.[257] In a postpneumonectomy patient, the bronchial stump is gently cleared of secretions and then probed to look for a source of air leak. Care must be taken to avoid overaggressive manipulation of the stump, thus creating a leak. Ventilation-perfusion scans have also been used to document a BPF. Radioactive xenon is inhaled; the appearance of the radionuclide in the postpneumonectomy air space is evidence of a fistula.[258] Other methods include instillation of methylene blue into the pleural space.[259] If the dye appears in the patient's sputum, then a BPF must be present. Thoracoscopy has also been used to diagnosis BPF.[260] If positive pressure is applied to the airway, bubbles can usually be seen at the site of air leak. Bronchography may be helpful in the diagnosis of late BPF.

Management of a BPF can be one of the most challenging feats in thoracic surgery. The sequence of therapies often depends on whether the BPF is an acute or chronic. In the acute setting, if the patient is coughing up copious secretions and contamination of the contralateral lung is a risk, then the patient is placed in a lateral decubitus position with the operated side down. Chest tube drainage is performed via tube thoracostomy. The most important principle in the treatment of BPF is obtaining adequate drainage. Adequate drainage alone results in closure of approximately 20% of patients.[261] In the remaining 80% of patients, surgical treatment is needed to take care of a large air leak, productive cough, and dyspnea. After adequate drainage is established, efforts are concentrated on closure of the fistula and obliteration of the residual pleural space.

Intraoperative management of a BPF depends on the cause of the fistula. If the fistula is secondary to an empyema, single-lung ventilation with a double-lumen endotracheal tube is used. Occasionally, a bronchial blocking tube is used to isolate the affected side. With either method, the contaminated side is separated from the uninvolved lung. By isolating the fistula, leakage of contaminated secretions into the healthy lung is prevented.[262]

Ventilatory support of the patient with a BPF can be a formidable challenge. If the air leak is small and there is little evidence to support an ongoing infection, conventional positive-pressure ventilation through a single-lumen endotracheal tube can be used. Increasing the tidal volume using pressure-supported ventilation or adding PEEP all encourage loss of air across the fistula.[263] To minimize the pressure gradient across the leak, airway pressures are kept to a minimum by using tidal volume settings less than those for standard mechanical ventilation. Adequate minute ventilation is approached by increasing respiratory rate rather than tidal volume. Of course, spontaneous ventilation, if adequate to sustain oxygenation and carbon dioxide removal, is encouraged. The use of intermittent mandatory ventilation at a low rate is preferable over assist-control mode to allow the greatest number of spontaneous breaths. Application of suction to a thoracostomy tube, if present, lessens the propensity of air leakage through the fistula. Placement of the thoracostomy tube to water seal is undertaken, and if the air space does not increase on the side of the BPF, the tube is kept off external suction.[264]

Some investigators have advocated measuring the so-called "critical opening pressure" of the BPF.[263] This pressure is the threshold airway pressure at which there is no leak across the fistula. To reduce fistula flow, attempts are made to keep the level of PEEP, CPAP, and pressure support below the critical opening pressure.

If the air leak is large and cannot be adequately controlled by the above measures, more aggressive interventions must be used. Often the patient is heavily sedated or paralyzed to reduce airway pressure as much as possible while on mechanical ventilation. Other maneuvers used with conventional positive-pressure ventilation include differential lung ventilation using a double-lumen endotracheal tube and two ventilators. With this method, the involved side may be ventilated with a very small tidal volume and low rate to decrease the amount of fistula leak. Respiratory systems to provide intermittent chest tube occlusion or PEEP via the water-seal chamber during positive-pressure inspiration have been designed; these lead to decreased air loss across the fistula.[265–267]

Much has been written about the use of high-frequency ventilation (HFV) in the setting of BPF. Unfortunately, its role has not been fully established. Potential advantages include lower airway pressures and tidal volumes leading to decrease air loss via the fistula.[268–271] Studies that have evaluated HFV in this setting have yielded mixed results with respect to gas exchange, fistula flow, and healing.[268,272,273] If the patient on conventional ventilation is failing, HFV should be considered.

Once the patient is stabilized from the ventilatory standpoint, attention is then given to surgical correction of the fistula. The surgical treatment of a BPF is performed by direct closure of the bronchial stump. Alternatively, indirect means that result in obliteration of the pleural cavity, cessation of purulent secretion production, and spontaneous closure of the fistula may also be used. Direct closure of a BPF is considered if the fistula occurs early in the postoperative course following pulmonary resection. Direct closure requires that sufficient length of residual bronchus be present to allow secondary closure. In addition, no residual proximal tumor or other obstructing lesions can be present. Direct closure is usually avoided in cases of active bronchial infection or empyema because of the failure rate of successful closure is extremely high. In some cases, the leak is substantial and may require attempts at direct closure even in the face of active inflammation or infection in the ipsilateral pleural space. Several approaches have been used to close the bronchial stump directly, including a contralateral thoracotomy[259] or a transsternal approach through the pericardium.[274–276] Once the bronchial stump is closed, it is usually covered with autologous tissue such as omentum, pericardial fat, or skeletal muscle.[243,249,277,278]

Since the majority of BPFs are associated with pleural empyemas, an indirect treatment approach allowing drainage, obliteration of the pleural space, and spontaneous closure of the leak is often first attempted. Following direct closure, if needed, the residual pleural space must obliterated. If percutaneous tube thoracostomy is unsuccessful or the patient presents in a moribund, septic condition open drainage of the pleural space has been accomplished by open window thoracostomy.[253,279,280] Granulation tissue forms at the site of the fistula and results in healing of the leak. Once the open thoracostomy is covered with granulation tissue, a secondary closure can be attempted, although the results have not been uniformly successful. Formal thoracoplasty with resection of three to five ribs and collapse of the thoracic cavity has also been used successfully.[281]

Endoscopic closure of a BPF has been performed with variable results. A fiberoptic bronchoscope is passed into the area of leak, and a sealant is applied via a small catheter. Several types of compounds have been used to try to seal the site of air loss including cyanoacrylate glue[282] and topical fibrin.[283,284] Although this approach is not uniformly successful, it may avoid a disfiguring and potentially debilitating thoracoplasty or more formal open thoracotomy.

Neurologic Injuries

Neurologic problems following thoracic surgery are a well-recognized complication. Nerve injuries following a thoracotomy and a median sternotomy, in particular, are relatively common. Although most such injuries are self-limited and usually manifest themselves in minor ways, some can have devastating consequences. Nerve injuries can be the result of patient positioning during the operation, and nerve damage may be caused by surgical disruption, compromise of the vascular supply, stretching, or direct compression.[285]

Intercostal Nerve Damage

Injury to the intercostal nerve is common.[286] Many operations require a posterolateral thoracotomy incision that routinely involves the division of the neurovascular bundle along with the superior rib. Division of the nerve in this manner may prevent its stretching and evulsion from the spinal cord and results in numbness in the associated dermatome. This is rarely a major problem and usually improves with time. Sensation to the dermatome probably returns as a result of the ingrowth of new sensory nerve fibers from adjacent dermatomes. The development of a neuroma at the site of transection has been reported, but is rare and usually is asymptomatic.

Direct trauma to the intercostal nerve can also occur during the placement of a thoracostomy tube. Although care is taken to pass the tube over the superior aspect of the rib, avoiding the neurovascular bundle that lies along the inferior margin, the intercostal nerve closest to the tube can be damaged occasionally. Local inflammation and infection that has traveled along the tube from the skin may also involve the intercostal nerve.

Long Thoracic and Thoracodorsal Nerves

The long thoracic and thoracodorsal nerves, which supply the serratus anterior and latissimus dorsi muscles, respectively, course through the axilla. When a surgical procedure involves dissection in the axillary region, such as with first rib removal, these nerves can be damaged. The result of injury to the long thoracic nerve is a "winged scapula," a deformity that is very difficult to treat. For the most part, injuries to these nerves are uncommon and related to the skill of the surgeon and to careful identification of these structures during surgical dissection.

Brachial Plexus Injury

Brachial plexus injuries have been recognized as a complication of median sternotomy since the early 1970s.[287] Many of the studies concerning this topic have been anecdotal in nature, and it is difficult to find exact data on incidence or severity. It appears that brachial plexus injury occurs in anywhere from 6% to 38% of all patients undergoing a median sternotomy incision, depending on how detailed the search for nerve injury is. Sensitive nerve conduction studies and electromyography identify many patients who are unaware of any deficit.

The mechanism of injury to the brachial plexus is thought to be related to compression by the first rib.[288] As the sternum is retracted, the first rib is forced upward because of its dorsal articulations, and it may impinge directly on the brachial plexus. In addition, the arms are usually pulled down and fixed toward the patient's sides. This pulls the clavicle inferiorly and may also cause impingement of the nerves as they are trapped between the clavicle and the first rib. The interscapular towel roll, which is often used, further accentuates the movement of the clavicle.

The usual deficit involves the C8-T1 root distribution. Morin[289] found that 6% of 958 patients undergoing sternotomy experienced postoperative neuropathy. Vander Salm[290] found an incidence of 15% in a study that looked at specific complaints, many which were minor. The most common symptoms involve paresthesias, usually of the small and ring fingers. Weakness and pain are seen less commonly. More than 90% of patients are asymptomatic three months after surgery. Since almost all of these patients experience full recovery, no specific treatment is needed. In the rare patient with prolonged symptoms, surgery involving resection of the first rib has been tried, but evidence supporting overall efficacy of this treatment is lacking.[291]

Ulnar Nerve Injury

The ulnar nerve is particularly susceptible to nerve damage from direct compression as it passes behind the medial epicondyle of the distal humerus. Here the nerve lies in a superficial position that is relatively unprotected from direct compression injuries. As the arm is held in pronation along the patient's side, the epicondylar area may come in direct contact with the hard surfaces of the operating table, causing compression of the nerve. Supination of the arm moves the epicondyle away from direct contact with the underlying surfaces. Ulnar nerve injury has also been reported from the use of automatically cycled blood pressure cuffs.[292] Most ulnar nerve injuries acquired in the perioperative period are usually self-limited, although they may take three to six months to resolve.

References

1. Matthay MA, Weiner-Kronish JP. Respiratory management after cardiac surgery. Chest 1989;95:424.
2. Hedley-Whyte J, Corning H, Laver MB, et al. Pulmonary ventilation-perfusion relationships after valve replacement or repair in man. J Clin Invest 1965; 44:406.
3. Dantzker DR, Cowenhaven WM, Willoughby WJ, et al. Gas exchange alterations associated with weaning from mechanical ventilation following coronary artery bypass surgery. Chest 1982;82:674.
4. Benumof JL, Wahrenbrock EA, Local effects of anesthetics on regional hypoxic vasoconstriction. Anesthesiology 1975;43:525.
5. Marshall E, Marshall C. Anesthesia and the pulmonary circulation In: Covina, BG, ed. Effects of anesthesia. Bethesda MD: American Physiology Society, 1985.
6. Meyers JR, Lembeck L, O'Kane M, et al. Changes in FRC of lung after operation. Arch Surg 1975;110: 576.
7. Don HF, Robson JG. The mechanics of the respiratory system during anesthesia. Anesthesiology 1965;26:168.
8. Ali J, Weisel RD, Layug AB, et al. Consequences of postoperative alterations in respiratory mechanics. Am J Surg 1974;128:376.
9. Hirschler-Schulte CJW, Hylkema BS, Meyer RW. Mechanical ventilation for acute postoperative respiratory failure after surgery for bronchial carcinoma. Thorax 1985;40:387.
10. O'Donohue WJ. Prevention and treatment of atelectasis. Chest 1985;87:1.
11. Shevland JE, Hirleman MT, Hoang KA, et al. Lobar collapse in the surgical intensive care unit. Br J Radiol 1983;56:531.
12. Braun SR, Birnbaum ML, Chopra PS. Pre- and postoperative pulmonary function abnormalities in coronary artery revascularization surgery. Chest 1973;73:316.
13. Tisi GM. State of the art: Preoperative evaluation of lung function. Am Rev Respir Dis 1979;119:293.
14. Olsen GN, Block AJ, Tobias JA. Prediction of postpneumonectomy pulmonary function using quantitative macroaggregate lung scanning. Chest 1974;66:13.

15. Marin T, Goldberg S, Mudge GH, et al. Factors contributing to altered left ventricular diastolic properties during angina pectoris. Circulation 1979;59:14.
16. Eichorn P, Grimm J, Koch R., et al. Left ventricular relaxation in patients with left ventricular hypertrophy secondary to aortic valve disease. Circulation 1982;65:1395.
17. Sharma B, Behrens TW, Erlein D, et al. Left ventricular diastolic properties and filling characteristics during spontaneous angina pectoris at rest. Am J Cardiol 1983;52:704.
18. Barry WH, Brooker JF, Alderman EL. Changes in diastolic stillness and tone of the left ventricle during angina pectoris. Circulation 1974;49:255.
19. Mammana RB. Inaccuracy of pulmonary artery wedge pressures when compared to left atrial pressure in the early postsurgical period. J Thorac Cardiovasc Surg 1982;84:420.
20. Harizi RC, Bianco JA, Alpert JS. Diastolic function of the heart in clinical cardiology. Arch Intern Med 1988;148:99.
21. Guyton AC, Lindsay AW. Effect of elevated left atrial pressure and decreased plasma protein concentration on the development of pulmonary edema. Circ Res 1959;7:649.
22. Rinaldo JE, Rogers RC, Riff E, et al. Medical progress: adult respiratory distress syndrome. Changing concepts of lung injury and repair. N Engl J Med 1982; 306:900.
23. Chenoweth DE. Complement activation during cardiopulmonary bypass. Evidence for generation of C3a and C5a anaphylatoxins. N Engl J Med 1981;304:497.
24. Moore FD, Warner KG, Assousa S, et al. The effects of complement activation during cardiopulmonary bypass. Ann Surg 1988;208:95.
25. Popovsky MA, Moore SB. Diagnostic and pathogenetic considerations in transfusion-related acute lung injury. Transfusion 1985;25:573.
26. Hollingsworth HM, Giansiracusa DF, Upchurch KS. Anaphylaxis. In: Rippe JM, Irwin RS, Alpert JS, et al, eds. Intensive care medicine, 2nd ed. Boston: Little, Brown, 1991:1771.
27. Ashbaugh DG, Bigelow DB, Petty TL, et al. Acute respiratory distress in adults. Lancet 1967;2:319.
28. Fowler AA, Hamman RF, Zerbe GO, et al. Adult respiratory distress syndrome: prognosis after onset. Am Rev Respir Dis 1985;132:472.
29. Montgomery BR, Stager MA, Carrico CJ, et al. Causes of mortality in patients with the adult respiratory distress syndrome. Am Rev Respir Dis 1985; 132:472.
30. Murray JF, Mathay MA, Luce JM, et al. An expanded definition of the adult respiratory distress syndrome. Am Rev Respir Dis 1988;138:720.
31. Brigham KL, Kariman K, Harris TR, et al. Correlation of oxygenation with vascular permeability-surface area but not with lung water in humans with acute respiratory failure and pulmonary edema. J Clin Invest 1983;72:339.
32. Rinaldo JE, Borovetz HS, Mancini MC, et al. Assessment of lung injury in the adult respiratory distress syndrome using multiple indicator dilution curves. Am Rev Resp Dis 1986;133:1006.
33. Melot C. Naeije R, Mols P, et al. Pulmonary tone improves pulmonary gas exchange in the adult respiratory distress syndrome. Am Rev Respir Dis 1987;136:1232.
34. Wright PE, Bernard GR. The role of airflow resistance in patients with the adult respiratory distress syndrome. Am Rev Respir Dis 1989;139:1169.
35. Martin WJ, Kuchel DL. Oxygen-mediated impairment of human endothelial cell growth: evidence for a specific threshold for toxicity. J Lab Clin Med 1989;113:412.
36. Witschi HR, Haschek WM, Klein-Szanto AJ, et al. Potentiation of diffuse lung damage by oxygen: determining variables. Am Rev Respir Dis 1981; 123:47.
37. Sassoon CSH. Positive pressure ventilation: alternate modes. Chest 1991;100:1421.
38. Garner W, Downs JB, Stock CM, et al. Airway pressure release ventilation (APRV). Chest 1988;94:779.
39. Hickling KG, Henderson SJ, Jackson R. Low mortality associated with low-volume pressure-limited ventilation with permissive hypercapnia in the severe respiratory distress syndrome. Intensive Care Med 1990;16:372.
40. Hickling KG. Low-volume ventilation with permissive hypercapnia in the adult respiratory distress syndrome. Clin Intensive Care 1992;3:67.
41. Zapol WM, Snider MT, Hill JD, et al. Extracorporeal membrane oxygenation in severe respiratory failure. JAMA 1979;242:2193.
42. Pesenti A, Pelizzola A, Mascheroni D, et al. Low-frequency positive-pressure ventilation with extracorporeal CO_2 removal (LFPPV-ECCO_2R) in acute respiratory failure (ARF) technique. Trans Am Soc Artif Intern Organs 1981;28:263.
43. Rinaldo JE. Adult respiratory distress syndrome. In: Rippe JM, Irwin RS, Alpert JS, et al, eds. Intensive care medicine. 2nd ed. Boston: Little, Brown, 1991:476.

44. Rinaldo JE. Prognosis of the adult respiratory distress syndrome: inappropriate pessimism? Chest 1986;90:470.
45. Matthay MA, Weiner-Kronish JP. Intact epithelial barrier function is critical for the resolution of alveolar edema in man. Am Rev Respir Dis 1990;141: 232.
46. Mills NL. Postoperative hemorrhage after cardiopulmonary bypass. Ann Thorac Surg 1982;34:100.
47. Petterfy A, Henze A. Hemorrhagic complications during pulmonary resections: a retrospective review of 1428 resections with 113 hemorrhagic episodes. Scand J Thorac Cardiovasc Surg 1983;17:283.
48. Wolk LA, Wilson RF, Burdick M, et al. Changes in antithrombin, antiplasmin, and plasminogen during and after cardiopulmonary bypass. Am J Surg 1985;51:309.
49. Bick RL. Alterations of hemostasis with cardiopulmonary bypass: pathophysiology, prevention, diagnosis, and management. Semin Thromb Hemost 1976;3:59.
50. Torosian M, Michelson EL, Morganroth J, et al. Aspirin- and coumadin-related bleeding after coronary artery bypass graft surgery. Ann Intern Med 1978;89:325.
51. McKenzie FN, Dhall DP, Arfors KE, et al. Blood platelet behavior during and after open-heart surgery. BMJ 1976;2:1125.
52. Czer LS, Bateman TM, Gray RJ, et al. Treatment of severe platelet dysfunction and hemorrhage after cardiopulmonary bypass: reduction in blood product usage with desmopressin. J Am Coll Cardiol 1987;9:1139.
53. Salzman EW, Weinstein MJ, Weintraub RM, et al. Treatment with desmopressin acetate to reduce blood loss after cardiac surgery. N Engl J Med 1986; 314:1402.
54. Rocha E, Llorens R, Paramo JA, et al. Does desmopressin acetate reduce blood loss after surgery in patients on cardiopulmonary bypass? Circulation 1988;77:1319.
55. Lacey JV, Penner JA. Management of idiopathic thrombocytopenic purpura in the adult. Semin Thromb Hemost 1977;3:160.
56. Sobel M, Salzman EW. Hemorrhagic and thrombotic complications of cardiac surgery. In: Baue AE, Geha AS, Hammond GL, et al, eds. Glenn's thoracic and cardiovascular surgery. 5th ed. Norwalk: Appleton & Lange, 1991:1547.
57. Cines DB, Kaywin P, Bina M, et al. Heparin-associated thrombocytopenia. N Engl J Med 1980;303: 788.
58. Hattersly PG. Heparin anticoagulation. In: Koepke JA, ed. Laboratory hematology. Vol. 2. New York: Churchill Livingstone: 1984:789.
59. Kapsch D, Silver D. Heparin-induced thrombocytopenia with thrombosis and hemorrhage. Arch Surg 1981;116:1423.
60. Pitney WR. Disseminated intravascular coagulation. Semin Hematol 1971;8:65.
61. Bachman F, McKenna R, Cole ER, et al. Hemostatic mechanism after open-heart surgery. Studies on plasma coagulation factors and fibrinolysis in 512 patients after extracorporeal circulation. J Thorac Cardiovasc Surg 1795;70:76.
62. Kalter RD, Saul CM, Wetstein L, et al. Cardiopulmonary bypass: associated hemostatic abnormalities. J Thorac Cardiovasc Surg 1979;77:427.
63. Milam JD, Austin SF, Martin RF, et al. Alteration of coagulation and selected clinical chemistry parameters in patients undergoing open heart surgery without transfusions. Am J Clin Pathol 1981;76: 155.
64. Bithell TC. The diagnostic approach to the bleeding disorders. In: Lee GR, Bithell TC, Foerster J, et al, eds. Wintrobe's clinical hematology. 9th ed. Philadelphia: Lea & Febiger, 1993:1301.
65. Spaethe R, Naumann M. Monitoring heparin during extracorporeal circulation in open-heart surgery. In: Witt I, ed. Heparin: new biochemical and medical aspects. New York: DeGruyton, 1983:329.
66. Bithell TC. Acquired coagulation disorders. In: Lee GR, Bithell TC, Foerster J, et al, eds. Wintrobe's clinical hematology. 9th ed. Philadelphia: Lea & Febiger, 1993:1473.
67. Umlas J, Taff RH, Gauvin G, et al. Anticoagulation monitoring and neutralization during open-heart surgery: a rapid method for measuring heparin and calculating safe protamine doses. Anesth Analg 1983;62:1095.
68. Gibbon JA, Camishion R. Problems in hemostasis with extracorporeal bypass. Ann N Y Acad Sci 1964; 115:195.
69. Bachmann F, MeKenna R, Cole ER, et al. The hemostatic mechanism after open-heart surgery: studies on plasma coagulation factors and fibrinolysis in 512 patients after extracorporeal circulation. J Thorac Cardiovasc Surg 1975;70:76.
70. Porter JM, Silver D, Durham NC. Alterations in fibrinolysis and coagulation associated with cardiopulmonary bypass. J Thorac Cardiovasc Surg 1968; 56:869.

71. DelRossi AJ, Cernaianu AC, Botros S, et al. Prophylactic treatment of postperfusion bleeding with EACA. Chest 1989;96:27.
72. Midel AI, Grady LH, Bloodwell RD, et al. Epsilon aminocaproic acid for bleeding after cardiopulmonary bypass. Ann Thorac Surg 1971;11:577.
73. Lambert CJ, Marengo-Row AJ, Leveson JE, et al. The treatment of postperfusion bleeding using epsilon-aminocaproic acid, cryoprecipitate, fresh-frozen plasma, and protamine sulfate. Ann Thorac Surg 1979;28:440.
74. Salm TJF, Ansell JE, Okike ON, et al. The role of epsilon-aminocaproic acid in reducing bleeding after cardiac operation: a double-blind randomized study. J Thorac Cardiovasc Surg 1988;95:538.
75. Ilbaca PA, Ochsner JL, Mills NL. Positive end-expiratory pressure in the management of the patient with a postoperative bleeding heart. Ann Thorac Surg 1980;30:281.
76. Hoffman WS, Tomasello DN, MacVaugh H. Control of post-cardiotomy bleeding with PEEP. Ann Thorac Surg 1982;34:71.
77. Zurick AM, Urzua J, Ghattas M, et al. Failure of positive end-expiratory pressure to decrease postoperative bleeding after cardiac surgery. Ann Thorac Surg 1982;34:608.
78. Mills NL. Postoperative hemorrhage after cardiopulmonary bypass. Ann Thorac Surg 1982;34:1.
79. Alajmo F, Calamai G, Perna AM, et al. High-dose aprotinin: Hemostatic effects in open-heart operations. Ann Thorac Surg 1989;48:536.
80. Benumof JL. Early serious complications specifically related to thoracic surgery. In: Anesthesia for thoracic surgery. Philadelphia: WB Saunders, 1987;434.
81. Cordel AR, Ellison RE. Postoperative hemorrhage. In: Complications of intrathoracic surgery. Boston; Little, Brown, 1979;240.
82. Mathisen DJ, Wain JC. Cardiac complications following pulmonary resection. Chest Surg Clin North Am 1992;2:793.
83. Craddock DR, Logan A, Fadali A. Reoperation for hemorrhage following cardiopulmonary bypass. Br J Surg 1968;55:17.
84. Engleman RM, Spencer FC, Reed GE, et al. Cardiac tamponade following open-heart surgery. Circulation 1970;41:165.
85. Weeks KR, Chattergee K, Block S, et al. Bedside hemodynamic monitoring. J Thorac Cardiovasc Surg 1976;71:250.
86. Bateman T, Gray R, Chaux A, et al. Right atrial tamponade caused by a hematoma complicating coronary artery bypass graft surgery: clinical hemodynamic and scintigraphic correlates. J Thorac Cardiovasc Surg 1982;84:413.
87. Jones MR, Vine DL, Attas M, et al. Late isolated ventricular tamponade: clinical, hemodynamic and echocardiographic manifestations of a previously unreported postoperative complication. J Thorac Cardiovasc Surg 1979;77:142.
88. Stevenson LW, Child JS, Laks H, et al. Incidence and significance of early pericardial effusions after cardiac surgery. Am J Cardiol 1984;54:848.
89. Kronzon I, Cohen MJ, Winer HE. Contribution of echocardiography to the understanding of the pathology of cardiac tamponade. J Am Coll Cardiol 1983;1:1180.
90. D'Cruz IA, Kensey K, Campbell C, et al. Two-dimensional echocardiography in cardiac tamponade after cardiac surgery. J Am Coll Cardiol 1985;5:1250.
91. Fowler NO, Gabel M, Buncher CR. Cardiac tamponade: A comparison of right versus left heart compression. J Am Coll Cardiol 1988;12:287.
92. Shebetai R. Changing concepts of cardiac tamponade. J Am Coll Cardiol 1988;12:194.
93. Bortolotti U, Livi U, Frugoni C, et al. Delayed cardiac tamponade following open-heart surgery: analysis of 12 patients. Thorac Cardiovasc Surg 1981;29:233.
94. Hardesty RL, Thompson M, Lerberg DB, et al. Delayed postoperative cardiac tamponade: Diagnosis and management. Ann Thorac Surg 1978;26:155.
95. Yacoub MH, Williams WG, Ahmad A. Strangulation of the heart following intrapericardial pneumonectomy. Thorax 1968;23:261.
96. Gates GF, Sette RS, Cope JA. Acute cardiac herniation with incarceration following pneumonectomy. Radiology 1970;94:561.
97. Takita H, Mijares WS. Herniation of the heart following intrapericardial pneumonectomy. Report of a case and review. J Thorac Cardiovasc Surg 1970; 59:443.
98. Beltrami V, Catenacci N. Cardiac herniation following intrapericardial pneumonectomy. Acta Chir Belg 1977;76:293.
99. Cassorla L, Katz JA. Management of cardiac herniation after intrapericardial pneumonectomy. Anesthesiology 1984;60:362.
100. Deiraniya AK. Cardiac herniation following intrapericardial pneumonectomy. Thorax 1974;29:545.
101. Wolodzko AA, Taff ML, Lukash LI. Herniation of the heart. Am J Med Path 1986;7:260.
102. Ginsburg M, Manganaro A, Weiner R. Herniation of

the heart: a complication of intrapericardial pneumonectomy. N Y State J Med 1984;84:401.
103. Gurney JW, Arnold S, Goodman LR. Impending cardiac herniation: the snow-cone sign. Radiology 1986;161:653.
104. Brady MB, Brogdon BG. Cardiac herniation and volvulus: radiographic findings. Radiology 1986; 161:657.
105. Tscherisch HU, Skorapa V. Fleming WH. Acute cardiac herniation following pneumonectomy. Radiology 1976;120:546.
106. Gergely M. Urban AE, Deverall PB, et al. Herniation of the heart after intrapericardial pneumonectomy. Acta Chir Hung 1977;18:129.
107. Wright MP, Nelson C, Johnson AM, et al. Herniation of the heart. Thorax 1970;25:656.
108. Michelson EL, Morganroth J, MacVaugh H. Postoperative arrhythmias after coronary artery and cardiac valvular surgery detected by long-term electrographic monitoring. Am Heart J 1979;97:442.
109. Kyosola K, Mattila T, Harjula A, et al. Life-threatening complications of cardiac operations and occurrence of myocardial catecholamine bombs. J Thorac Cardiovasc Surg 1988;95:334.
110. Vozeh S, Kewitz G, Perruchoud A. Theophylline serum concentrations and therapeutic effect in severe acute bronchial obstruction. The optimal use of intravenously administered aminophylline. Am Rev Respir Dis 1982;125:181.
111. Smith PK, Burhman WC, Levett JL, et al. Supraventricular conduction abnormalities following cardiac operations: a complication of inadequate atrial preservation. J Thorac Cardiovasc Surg 1983; 85:105.
112. Douglas P, Hirshfeld JW, Edmunds LH. Clinical correlates of postoperative atrial fibrillation. Circulation 1984;70(Suppl II):165.
113. Mowry F, Reynolds E. Cardiac rhythm disturbances complicating resectional surgery of the lung. Ann Intern Med 1964;61:688.
114. Shields TW, Ujiki G. Digitalization for the prevention of arrhythmias following pulmonary surgery. Surg Gynecol Obstet 1968;126:743.
115. Smith PK, Burhman WC, Ferguson TB, et al. Relationship between atrial hypothermia and cardioplegic solution potassium concentration to postoperative conduction defects. Surg Forum 1983; 34:304.
116. Silverman NA, DuBrow I, Kohler J, et al. Etiology of atrioventricular conduction abnormalities following cardiac surgery. J Surg Res 1984;36:198.
117. Ellis RJ, Mavroudis C, Gardner C, et al. Relationship between atrioventricular arrhythmias and the concentration of potassium ion in cardioplegic solution. J Thorac Cardiovasc Surg 1980;80:517.
118. Page PL, Plumb VJ, Okumara K, et al. A new animal model of atrial flutter. J Am Coll Cardiol 1986; 8:872.
119. Angelini GD, Penny WJ, El-Chamaray F, et al. The incidence of significance of early pericardial effusion after open-heart surgery. Eur J Cardio thorac Surg 1987;1:165.
120. Ormerod OM, McGregor CG, Stone DL, et al. Arrhythmias after coronary bypass surgery. Br Heart J 1984;51:618.
121. Smith EE, Shore DF, Monro JJ, et al. Oral verapamil fails to prevent supraventricular tachycardia following coronary artery surgery. Int J Cardiol 1985; 9:37.
122. Nayler WG, Szeto J. Effect of verapamil on contractility, oxygen utilization, and calcium exchangeability in mammalian heart muscle. Cardiovasc Res 1972;6:120.
123. Johnson LW, Dickstein RA, Fruehan T, et al. Prophylactic digitalization for coronary artery bypass surgery. Circulation 1976;53:819.
124. Csicsko JF, Schaatzlein MH, King RD. Immediate postoperative digitalization in the prophylaxis of supraventricular arrhythmias following coronary artery bypass. J Thorac Cardiovasc Surg 1981;81: 419.
125. Tyras DH, Stothert JC, Kaiser GC, et al. Supraventricular arrhythmias after myocardial revascularization: a randomized trial of prophylactic digitalization. J Thorac Cardiovasc Surg 1979;77:310.
126. Juler GL, Stemmer EA, Connolly JE. Complications of prophylactic digitalization in thoracic surgical patients. J Thorac Cardiovasc Surg 1969;58:352.
127. Ritchie AJ, Bowe P, Gibbons JRP. Prophylactic digitalization for thoracotomy: A reassessment. Ann Thorac Surg 1990;50:86.
128. Mohr R, Smolinsky A, Goor DA. Prevention of supraventricular tachyarrhythmia with low-dose propranolol after coronary bypass. J Thorac Cardiovasc Surg 1981;81:840.
129. Matangi MF, Neutze JM, Graham KJ, et al. Arrhythmia prophylaxis after aorto-coronary bypass. J Thorac Cardiovasc Surg 1983:85:105.
130. Stephenson LW, MacVaugh H, Tomasello DN, et al. Propranolol for prevention of postoperative cardiac arrhythmias: a randomized study. Ann Thorac Surg 1980;29:113.

131. Williams J, Stephenson LW, Holford FD, et al. Arrhythmia prophylaxis using propranolol after coronary artery surgery. Ann Thorac Surg 1982;34:435.
132. Roffman JA, Fieldman A. Digoxin and propranolol in the prophylaxis of supraventricular tachydysrhythmias after coronary artery bypass surgery. Ann Thorac Surg 1981;31:496.
133. Mills SA, Poole GV, Breyer RH, et al. Digoxin and propranolol in the prophylaxis of dysrhythmias after coronary artery bypass grafting. Circulation 1982;68(Suppl II):222.
134. Gray RJ, Bateman TM, Czer LSC, et al. Esmolol: a new ultrashort-acting beta-adrenergic blocking agent for rapid control of heart rate in postoperative supraventricular tachyarrhythmias. J Am Coll Cardiol 1985;5:1451.
135. Falk RH, Knowlton AA, Bernard SA, et al. Digoxin for converting recent-onset atrial fibrillation to sinus rhythm. Ann Intern Med 1987;106:503.
136. Smith TW. Drug therapy: digitalis glycosides. N Engl J Med 1973;288:719.
137. Haft JI, Habbab MA. Treatment of atrial arrhythmias. Arch Intern Med 1986;146:1085.
138. Betriu A, Chaitman BR, Bourassa MG, et al. Beneficial effect of intravenous diltiazem in the acute management of paroxysmal supraventricular tachyarrhythmias. Circulation 1983;67:88.
139. Ellenbogen KA, Dias VC, Plumb VJ, et al. A placebo-controlled trial of continuous intravenous diltiazem infusion for 24-hour heart rate control during atrial fibrillation and atrial flutter: a multicenter study. J Am Coll Cardiol 1991;18:891.
140. Michelson EL, Sawin HS, MacVaugh H. Esmolol: safety and efficacy in postoperative cardiothoracic patients with supraventricular tachyarrhythmias. Chest 1988;93:705.
141. Platia EV, Michelson EL, Porterfield JK, et al. Esmolol versus verapamil in the acute treatment of atrial fibrillation or atrial flutter. Am J Cardiol 1989;63:925.
142. Simpson RJ, Foster JR, Woelfel AK, et al. Management of atrial fibrillation and flutter—a reappraisal of digitalis therapy. Postgrad Med 1986;79:241.
143. Halpern S, Ellrodt AG, Singh BN, et al. Efficacy of intravenous procainamide infusion in converting atrial fibrillation to sinus rhythm. Br Heart J 1980; 44:589.
144. Rankin AC, Brooks R, Ruskin JN, et al. Adenosine in the treatment of supraventricular tachycardia. Am J Med 1992;92:655.
145. DiMarco JP, Sellars D, Belardinelli L. Rapid termination of supraventricular tachycardia by intravenous adenosine. Circulation 1983;68(Suppl III):358.
146. Belhassen B, Pelleg A, Shoshasni D, et al. Electrophysiologic effects of adenosine triphosphate in AV reentrant tachycardia. Circulation 1983;68(Suppl III):358.
147. Vine DL. Adenosine for diagnosing wide-complex tachycardias. Kans Med 1990;91:304.
148. Stewart RB, Bardy GH, Greene HL. Wide-complex tachycardia: misdiagnosis and outcome after emergent therapy. Ann Intern Med 1986;104:766.
149. Douglas P, Hirschfield JW, Edmunds LH. Clinical correlates of post-operative atrial fibrillation. Circulation 1984;70(Suppl II):165.
150. Arnold AZ, Mick MJ, Mazurek RP, et al. Role of prophylactic anticoagulation for direct-current cardioversion. J Am Coll Cardiol 1992;19:851.
151. DiMarco JP. Further evidence in support of anticoagulant therapy before elective cardioversion of atrial fibrillation. J Am Coll Cardiol 1992;19:856.
152. Weinberg DM, Mancini J. Anticoagulation for cardioversion of atrial fibrillation. Am J Cardiol 1989; 63:745.
153. Ewy GA. Optimal technique for electrical cardioversion of atrial fibrillation. Circulation 1992;86:1645.
154. Cooper TB, MacLean WAH, Waldo AL. Overdrive pacing for supraventricular tachycardia. A review of theoretical implications and therapeutic techniques. PACE 1978;1:196.
155. Von Knorring J, Lepantalo M, Lindgren L, et al. Cardiac arrhythmias and myocardial ischemia after thoracotomy for lung cancer. Ann Thorac Surg 1992;53:642.
156. Rubin DA, Nieminski KE, Monteferrante JC, et al. Ventricular arrhythmias after coronary artery bypass surgery: incidence, risk factors and long-term prognosis. J Am Coll Cardiol 1985;6:307.
157. Gray RJ, Mandel WJ. Management of common postoperative arrhythmias. In: Gray RJ, Matloff JM, eds. Medical management of the cardiac surgical patient. Baltimore: Williams & Wilkins, 1990:208.
158. Adult advanced cardiac life support. JAMA 1992; 268:2199.
159. Reed CE, Spinale FG, Crawford FA. Effect of pulmonary resection on right ventricular function. Ann Thorac Surg 1992;53:578.
160. Kaul KB, Bain WH, Jones JV, et al. Mitral valve replacement in the presence of severe pulmonary hypertension. Thorax 1976;31:332.
161. Deeb GM, Bolling SF, Guynn TP, et al. Amrinone versus conventional therapy in pulmonary hyper-

tensive patients awaiting cardiac transplantation. Ann Thorac Surg 1989;48:665.
162. Lappas DG, Powell WJ, Daggett WM. Cardiac dysfunction in the perioperative period: pathophysiology, diagnosis and treatment. Anesthesiology 1977;47:117.
163. D'Ambra MN, LaRaia PJ, Philbin DM, et al. Prostaglandin E: a new therapy for refractory right ventricular failure and pulmonary hypertension after mitral valve replacement. J Thorac Cardiovasc Surg 1985;89:567.
164. Mills NL, Ochsner JL. Right ventricular failure: observations of the interrelationships affecting RV failure after aortocoronary bypass, valve surgery, and congenital heart defect repair. Cardiovasc Clin 1987;17:45.
165. Spense PA, Weisel RD, Easdown JA, et al. The hemodynamic effects and mechanism of action of pulmonary artery balloon counterpulsation in the treatment of right ventricular failure during left heart bypass. Ann Thorac Surg 1985;39:329.
166. Gillinov AM, Davis EA, Alberg AJ, et al. Pulmonary embolism in the cardiac surgical patient. Ann Thorac Surg 1992;53:988.
167. Dismuke SE, Wagner EH. Pulmonary embolism as a cause of death, the changing mortality in hospital patients. JAMA 1986;255:2039.
168. Virchow R. Die cellular pathologie in ihere begrundung auf physiologische and pathologische gewebelehre. Berlin: A Hirschwald, 1858.
169. Risberg B. Surgery and fibrinolysis. J Surg Res 1979;26:698.
170. Coon WW, Coller FA. Clinicopathologic correlation in thromboembolism. Surg Gynecol Obstet 1959;109:259.
171. Goodall RJR, Greenfield LJ. Clinical correlation in the diagnosis of pulmonary embolism. Ann Surg 1980;191:219.
172. Allgood RJ, Wolfe WG, Ebert PA, et al. Effects of carbon dioxide on bronchoconstriction after pulmonary artery occlusion. Am J Physiol 1968;214: 772.
173. Greenfield LJ. Surfactant in surgery. Surg Clin North Am 1974;54:979.
174. Wilson JE, Pierce AK, Johnson RL, et al. Hypoxemia in pulmonary embolism, a clinical study. J Clin Invest 1971;:50:481.
175. Dontzker DR, Bower JS. Alterations in gas exchange following pulmonary thromboembolism. Chest 1982;81:495.
176. Moser KM. Pulmonary embolism. Am Rev Respir Dis 1977;115:829.
177. Greenfield LJ Baue AE, Geha AS, Hammond GL, Laks H, Naunheim KS, eds. Pulmonary embolism: pathophysiology and treatment. In: Glenn's thoracic and cardiovascular surgery. 5th ed. Norwalk: Appleton & Lange, 1991:1561.
178. Gurewich V. Cohen ML, Thomas DP. Humoral factors in massive pulmonary embolism: an experimental study. Am Heart J 1968;76:784.
179. McIntyre KM, Sasahara AA. Determination of the cardiovascular responses to pulmonary embolism. In: Moser KM, Stein M, eds. Pulmonary thromboembolism. Chicago: Yearbook Medical 1973:144.
180. McIntyre KM, Sasahara AA. Determinants of right ventricular function and hemodynamics in pulmonary embolism. Chest 1974;65:534.
181. Urokinase pulmonary embolism trial: a national cooperative study. Circulation 1973;47(Suppl II):60.
182. Dalen JE, Haffajee CI, Alpert JS, et al. Pulmonary embolism, pulmonary hemorrhage, and pulmonary infarction. N Engl J Med 1977;296:1431.
183. Parker BM, Smith JR. Pulmonary embolism and infarction. Am J Med 1958;24:402.
184. Gilday DL, Roulose KP, DeLand F. Accuracy of detection of pulmonary emboli by lung scanning correlated with pulmonary angiography. Am J Roentgenol Radium Ther Nucl Med 1972;115:732.
185. McIntyre KM, Sasahara AA. Pulmonary angiography, scanning, and hemodynamics in pulmonary embolism: a critical review and correlations. Crit Rev Radiol Sci 1972;3:489.
186. Prescott SM, Richard KL, Tikoff G, et al. Venous thromboembolism in decompensated chronic obstructive pulmonary disease. Am Rev Respir Dis 1981;123:32.
187. Hull RD, Hirsch J, Carter CJ, et al. Pulmonary angiography, ventilation lung scanning, and venography for clinically suspected pulmonary embolism with abnormal perfusion scan. Ann Intern Med 1983;98:891.
188. Kahn D, Bushnell DL, Dean R, et al. Clinical outcome of patients with "low-probability" of pulmonary embolism on ventilation-perfusion lung scan. Arch Intern Med 1989;149:377.
189. Kelly MA, Carson JL, Palewvsky HI, et al. Diagnosing pulmonary embolism: new facts and strategies. Ann Intern Med 1991;114:300.
190. Israeli D, Kalhorn A, Menzoian JO. Physician practices in the diagnosis and management of patients with pulmonary embolism. Ann Vasc Surg 1991; 5:337.

191. Greenfield LJ, Zocco J, Wilk JD, et al. Clinical experience with the Kim-Ray Greenfield vena caval filter. Ann Surg 1977;185:692.
192. Mobin-Uddin K, McLean R, Bolooki H, et al. Caval interruption for prevention of pulmonary embolism: long-term results of a new method. Arch Surg 1969;99:711.
193. Carabasi RA, Moritz MJ, Jarrell BE. Complications encountered with the use of the Greenfield filter. Am J Surg 1987;154:163.
194. Turnier E, Hill JD, Kerth WJ, et al. Massive pulmonary embolism. Am J Surg 1973;125:611.
195. Robinson RJ, Fehrenbacher J, Brown JW, et al. Emergent pulmonary embolectomy: the treatment for massive pulmonary embolus. Ann Thorac Surg 1986;42:52.
196. Hietala SO, Greenfield LJ. Percutaneous pulmonary embolectomy on the transvenous route. Eur Soc Cardiovasc Radiol 1979;23:325.
197. Centers for Disease Control. Nosocomial infection surveillance, 1984. MMWR 1986;35:17SS.
198. Gross PA. Deaths from nosocomial infections: experience in a university hospital and a community hospital. Am J Med 1980;68:219.
199. Feely TW. Aerosol polymixin and pneumonia in seriously ill patients. N Engl J Med 1975;293:471.
200. du Moulin GC. Aspiration of gastric bacteria in antacid-treated patients: a frequent cause of postoperative colonization of the airway. Lancet 1982;1:242.
201. Johanson WG, Pierce AK, Sanford JP, et al. Nosocomial respiratory infections with Gram-negative bacilli. The significance of colonization of the respiratory tract. Ann Intern Med 1072;77:701.
202. Sanderson PJ. The sources of pneumonia in ICU patients. Infect Control Hosp Epidemiol 1986;7:104.
203. Johanson WG, Pierce AK, Sanford JP. Changing pharyngeal bacterial flora of hospitalized patients. Emergence of gram-negative bacilli. N Engl J Med 1969;281:1137.
204. Johanson WG, Higuchi JH, Chaudhuri TR, et al. Bacterial adherence to epithelial cells in bacillary colonization of the respiratory tract. Am Rev Respir Dis 1980;121:55.
205. Tobin M, Grenvik A. Nosocomial lung infection and its diagnosis. Crit Care Med 1984;12:199.
206. Craven DE. Nosocomial pneumonia: new concepts of an old disease. Infect Control Hosp Epidemiol 1988;9:57.
207. Pingleton SK, Hinthorn DR, Chien L. Enteral nutrition in patients receiving mechanical ventilation. Am J Med 1986;80:827.
208. Atherton ST, White DJ. Stomach as a source of bacteria colonizing respiratory tract during artificial ventilation. Lancet 1978;2:968.
209. Driks MR, Craven DE. Nosocomial pneumonia in intubated patients given sucralfate as compared with antacids or histamine type 2 blockers. N Engl J Med 1987;317:1376.
210. Daschner F. Stress ulcer prophylaxis and ventilation pneumonia: prevention by antibacterial cytoprotective agents? Infect Control Hosp Epidemiol 1988;9:59.
211. Cook DJ, Laine LA, Guyatt GH, et al. Nosocomial pneumonia and the role of gastric pH. Chest 1991;91:519.
212. Pingleton SK. Commentary on stress ulcer prophylaxis and nosocomial pneumonia. Ann Intern Med 1992;116(Suppl I):8.
213. Chauncey JB, Lynch JP, Hyzy RC, et al. Invasive techniques in the diagnosis of bacterial pneumonia in the ICU. Semin Infect Dis 1990;5:215.
214. Downs JB. Postoperative respiratory care. In: Kaplan JA, ed. Thoracic anesthesia. New York: Churchill Livingstone, 1983:635.
215. Gale GD, Teasdale SJ, Sanders DE, et al. Pulmonary atelectasis and other complications after cardiopulmonary bypass and investigation of aetiologic factors. Can J Anaesth 1979;26:15.
216. Brismar B, Hedensteirna G, Lundquist H, et al. Pulmonary densities during anesthesia with muscular relaxation—a proposal for atelectasis. Anesthesiology 1985;62:422.
217. Tokics L, Hedensteirna G, Strandberg A, et al. Lung collapse and gas exchange during general anesthesia: effects of spontaneous breathing, muscle paralysis, and positive end-expiratory pressure. Anesthesiology 1987;66:157.
218. Nunn JF, Bergman NA, Coleman AJ. Factors influencing the oxygen tension during anesthesia with artificial ventilation. Br J Anaesth 1965;37:898.
219. Rehder K, Sessler AD, Marsh HM. General anesthesia and the lung. Am Rev Respir Dis 1975;112:545.
220. Covino B, Fozzard H, Rehder K, eds. Effects of anesthesia. Bethesda MD: American Physiology Society, 1985.
221. Good JT, Wolz JF, Andersen JT, et al. The routine use of positive end-expiratory pressure after open heart surgery. Chest 1979;76:397.
222. Markand ON, Moorthy SS, Mahomed Y, et al. Postoperative phrenic nerve palsy in patients with open-heart surgery. Ann Thorac Surg 1985;39:68.

223. Benjamin JJ, Cascade PN, Rubebenfire M, et al. Left lower lobe atelectasis and consolidation following cardiac surgery: the effect of topical cooling on the phrenic nerve. Radiology 1982;142:11.
224. Marco JC, Hahn JW, Barner HB. Topical cardiac hypothermia and phrenic nerve injury. Ann Thorac Surg 1977;23:235.
225. Wilcox P, Baile E, Hards J, et al. Phrenic nerve function and its relationship to atelectasis after coronary artery bypass surgery. Chest 1988;93:693.
226. Meyers JR, Lembeck L, O'Kane H, et al. Changes in functional residual capacity of the lung after operation. Arch Surg 1975;110:576.
227. Strandberg A, Tokics L, Brismar B, et al. Atelectasis during anesthesia and in the postoperative period. 1986;30:154.
228. Tobin MJ, Dantzker DR. Mechanical ventilation and weaning. In: Dantzker DR, ed. Cardiopulmonary critical care. Orlando: Grune & Stratton, 1986: 203.
229. Scholten DJ, Novak R, Snyder JV. Directed manual recruitment of collapsed lung in intubated and non-intubated patients. Am J Surg 1985;51:330.
230. O'Donohue WJ. National survey of the usage of lung expansion modalities for the prevention and treatment of postoperative atelectasis following abdominal and thoracic surgery. Chest 1985;87:76.
231. Covelli HD, Weled BJ, Beekman JF. Efficacy of continuous positive airway pressure administered by face mask. Chest 1982;81:147.
232. Katz JA. PEEP and CPAP in perioperative respiratory care. 1984;29:614.
233. Stock MC, Downs JB, Corkran ML. Pulmonary function before and after prolonged continuous positive airway pressure by mask. Crit Care Med 1984; 12:973.
234. Jenkins SC, Soutar SA, Loukota JM, et al. Physiotherapy after coronary artery surgery: are breathing exercises necessary? Thorax 1989;44:634.
235. Dull JL, Dull WL. Are maximal breathing exercises or incentive spirometry better than early mobilization after cardiopulmonary bypass? Phys Ther 1983;63:655.
236. O'Donohue WJ. Prevention and treatment of postoperative atelectasis. Chest 1985;87:1.
237. Fraser RG, Pare JAP, Pare JD, et al, eds. Diseases of the thorax caused by external physical agents. In: Diagnosis and diseases of the chest. 3rd ed. Philadelphia: WB Saunders, 1991:2523.
238. Brewer LA. Bronchopleural fistula: management. In: Grillo HC, Eschapasse H, eds. International trends in general thoracic surgery. Vol. 2. Philadelphia: WB Saunders, 1987:398.
239. Franz BJ, Murphy JD. The masked bronchopleural fistula. J Thorac Surg 1955;29:512.
240. Malave G, Foster ED, Wilson JA, et al. Bronchopleural fistula—present day study of an old problem. A review of 52 cases. Ann Thorac Surg 1971;11:1.
241. Williams NS, Lewis CT. Bronchopleural fistula: a review of 86 cases. Br J Surg 1976;63:520.
242. Bjork VO. Suture material and technique for bronchial closure and bronchial anastomosis. J Thorac Surg 1956;32:22.
243. Mathisen DJ, Grillo HC, Vlahakes GJ, et al. The omentum in the management of complicated cardiothoracic problems. J Thorac Cardiovasc Surg 1988;95:677.
244. Pairolero PC, Arnold PG, Trastek VF, et al. Postpneumonectomy empyema. The role of intrathoracic muscle transposition. J Thorac Cardiovasc Surg 1983;99:958.
245. Hoier-Madsen K, Schulze S, Pedersen VM, et al. Management of bronchopleural fistula following pneumonectomy. Scand J Thor Cardiovasc Surg 1984;18:263.
246. Ellis LH, Grindley JH, Edwards JE. The bronchial arteries. Experimental occlusion. Surgery 1951; 30:810.
247. Wilkins EW. Bronchopleural fistula: prophylaxis. In: Grillo HC, Eschapasse H, eds. International trends in general thoracic surgery. Philadelphia: WB Saunders 1987:394.
248. Smith DE, Karish AK, Chapman JP. Healing of the bronchial stump after pulmonary resection. J Thorac Cardiovac Surg 1963;46:548.
249. Iverson LG, Young JN, Ecker RR, et al. Closure of bronchopleural fistulas by an omental pedicle flap. Am J Surg 1988;152:40.
250. Demos NJ, Timmes JJ. Myoplasty for closure of tracheobronchial fistula. Ann Thorac Surg 1973;15:88.
251. Icenogle TB, Levinson MM, Copeland JG, et al. Use of pericardial fat pad flap to prevent bronchopleural fistula. Ann Thorac Surg 1986;42:216.
252. Rice T, Kirby TJ. Prolonged air leak. Complications of pulmonary surgery. Ch Surg CIN Am 1992;2:803.
253. Maeseneer MD, VanHee R, Schoofs E, et al. The management of bronchopleural fistulas. Acta Chir Belg 1987;87:269.
254. Virkkula L, Eerola S. Treatment of postpneumonectomy empyema. Scand J Thorac Cardiovasc Surg 1974;8:133.
255. Christianson KH, Morgan SW, Karich AF, et al.

Pleural space following pneumonectomy. Ann Thorac Surg 1965;1:298.
256. Lauckner ME, Beggs I, Armstrong RF. The radiologic characteristics of bronchopleural fistula following pneumonectomy. Anaesthesia 1983;38:452.
257. York EL, Lewall DB, Hirji M, et al. Endoscopic diagnosis and treatment of postoperative bronchopleural fistula. Chest 1990;97:1390.
258. Friedman PJ, Hellekant CAG. Radiologic recognition of bronchopleural fistula. Radiology 1977; 124:289.
259. Bruni F. Bronchopleural fistula: treatment of long stump after pneumonectomy. In: Grillo HC, Eschapasse H, eds. International trends in general thoracic surgery. Vol. 2. Philadelphia: WB Saunders, 1987:413.
260. Chowdery JK. Percutaneous use of fiberoptic bronchoscope to investigate bronchopleurocutaneous fistula. Chest 1979;75:203.
261. Kirsch MM, Rotman H, Behrendt DM, et al. Complications of pulmonary resection. Ann Thorac Surg 1975;20:215.
262. Steiger Z, Wilson RF. Management of bronchopleural fistulas. Surg Gynecol Obstet 1984;158:267.
263. Ronan KP, Murray MJ. Perioperative assessment and mechanical ventilation. Ch Surg Cl N Am 1992;2:745.
264. Powner DJ, Cline CD, Rodman GH. Effect of chest-tube suction on gas flow through a bronchopleural fistula. Crit Care Med 1985;13:99.
265. Blanch PB, Koens JC, Layon AJ. A new device that allows synchronous intermittent inspiratory chest tube occlusion with any mechanical ventilator. Chest 1990;97:1426.
266. Gallagher TJ, Smith RA, Kirby RR, et al. Intermittent inspiratory chest tube occlusion to limit bronchopleural cutaneous airleaks. Crit Care Med 1976;4:328.
267. Phillips YY, Lonigan RM, Joyner LR. A simple technique for managing a bronchopleural fistula while maintaining positive pressure ventilation. Crit Care Med 1979;7:351.
268. Bishop MJ, Benson MS, Sato P, et al. Comparison of high-frequency jet ventilation with conventional mechanical ventilation for bronchopleural fistula. Anesth Analg 1987;66:833.
269. Carlon GC, Ray C, Klain M, et al. High-frequency positive pressure ventilation in management of a patient with bronchopleural fistula. Anesthesiology 1980;52:160.
270. Poelart J, Mortier E, De Deyne C, et al. The use of combined high-frequency jet ventilation and intermittent positive pressure ventilation in bilateral bronchopleural fistulae. Acta Anaesthiol Belg 1987;38:225.
271. Rubio JJ, Algora-Weber A, Dominguez-de Villota E, et al. Prolonged high-frequency jet ventilation in a patient with bronchopleural fistula. An alternative mode of ventilation. Intensive Care Med 1986; 12:161.
272. Albelda SM, Hansen-Flaschen JH, Taylor E, et al. Evaluation of high-frequency jet ventilation in patients with bronchopleural fistulas by quantitation of the air leak. Anesthesiology 1985;63:551.
273. Mayers I, Mink JT. High-frequency oscillatory ventilation of a canine bronchopleural fistula. Crit Care Med 1989;17:58.
274. Baldwin JC, Mark JBD. Treatment of bronchopleural fistula after pneumonectomy. J Thorac Cardiovasc Surg 1985;90:813.
275. Perelman MI, Rymko LP, Ambatiello GP. Bronchopleural fistula: surgery after pneumonectomy. In: Grillo HC, Eschapasse H, eds. International trends in general thoracic surgery. Philadelphia: WB Saunders, 1987:407.
276. Beltrami V. Surgical transsternal treatment of bronchopleural fistula postpneumonectomy. Chest 1989;95:379.
277. Chicarilli ZN, Ariyan S, Glenn WWL, et al. Management of recalcitrant bronchopleural fistulas with muscle flap obliteration. Plast Reconstr Surg 1985; 75:882.
278. Meland NB, Arnold PG, Pairolero PC, et al. Refinements in intrathoracic use of muscle flaps. Clin Plast Surg 1990;17:697.
279. Dorman JP, Campbell D, Grover FL, et al. Open-thoracostomy drainage of postpneumonectomy empyema with bronchopleural fistula. J Thorac Cardiovasc Surg 1973;66:979.
280. Weissberg D. Empyema and bronchopleural fistula: experience with open-window thoracostomy. Chest 1982;82:447.
281. Steiger Z, Wilson RF. Management of bronchopleural fistulas. Surg Gynecol Obstet 1984;158:267.
282. Torre G, Chiesa G, Ravini M, et al. Endoscopic gluing of bronchopleural fistula. Ann Thorac Surg 1987;43:295.
283. Fleisher AG, Evans KG, Nelems B, et al. Effect of routine fibrin glue use on the duration of airleaks after lobectomy. Ann Thorac Surg 1990;49:133.

284. McCarthy PM, Trastek VF, Bell DG, et al. The effectiveness of fibrin glue sealant for reducing experimental air leak. Ann Thorac Surg 1988;45:203.
285. Thompson GE, Lui ACP. Perioperative nerve injury. In: Benumof JL, Saidman LJ, eds. Anesthesia and perioperative complications. St. Louis: Mosby-Year Book, 1992:160.
286. McLaughlin JS. Positional and incisional complications of thoracic surgery. In: Waldhausen JA, Orringer MB, eds. Complications of cardiothoracic surgery. St. Louis: Mosby Year Book, 1991:20.
287. Kirsch MM, Magee KR, Gagot O, et al. Brachial plexus injury following median sternotomy incision. Ann Thorac Surg 1971;11:315.
288. Hanson MR, Breuer AC, Furlan AJ, et al. Brachial plexus lesions following open heart surgery: a prospective analysis and possible new mechanism of injury. Neurology 1980;30:441.
289. Morin JE, Long R, Elleker MG, et al. Upper extremity neuropathies following median sternotomy. Ann Thorac Surg 1982;34:181.
290. Vander Salm TJ, Cereda JM, Cutler BS. Brachial plexus injury following median sternotomy. J Thorac Cardiovasc Surg 1982;83:914.
291. Salvador JD. Upper extremity neuropathies following median sternotomy. Ann Thorac Surg 1982; 34:185. Editorial.
292. Sy WP. Ulnar nerve palsy possibly related to use of automatically cycled blood pressure cuff. Anesth Analg 1981;60:687.

CHAPTER

16

Postoperative Pain Management

James C. Crews
Phillip O. Bridenbaugh

In the past 15 years, several reviews have reported that historically, postoperative pain has been mismanaged. This mismanagement has been related to a combination of factors including the lack of knowledge and skill of physicians and nurses the counterproductive attitudes of physicians, nurses, patients, and the health care system.[1–8]

In response to this historical perspective, recent advances in the management of postoperative pain have combined several features to improve this aspect of patient care: (1) the development of postoperative pain management services, (2) the use of scientific principles in the prescription of analgesic medications, (3) the administration of analgesics by new techniques and routes, and (4) a change in the philosophy of postoperative pain management. The treatment of postoperative pain should be approached as an integral component of the routine surgical and anesthetic management of each patient and based on consideration of specific perioperative, anesthetic, surgical, physiological, and pharmacological factors.

Perioperative Considerations

Patient-related Considerations

Postoperative pain following thoracic surgery can complicate the pulmonary and general physical recovery. The majority of thoracic surgery patients have some degree of preoperative alteration in cardiopulmonary physiology resulting from the nature of the associated disease processes (bronchitis, emphysema, infection; or airway, parenchymal, mediastinal, or chest wall masses). Preexisting abnormalities of pulmonary function are exacerbated in the postoperative period because of the effects of the surgical procedure on respiration and ventilation. Although aggressive pulmonary and physical rehabilitation is necessary to prevent or treat the potential postoperative pulmonary complications, therapy may be hindered by insufficient effort in the patient with inadequate postoperative analgesia. In addition to the problems associated with inadequate postoperative analgesia, the undesirable effects of analgesic medications and pain management techniques must also be considered.

Patients demonstrate a high degree of variability in their perception and response to postoperative pain. Previous painful experiences, emotional and psychological characteristics, and individual expectations are important considerations in the management of patients with pain following major surgical procedures. A thorough discussion of the anticipated anesthetic and surgical procedures with the patient should take place preoperatively. A discussion of available options for the management of postoperative pain, and an understanding of the importance of postoperative rehabilitation efforts (e.g., incentive spirometry, deep breathing, coughing, early ambulation) inform and prepare the patient for the postsurgical period. This preoperative preparation and reassurance may decrease perioperative anxiety and reduce analgesic requirements in the postoperative period.[9,10]

Anesthetic Considerations

The intraoperative anesthetic technique may also affect the severity of postoperative pain. Studies have demonstrated that intraoperative anesthetic techniques that are directed at the prevention of postoperative pain are more effective than techniques that involve the management of pain once present in the postoperative period.[11,12] An improvement in postoperative analgesic efficacy and pulmonary function is noted when neural blockade or nociceptive modulating techniques are used in combination with general anesthesia during the surgical procedure.[13,14] The judicious intraoperative administration of intravenous opioids has been associated with increased postoperative analgesic efficacy as compared to the intraoperative administration of inhalation anesthetics alone.[15] The improvements in postoperative analgesia associated with these intraoperative techniques directed toward prevention of postoperative pain are thought to be related to activation of psychological and neurohumoral stress responses by the nociceptive stimulus.

Surgical Considerations

Certain surgical considerations also affect the intensity and severity of postoperative pain. Posterolateral thoracotomy incisions and extensive midline upper abdominal incisions are generally considered to be the most painful of surgical approaches to the thorax or upper abdomen. Midline sternotomy has been reported to be associated with less postoperative pain and impairment of respiratory function than posterolateral thoracotomy.[16,17] Factors such as the nature of the incision (does the procedure involve an incision through the serratus anterior muscle or require rib resection), the extent of surgical exposure, the duration of surgical procedure, the type of wound closure, and the size and placement of thoracostomy drainage tubes all affect the nature and intensity of postoperative pain.

Physiologic and Pharmacologic Considerations

Postoperative pain involves several anatomical structures and neural pathways that must be taken into consideration for effective patient management. Pain following thoracic surgical procedures is the result of neural activation in somatic afferent fibers from the chest wall musculature, surgical incision, and thoracostomy drainage tube sites. Visceral afferent neural stimulation related to pleural and parenchymal resection, thoracostomy drainage tubes, and mediastinal and diaphragmatic irritation is also involved. Nociceptive stimulation associated with respiratory excursions, coughing, or patient movement can be associated with muscle splinting and impairment of respiratory effort.

In the immediate postoperative period, pain can increase the likelihood for worsening atelectatic changes in the lung and impairment of gas exchange.

The selection of analgesic modality should consider the contribution and effects of the various anatomical structures responsible for nociceptive stimuli and the involved afferent neural pathways. Various analgesic modalities are available for altering the flow of nociceptive information from the periphery to cortex. These mechanisms of producing analgesia may affect (1) the transduction of nociceptive information at the peripheral receptor (local anesthetics, nonsteroidal anti-inflammatory analgesics); (2) the transmission of nociceptive information along the afferent sensory neural pathways (peripheral, epidural, or intrathecal local anesthetics), or (3) the modulation of nociceptive input at the level of the dorsal horn of the spinal cord (epidural and intrathecal opioids, spinal α_2-adrenergic receptor agonists, transcutaneous electrical nerve stimulation) or the brain (systemic opioids) (Fig. 16-1).

The complete abolition of pain in the postoperative period does not restore postoperative pulmonary function to preoperative levels, thus indicating that pain is but one of several factors related to the mechanical respiratory abnormalities following thoracic surgery.[18] The goals of pain management in the patient following thoracic surgery should be directed toward sufficient analgesia to allow efficient postsurgical rehabilitation efforts and maintain a satisfactory level of patient comfort without adverse circulatory, respiratory, or neurological complications. Tailoring therapy to the specific analgesic requirements of the individual patient is imperative. Various types of postoperative analgesia management have been described, including the systemic administration of analgesics, neural blockade procedures, electrical stimulation analgesia, and the administration of spinal/epidural analgesics. This chapter will provide a review of these modalities with an emphasis on the role each provides in achieving the management goals outlined above.

Figure 16-1. Sites of antinociceptive effects of various pharmacologic substances.

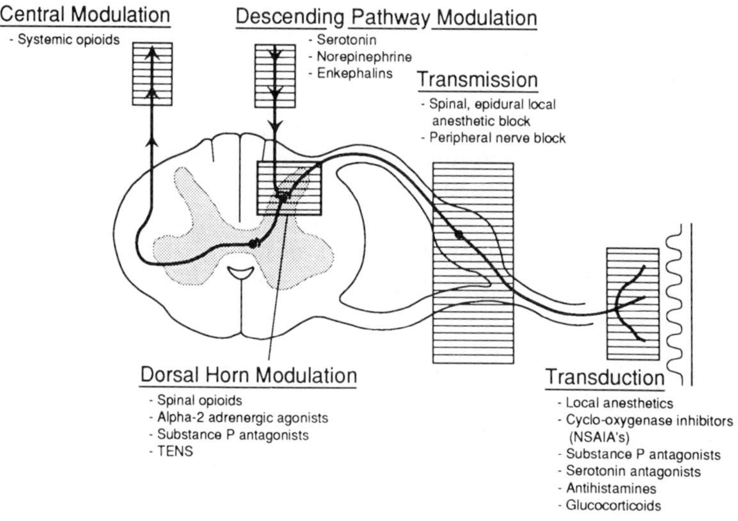

Systemic Opioid Analgesia

The intermittent intramuscular administration of opioids on an "as needed" basis is considered to be the conventional analgesic regimen for the management of postoperative pain. Several reviews of the efficacy of such treatment have described the inadequacies and technical difficulties associated with this analgesic method.[19–21] Studies of plasma concentration-response relationships in postoperative patients have demonstrated that the basal analgesic requirements show a high degree of intrapatient consistency and interpatient variability.[22–24] The ineffectiveness of intramuscular opioid analgesia is attributed partly to the plasma concentration peak and trough effects associated with the intermittent intramuscular administration of relatively large doses of opioid and to the intrapatient and interpatient variability in absorption and site of injection. More important, however, is the fact that conventional intramuscular opioid analgesia fails to focus on the prevention of postoperative pain; historically, this method has lacked adequate ongoing assessment of analgesic efficacy and titration of analgesia to patient-specific requirements. These factors should be considered in the development of alternative analgesic modalities.

The ideal systemic opioid analgesic method for postoperative pain would provide continuous analgesia with titration to patient-specific requirements sufficient to allow patient comfort during vigorous respiratory efforts, ambulation, and other activities. The complete absence of side effects would be equally ideal. This scheme could be achieved through the intermittent administration of opioids with a relatively long duration of action, the use of frequent incremental doses of opioids with a relatively short duration of action, or by the administration of a continuous opioid infusion; in each scheme, the opioid could be administered to maximum analgesic effect. If additional analgesia is required for intermittent activity-related pain, these needs could be met by the administration of an opioid with a relatively rapid onset of analgesia and a short-to-intermediate duration of action.

Most patients are unable to tolerate oral administration of medications in the immediate postoperative period. In addition to the previously discussed intramuscular route, other routes of administration for systemic opioid analgesia have included subcutaneous and intravenous methods. The intravenous route has several advantages in the postoperative patient, two of which are particularly notable: (1) uniform availability and accessibility, especially in the immediate and intermediate postoperative period, and (2) more rapid and predictable absorption and distribution as compared to subcutaneous and intramuscular routes of administration. Rectal, intranasal, sublingual, and transdermal routes may also be used for systemic opioid administration.

Intravenous Opioid Administration

Due to the rapid absorption and distribution of intravenous opioids, an opioid of relatively short duration can be used for intermittent activity-related pain stimuli. For prolonged analgesia, however, intravenous opioids must be administered on a frequent basis or must have a long duration of action.

The use of methadone, an opioid with a relatively long duration of action, for the management of postoperative pain in adults following abdominal surgery was reported to have an average duration of approximately 20 hours following the intraoperative administration of a 20-mg dose.[23–26] No patients required naloxone to initiate postanesthetic spontaneous ventilation. Immediately postoperatively, patients received additional methadone in 5-mg increments with titration to individual analgesic requirements. Supplemental basal analgesic requirements were provided by additional 5-mg doses of methadone throughout the 60-hour study period.[25] The long duration of analgesia following methadone administration is due to a gradual decline in plasma concentration resulting from the relatively low clearance (long half-life) of the drug.[24] The cautious intraoperative titration of methadone in patients undergoing thoracic surgery can provide prolonged basal analgesia postoperatively.

Patient-Controlled Analgesia

In 1968, Sechzer described the administration of repeated, small, intermittent, intravenous doses of morphine and meperidine to postoperative patients following thoracic or abdominal surgical procedures.[27] The medication was administered in response to patient request by a constantly available nurse-observer upon activation of a hand-held, analgesic-demand button. This method of analgesia delivery was found to be highly effective in managing postoperative pain but was extremely time-consuming for nursing personnel. More practical patient-controlled, analgesic-demand systems were developed and described in the early 1970s.[28–30] These systems were the predecessors of the microprocessor-controlled, patient-activated analgesia delivery systems in use today (so-called patient-controlled analgesia systems, or PCAs). These allow patients to self-administer a prescribed intravenous dose of opioid analgesic via a hand-held triggering device. The risk of overmedication is reduced by limiting the frequency of patient-activated medication deliveries by programming a minimum lockout interval. Theoretical advantages to PCA include (1) the ability to titrate opioid to individual analgesic requirements and adjust for changes in pain intensity associated with activity is patient-controlled, (2) analgesic response to a dose is rapid, (3) plasma concentration of opioid can be maintained within a fairly narrow range by the intermittent administration of small doses over time, and (4) nursing time is saved as compared to conventional intramuscular opioid analgesia. Theoretical disadvantages to PCA include (1) the need for sophisticated microprocessor-controlled pumps and (2) the requirement that patients understand the concept of PCA and use the medication effectively to maintain adequate analgesia to perform the necessary postoperative activities including respiratory therapy and ambulation.

Analgesic efficacy of PCA in other postoperative patient populations has been demonstrated to be superior to the intermittent, intramuscular administration of opioids.[31,32] Despite a lack of published data from similar comparative studies in patients following major thoracic or abdominal surgical procedures, PCA should theoretically provide improved analgesic efficacy in these patient populations as well. Some patients may not be adequately managed with PCA because psychological factors limiting its effective use[33] or because pain intensity-systemic side effect relationships limit the ability of patients to maintain adequate analgesia without excessive central nervous system effects (eg, respiratory depression, somnolence, nausea, vomiting, pruritus).

Dosing parameters must be individualized for each patient. Analgesic efficacy must be frequently assessed and subsequent adjustments in dosing parameters should be made on the basis of analgesia, frequency of patient demands, and side effects. An improvement in the efficacy of PCA therapy occurs if the patient receives an adequate amount of opioid before the initiation of PCA.[34] The patient is more likely to be able to maintain sufficient analgesia with smaller doses of opioid if an adequate plasma concentration is first established. The amount of opioid required to obtain analgesia initially may also provide some indication of the subsequent opioid requirements of the patient. Suggested starting dosage guidelines and lockout intervals for various opioid analgesics in the management of postoperative pain are provided in Table 16-1.[35]

Continuous Intravenous Infusion

Continuous intravenous infusion of opioid can also provide basal analgesia in the management of postoperative pain. Desirable pharmacokinetic and pharmacodynamic characteristics for continuous intravenous infusion in the postoperative period are a relatively rapid onset of analgesic action, a high degree of efficacy without undesirable side effects, a short-to-intermediate duration of action to allow rapid adjustment of plasma concentration to improve analgesia or reduce side effects without excessive accumulation of drug over time, and a low incidence of development of tolerance.

Although this modality can provide a theoretically constant level of basal analgesia, it has several potential drawbacks: (1) the titration of opioid dose to analgesic requirements of the individual patient may be difficult without the benefit of previous determination of patient-specific pharmacokinetic parameters (eg, clearance, volume of distribution), (2) the level of analgesia at rest may not provide adequate analgesia during periods of activity, and (3) tolerance may develop more rapidly in patients with continuous opioid infusions as compared to patients receiving intermittent dosing.[36]

A combination of modalities incorporating PCA and continuous low-dose opioid infusion has been developed to give the theoretical advantage of maintenance of a basal level of analgesia in addition to patient-activated intermittent doses when necessary for activity-related pain or inadequate basal analgesia. Such a combination should also improve patient sleep patterns by maintaining an effective plasma opioid concentration during sleep, when the patient is not activating the demand device. However, in clinical practice, these theoretical advantages have not been well-documented.[37] In comparative studies of PCA plus concurrent infusion versus PCA only, researchers have reported increased opioid administration in the patients with PCA plus concurrent infusion with no subjective improvement in pain scores, patient satisfaction, or sleep patterns.[38] In selected patients, a concurrent infusion may be beneficial when necessary for rest pain or periods of sleep, as during the first 12–24 hours postoperatively. The contribution of opioid supplied by the continuous infusion should be maintained at a fraction of the patient's hourly opioid requirement. The continuous infusion component if needed at all, can usually be discontinued fairly early in the postoperative period. The risks of

Table 16-1. Intravenous Opioid Dosing Guidelines for Patient-Controlled Analgesia*

Opioid	Dose	Lockout Interval (min)	4-hour Dose Limit
Morphine (1 mg/mL)	0.5–2.0 mg	5–20	20 mg
Meperidine (10 mg/mL)	5–20 mg	5–20	200 mg
Hydromorphone (0.2 mg/mL)	0.1–0.4 mg	5–15	4 mg
Fentanyl (50 μg/mL)	25–50 μg	5–15	400 μg

* These dosages are recommendations only and should be adjusted to individual patient requirements.

excessive sedation and respiratory depression are increased with the use of the combination of PCA and concurrent continuous intravenous infusion.

Systemic opioid analgesia with careful titration of medication dose to individual patient requirements can provide adequate analgesia for patients following thoracic surgery. The frequent association of the level of analgesia required for activity-related periods with undesirable side effects such as respiratory depression or excessive sedation in thoracic surgery patients limits the clinical use of this method. Superior analgesia and fewer side effects may be possible with modalities that demonstrate a more favorable therapeutic index.

Alternate Methods of Systemic Opioid Administration

Several other methods of postoperative opioid administration besides the intravenous route have been explored. These include transdermal delivery systems and sublingual, intranasal, rectal, and oral dosing preparations. Some of these modalities offer significant advantage to the patient because of sustained duration of action, as well as ease and convenience of administration.

Gourlay and coworkers have reported clinical trials of the transdermal administration of the opioid fentanyl for the management of postoperative pain.[39,40] These studies reported analgesia in the group of patients administered transdermal fentanyl as evidenced by a reduction in supplementary meperidine requests as compared to the control group. A delay of 12–16 hours before the achievement of minimum effective plasma fentanyl concentrations was a disadvantage. Patients receiving either fentanyl or placebo (supplementary meperidine was administered in both groups) had a similar incidence of side effects. Despite the long delay time before achievement of appreciable analgesia and the need for supplementation of analgesia for activity-related pain, the authors concluded that this delivery system provides effective postoperative analgesia in patients following abdominal surgical procedures. A similar study of patients following thoracic surgery is needed.

The sublingual route has been explored because of the convenience of administration and the absence of first-pass hepatic metabolism associated with the oral route. Buprenorphine, the partial μ-opioid receptor agonist, has been studied most extensively[41–43] because of its high lipid solubility (promoting sublingual absorption) and absence of unpleasant taste and mucosal irritation. Preliminary studies indicate that the transnasal-metered administration of the opioid receptor agonist-antagonist butorphanol may be safe and efficacious in the control of postoperative pain.[44]

The rectal and oral routes of administration are also being explored for possible increased utilization for postoperative analgesia. Sustained-release preparations of morphine that provide prolonged analgesia allowing less frequent dosing have been developed. In patients unable to tolerate oral intake due to vomiting or gastric suctioning in the immediate postoperative period, the oral administration of opioids may not be feasible. This route of administration is extensively utilized as patients begin to recover and can tolerate oral intake, however. Perhaps the oldest and simplest example of PCA is still the self-administration of oral opioid compounds by patients in response to postoperative pain.

These alternate methods of systemic opioid administration may hold future promise but await investigation for use in patients following thoracic surgery. Without regard to the route of administration, the clinical efficacy of systemic opioid analgesia for the management of postoperative pain is limited by the undesirable side effects to the central nervous system and gastrointestinal and urinary systems that are associated with systemic administration.

Intercostal and Interpleural Analgesia

Intercostal Analgesia

In an attempt to provide profound postoperative analgesia following thoracic surgery while minimizing the undesirable systemic side effects associated with opioid analgesia, neural blockade procedures have been applied perioperatively. Neural blockade techniques are efficacious and reproducible in producing intraoperative analgesia; use of these techniques in the postoperative management of patients can provide significant adjunctive analgesia, thus reducing or eliminating the need for opioid analgesics.

Intercostal nerve blockade with local anesthesia has been used extensively in the immediate postoperative period for the management of pain following thoracic and upper abdominal surgery. In a 1975 review of the use of this method, Moore described this procedure as "having no therapeutic equal in eliminating somatic pain resulting from surgery of the thorax and upper abdomen."[45] Principal advantages of intercostal nerve blockade include (1) profound relief of somatic pain and muscle spasm in the distribution of the block; (2) lack of significant central nervous system or cardiovascular effects such as respiratory depression, sedation, or hypotension; (3) relatively long duration of analgesia (up to 12 hours) with the use of local anesthetics such as bupivacaine or etidocaine; and (4) technical ease of performance in the perioperative period. A potential disadvantage of this procedure is the risk of pneumothorax; however, the incidence of this complication is reported as less than 0.1% in experienced hands.[45] Many excellent discussions of the technical aspects of intercostal nerve blockade have been previously published.[46]

Faust and Nauss published a randomized study of 34 thoracic surgery patients who were to receive either intercostal nerve block (ICB) or intramuscular meperidine. The ICB group demonstrated a smaller decline in postoperative vital capacity measurement (60% versus 78% change from preoperative values) and a smaller increase in postoperative $PaCO_2$ tension, as compared to the intramuscular meperidine group.[47]

Crawford and coworkers published the results of a double-blind, randomized study of 30 patients undergoing a rib-resecting thoracoabdominal incision to determine the effect of intraoperative intercostal nerve block with bupivacaine versus saline on postoperative pain and complications, day of ambulation, and day of fluid intake. Patients in both groups were allowed to have postoperative intramuscular opioid analgesia on request. The authors reported a significant reduction in the mean total dose of morphine required in the bupivacaine group (133 mg) versus the saline group (234 mg). Three patients in the saline group had postoperative atelectasis; one patient in the bupivacaine group had this condition. No intergroup differences in day of ambulation or fluid intake were noted.[48]

Willdeck-Lund and Edstrom compared the efficacy and duration of postoperative analgesia of 2 mL 0.5% bupivacaine with those of 1.0% etidocaine for intercostal blockade following thoracotomy. Patients in the etidocaine group received approximately six hours of postoperative analgesia compared to five hours in the bupivacaine group. Patients in both groups reported comparable analgesia with no significant difference in duration; Reports of shoulder pain in both groups led these authors to conclude that these methods of postoperative analgesia are beneficial for incisional pain but cannot provide complete pain relief after thoracotomy. Possible explanations of the etiology of shoulder pain include referred visceral pain from diaphragmatic irritation, percutaneous thoracostomy drainage tubes, and intraoperative overextension of the shoulder.[49] An explanation for the difference in duration of analgesia between this study and that reported by Moore and other investigators[45,50] may relate to the volume of local anesthetic injected (2 mL versus 3–5 mL).

Most authors recommend the routine addition of epinephrine in a concentration of 1:200,000 to local anesthetic solutions for intercostal blockade, because the plasma concentrations of local anesthetic following ICB are higher than most other regional anesthetic procedures. The addition of epinephrine markedly decreases the vascular absorption of the local anesthetic and prolongs the duration of analgesia.[51]

In an effort to extend the duration of postoperative analgesia beyond 12 hours following a single intercostal block procedure, Kaplan and coworkers evaluated the duration of analgesia with the addition of dextran versus saline to bupivacaine. These investigators reported a mean duration of analgesia of less than 12 hours with bupivacaine and saline, as compared to 36 hours for patients receiving bupivacaine and low-molecular-weight dextran 40.[50] The suggested mechanism of action responsible for the prolonged analgesia with the combination of bupivacaine and dextran 40 was the formation of a complex that decreased the rate of absorption of the local anesthetic.[52] A control group of patients receiving dextran 40 and saline was included; no analgesia to pinprick was noted in these patients. Significant improvements in PaO_2, $PaCO_2$, vital capacity, forced expiratory flow rates, analgesic requirements, and patient comfort compared to controls were apparent in both groups of patients.

Intercostal blockade may be performed in the preoperative, intraoperative, or immediate postoperative period. Blockade procedures in the preoperative period can decrease intraoperative anesthetic requirements by providing profound adjunctive somatic analgesia. Postoperative analgesia may be supplemented with repeated blockade every 6–12 hours as necessary. The intraoperative blockade of intercostal nerves from within the thoracic cavity may be performed under direct vision.[53] Several case reports describing hypotensive complications following the intraoperative blockade of intercostal nerves with local anesthetic under direct vision have been published.[54–56] Explanations of the etiology of these hypotensive complications have included injection of local anesthetic into a peripheral extension of a dural sheath producing total spinal anesthesia, paravertebral spread of local anesthetic resulting in blockade of thoracic sympathetic fibers, and direct intravascular injection of local anesthetic. The onset of profound somatic intercostal blockade during general anesthesia resulting in an abrupt decrease in anesthetic requirement may contribute to the hypotension.

In an attempt to produce a greater duration of postoperative analgesia following intercostal blockade, intermittent injection or continuous infusions of local anesthetics via catheters has been described.[57–62] The catheter is placed intraoperatively in the subpleural intercostal space or in the ipsilateral paravertebral space. Results of efficacy are variable, but most studies indicate an adjunctive opioid-sparing analgesic effect in the postoperative period. Catheter placement by the surgical team may prolong the duration of the surgical procedure depending on the location of placement and the number of catheters used. Most approaches depend on a rather large volume of local anesthetic to achieve the desired analgesic effect, and the dermatomal distribution of analgesia is inconsistent. In one rather aggressive approach to the enhancement of analgesic duration, a series of cases was published supporting the intraoperative neurolysis of intercostal nerves with phenol. Patients in the phenol group were reported to have superior analgesia and improved postoperative respiratory parameters as compared to the control group of patients. No "disagreeable collateral effects" were noted in the 32 patients, and analgesic duration ranged from 6 to 18 weeks with a reported mean duration of 13 weeks.[63]

Interpleural Analgesia

Reiestad and Stromskag developed and originated postoperative analgesia which is produced by the intermittent administration of local anesthetic into the pleural space through an interpleural catheter. They reported its use following subcostal cholecystectomy, renal surgery, and unilateral breast operations. Twenty milliliters of 0.5% bupivacaine with epinephrine was reported to provide an average duration of 10 hours of analgesia; no complications were reported in all 81 patients. The addition of radiopaque contrast material to local anesthetic filled the entire interpleural space within 30 seconds in patients following nonpulmonary procedures. The technique was described as relatively simple to perform and capable of producing unilateral analgesia over a wide thoracic dermatomal distribution without the hypotension associated with epidural administration of local anesthetics.[64] The technique was subsequently investigated as a possible modality for analgesia following thoracic surgery.[65–69]

The mechanism of analgesia following interpleural administration of local anesthetic is unknown. Theoretical mechanisms, include thoracic sympathetic blockade, vagal or phrenic blockade, or somatic intercostal neural blockade resulting from diffusion of local anesthetic across the parietal pleura have been proposed. The ability to produce somatic analgesia to pinprick appears related to the dosage of local anesthetic or concentration; reproducible somatic blockade occurs after administration of 0.5% bupivacaine but not after administration of 0.25% bupivacaine.[70] The duration of pain relief resulting from interpleural analgesia also appears to be somewhat related to total dose of local anesthetic.[71]

Administration of the relatively large volumes of bupivacaine required for interpleural analgesia causes concern related to peak plasma concentrations of local anesthetic. Most investigators recommend administration of bupivacaine with the addition of epinephrine in an effort to decrease the maximum plasma concentration of bupivacaine following interpleural administration. One study reports an average arterial plasma concentration of bupivacaine of 1.2 μg/mL following the interpleural administration of 100 mg of bupivacaine with epinephrine for pain following cholecystectomy.[71] Seltzer and coworkers reported a mean maximal plasma concentration of 2.07 μg/mL following interpleural administration of 150 mg of bupivacaine with epinephrine in a similar patient population.[72] Both of these studies suggest that interpleural administration of 100–150 mg of bupivacaine with epinephrine produce peak plasma bupivacaine concentrations below the level of 2–4 μg/mL, which are associated with increasing toxicity.

Although reports indicate that interpleural analgesia is generally effective in reducing postoperative opioid requirements following nonpulmonary surgical procedures, studies of analgesic efficacy following thoracic surgery have had inconsistent results that range from disappointing to efficacious.[65–69] Several possible technical factors may be responsible for the disparity in analgesic efficacy between pulmonary and nonpulmonary surgical procedures and the variability in efficacy of interpleural analgesia for pain in patients following thoracotomy. Loss of interpleurally administered local anesthetic in thoracostomy drainage tubes, dilution of local anesthetic in extravasated blood or pleural fluid, and inadequate interpleural spread of local anesthetic as a result of restricted motion of an operated lung are theoretical considerations.

Symreng and colleagues[69,74] compared the effects of interpleural 0.5% bupivacaine (1.5 mg/kg) versus saline in a double-blind study of analgesia, opioid requirement, and pulmonary function in 15 patients following thoracotomy. The results demonstrated a decrease in opioid requirement and pain score and a significant improvement in pulmonary function tests in patients receiving interpleural bupivacaine; no changes occurred in patients receiving interpleural saline. Thoracostomy drainage tubes were disconnected from suction and placed to water seal for 15 minutes following interpleural injection. The duration of analgesia was only two to five hours. The authors believed that the effect was short-lived because of possible loss of bupivacaine in the chest drains. Maximum peak plasma bupivacaine concentrations were less than 1.5 μg/mL.

Kambam and coworkers compared analgesic efficacy and the peak plasma concentration of bupivacaine following the interpleural administration of 20 mL of 0.5% bupivacaine with and without epinephrine 1:200,000. In this study, thoracostomy drainage tubes were clamped for five minutes after bupivacaine administration. No intergroup differences in analgesic efficacy were evident. The mean peak plasma concentration was 0.32 μg/mL following the administration of bupivacaine with epinephrine as compared to 1.28 μg/mL for bupivacaine without epinephrine.[65] In a similar study, Ferrante and coworkers evaluated the roles of epinephrine, thoracostomy drainage, and a double- versus single-catheter technique on analgesic efficacy of interpleural analgesia after thoracotomy. The addition of epinephrine to bupivacaine neither influenced analgesic efficacy nor resulted in a decrease in peak plasma bupivacaine concentration. Approximately 30%–40% of the administered bupivacaine dose was lost via the thoracostomy tube in a four-hour period. Use of two catheters, with one catheter tip placed in the paravertebral and one in the lateral thoracic wall location, resulted in a greater reduction in opioid analgesic requirements. Patients consistently complained of ipsilateral paravertebral pain despite interpleural bupivacaine administration.[73]

Potential complications associated with interpleural analgesia include toxicity to the local anesthetic and pneumothorax. Higher-than-expected plasma bupivacaine levels (>2–4 μg/mL are associated with increasing toxicity) have been reported in patients with recent pneumonia (pleural inflammation)[72] and following the inadvertent placement of an interpleural catheter in lung tissue.[74] Percutaneous placement of catheters through the thoracic wall prior to wound closure in patients undergoing thoracic surgical procedures eliminates the risk of pneumothorax reported with preoperative placement or with percutaneous placement in patients undergoing extrathoracic surgical procedures.[69]

In review, interpleural analgesia with bupivacaine produces rapid-onset adjunctive analgesia with an effective duration of approximately four hours in patients following thoracic surgery. This analgesia is associated with an improvement in pulmonary function and a reduction in postoperative opioid requirements. The interpleural administration of 20 mL of 0.5% bupivacaine produces plasma bupivacaine levels below the level associated with local anesthetic toxicity. Intermittent reinjection of the interpleural catheter with local anesthetic can provide prolonged analgesia if administered every four hours. The use of two interpleural catheters to provide a better distribution of local anesthetic within the pleural space following thoracic surgical procedures may be associated with better analgesia than a single catheter. Continuous infusion of local anesthetic via an interpleural catheter has not demonstrated adequate analgesic efficacy in adult patients following thoracotomy. Investigations of the analgesic effect of a multiple orifice catheter technique that is theoretically capable of distributing local anesthetic over a wide interpleural area and comparative studies of analgesia and effects on postoperative pulmonary function of interpleural versus epidural analgesia are both needed.

Transcutaneous Electrical Stimulation Analgesia and Cryoanalgesia

Transcutaneous Electrical Nerve Stimulation

Transcutaneous electrical nerve stimulation (TENS) is a noninvasive analgesic modality used in the adjunctive management of various acute and chronic pain syndromes, especially chronic benign pain. The application of TENS in the management of acute postoperative pain was described by Hymes and colleagues as being potentially beneficial in reducing postoperative opioid requirements following general surgical procedures.[75] As proposed in the gate control theory of pain developed by Melzack and Wall,[76] the mechanism of analgesia produced by the transcutaneous electrical stimulation of peripheral nerves is based on the modulation of nociceptive input in the dorsal horn of the spinal cord by peripheral stimulation of large sensory afferent fibers. An alternative mechanism involves the release of endorphins as a result of the peripheral afferent fiber stimulation.[77]

The use of TENS as an adjunctive analgesic modality following thoracic surgery has been described as potentially beneficial in reducing postoperative opioid requirements[78] and improving postoperative pulmonary function[79,80] as compared to patients who receive only systemic opioids. Sterile electrodes may be placed on each side of the surgical incision following wound closure, connected to the TENS unit, and covered by a sterile dressing. Stimulation may be initiated in the recovery room and maintained on a continuous basis during the postoperative period.

These authors believe that the use of TENS is more efficacious in more highly motivated patients with an internal locus of control and less effective in anxious patients with an external locus of control and a dependent personality. With appropriate patient selection, TENS may provide adjunctive analgesia and a reduction of postoperative opioid requirements in patients following thoracic surgery. However, establishing the potential utility of this modality as compared to other forms of postoperative analgesia management requires additional controlled investigations.

Cryoanalgesia

Cryoanalgesia, a neurolytic technique, produces neural blockade for a period ranging from several days to weeks. The technique is based on the freezing of a small nerve segment with a small-diameter cryoprobe (approximately 2 mm) cooled to −60°C by the rapid expansion of pressurized gas in the tip. The probe is left in contact with the nerve for 30–60 seconds, and a 2–4-mm ice ball is formed that freezes the nerve and damages the nerve fiber, thus inhibiting neural function. This process is followed by wallerian degeneration of the distal nerve fibers. Although the freezing process causes acute destruction of the nerve fiber, the Schwann cell basal lamina is preserved and provides a conduit for the process of regeneration and subsequent reinnervation of distal structures.

The neurolysis of intercostal nerves within the pleural cavity by the application of a cryoprobe at the time of thoracotomy has been described by various authors as a beneficial analgesic technique in the management of postoperative pain. Glynn and coworkers reported the use of intraoperative cryoanalgesia in a group controlled study of patients who underwent thoracotomy. These investigators reported that the 29 patients who received cryoanalgesia required significantly lower total dosages of opioid analgesics in the postoperative period than the 29 control patients. A subjective improvement in patient compliance with postoperative respiratory physiotherapy was also suggested.[81] In a similar study reported by Katz and coworkers, patients who received cryoanalgesia had lower postoperative pain scores and an approximately 50% lower total dose requirement for opioid analgesics than the control patients.[82] Joucken and colleagues described a study designed to assess the efficacy of cryoanalgesia versus intrathoracic intercostal nerve block with bupivacaine for the relief of postoperative pain following thoracotomy. The patients who received cryoanalgesia required a significantly lower amount of opioid analgesics in the 36-hour postoperative study period. Patients who received intraoperative intercostal nerve blocks with bupivacaine had no subsequent postoperative percutaneous intercostal blocks. They did not demonstrate a reduction in postoperative opioid requirements when compared to control patients in the first 36 hours postoperatively.[83] Adjunctive analgesia of cryoanalgesia was also reported by Brynitz and Schroder.[84]

More recent studies, however, have not demonstrated a significant difference in opioid requirements or pain scores with cryoanalgesia versus control groups of patients.[85,86] Roxburgh and coworkers have reported an increase in long-term postoperative morbidity as defined by persistent neuralgic pain in the distribution of the peri-incisional intercostal nerves associated with intraoperative cryoanalgesia.

An increase in postprocedural neuralgic pain complaints may possibly be related to technical aspects of the cryoanalgesia procedure. Dissection of the intercostal nerve and isolation of the nerve from surrounding tissues with a nerve hook or forceps prior to application of the cryoprobe has been described. Application of the cryoprobe to the intrathoracic subpleural intercostal nerve without dissection of the nerve from the surrounding tissue is a more simple, less traumatic, and equally effective technique. The removal of perineurium in peripheral nerves has been associated with the development of neuroma formation.

Another technical aspect that should be considered in the cryoanalgesia procedure is allowance of an appropriate *thaw* period following the *freeze* period prior to removing the cryoprobe from the area of the nerve. In the author's institution, the thaw period is the same length (30–60 seconds) as the freeze period. This ensures that the ice ball at the tip of the cryoprobe thaws before the probe is removed from the tissue, which reduces trauma to the nerve.

In addition to a potentially increased likelihood for the development of postoperative intercostal neuropathic complications, other potential disadvantages of cryoanalgesia include the additional operative time (approximately 15 minutes) required for the performance of the technique prior to wound closure and occasional production of appreciable chest wall bleeding (approximately 5% of cases).[86]

Although blockade of intercostal nerves with cryoanalgesia does have demonstrable analgesic benefits in the management of postoperative pain following thoracic surgical procedures, this author believes that many of the other analgesic modalities discussed in this chapter are capable of achieving nearly equal or superior analgesia without the risk of long-term neuralgic complications.

Epidural and Intrathecal Analgesia

The localization of opioid receptors in the substantia gelatinosa of the spinal cord[87,88] and the demonstration that analgesia could be obtained in animals by the intrathecal administration of opioids[89] led to the description of potent analgesia produced by the intrathecal and epidural administration of opioids in humans.[90] The epidural administration of analgesic concentrations of local anesthetic solutions to provide regional analgesia has classically been considered by many to be the most effective method of managing acute postoperative pain. The intrathecal or epidural administration of analgesic medications is based on the principle of interruption or modulation of nociceptive input at the level of a nerve root or spinal cord. Total doses are less than those associated with undesirable central systemic effects such as sedation and respiratory depression. Intrathecal and epidural opioid analgesia with or without the combination of analgesic concentrations of local anesthetic solutions has become an important method in the delivery of postoperative analgesia to patients following major thoracic and upper abdominal surgery.

Analgesic concentrations of local anesthetic solutions administered into the epidural space produce interruption of afferent nociceptive input at the level of the intradural spinal nerve roots.[91] The analgesic activity of the spinal administration of opioids involves binding to opioid receptors in the substantia gelatinosa of the dorsal horn of the spinal cord and modulation of activity associated with the transmission of nociceptive information.[92]

Spinal analgesia refers to the use of opioids or analgesic concentrations of local anesthetics to produce analgesia by either intrathecal or epidural administration. The term *spinal* (analgesia or administration) is used in this chapter to refer to both intrathecal and epidural collectively. Spinal analgesia produced by opioids has been referred to as *selective analgesia*[34]; the analgesia is produced by modulation of nociceptive input at the level of the spinal cord in the absence of other sensory, motor, or sympathetic blockade. Analgesia produced by the epidural administration of local anesthetics or opioids has also been referred to as *segmental analgesia*, because the extent of analgesia spread is related to the spinal segmental level of administration and the volume of local anesthetic or opioid administered. By selection of an appropriate spinal level and manipulation of local anesthetic concentration and volume, analgesia may be limited to a relatively specific dermatomal distribution. The distinct mechanisms of action of intrathecal or epidural opioids or local anesthetics are each associated with inherent physiologic effects, advantages and disadvantages, and risks and benefits. These must all be considered in the prudent application of these techniques to the management of postoperative pain.

Pharmacokinetics and Pharmacodynamics

Intrathecal opioid or local anesthetic administration places the drug in the cerebrospinal fluid (CSF) with direct access to the sites of action at the neural axis. The onset of analgesia is rapid and obtained at a much lower total dose than with epidural administration. The duration of analgesic effect following a single lumbar intrathecal dose of 10 μg/kg of morphine has been reported to range from 12 to 26 hours following thoracotomy.[93]

Opioid or local anesthetic administered into the epidural space is distributed via three different pathways: (1) penetration of the dural membrane to gain access to the CSF, nerve roots, and spinal cord; (2) vascular uptake according to a concentration gradient involving the spinal radicular arteries and the epidural venous plexi; and (3) deposition into the inert, lipid-rich structures in the epidural space. The physicochemical properties of the local anesthetics and opioids are important determinants of dural penetration; nerve, spinal cord, and opioid receptor binding; vascular absorption; onset and duration of analgesia; and systemic absorption of these agents. The physicochemical characteristics believed to be most important in the determination of these pharmacokinetic and pharmacodynamic properties appear to be lipid solubility, pKa, and opioid receptor-binding affinities. A detailed description is beyond the scope of this chapter; for detailed discussion of this subject, the reader is referred to more comprehensive reviews.[94–98] Selected physicochemical and pharmacokinetic properties of epidural opioids are shown in Table 16-2.

Pharmacokinetic analysis of specific opioid and local anesthetic uptake, distribution, and elimination into the relatively isolated CSF compartment following intrathecal or epidural administration is understandably difficult to assess. The most definitive study of CSF and plasma pharmacokinetics following epidural administration of opioids was reported by Sjostrom and coworkers. Following the epidural injection of 3 mg of morphine or 30 mg of meperidine, peak CSF concentrations were reported for morphine at 21.7 minutes and for meperidine at 7.6 minutes. Morphine appeared rapidly in the plasma, with maximal plasma concentrations within five minutes of injection, whereas meperidine appeared in the plasma at maximal concentrations 10–15 minutes after injection.[98]

Gourlay and associates studied the relative differences in the cephalad migration of morphine and meperidine in CSF. Lipid affinity was reported to be the physicochemical property that determined the degree of CSF migration exhibited by these two drugs. In this investigation, morphine (10 mg) and meperidine (50 mg) were administered simultaneously into the lumbar epidural space of each subject. CSF samples were obtained at the C7-T1 interspace and analyzed for opioid concentration at one of the following times: 10, 30, 60, 120, 180, and

Table 16-2. Physicochemical and Pharmacokinetic Properties of Opioids

Opioid	Molecular Weight	pKa	Partition Coefficient	Dose (mg)	Onset (min)	Duration (min)	Chapter Reference
Hydromorphone	285	9.5	0.307	1	10–15	660	11
Morphine	285	7.9	1.42	6	. . .	740	132
				6	30–60	938	93
				5	20–40	1100	11
Meperidine	247	8.5	38.8	60	. . .	400	132
				100	5–30	360	45
Methadone	309	9.3	116	6	. . .	525	132
				5	12–17	432	11
Fentanyl	336	8.4	813	0.06	. . .	345	132
				0.10	4–20	200–240	145

240 minutes postinjection. Peak cervical CSF morphine concentrations were noted at 120 minutes postinjection; in contrast, peak cervical CSF meperidine concentrations were found to occur between 10 and 60 minutes. The ratio of the peak meperidine to peak morphine CSF concentrations was 1:6, which is significantly less than the concentration ratio of the two opioids in the injected solution. This result indicates that (1) meperidine is absorbed more rapidly than morphine into the CSF following lumbar epidural administration and (2) proportionately less meperidine reached the cervical level where the CSF samples were obtained.[97]

The effect of lipid-solubility on the distribution of analgesia following intrathecal or epidural administration has been less clearly defined. Theoretically the more lipid-soluble opioids should produce a more segmental distribution of analgesia as a consequence of more rapid diffusion into the spinal cord and reduced drug availability in the aqueous phase (CSF) for distant migration. The ability of morphine, a hydrophilic drug, to produce analgesia in levels distant from the site of injection is well established. Several studies report good-to-excellent analgesia for postoperative pain following thoracic and upper abdominal surgery with lumbar administration.[99–102] Hydromorphone, another hydrophilic opioid, exhibits an extensive distribution of analgesia clinically despite earlier reports to the contrary.[103–105] The more lipophilic agents such as meperidine and fentanyl are clinically associated with a more segmental distribution of analgesia concentrated near the level of administration.

Multiple factors affect the duration of analgesia following the spinal administration of opioids. In general, the duration of analgesia is dose-dependent; duration is shorter with the more lipophilic agents such as meperidine and fentanyl than the more hydrophilic agents such as morphine and hydromorphone. It is suggested that opioid receptor-binding affinity is responsible for the prolonged duration of analgesia associated with the drugs sufentanil, lofentanil, and buprenorphine. The duration of analgesia following spinal administration is physically determined by removal of the drug from the CSF and redistribution into the systemic circulation.[106]

Technical Considerations

Intrathecal analgesia for the management of postoperative pain has primarily involved the single-dose administration of morphine or a combination of morphine and another opioid. This type of analgesia is usually initiated in the preoperative or intraoperative period with or without the coadministration of local anesthetic. The ability of intrathecal morphine (ITM) given prior to skin incision to reduce the anesthetic requirements during thoracotomy and its effect on postoperative meperidine requirements were investigated by Cohen and Neustein.[106A] In the first part of the study, 24 patients scheduled for thoracic surgery were induced with thiamylal and 100 mcg fentanyl. Prior to skin incision, 12 patients received intrathecal injection of 12 mcg/kg preservative-free undiluted morphine sulfate at the L3-4 or L4-5 level while the remaining 12 patients served as controls. Anesthesia was maintained solely with enflurane and vecuronium. No additional narcotics were administered. The intraoperative mean end-tidal (ET) of enflurane was significantly reduced in the intrathecal morphine group, beginning 1 hour after the injection of ITM (1.19 ± .45% in the control group versus 0.73 ± 0.08% in the intrathecal group) (Fig. 16-2). The enflurane requirements, expressed as % end-tidal enflurane/hour, were significantly less in the intrathecal morphine group for the duration of the procedure.

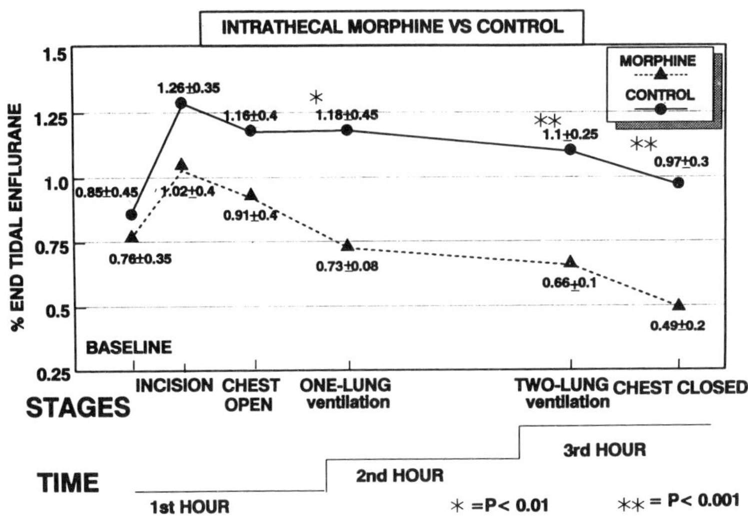

Figure 16-2. The percentage of end-tidal enflurane (mean ± standard deviation) at various stages of the procedure. Reprinted with permission from Cohen E, Neustein SM. Intrathecal morphine during thoracotomy, Part I: effect on intraoperative enflurane requirements. J Cardiothorac Anesth 1993;7,155.

In the second part of the study, the ability of ITM to reduce post-thoracotomy pain and meperidine requirements was investigated. Patients were evaluated postoperatively for the total doses of meperidine required over 24 hours and pain scores. Meperidine was given in 12.5 mg incremental doses and the nurses caring the patients were blinded to the presence or absence of ITM. The patients in the ITM group required significantly less meperidine compared to the control group and had lower pain scores (See Fig. 16-3 and Table 16-3). There were no serious side effects attributable to ITM. Intrathecal morphine is an effective treatment for control of post-thoracotomy pain. It is simple, less time consuming, and is a good alternative in cases where epidural administration is not possible. However, some anesthesiologists may feel uncomfortable with a single-dose technique which can be unpredictable, have a limited duration, and potentially increase the incidence of respiratory depression.

The prolonged administration of intermittent or continuous analgesia through placement of a subarachnoid catheter has not achieved the widespread application associated with epidural analgesia. The risk of late respiratory depression or introduction of infection into the subarachnoid space, the inability to titrate analgesia to individual patient requirements, and concern about the issue of postdural puncture headache has contributed to the limited use of intrathecal analgesia.

The techniques of epidural analgesia administration may include intermittent dosing, continuous infusion, or application of PCA technology. Adequate analgesia is possible with any of these techniques. The choice is usually made on the basis of the specific needs of the

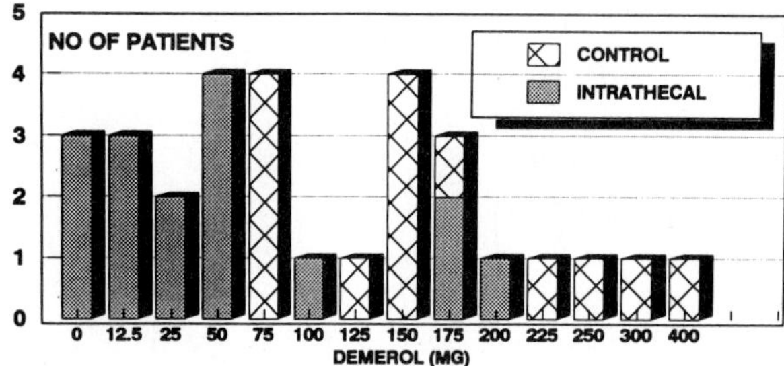

Figure 16-3. Patient distribution of total 24 hour meperidine requirements. Seventy-five percent of patients in the ITM group required less than 50 mg of meperidine, compared to no patients in the control group that needed less than 75 mg of meperidine. Reprinted with permission from Cohen E, Neustein SM. Intrathecal morphine during thoracotomy, Part II: effect on postoperative meperidine requirements and pulmonary function tests. J. Cardiothorac Anesth 1993;7,158.

patient or the judgment of the pain management team.

Administration of epidural opioid by intermittent dosing is probably the simplest, most widely used technique. The repeat doses can be delivered either on an "as needed" basis by patient demand or on a time-scheduled dosing interval. Potential disadvantages include the necessity of personnel to be available for drug administration and the variability in analgesia associated with dosing intervals. Opioid administered in incremental epidural doses is associated with significant fluctuations in plasma and CSF concentrations, and the potential for adverse effects following the dose related to peak concentration effects must be considered. Opioid concentrations and diluent volumes, as well as total dose, may be adjusted to provide optimal analgesic efficacy and duration.[107]

Table 16-3. Total 24 hour Meperidine Requirement, Pain Scores, and Level of Consciousness in the ITM and Control Group

Groups	ITM	Control
Meperidine requirements (mg)	59 + 68 (37)	167 + 97* 143
Pain score	1.4 + 1.1 (1.0)	2.4 + 0.9† (2.5)
Consciousness level	2.7 + 0.6 (3.0)	1.2 + 0.5* (1.0)

Reprinted with permission from Cohen E and Neustein SM. Intrathecal morphine during thoracotomy, Part II: effect on postoperative meperidine requirements and pulmonary function tests. J Cardiothorac Anesth 1993;7,158.

NOTE. Mean + SD. ( ) = Median. The assessment of pain was 0 = pain free; 1 = mild; 2 = moderate; 3 = severe; 4 + unbearable. The level of consciousness was 0 = unarousable; 1 = responsive to tactile stimulation; 2 = responsive to verbal command; and 3 = awake.
* $P < 0.001$.
† $P < 0.02$.

Compared to intermittent dosing, the use of continuous opioid infusion delivery systems has several potential advantages. Although this technique does require a volumetric infusion pump capable of fairly high infusion pressures to overcome the resistance of the epidural catheter, the analgesia provided is more consistent and is associated with more constant plasma and CSF opioid concentrations. Avoidance of large single doses, long dosing intervals, and fluctuations in opioid concentration reduces the incidence of adverse effects.[13]

Continuous epidural opioid infusion allows a more selective titration of analgesia to patient requirements via manipulation of opioid concentration and infusion rate as compared to intermittent dosing. The use of combinations of local anesthetic and opioid infusions is accomplished more safely because the level of sympathetic blockade associated with continuous infusion is relatively consistent.[108] More lipophilic opioids (meperidine) can be administered with continuous infusion systems with less intrinsic risk of respiratory depression associated with cephalad spread in CSF and with no concern about the shorter duration of action of the drug (compared to the more hydrophilic morphine).[109] In the author's institution, continuous epidural infusion of opioid with or without local anesthetic is the preferred method of delivery. Suggested starting doses for various epidural opioid analgesics in the management of postoperative pain are provided in Table 16-4.

Studies of CSF opioid concentration and cephalad migration of opioid in the CSF indicate that the highest concentrations of opioid and therefore the most rapid onset of analgesia occurs at the level of epidural opioid administration.[95,110] Consequently, the most intense distribution of analgesia is near the level of the epidural catheter tip, especially with continuous infusion of opioid. Thus the most efficacious location for the epidural catheter is at the level of the spinal cord corresponding to the segmental dermatomal distribution of the pain stimulus. Such placement allows the use of the lowest possible dose and infusion volume to maintain adequate analgesia and titration of analgesia by manipulation of dose or infusate volume. Such placement may be even more important if combinations of local anesthetics and opioids are used. One study has shown that the lumbar epidural administration of morphine provides analgesia comparable to thoracic epidural morphine administration for the relief of postthoracotomy pain, however.[99] The lumbar epidural administration of morphine may be a consideration in situations where thoracic administration is not possible.

Table 16-4. Epidural Opioid Dosing Guidelines*

Opioid	Initial Dose	Infusion Rate
Morphine	2–3 mg	0.25–0.5 mg/h
Hydromorphone	0.5–0.75 mg	0.1–0.2 mg/h
Meperidine	20–40 mg	10–15 mg/h
Fentanyl	50–100 μg	50–75 μg/h

* The dosages are recommendations only and should be adjusted to individual patient requirements. Lower dosages are suggested for elderly patients or for those who have received other opioid agonists.

PCA pumps are being investigated with great interest for the intermittent epidural administration of opioids.[111,112] The use of PCA systems for opioid administration via the epidural route is being explored as a method for allowing the patient to self-administer intermittent doses as needed to supplement continuous epidural infusions. The physicochemical and pharmacokinetic characteristics of the rapid-acting, lipophilic opioids provide advantages for their use in this application.

Analgesic Efficacy

The analgesic efficacy of spinal analgesia as compared to other postoperative pain management techniques has been documented. Interstudy comparisons are difficult because of differences in study design, definition of analgesia, and choice of drugs. In general, however, spinal analgesia has been demonstrated to be superior or equal to other parenteral opioid techniques (intramuscular, intravenous, PCA) in significantly smaller doses.[93,95,113–115] Spinal analgesia has been associated with less sedation, greater improvement in postoperative pulmonary function, and earlier ambulation compared to other parenteral analgesia techniques.[116–120]

In a comparison of five different analgesic methods for controlling pain in 51 patients after thoracotomy, epidural analgesia with bupivacaine or morphine was demonstrated to be more favorable than an intramuscular opioid alone or a intercostal nerve block and intramuscular opioid in combination.[113] Hypotension was not found to be a problem in patients receiving 0.25% epidural bupivacaine by continuous infusion in this study, despite previous reports to the contrary.[118] In a similar study, Logas and coworkers reported that in patients who received either continuous epidural analgesia with bupivacaine only, morphine only, or a combination of bupivacaine and morphine, analgesia was superior to that resulting from intermittent intramuscular opioid administration. Epidural morphine was found to produce better analgesia than epidural bupivacaine, but the combination of epidural bupivacaine and morphine was superior to either drug alone.[115]

In patients undergoing thoracic surgery, the initiation of epidural analgesia during the operative procedure and then continued into the postoperative procedure results in a significant improvement in analgesia.[13] The authors' preferred technique involves preoperative placement of the epidural catheter and initiation of epidural opioid analgesia (with or without local anesthetic) by continuous infusion during the intraoperative period, thus producing a balance between inhalation anesthesia and epidural analgesia. Continuation of the analgesia into the postoperative period by continuous epidural infusion of opioid is associated with a remarkably pain-free recovery from anesthesia and greatly improved analgesia.

Additional Therapeutic Benefits

The analgesia produced by the spinal administration of opioid or analgesic concentrations of local anesthetics has been described in the previous section. As a result of the improved analgesia and less sedation associated with spinal analgesia, other therapeutic benefits of this analgesic method include improvement in pulmonary function, modification of the endocrine stress response, improvement in time to ambulation, decreased morbidity, and shorter hospital stay.

Significant alterations in pulmonary function occur following thoracotomy. Recovery of pulmonary function to preoperative baseline levels may be delayed for days or weeks. Characteristic mechanical abnormalities include reductions in inspiratory capacity (IC), vital capacity (VC), and functional residual capacity (FRC), resulting in a restrictive pattern of pulmonary function. Following upper abdominal and thoracic surgical procedures VC is reduced to approximately 40% and FRC to approximately 70% of preoperative values. Patients are unable or unwilling to inspire deeply, and they attempt to compensate for the reduction in tidal volume by increasing respiratory rate. Pain resulting from upper abdominal or thoracic surgical procedures enhances the tachypnea; muscle splinting as a result of pain may further interfere with pulmonary mechanics by affecting chest wall function.[18] Shulman and coworkers reported results of a randomized, double-blind trial of 30 patients undergoing thoracotomy for lung resection. They compared the effects of epidural versus intravenous morphine on postoperative pain and pulmonary function.[120] Patients who received epidural morphine analgesia had significantly less pain at the 2-hour and 8-hour measurement times and significantly less decrease in both forced vital capacity (FVC) and forced expiratory volume in 1 second (FEV_1) at 2, 8, and 24 hours, and peak expiratory flow rate (PEFR) at 24 hours postoperatively (Figs. 16-4, 16-5, and 16-6). In a similar study, Welchew and Thorton compared the analgesia and side effects of epi-

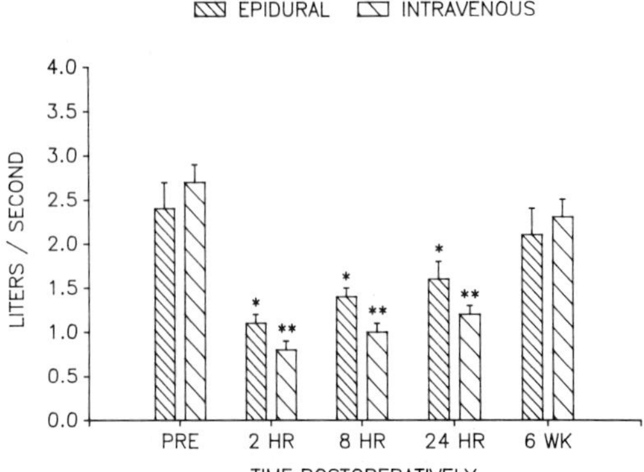

Figure 16-4. Forced expiratory volume (FEV). Comparison of preoperative and postoperative FEV_1 following thoracic surgery in patients receiving epidural versus intravenous morphine; (*) indicates statistical significance from preoperative value within groups (*P*<.05). (**) indicates statistical significance in between-group comparison (*P*<.05). (Data from Shulman M, Sandler AN, Bradley JW, et al.[118])

Figure 16-5. Forced vital capacity (FVC). Comparison of preoperative and postoperative FVC following thoracic surgery in patients receiving epidural versus intravenous morphine; (*) indicates statistical significance from preoperative value within groups (*P*<.05), and (**) indicates statistical significance in between-group comparison (*P*<.05). (Data from Shulman M, Sandler AN, Bradley JW, et al.[118])

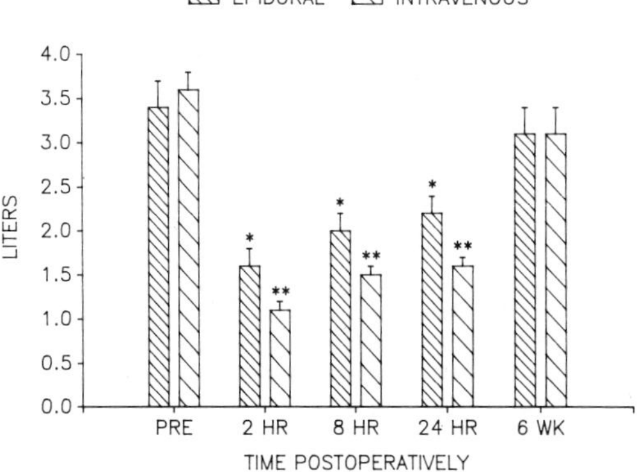

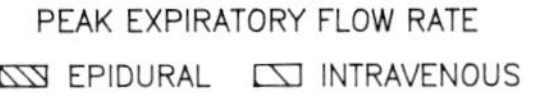

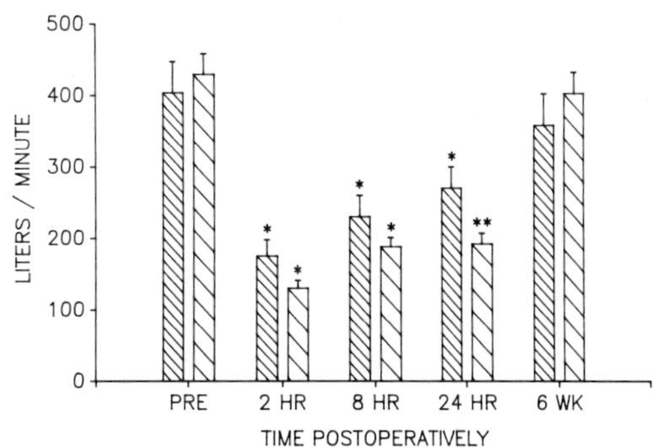

Figure 16-6. Peak expiratory flow rate (PEFR). Comparison of preoperative and postoperative PEFR following thoracic surgery in patients receiving epidural versus intravenous morphine; (*) indicates statistical significance from preoperative value within groups (*P*<.05), and (**) indicates statistical significance in between-group comparison (*P*<.05). (Data from Shulman M, Sandler AN, Bradley JW, et al.[118])

dural fentanyl infusion versus intramuscular papaveretum, in patients following major upper abdominal surgery.[121] During the first 24 hours after surgery, thoracic epidural fentanyl produced better analgesia with less sedation than intramuscular papaveretum. Postoperative respiratory function tests (FEV_1, FVC, and PEFR) were significantly better in those patients who received epidural fentanyl. Improvement in postoperative pulmonary function as a result of more effective analgesia with epidural opioids has been supported in other similar studies.[122]

Elevation of plasma levels of cortisol, catecholamines, antidiuretic hormone (ADH), and other hormones, is noted in the postoperative period; such increases are indicative of the neuroendocrine response to stress. Effective analgesia can reduce the magnitude of this response, as demonstrated by lower plasma levels of these stress response markers, although it does not entirely eliminate this reaction to stress.[123] Several extensive reviews of the subject of post-injury stress responses and the modifying effect of anesthesia and analgesia have been published.[124–126]

The role of techniques used for management of perioperative pain on plasma levels of ADH has been evaluated in patients undergoing upper abdominal and thoracic surgical procedures. One group had general neuroleptanesthesia intraoperatively followed by intramuscular piritramide for relief of postoperative pain, and another group received a combination of epidural and general anesthesia intraoperatively followed by epidural fentanyl. All patients had daily measurements of serum levels of potassium and sodium, plasma levels of ADH, and plasma osmolality for the first five postoperative days. This study demonstrated that the endocrine-metabolic stress response was less pronounced (as evidenced by influence on ADH secretion) when epidural fentanyl was used for the relief of postoperative pain than when intramuscular narcotic analgesia was used. This result indicates that more effective postoperative analgesia can attenuate the metabolic reaction after major surgery.[127] The indication that epidural opioid analgesia can attenuate the endocrine stress response to postoperative pain has also been demonstrated in other studies.[128]

The effects of perioperative anesthesia and analgesia on postoperative morbidity and operative outcome in high-risk surgical patients were evaluated by Yeager and coworkers.[129] In a randomized, controlled clinical trial, the effect of epidural anesthesia and postoperative epidural analgesia in one group of patients was compared to a control group of patients who received general anesthesia and postoperative parenteral analgesia. Preoperatively, patients were determined to be at high-risk for perioperative morbidity on the basis of preexisting systemic disease or the magnitude of the anticipated surgical procedure. Major outcome variables selected for analysis were (1) clinical outcome, (2) endocrine response, and (3) cost utilization. When compared to the control group, patients who received epidural anesthesia and analgesia (local anesthetics or opioids) had a reduced overall postoperative complication rate, the incidence of cardiovascular failure, and number of major infectious complications. Hospital costs were significantly less in patients who received epidural anesthesia and analgesia. The authors concluded that epidural anesthesia and analgesia had a significant beneficial effect on operative outcome in a group of high-risk surgical patients.

Side Effects and Complications

Intrathecal and epidural analgesia produce safe, effective pain relief that is superior to that of conventional analgesic techniques. Such effective analgesia is associated with potential side effects and complications, however. The most serious of these problems is the respiratory depression associated with the cephalad migration of spinal opioids and the hypotension associated resulting from the epidural administration of analgesic concentrations of local anesthetics. Other opioid-related side effects of spinal analgesia are, for the most part, also associated with opioid analgesia using other routes of administration; these effects include nausea, vomiting, pruritus, urinary retention, and changes in gastrointestinal motility and thermoregulation. Potential complications related specifically to the spinal route of administration include dural puncture headache, catheter migration, infection, and epidural hematoma. Fortunately, these potential complications and problems occur rarely or are either controllable or preventable with appropriate patient selection and management.

The risk of respiratory depression is the dose-limiting and therefore the analgesia-limiting factor associated with opioid administration by any route. Early reports suggested that the analgesia produced by spinal opioids led to less respiratory depression than other parenteral routes of administration.[104, 130] However, it was soon recognized that the long duration of analgesia associated with spinal opioid administration, especially morphine, carried a risk of a delayed, profound respiratory depression.[131–133] Researchers hypothesized that this risk resulted from occupation of opioid receptors in the brainstem. A biphasic depression of central control of ventilation following epidural morphine administration (especially in higher doses) has been described. Two distinct mechanisms are believed to be involved: (1) an early depression resulting from absorption into the epidural veins and circulatory redistribution to the brain and (2) a late phase associated with a rise in the segmental level of analgesia, which is the result of cephalad movement and high concentration of morphine in the CSF.

Several risk factors for severe respiratory depression have been identified, including advanced age, impaired respiratory function, and the coadministration of parenteral sedatives. In a large retrospective review, the overall incidence of respiratory depression requiring opioid antagonist administration following epidural morphine administration was less than 0.25%.[134] Opioid administration by any route is associated with dose-related respiratory depression. Avoidance of large doses of spinal opioids, awareness of potential risk factors associated with severe respiratory depression, and titration of analgesia to individual patient requirements can significantly increase the margin of safety.

Hypotension following the epidural administration of local anesthetic solutions as a result of the blockade of thoracic sympathetic fibers presents a management dilemma in patients following major thoracic surgery. As previously discussed, reports indicate that analgesia resulting from the combination of epidural opioid and local anesthetic administration is superior to either agent when used alone. Despite satisfactory analgesia in 70% of the patients receiving a continuous postoperative infusion, Conacher and colleagues reported an 80% incidence of hypotension that required intravenous fluid administration of 5–10 mL/kg body weight and use of sympathomimetic agents in refractory cases.[135] Although the incidence of hypotension associated with epidural administration of local anesthetic solutions may be decreased by fluid expansion of intravascular volume, there is the potential for extravasation of intravascular fluids in lung tissue contused as a result of surgical manipulation and pulmonary resection. A increase in lung water could predispose high-risk patients to postoperative pulmonary dysfunction. A low-dose, intravenous infusion of dopamine (4 μg/kg/min) has been reported to reverse the hypotension and negative inotropism associated with epidural local anesthetic administration effectively. Intravenous dopamine should be considered as an alternative to intravascular volume loading in appropriate patients.[136]

The effect of spinal analgesia on gastrointestinal function is complex. Local anesthetic administration is associated with sympathetic blockade of visceral afferents, thus resulting in unopposed parasympathetic stimulation of gastrointestinal motility. In comparison to conventional opioid analgesia, spinal opioid administration reportedly improves motility indirectly by improving analgesia and allowing earlier postoperative ambulation, which tends to stimulate postoperative return of gastrointestinal function. In contrast, morphine administered via the epidural route has been postulated to have an inhibitory effect on gastrointestinal function by a nonsystemic mechanism.[137]

The urinary retention that occurs with systemic opioid administration is the result of effects on peripheral and central neurogenic control of the micturition reflex.[138] Opioid-related urinary retention has been postulated to be associated with two independent mechanisms: (1) blockade of the periodic volume-evoked contractions of the bladder and (2) blockade of the vesical somatic reflex on which external sphincter relaxation depends.[139] The reported incidence of urinary retention following spinal opioid administration that requires bladder catheterization has been reported to be in the range of 40%.[140] The significance of this complication is minimized following major thoracic surgery in patients who require bladder catheterization for reasons other than urinary retention. The effect of local anesthetic-related urinary retention is reduced more by thoracic catheter placement than lumbar placement.

Itching is a known side effect of systemic opioid administration and is usually a generalized phenomenon. Itching, which seems to occur more commonly after epidural or intrathecal opioid administration than systemic administration, is typically noted in a segmental distribution near the site of injection or localized to the face. In a review of the incidence of itching in published reports of epidural opioid administration, the overall incidence of the condition is 8.5%. This compares with a 46% incidence of itching following intrathecal opioid administration and a 1% incidence following systemic administration of morphine. Therefore it is speculated that the mechanism involves the spinal cord; epidural opioids may have a direct excitatory effect on dorsal or ventral neurons, thus producing the itching sensation.[141] Naloxone administration has been reported to relieve the sensation of itching effectively within a few minutes without antagonism of analgesia with titration of the drug to effect.[142] Systemic or epidural administration of opioid agonist-antagonist agents also appears to decrease the incidence of pruritus in preliminary clinical observations; controlled studies are lacking, however. At this point, if analgesia is adequate, the most prudent management should begin with a reduction in opioid dose. Histamine release, Antihistamine administration is usually effective as well, the mechanism is probably unrelated to histamine release.

The incidence of nausea and vomiting in the postoperative period has been reported to be as high as 30% with the routine use of parenteral opioids. Studies of spinal versus systemic administration with respect to the incidence of nausea have yielded comparable results. The incidence of nausea may be opioid-specific in some cases, and therefore consideration of an alternate opioid is justified.[143]

Complications and contraindications for spinal analgesia relate to the considerations for dural puncture or epidural catheterization. Potential complications associated with epidural catheter-related problems include infection, catheter migration, occlusion, or displacement; epidural hematoma may be a problem in patients receiving anticoagulant therapy. As with any invasive procedure with potential complications, the risks must be considered in light of the potential benefits.

Present and Future Considerations

As evidenced by the previous discussion, several techniques may provide superior analgesia when compared to conventional intermittent, intramuscular opioid administration. The technique must be individualized on the basis of patient-related indications and management capabilities of the postoperative patient care team. The technique that a single author or institution prefers may not be directly applicable to all patients or institutions.

The authors' preferred management of thoracic surgery patients is based on patient safety, analgesic efficacy, and optimization of postoperative recovery. Patients are assessed preoperatively, and postoperative management is discussed with the patient by the surgical and anesthesia care team. Preoperatively a thoracic epidural catheter is placed in the region of T5-T6 using a paramedian approach from the contralateral side with respect to the operative site. Catheter placement is tested to rule out subarachnoid or intravenous placement. The catheter is then tunneled subcutaneously for a distance of 4–5 cm in the paravertebral region to remove the catheter and its dressing from the operative site and wound dressing.[144] The catheter is secured to the skin with Steri-strips, and a sterile plastic occlusive dressing is applied.[145] Intraoperative anesthesia is maintained by a combination of inhalation anesthesia and epidural analgesia with bupivacaine and morphine.

Patients are routinely extubated at the completion of the surgical procedure and are taken to the intensive care unit overnight. A continuous epidural infusion of morphine at a rate of less than 0.5 mg/h is started upon arrival to the unit. Patients are actively encouraged to perform regular pulmonary physiotherapy within one to two hours after completion of the surgical procedure and are allowed to sit in a bedside chair the afternoon of surgery. Most patients are able to tolerate a regular diet on the first postoperative day. The epidural opioid infusion is continued for 48–96 hours until patients have demonstrated the ability to ambulate without assistance and tolerate oral opioid analgesics. In general, this management approach allows adequate analgesia to support early postoperative recovery of pulmonary and gastrointestinal function and ambulation.

A consideration for adjunctive analgesia in the above management approach includes the perioperative administration of systemic nonsteroidal anti-inflammatory analgesics (NSAIDs). Reports demonstrating improvement of analgesic efficacy with the combination of epidural analgesia and NSAIDs via a mechanism involving reduction in peripheral anti-inflammatory response to surgical trauma have been recently published.[123, 146] Administration of NSAIDs beginning in the preoperative period and extending 72–96 hours into the postoperative period is possible through the use of oral agents and rectal (indomethacin, piroxicam) or parenteral agents (ketorolac). Preliminary clinical impressions suggest improvement in analgesia following thoracotomy in patients who receive a combination of epidural morphine and NSAIDs rather than epidural morphine alone; prospective, controlled studies are currently underway.

The prevention of postoperative pain through the expanded use of balanced analgesia techniques involving inhibition on the peripheral transduction, neural transmission, and spinal modulation of nociceptive stimulation provide the foundation for future directions in postoperative patient management. A greater understanding on the part of patients and health care professionals of the importance of pain management in postoperative rehabilitation following major surgical procedures is needed. New analgesic medications such as the α_2-adrenergic agonist agents (eg, clonidine) are currently under investigation for use in the management of postoperative pain.[147] New analgesia delivery techniques, including patient-controlled epidural opioid administration and patient-controlled infusion analgesia are being explored as potential management techniques to allow better adaptation to individual patient requirements.

Efficient postoperative management of the patient following major thoracic surgery must be directed toward effective pulmonary and general physical rehabilitation in an effort to decrease postoperative morbidity. Rehabilitation efforts can be hindered by several factors, including inadequate postoperative analgesia. The application of effective postoperative pain management techniques, which allow the patient more rapid postoperative recovery, can contribute to improvement in perioperative outcome. The goals of postoperative pain management in the patient following thoracic surgery should be directed toward sufficient perioperative analgesia to allow compliance with postsurgical rehabilitation efforts and maintain a satisfactory level of patient comfort without adverse circulatory, respiratory, or neurological complications. Therapy must be tailored to the specific analgesic requirements of the individual patient. Through a knowledge of the various modalities of postoperative analgesia management and appropriate application of these techniques in the individualization of therapy, effective and safe postoperative pain management can be accomplished.

References

1. Donovan M, Dillon P, McGuire L. Incidence and characteristics of pain in a sample of medical-surgical inpatients. Pain 1987;30:69.
2. Grossman SA, Sheidler VR. Skills of medical students and house officers in prescribing narcotic medications. Med Educ 1985;60:552.
3. Iafrati NS. Pain on the burn unit: patient vs. nurse perceptions. J Burn Care Rehabil 1986;7:413.
4. Ketovuori H. Nurses' and patients' conceptions of wound pain and the administration of analgesics. J Pain Symp Manag 1987;2:213.
5. Marks RM, Sachar EJ. Undertreatment of medical inpatients with narcotic analgesics. Ann Intern Med 1973;78:172.
6. Melzack R, Abbott FV, Zackon W, et al. Pain on a surgical ward: a survey of the duration and intensity of pain and the effectiveness of medication. Pain 1987;29:67.
7. Watt-Watson JH. Nurses' knowledge of pain issues: a survey. J Pain Symp Manag 1987;2:207.
8. Weis OF, Sriwatanakul K, Alloza JL, et al. Attitudes of patients, housestaff, and nurses toward postoperative analgesic care. Anesth Analg 1983;62:70.
9. Egbert LD, Battit GE, Welch CE, et al. Reduction of postoperative pain by encouraging and instruction of patients: a study of doctor-patient rapport. N Engl J Med 1964;270:825.
10. Wallace PGM, Norris W. The management of postoperative pain. Br J Anaesth 1975;47:113.
11. Coderre TJ, Melzack R. Cutaneous hyperalgesia: contributions of the peripheral and central nervous systems to the increase in pain sensitivity after injury. Brain Res 1987;404:95.
12. Tverskoy M, Cozacov C, Ayache M, et al. Postoperative pain after inguinal herniorrhaphy with different types of anesthesia. Anesth Analg 1990;70:29.
13. El-Baz N, Farber L, Jensik R. Continuous epidural infusion of morphine for treatment of pain after thoracic surgery: a new technique. Anesth Analg 1984;63:757.
14. Sydow FW. The influence of anesthesia and postoperative analgesic management on lung function. Acta Chir Scand Suppl 1988;550:159.
15. Cousins MJ. Acute pain and the injury response: immediate and prolonged effects. Reg Anaesth 1989;14:162.
16. Asaph JW, Keppel JF. Midline sternotomy for the treatment of primary pulmonary neoplasms. Am J Surg 1984;147:589.
17. Bonica JJ. Postoperative pain. In: Bonica JJ. The management of pain. Philadelphia: Lea & Febiger, 1990:461.
18. Craig DB. Postoperative recovery of pulmonary function. Anesth analg 1981;60:46.
19. Austin KL, Stapleton JV, Mather LE. Multiple intramuscular injections: a major source of variability in analgesic response to meperidine. Pain 1980;8:47.
20. Grabinski PY, Kaiko RF, Rogers AG, et al. Plasma levels and analgesia following deltoid and gluteal injections of methadone and morphine. J Clin Pharmacol 1983;23:48.

21. Rigg JRA, Browne RA, Davis C, et al. Variation in the disposition of morphine after administration in surgical patients. Br J Anaesth 1978;50:1125–1130.
22. Austin KL, Stapleton JV, Mather LE. Relationships between blood meperidine concentrations and analgesic response: A preliminary report. Anesthesiology 1980;53:460.
23. Gourlay GK, Willis RJ, Wilson PR. Postoperative pain control with methadone: influence of supplementary methadone doses and blood-concentration-response relationships. Anesthesiology 1984; 61:19.
24. Gourlay GK, Wilson PR, Glynn CJ. Pharmacodynamics and pharmacokinetics of methadone during the perioperative period. Anesthesiology 1982;57:458.
25. Gourlay GK, Willis RJ, Lamberty J. A double-blind comparison of the efficacy of methadone and morphine in postoperative pain control. Anesthesiology 1986;64:322.
26. Gourlay GK, Wilson PR, Glynn CJ. Methadone produces prolonged postoperative analgesia. BMJ 1982;284:630.
27. Sechzer PH. Objective measurement of pain. Anesthesiology 1968;29:209.
28. Forrest WH Jr, Smethurst PWR, Kienitz ME. Self-administration of intravenous analgesics. Anesthesiology 1970;33:363.
29. Kerri-Szanto M. Apparatus for demand analgesia. Can J Anaesth 1971;18:581.
30. Sechzer PH. Studies in pain with analgesic demand system. Anesth Analg 1971;50:1.
31. Eisenach JC, Grice SC, Dewan DM. Patient-controlled analgesia following cesarean section: a comparison with epidural and intramuscular narcotics. Anesthesiology 1988;68:444.
32. Harrison DM, Sinatra R, Morgese L, et al. Epidural narcotic and patient-controlled analgesia for post-cesarean section pain relief. Anesthesiology 1988; 68:454.
33. Ferrante FM, Orav EJ, Rocco AG, et al. A statistical model for pain in patient-controlled analgesia and conventional intramuscular opioid regimens. Anesth Analg 1988;67:457.
34. Cousins MJ, Mather LE, Glynn CJ, et al. Selective spinal analgesia. Lancet 1979;1:1141.
35. White PF. Patient-controlled analgesia: a new approach to the management of postoperative pain. Semin Anesth 1985;4:255–266.
36. Marshall H, Porteous C, McMillan I. Relief of pain by continuous infusion of morphine after operation: Does tolerance develop? BMJ 1985;291:19.
37. Mather LE, Owen H. The scientific basis of patient-controlled analgesia. Anaesth Intensive Care 1988; 16:427.
38. Owen H, Szekely SM, Plummer JL, et al. Variables of patient-controlled analgesia. 2. concurrent infusion. Anaesthesia 1989;44:11.
39. Gourlay GK, Kowalski SR, Plummer JL, et al. The transdermal administration of fentanyl in the treatment of postoperative pain: pharmacokinetics and pharmacodynamic effects. Pain 1989;37:193.
40. Gourlay GK, Kowalski SR, Plummer JL, et al. The efficacy of transdermal fentanyl in the treatment of postoperative pain: a double-blind comparison of fentanyl and placebo systems. Pain 1990;40:21.
41. Bullingham RES, McQuay HJ, Porter EJB, et al. Sublingual buprenorphine used postoperatively: ten-hour plasma drug concentration analysis. Br J Clin Pharmacol 1982;13:665.
42. Maunuksela EL, Korpela R, Olkkola KT. Comparison of buprenorphine with morphine in the treatment of postoperative pain in children. Anesth Analg 1988;67:233.
43. Sjogren P, Laub M, Gronnebech H, et al. Sublingual buprenorphine on regular intervals in postoperative pain due to total hip replacement. Pain 1990;Suppl 5:S144. Abstract.
44. Harshaw DH, Schwesinger WH, Reynolds JC, et al. Transnasal butorphanol vs. intramuscular meperidine in the treatment of postoperative pain. Pain 1990;Suppl 5:S153. Abstract.
45. Moore DC. Intercostal nerve block for postoperative somatic pain following surgery of thorax and upper abdomen. Br J Anaesth 1975;47:284.
46. Thompson GC, Moore DC. Celiac plexus, intercostal, and minor peripheral blockade. In: Cousins MJ, Bridenbaugh PO, eds. Neural blockade in clinical anesthesia and management of pain. 2nd Ed. Philadelphia: JB Lippincott, 1988:510.
47. Faust RJ, Nauss LA. Postthoracotomy intercostal block: comparison of its effects on pulmonary function with those of intramuscular meperidine. Anesth Analg 1976;55:542.
48. Crawford ED, Skinner DG, Capparell DB. Intercostal nerve block with thoracoabdominal incision. J Urol 1979;121:290.
49. Willdeck-Lund G, Edstrom H. Etidocaine in intercostal nerve block for pain relief after thoracotomy; a comparison with bupivacaine. Acta Anaesth Scand 1975;60:33.
50. Kaplan JA, Miller ED, Gallager EG. Postoperative analgesia for thoracotomy patients. Anesth Analg 1975;54:773.

51. Thompson GC, Moore DC. Celiac plexus, intercostal, and minor peripheral blockade. In: Cousins MJ, Bridenbaugh PO, eds. Neural blockade in clinical anesthesia and management of pain. 2nd Ed. Philadelphia: JB Lippincott, 1988:508.
52. Chinn MA, Wirjoatmadja K. Prolonging local anesthesia. Lancet 1967;2:835.
53. Loder RE. A long-acting local anesthetic solution for the relief of pain after thoracotomy. Thorax 1962; 17:375.
54. Benumof JL, Semenza J. Total spinal anesthesia following intrathoracic intercostal nerve blocks. Anesthesiology 1975;43:124.
55. Gallo JA, Lebowitz PW, Battit GE, et al. Complications of intercostal nerve blocks performed under direct vision during thoracotomy: a report of two cases. J Thorac Cardiovasc Surg 1983;86:628.
56. Skretting P. Hypotension after intercostal nerve block during thoracotomy under general anesthesia. Br J Anaesth 1981;53:527.
57. Conacher ID, Kokri M. Postoperative paravertebral blocks for thoracic surgery: a radiological approach. Br J Anaesth 1987;59:155.
58. Kolvenbach H, Lauven PM, Schneider B, et al. Repetitive intercostal nerve block via catheter for postoperative pain relief after thoracotomy. Thorac Cardiovasc Surg 1989;37:273.
59. Olivet RT, Nauss LE, Payne WS. A technique for continuous intercostal nerve block analgesia following thoracotomy. J Thorac Cardiovasc Surg 1980;80:308.
60. Sabanathan S, Smith PJB, Pradhan GN, et al. Continuous intercostal nerve block for pain relief after thoracotomy. Ann Thorac Surg 1988;46:425.
61. Safran D, Kulhman G, Orhant RR, et al. Continuous intercostal blockade with lidocaine after thoracic surgery: clinical and pharmacokinetic study. Anesth Analg 1990;70:345.
62. Wolfe MJ, Nicholas ADG. Selective epidural analgesia. Lancet 1979;2:150.
63. Roviaro GC, Varoli F, Fascianella A, et al. Intrathoracic intercostal nerve block with phenol in open chest surgery: a randomized study with statistical evaluation of respiratory parameters. Chest 1986;90:64.
64. Reiestad F, Stromskag KE. Interpleural catheter in the management of postoperative pain: a preliminary report. Reg Anaesth 1986;11:89.
65. Kambam JR, Hammon J, Parris WCV, et al. Intrapleural analgesia for postthoracotomy pain and blood levels of bupivacaine following intrapleural injection. Can J Anaesth 1989;36:106.
66. McIlvaine WB, Knox RF, Fennessey PV, et al. Continuous infusion of bupivacaine via intrapleural catheter for analgesia after thoracotomy in children. Anesthesiology 1988;69:261.
67. Rosenberg PH, Scheinin BMA, Lepantalo MJA, et al. Continuous intrapleural infusion of bupivacaine for analgesia after thoracotomy. Anesthesiology 1987;67:811.
68. Scheinin B, Lindgren L, Rosenberg PH. Treatment of postthoracotomy pain with intermittent instillations of intrapleural bupivacaine. Acta Anaesthesiol Scand 1989;33:156.
69. Symreng T, Gomez MN, Rossi N. Intrapleural bupivacaine vs. saline after thoracotomy—Effects on pain and lung function - A double-blind study. J Cardiothorac Anesth 1989;3:144.
70. Rocco A, Reiestad F, Gudman J, et al. Intrapleural administration of local anesthetics for pain relief in patients with multiple rib fractures. Reg Anaesth 1987;12:10.
71. Stromskag KE, Reiestad F, Holmqvist ELO, et al. Intrapleural administration of 0.25%, 0.375%, and 0.5% bupivacaine with epinephrine after cholecystectomy. Anesth Analg 1988;67:430.
72. Seltzer JL, Larijani GE, Goldberg ME, et al. Intrapleural bupivacaine—A kinetic and dynamic evaluation. Anesthesiology 1987;67:798.
73. Ferrante FM, Chan VWS, Arthur GR, et al. Interpleural analgesia after thoracotomy. Anesth Analg 1991;72:105.
74. Symreng T, Gomez MN, Johnson B, et al. Intrapleural bupivacaine—Technical considerations and intraoperative use. J Cardiothorac Anesth 1989;3:139.
75. Hymes AC, Raab DE, Yonehiro EG, et al. Electrical surface stimulation for control of acute postoperative pain and prevention of ileus. Surg Forum 1973;24:447.
76. Melzack R, Wall PD. Pain mechanisms: a new theory. Science 1965;150:971.
77. Tyler E, Caldwell C, Ghia J. Transcutaneous electrical nerve stimulation: an alternative approach to the management of postoperative pain. Anesth Analg 1982;61:449.
78. Rooney S-M, Jain S, Goldiner PL. Effect of transcutaneous nerve stimulation on postoperative pain after thoracotomy. Anesth Analg 1983;62:1010.
79. Rooney S-M, Jain S, McCormack P, et al. A comparison of pulmonary function tests for postthoraco-

tomy pain using cryoanalgesia and transcutaneous nerve stimulation. Ann Thorac Surg 1986;41:204.
80. Warfield CA, Stein JM, Frank HA. The effect of transcutaneous electrical nerve stimulation on pain after thoracotomy. Ann Thorac Surg 1985;39:462.
81. Glynn CJ, Lloyd JW, Barnard JDW. Cryoanalgesia in the management of pain after thoracotomy. Thorax 1980;35:325.
82. Katz J, Nelson W, Forest R, et al. Cryoanalgesia for postthoracotomy pain. Lancet 1980;1:512.
83. Joucken K, Michel L, Schoevaerdts J-C1, et al. Cryoanalgesia for postthoracotomy pain relief. Acta Anaesthesiol Belg 1987;38:179.
84. Brynitz S, Schroder M. Intraoperative cryolysis of intercostal nerves in thoracic surgery. Scand J Thorac Cardiovasc Surg 1986;20:85.
85. Muller LCh, Salzer GM, Ransmayr G, et al. Intraoperative cryoanalgesia for postthoracotomy pain relief. Ann Thorac Surg 1989;48:15.
86. Roxburgh JC, Markland CG, Ross BA, et al. Role of cryoanalgesia in the control of pain after thoracotomy. Thorax 1987;42:292.
87. Atweh S, Kuhar M. Autoradiographic localization of opiate receptors in rat brain. 1. Spinal cord and lower medulla. Brain Res 1977;124:53.
88. Snyder SH. Opiate receptors and internal opiates. Sci Am 1977;236:44.
89. Yaksh TL. Spinal opiate analgesia: characteristics and principles of action. Pain 1981;11:293.
90. Behar M, Olshwang D, Magora F, et al. Epidural morphine in the treatment of pain. Lancet 1979; 1:527.
91. Cousins MJ, Bromage PR. Epidural neural blockade. In: Cousins MJ, Bridenbaugh PO, eds. Neural blockade in clinical anesthesia and management of pain. 2nd Ed. Philadelphia: JB Lippincott, 1988:306–308.
92. Yaksh TL, Rudy TA. Analgesia mediated by a direct spinal action of narcotics. Science 1976;192:1357.
93. Gray JR, Fromme GA, Nauss LA, et al. Intrathecal morphine for postthoracotomy pain. Anesth Analg 1986;65:873.
94. Cousins MJ, Bromage PR. Epidural neural blockade. In: Cousins MJ, Bridenbaugh PO, eds. Neural blockade in clinical anesthesia and management of pain. 2nd Ed. Philadelphia: JB Lippincott, 1988:253.
95. Cousins MJ, Mather LE. Intrathecal and epidural administration of opioids. Anesthesiology 1984; 61:276.
96. Crews JC. Epidural opioid analgesia. In: Hoyt JW, ed. Pain management in the ICU. Crit Care Clin 1990;6:315.
97. Gourlay GK, Cherry DA, Plummer JL, et al. The influence of drug polarity on the absorption of opioid drugs into CSF and subsequent cephalad migration following lumbar epidural administration: application to morphine and pethidine. Pain 1987;31:297.
98. Sjostrom S, Hartvig P, Persson P, et al. Pharmacokinetics of epidural morphine and meperidine in humans. Anesthesiology 1987;67:877.
99. Fromme GA, Steidl LJ, Danielson DR. Comparison of lumbar and thoracic epidural morphine for relief of postthoracotomy pain. Anesth Analg 1985; 64:454.
100. Larsen VH, Iversen AD, Christensen P, et al. Postoperative pain treatment after upper abdominal surgery with epidural morphine at thoracic or lumbar level. Acta Anaesthesiol Scand 1985;29:566.
101. Nordberg G, Hedner T, Mellstrand T, et al. Pharmacokinetic aspects of epidural morphine analgesia. Anesthesiology 1983;58:545.
102. Parab PV, Coyle DE, Streng WH, et al. Biopharmaceutic parameters of hydromorphone and in vitro evaluation of its tablet and suppository dosage form. Pharm Ind 1987;49:951.
103. Bromage PR, Camporesi EM, Chestnut D. Epidural narcotics for postoperative analgesia. Anesth Analg 1980;59:473.
104. Bromage PR, Camporesi E, Leslie J. Epidural narcotics in volunteers: sensitivity to pain and carbon dioxide. Pain 1980;9:145.
105. Horan CT, Beeby DG, Brodsky JB, et al. Segmental effect of lumbar epidural hydromorphone: a case report. Anesthesiology 1985;62:84.
106. Woltering EA, Flye MW, Huntley S, et al. Evaluation of bupivacaine nerve blocks in the modification of pain and pulmonary function changes after thoracotomy. Ann Thorac Surg 1980;30:122.
106A. Cohen E, Neustein SM. Intrathecal morphine during thoracotomy, Part I: effect on intraoperative enflurane requirements. Part II: effect on postoperative meperidine requirements and pulmonary function tests. J Cardiothorac Anesth 1993;7:154.
107. Welchew EA. The optimum concentration for epidural fentanyl. Anaesthesia 1983;38:1037.
108. Griffiths DPG, Diamond AW, Cameron JD. Postoperative extradural analgesia following thoracic surgery: a feasibility study. Br J Anaesth 1975;47:48.
109. Fischer RL, Lubenow TR, Liceaga A, McCarthy RJ, et al. Comparison of continuous epidural infusion of fentanyl-bupivacaine and morphine-bupivacaine in management of postoperative pain. Anesth Analg 1988;67:559.

110. Bromage PR, Camporesi EM, Durant PAC, et al. Rostral spread of epidural morphine. Anesthesiology 1982;56:431.
111. Lysak SZ, Eisenach JC, Dobson CE. Patient-controlled epidural analgesia (PCEA) during labor: a comparison of three solutions with continuous epidural infusion (CEI) control. Anesthesiology 1988;69:A690. Abstract.
112. Sjostrom S, Hartvig D, Tamsen A. Patient-controlled analgesia with extradural morphine or pethidine. Br J Anaesth 1988;60:358.
113. Asantila R, Rosenberg PH, Scheinin B. Comparison of different methods of postoperative analgesia after thoracotomy. Acta Anaesthesiol Scand 1986;30:421.
114. Hasenbos M, van Egmond J, Gielen M, et al. Postoperative analgesia by epidural versus intramuscular nicomorphine after thoracotomy. Part I. Acta Anaesthsiol Scand 1985;29:572.
115. Logas WG, El-Baz N, El-Ganzouri A, et al. Continuous thoracic epidural analgesia for postoperative pain relief following thoracotomy: a randomized prospective study. Anesthesiology 1987;67:787.
116. Hasenbos M, Simon M, van Egmond J, et al. Postoperative analgesia by nicomorphine intramuscularly versus high thoracic epidural administration. Acta Anaesthesiol Scand 1986;30:426.
117. Hasenbos M, van Egmond J, Gielen M, et al. Postoperative analgesia by epidural versus intramuscular nicomorphine after thoracotomy. Part II. Acta Anaesthsiol Scand 1985;29:577.
118. James EC, Kolberg HL, Iwen GW, et al. Epidural analgesia for postthoracotomy patients. J Thorac Cardiovasc Surg 1981;82:898.
119. Rawal N, Sjostrand U, Dahlstrom B. Postoperative pain relief by epidural morphine. Anesth Analg 1981;60:726.
120. Shulman M, Sandler AN, Bradley JW, et al. Post-thoracotomy pain and pulmonary function following epidural and systemic morphine. Anesthesiology 1984;61:569.
121. Welchew EA, Thornton JA. Continuous thoracic epidural fentanyl. Anaesthesia 1982;37:309.
122. Rybro L, Schurizek BA, Petersen TK, et al. Postoperative analgesia and lung function: a comparison of intramuscular with epidural morphine. Acta Anaesthesiol Scand 1982;26:514.
123. Schulze S, Roikjaer O, Hasselstrom L, et al. Epidural bupivacaine and morphine plus systemic indomethacin eliminates pain but not systemic response and convalescence after cholecystectomy. Surgery 1988;103:321.
124. Kehlet H. The stress response to surgery: release mechanisms and the modifying effect of pain relief. Acta Chir Scand Suppl 1988;550:22.
125. Kehlet H. Surgical stress: the role of pain and analgesia. Br J Anaesth 1989;63:189.
126. Pflug AN, Halter JB, Tolas AG. Plasma catecholamine levels during anesthesia and surgical stress. Reg Anaesth 1982;7:S49.
127. Von Bormann B, Weidler B, Dennhardt R, et al. Influence of epidural fentanyl on stress-induced elevation of plasma vasopressin (ADH) after surgery. Anesth Analg 1983;62:727.
128. Rutberg H, Hakanson E, Anderberg B, et al. Effects of the extradural administration of morphine, or bupivacaine, on the endocrine response to upper abdominal surgery. Br J Anaesth 1984;56:233.
129. Yeager MP, Glass DD, Neff RK, et al. Epidural anesthesia and analgesia in high-risk surgical patients. Anesthesiology 1987;66:729.
130. Torda TA, Pybus DA, Liberman H, et al. Experimental comparison of extradural and intramuscular morphine. Br J Anaesth 1980;52:939–943.
131. Bromage PR. The price of intraspinal narcotic analgesia: basic constraints. Anesth Analg 1981;60:461.
132. Knill RL, Clement JL, Thompson WR. Epidural morphine causes delayed and prolonged ventilatory depression. Can J Anaesth 1981;28:537.
133. Reiz S, Westberg M. Side effects of epidural morphine. Lancet 1980;II:203–204.
134. Gustafsson LL, Schlidt B, Jacobsen K. Adverse effects of extradural and intrathecal opiates: report of a nationwide survey in Sweden. Br J Anaesth 1982; 54:479.
135. Conacher ID, Paes ML, Jacobson L, et al. Epidural analgesia following thoracic surgery: a review of two years experience. Anaesthesia 1983;38:546.
136. Lundberg J, Norgren L, Thomson D, et al. Hemodynamic effects of dopamine during thoracic epidural analgesia in man. Anesthesiology 1987;66:641.
137. Thoren T, Tanghoj H, Wattwil M, et al. Epidural morphine delays gastric emptying and small intestinal transit in volunteers. Acta Anaesthesiol Scand 1989;33:174.
138. Dray A. Epidural opiates and urinary retention: new models provide new insights. Anesthesiology 1988;68:323.
139. Durant PAC, Yaksh TL. Drug effects on urinary bladder tone during spinal morphine-induced inhibition of the micturition reflex in unanesthetized rats. Anesthesiology 1988;68:325.

140. Stenseth R, Sellevold O, Breivik H. Epidural morphine for postoperative pain: experience with 1085 patients. Acta Anaesthesiol Scand 1985;29:148.
141. Ballantyne JC, Loach AB, Carr DB. Itching after epidural and spinal opiates. Pain 1988;33:149.
142. Bromage PR, Camporesi EM, Durant PAC, et al. Nonrespiratory side effects of epidural morphine. Anesth Analg 1982;61:490.
143. Lanz E, Theiss D, Riess W, et al. Epidural morphine for postoperative analgesia: a double-blind study. Anesth Analg 1982;61:236.
144. Hord AH. An improved method for subcutaneous tunneling of epidural catheters. Reg Anaesth 1988; 13:S50. Abstract.
145. Raj PP, Denson DD. Prolonged analgesia technique with local anesthetics. In: Raj PP. Practical management of pain. Chicago: Year Book Medical Publishers, 1986:692.
146. Dahl JB, Rosenberg J, Dirkes WE, et al. Prevention of postoperative pain by balanced analgesia. Br J Anaesth 1990;64:518.
147. Eisenach JC, Lysak SZ, Viscomi CM. Epidural clonidine analgesia following surgery: phase I. Anesthesiology 1989;71:640.

SECTION

V

Anesthetic Management for Special Procedures

CHAPTER

17

Endoscopic Procedures of the Airways, Lungs, and Pleurae

Charles B. Watson

Endoscopic procedures on the airways, lungs, and pleurae have dramatically evolved in recent years. In the past years, thoracic surgeons routinely performed rigid bronchoscopy as a diagnostic procedure prior to open thoracotomy. Now an increasing number of problems that used to require open thoracotomy are being managed endoscopically. Both technical and conceptual advances have increased the number of diagnostic possibilities and enhanced the therapeutic and surgical capabilities of modern endoscopes. Recent advances include laser bronchoscopy and thoracoscopic biopsy with lung resection. The success of each technique followed development of new endoscopes, light sources, and transendoscopic equipment. Newer anesthetic approaches have developed along with newer surgical procedures. In some cases (eg, laser surgery *via* a bronchoscope versus hot wire cautery *via* a bronchoscope), anesthesiologists have rediscovered old principles through use of new monitors and agents. In others, such as thoracoscopy, new physiologic problems have required the anesthesiologist to develop new management principles.

History

Use of a rigid esophagoscope for bronchoscopy was first described around 1900 (Table 17-1). Early bronchoscopes were esophagoscopes perforated along the distal third of the tube to allow effective ventilation of contralateral airways when an instrument was advanced down one bronchus or the other. All variations were hollow tubes through which one could advance and withdraw differently angled optic telescopes, biopsy forceps, or suction cannulae. Thoracic surgeons used the bronchoscope largely as a diagnostic instrument until newer devices allowed the operator to expand the therapeutic indications.

Fiberoptic technology, which was developed in the 1960s, allowed improved design for rigid equipment and led to the development of flexible telescopes. Murphy is credited with the first use of a flexible fiberoptic instrument (a choledochoscope) as an intubation guide in 1967. Ikeda first described use of the flexible bronchoscope for surgical evaluation of smaller airways in 1968. As with rigid bronchoscopy, flexible equipment became widely used upon anesthetized patients following its intro-

Table 17-1. Historical Milestones

Method	Use	Author
Endoscopy concept	Cylindrical tube and illumination	Bozzini 1807
Autoscope	Direct exam of larynx and trachea via mouth	Kirstein 1896[1]
Bronchoscopy	ENT and thoracic practice	Jackson and Negus 1900
Thoracoscopy	Pleural effusions in TB	Jacobaueus 1910[2]
Intubating bronchoscope	Rigid optical stylette	Magill 1936
Apneic oxygenation	Replaced intermittent ventilation	Draper 1947
Ventilating bronchoscope	Continuous ventilation throughout procedure	Mansfield 1956
Venturi injector bronchoscope	Reduced difficulty interrupted vent	Sanders 1967
Fiberoptics (rigid) and light source	Direct light taken to specific field in view	Storz c.1960
Flexible fiberoptic endoscopes	Ability to flex fibers and follow anatomy	Machida and Olympus c.1966
Fiberoptic bronchoscope	Flexible, less traumatic	Ikeda 1968
EBT placement for OLA	Fiberoptic position endobronchial tube	Raj. et al 1975[3]
Pediatric Bronchoscopy	Diameter < 4 mm	Olympus. etc. 1979
Pediatric FFB EBT for OLA	Age 2, OLA in thoracic surgery	Vale, 1970[4] Watson, etc, 1983[5]
Bronchoscopy for BPF	Fibrin glue applied via flexible scope for BPF	Glover. et al 1987[6]
Video endoscopy	High-resolution monitors and mini-cameras in field	Olympus, Storz 1980s
Thoracoscopic pleurodesis	Lung biopsy and resection	Torre and Belloni[7] 1989
Thoracoscopic lung resection	Endoscopic stapling instruments	Krasna and Nazem 1991[8]

duction. Nonsurgical specialists discovered the relative safety of "noninvasive" flexible bronchoscopy throughout the 1970s. By the mid-1980s, anesthesiologists, otolaryngologists, pulmonologists, and radiologists, as well as thoracic and general surgeons, were using the flexible bronchoscope for a wide range of diagnostic and therapeutic applications.

Jacobaueus first described thoracoscopy after the turn of the century for the management of pleural adhesions following tuberculosis. Morton and Guinn reviewed the role of thoracoscopy in the modern surgical literature as a local or topical procedure for evaluating the pleurae and chest wall in 1971. During the 1970s, the laparoscopes and mediastinascopes that were occasionally used for thoracoscopy gave way to specifically designed rigid and flexible thoracoscopes. Indications for thoracoscopy have gradually expanded from examination of the pleurae and chest wall to lung biopsy and, more recently, resection. Initially thoracoscopy was widely practiced only in Europe and major thoracic referral facilities in the United States. Use of new high-resolution video systems together with new stapling devices that can be passed through the rigid thoracoscope has expanded the capabilities of the endoscopic technique. Surgical interest in "noninvasive" wedge or lung segment resection has paralleled the greater public demand for noninvasive surgery.

Anesthetic approaches are evolving rapidly to meet the increased demand. As with laparoscopic cholecystectomy, it can be anticipated that thoracoscopic resection may be proposed for a group of patients who were once thought to be too sick for open surgery. The anesthetic story continues to develop in 1995.

Evolution and Impact of Closed Interventions

For the most part, endoscopes were designed for very specific indications; they first gained acceptance among thoracic and other surgeons in that context. Innovative clinicians who encountered unusual circumstances devised new thoracoscopic applications. Procedures such as foreign body removal, lung isolation, biopsy, and, eventually, lung resection via endoscope followed diagnostic airway endoscopy as a means to avoid more traumatic, open, procedures. In almost every case, experience with endoscopy in one body cavity allowed the application of the concept to another (eg, airway endoscopy was created by extension of the principles of laparoscopy). Mediastinoscopy and thoracoscopy evolved from airway endoscopy in similar fashion. The first flexible fiberoptic instruments were designed for gastrointestinal (GI) endoscopy. After successful use of GI endoscopes in the airway, flexible bronchoscopes followed.

Improvements in light sources, light carrying bundles, suction, ventilation, patient monitoring, and tissue handling equipment have allowed more innovative procedures in recent years. Sometimes the evolution of technique has gone hand-in-hand with modifications of equipment. At other times, a growing clinical demand provided the impetus for industry to overcome its reservations about need versus profit and to develop equipment for which a previously undiscovered market existed (eg, the creation of pediatric endoscopes).

The history of these procedures as surgical innovations is important to anesthesiologists because evolution of anesthetic approaches for airway-sharing procedures teaches lessons that apply when the next technical wrinkle is introduced. Despite newer techniques and agents, the problems of a shared airway and the need to ensure effective ventilation and oxygenation with acceptable surgical conditions and control of noxious "protective" reflexes have not changed. Even the fear of airway fires—long thought to be relegated to a historical dust bin following the introduction of newer, nonflammable anesthetic agents—has resurfaced with the introduction of bronchoscopic laser resection techniques. Those anesthesiologists who have seen or feared this dreaded complication have not been surprised to see that patient management and prevention principles remain much the same.

The impact of closed techniques on the evolution of medical practice can be demonstrated through the anesthesiologist's experience with flexible bronchoscopy. As the diagnostic and therapeutic benefits of newer endoscopes were made clear to nonsurgical physicians like pulmonologists, intensivists and general internists, these newer instruments were used outside of the operating room environment under "awake sedation" and topical or local anesthesia. In general thoracic surgeons were not pleased by this trend, arguing that bleeding caused by airway biopsy might require thoracotomy. In other words, no one should perform a procedure unless he or she could treat each complication. Many anesthesiologists agreed, especially since they had experienced physiologic problems associated with endoscopic procedures in the operating room, and expected that the unmonitored procedure would be more dangerous in the hands of nonsurgeons. In some areas of the United States access to the operating room was used as a means to limit the spread of these procedures to other clinicians. No one but a surgeon could obtain operating privileges. Quality of care was cited as the reason, using the logical observation that the combination of diminished airway reflexes and the shared airway can lead to disaster without good anesthesia care. In fact, the literature of fiberoptic endoscopy for unanesthetized patients documented low complication rates in large series of patients, many of whom were high risk. Soon after pulmonologists established their ability with the flexible bronchoscope, anesthesiologists found that they needed to add flexible endoscopes to their technical armamentarium. The tools were simply too valuable for anesthetic management of the difficult airway and, ironically, for the placement of endobronchial tubes in thoracic anesthesia practice. Thus the safety of airway endoscopes has been proved to a hesitant anesthesia community. It is not uncommon for the anesthesiologist, pulmonologist, and thoracic surgeon to perform simultaneous bronchoscopy, each for a different purpose during the surgical period.

The important principle that someone must monitor and manage an anesthetized or sedated patient while the endoscopist works applies to the anesthesiologist as an endoscopist as much as it does to the surgeon. Although a historical circle has been completed, underlying principles of patient management have not changed.

Role of Anesthesia

Although many popular endoscopic procedures were introduced in the operating room under general anesthesia, they became successful partly because the operator could avoid general anesthesia. Modern endoscopic procedures are most often performed with sedation, good patient rapport and local analgesia. Endoscopy is performed under general anesthesia when a surgical procedure that requires general anesthesia is either planned or highly probable. More rarely anesthesia may be necessary for optimal surgical conditions or patient comfort when difficult surgery or prolonged endoscopy is necessary. Monitored anesthesia care is commonly requested when patients are extremely anxious, when patients are at greater than average risk of organ system decompensation during sedation and endoscopy, and when the surgeon does not know whether general anesthesia and a more extensive procedure will be necessary.

Monitoring Ventilation and Oxygenation

The primary goal of anesthesia care in any of the above circumstances is to ensure adequate ventilation and oxygenation. The challenge is very real: all anesthetic techniques limit or modify physiologic reserve to some extent. Newer respiratory and cardiovascular monitoring modes give the surgeon and anesthesiologist an early warning when organ failure is likely.

End-tidal carbon dioxide is the most important monitor of the adequacy of gas exchange under anesthesia. Good clinical practice dictates that an arterial blood gas "calibrate" the capnograph so that an arterial to end-tidal gradient can be defined. Unfortunately, many endoscopic procedures are brief; by the time arterial blood gasses have returned from a clinical laboratory, the procedure may have ended. A clinically valid end-tidal check can be made against the operator's exhalation prior to induction of anesthesia.

Pulmonary patients with significant obstructive airway disease or ventilation/perfusion (V/Q) mismatching (increased deadspace to tidal volume ratios) often have large arterial to end-tidal tension discrepancies. Baseline pulmonary function tests can help predict discrepancies but are not often obtained in the current cost-conscious health care climate. The most recent generation of anesthesia machines and continuous ventilators combines the capnograph with a graphic display of exhaled tidal volume, gas flow, and airway pressures. This provides a powerful tool for the clinician who wishes to adjust inspiratory to expiratory time ratios, tidal volume, and inspiratory gas flow from moment-to-moment during endoscopy for optimal gas exchange because such systems allow the anesthetist or anesthesiologist to obtain a baseline ventilatory profile for comparison with changes noted during anesthesia and endoscopy.

A specific limitation of capnography is obvious when ventilatatory patterns fluctuate. Tidal volumes just at or near dead anatomic and physiologic space volumes reach an exhaled plateau that may be far below actual alveolar levels. Tachypnea cuts exhalation short so that exhaled levels do not approximate an exhaled plateau, and the open airway or intermittant suction disrupts the orderly level of tidal exchange so that no end-tidal plateau is consistent. Capnographic and ventilatory wave form displays can help the experienced clinician to identify such problematic readings.

Transient disturbances of tidal gas exhange as a result of airway obstruction or lung compression during inhalation and exhalation are less significant than the ensuing V/Q mismatch and hypoxemia. The pulse oximeter has revolutionized monitoring of patients who are at risk. Technical problems with probe placement (eg, site of procedure, poor fit, position versus the blood pressure cuff, on the ear next to the endoscopist's hand, etc.) can be overcome by advance planning. It is important to have a good baseline value prior to induction of anesthesia or the start of an endoscopic procedure because the incidence of transient abnormalities is so high. One cannot expect one's ambulatory endoscopy patients to have better lung function postoperatively. Since it is now a standard of care that postprocedure levels be recorded, most Post-Anesthetic Care Units (PACU's) and ambulatory units document oxygen saturation during recovery and at discharge. Persistent hypoxemia following a procedure may be the first definite clinical indicator of hypoventilation and lung volume loss, atalectasis, or pneumothorax. Although the value of the measurement as an outcome indicator is doubtful, peri-anesthetic events influencing oxygenation can be identified and corrected before sustained hypoxemia injures the patient.

Problems with Anesthetic Approaches

Although many anesthesia personnel use a "routine" anesthetic for specific types of endoscopy, the technique should be matched to each patient's problems and surgical requirements. For example, although muscle relaxation may assist the rigid bronchoscopist in passing the instrument, it may be a therapeutic necessity that the patient cough during and after the procedure; the fiberoptic operator may wish to observe dynamic compression of the airways during spontaneous breathing to assess a region of tracheomalacia; or the thoracoscopist may need to assess a bronchopleural fistula (BPF) with spontaneous breathing before sealing it with topical glue. Since surgical requirements may change during endoscopy, the anesthesiologist must be an effective communicator and select a versatile technique. In our experience, a diagnostic operative bronchoscopy as part of a scheduled bronchoscopy and thoracotomy for biopsy that contraindicates thoracotomy poses a not uncommon communications problem. When long-acting muscle relaxants have been given, the anesthesiologist has little choice in this case other than post-procedure ventilation. Arterial or central venous monitoring catheters should not be placed until it is known whether an open procedure will follow.

Succinyl choline is often given by infusion for bronchoscopy in children and adults so that the level of muscle relaxation needed can be acutely titrated and procedures will not be delayed for reversal. With this versatile technique, the patient can be made to cough vigorously one minute while cadavorously paralysed the next. An overly long procedure can put such patients at risk for "dual" block. Conversion from the infusion approach to use of a nondepolarizing agent may complicate the clinical picture and delay effective reversal. For this reason, monitoring the neuromuscular junction is always indicated. The clinical decision of which technique to use at the start is less important than anticipating a necessary change of technique or ensuring that problems are recognized and managed properly.

A unique feature of endoscopic procedures is that they produce intense stimulation with little or no transition warning. Anesthetic techniques designed to titrate the anesthetic dose according to the level of pain or reflex response must adapt to sudden shifts. While the endoscopist may be casually draping at one moment, the patient may experience a maximal stimulus deep in the airway or an iatrogenic pneumothorax within a few seconds. The anesthesiologist can also be caught with a deeply anesthetized patient who is slow to emerge when a procedure ends suddenly. These anesthetic transitions explain why endoscopy can be so challenging. Rapid changes during rather short procedures provide many opportunities for a relative under- or overdose of anesthetic and the potential for sudden hemodynamic compromise. Furthermore, the patient and his endoscopist expect a rapid, uneventful emergence and "street readiness" after a brief stay in the recovery area. This is not always compatable with a need for deep anesthesia moments before the completion of endoscopy.

Such problems also provide the basis for a long-running clinical argument between those who advocate a total intravenous technique and those who champion inhalational anesthesia. Intravenous, or balanced, anesthesia with a drip infusion or bolus of narcotics and sedatives and an infusion of succinylcholine is relatively easy to reverse or discontinue for most patients, especially if the patient is kept "light." A few patients become hypotensive following small doses of narcotics and sedatives. Time is required to prevent this with fluid loading or to restore effective blood volume as the venous capacitance changes. On the other hand, hypertensive, tachycardiac, paralyzed patients may appear well anesthetized only to the endoscopist and have more difficulty with dysrhythmias or myocardial ischemia. When inhalational techniques are chosen over "balanced" techniques to ensure an adequate depth of anesthesia and the ability to use high inspired oxygen tensions, some patients do not tolerate the anesthetic depth before endoscopy begins. Others may demonstrate dramatic, breakthrough autonomic responses, just as during "balanced" techniques. Perhaps a greater number of patients manifest vasodilation and hypotension with inhaled techniques, but this is seen often enough with either approach and neither technique is ideal. After longer procedures, residual effects of narcotics and sedatives are as likely to impair effective ventilation and resumption of airway reflexes as waning concentrations of specific anesthetic agents can. Either approach can be chancey when anesthetic requirements change rapidly.

An intermediate anesthetic approach uses small increments of potent, short-acting narcotics, major tranquilizers, and low concentrations of an inhaled volatile agent together with either succinylcholine by bolus or infusion of a short-to-intermediate-acting nondepolarizing relaxant (ie, vecuronium, atracurium, rocuronium, or mivicurium). The art of safe anesthesia lies in determining the specific dose and timing of each drug as the patient's needs change. This requires good communication skills, experience, and close attention to detail.

Rigid Bronchoscopy

History

The rigid bronchoscope was designed following successful use of an esophagoscope for translaryngeal removal of an endobronchial foreign body by Killian about 1900. Early procedures were performed under topical and local anesthesia with sedation or during spontaneous ventilation with ether in oxygen. After initial case reports, the bronchoscope was widely used for diagnostic and therapeutic indications as an emergency airway management resource and for elective care as an alternative to thoracotomy. The Negus design allowed continuous insufflation of an anesthetic gas mixture during endoscopy. The rigid instrument was used as a means for dealing with the difficult intubation by Magill in 1936. The elucidation of apneic oxygenation by Draper in the 1940s justified periods of apnea under anesthesia and provided a quiet field for delicate maneuvers.

After the introduction of lidocaine in the 1960s, new topical and local anesthetic agents from both the ester and amide pharmacologic groups supplanted older agents (eg, cocaine, benzocaine, and tetracaine) and increased the safety of bronchoscopic procedures performed with sedation and monitored anesthesia care (MAC). Whether improved understanding of the determinants of local anesthetic toxicity or the more broad therapeutic index provided by newer agents played the major role, the incidence of local agent toxicity reported has decreased over the past three decades.

Mansfield's modification of the rigid bronchoscope allowed intermittant ventilation with the objective lens in place on the proximal end of the telescope. The ventilating bronchoscope allowed longer procedures and decreased risk to the patient as well as better surgical conditions. These instruments could be distinguished from the modified esophagoscopes that had been previously used by the side holes along the shaft of the tube and a side-arm connector for anesthesia circuit ventilating adaptors. Instead of alternating brief periods of mask-assisted or controlled ventilation with recurrent passage of the bronchoscope or spontaneous ventilation with gas insufflation, anesthesia and ventilation could be provided simultaneously through the endoscope. The airway was, therefore, shared by the endoscopist and the anesthetist. This modification also enhanced use of the bronchoscope as an emergency airway.

Many surgeons welcomed the Sander's injector in 1967.[9] Low frequency jet ventilation allowed more effective gas movement in a shorter time, thus decreasing the surgeon's "down" time for intermittant ventilation during procedures. Modifications such as the Carden apparatus and Carden tube allowed automatic control or ventilation from a small-diameter, external jet source within the trachea or larynx. The anesthesia community accepted jet ventilation with mixed emotions. Hypoxemia, hypoventilation, barotrauma, foreign body injection further down the airway, inspissation of secretions, and damage to the mucosa were all reported. Assessment of ventilatory adequacy or oxygenation with any technique was a matter of educated guessing—anything that went wrong with the patient during endoscopy was assumed to be a result of hypoxemia. At least when using a ventilating bronchoscope, the anesthetist could see and hear the chest rise and fall and use this evidence as a clinical guide.

In the mid 1970s Sjöstrand and colleagues popularized a form of high-frequency jet ventilation during airway endoscopy that they called high frequency positive pressure ventilation (HFPPV).[10] They developed a specific jet ventilator for the purpose and publicized their experience with various rate settings, driving pressures, and cannula diameters as a guide for other clinicians. Later, Miroslav Klain and colleagues demonstrated that percutaneous (ie, transtracheal) jet ventilation (HFJV)[11] provides a viable option. Of the various high frequency ventilation modalities introduced for rigid and flexible endoscopy, HFJV has proven most appropriate in open systems. Gas flows of up to 100–200 liters per minute can be achieved with a driving pressure of 50 psi, an 18 gauge orifice, and distal airway pressures that generally range from 25 to 30 cm H_2O.

The introduction of the pulse oximeter and capnometer into clinical anesthesia practice has resolved some of the controversy surrounding ventilatory modes employed for bronchoscopy under anesthesia or sedation. No matter whether the surgical preference is for apnea, HFJV, or intermittant ventilation, the anesthetist can periodically assess ventilation by closing the system and measure exhaled carbon dioxide after inserting a large manual breath. Continuous oximetry offers an unarguable physiologic endpoint that both the endoscopist and the anesthetist easily recognize. The intensity of many anesthesiologists' preferences has diminished as new monitoring modalities have removed the historical "seat of the pants" approach to ventilatory adequacy. Consequently, larger centers now offer a range of equipment and technique possibilities that can be adapted to most clinical situations—whether adult or pediatric.

Indications

Bronchoscopy is performed for a range of diagnostic and therapeutic indications (Table 17-2) that can be classified into three groups.[12] One, some chronic medical symptoms such as wheezing and cough that do not respond to other therapy suggest an anatomic process that could be treated via the bronchoscope. Two, bronchoscopy has an established role in a clinical work up before thoracotomy, where it helps clarify the anatomy associated with surgical disease. Three, the procedure is widely accepted in the emergency diagnosis or management of anatomic airway problems whether they are intrinsic (eg, burns, bleeding, foreign body, stenosis, malacia) or extrinsic (eg rupture, compression). These indications overlap with those for flexible fiberoptic bronchoscopy. To some extent, use of the flexible instrument has overtaken use of the rigid bronchoscope, but the rigid endoscope allows such direct access for suction and large instruments that it continues to have a well-established place in surgical practice.

Table 17-2. Indications for Rigid Bronchoscopy

Emergent	Elective	Operative
Foreign body	Cough	Endobronchial tumor
Critical atelectasis	Hemoptysis	Metastatic workup
Aspiration	Wheezing	Define compression
Airway compression	Atelectasis	Identify distortion
Acute obstruction	Chronic infection	Endobronchial blockade
Inhalation injury	Bronchography	One-lung anesthesia
Laryngeal obstruction	Biopsy lesion	Stent compressed airway
Secretion management		

Types of Anesthesia for Rigid Bronchoscopy

Emergency Bronchoscopy

Emergency procedures are most commonly requested for foreign body, secretion plugging or airway cast (burns) removal. Patients with sudden airway obstruction due to extrinsic compression of the upper or lower airway present rarely; but a rigid endoscope may be the only airway that is sufficiently stiff or extends far enough to relieve obstruction and allow the surgical and anesthesia team time to assess and further treat the underlying cause. In addition, a rigid endoscope and skilled endoscopist should always be available during anesthesia for patients with large anterior mediastinal mass or suspected epiglottitis. In the former situation, the endoscope may be passed to or below the carina, if necessary, to establish an airway. With epiglottitis, the rigid instrument has been used to force through the swollen glottis when a styletted endotracheal tube does not pass.

The emergency patient is rarely NPO; and the risk of aspiration must always be considered. In most cases there is not time for an adequate preanesthetic evaluation. GI prophylaxis with H_2 blockers and metoclopramide is not likely to be effective, given a short lead time and the stress associated with hypoxemia or respiratory distress. NPO status and associated comorbid factors such as coronary artery disease or chronic obstructive pulmonary disease are usually less important than correction of the threatening process that indicates endoscopy. Key issues include the patient's state of circulation, hydration, adequacy of ventilation and oxygenation and the presence of associated insults like pneumothorax. Since the reason for urgent endoscopy may be the underlying cause of circulatory and ventilatory disorders, preanesthetic preparation must be brief and may not fully correct the problem. The anesthesiologist must be certain that all necessary ventilating equipment and adaptors are present and checked; basic anesthetic life support should be set up prior to the procedure. Moments lost trying to identify the appropriate connector for the endoscope could be vital to a safe, successful bronchoscopy.

The anesthesiologist should establish and manage the best airway possible with 100% oxygen during the preanesthetic evaluation. Not infrequently, patients markedly improve when given oxygen and assisted ventilation by a bag-valve-mask system after obstruction or other problems have limited oxygenation with various oxygen therapy devices (including a 100% nonrebreathing mask system). Those patients who are intubated may improve when a clinician who is more attentive to respiratory problems than a referring surgeon, intensive care nurse, or primary physician, substitutes a knowing hand for the mechanical ventilator. The significant exceptions are the patients with noncompliant lungs whose oxygenation immediately deteriorate when airway pressure therapy (continuous positive airway pressure [CPAP], reverse inspiration to expiration ratio ventilation, HFJV, etc) is interrupted. With pulmonary edema, adult respiratory distress syndrome and related pathology, the anesthesiologist does well to inquire whether flexible fiberoptic bronchoscopy (FFB) would be better than rigid endoscopy because FFB can be used with minimal interruption of barotherapy.

Patients in extremis or with circulatory collapse should have emergent procedures performed without anesthesia during other resuscitation efforts. Although glycopyrrolate has a less central effect and is a relatively more potent antisialogogue than atropine, the latter drug is important because compromised ventilation (acidosis) and hypoxemia commonly cause bradycardia or sinus arrest that may exacerbate the ongoing respiratory insult. A muscle relaxant may be necessary to allow the endoscopist access to the airway, but sedatives and narcotics can provide the coup de grace that converts shock to frank cardiorespiratory arrest. Regardless of the routine practice or the aesthetic demands of an endoscopist or other health professionals, the anesthesiologist or nurse anesthetist who gives general anesthesia to a patient in prearrest condition is on unsteady ground. An acute, curative endoscopic intervention that stabilizes the situation may allow use of agents such as midazolam, ketamine, and lorazepam that impart some retrograde amnesia. With resolution of the emergency one can convert the technique to a general or topical approach. The anesthesiologist should remember that sedation with as little as one or two milliliters of fentanyl citrate, or the equivalent, is as effective in blocking protective laryngeal reflexes as topical anesthesia. Two large-diameter suction systems should be available. Often an emergency procedure is completed so rapidly that the issue of anesthesia is moot.

For less emergent patients in distress, a "rapid sequence" intravenous induction technique is used. Succinylcholine by bolus and infusion remains the relaxant of choice when time is a critical factor, except for the severely burned or crush injury patients at risk for rhabdomyolysis and hyperkalemic cardiac arrest. Under these circumstances, a larger than usual dose of short (mivicurium) or intermediate (rocuronium or vecuroneum) duration nondepolarizing agent should be substituted. Small doses of intravenous agents that have a short duration of action (eg, pentothal, propofol, midazolam) are preferable to longer lasting, less predicatable sedatives, such as diazepam. Narcotics are ill-advised, since there is little pain after endoscopy and the patient's protective airway reflexes may be crucial for continued well-being. Cricoid pressure with neck extension should be provided by an assistant throughout induction, endoscopy, and emergence.

Foreign Body Removal

Patients with foreign bodies (FB) can present with asymptomatic, complete, or partial airway obstruction. The rigid bronchoscope is commonly used when the FB can be withdrawn in toto through the instrument under direct vision or when the FB is so large that larger forceps are needed to remove it. A chest film should be obtained in order to locate the level of the FB before endoscopy. Even if the FB is not radioopaque, the film may reveal distal atelectasis or air trapping and hyperinflation. Laryngoscopy and direct tracheal intubation is not wise prior to endoscopy unless the FB is known to be quite distal. Nitrous oxide should be avoided when obstruction is associated with air trapping because further hyperinflation can worsen V/Q mismatching or lead to pneumothorax with adverse circulatory and ventilatory consequences.

Some anesthesiologists have advocated use of helium-oxygen mixtures for ventilation during FB removal because significant improvement in air flow can be achieved when gas viscosity decreases. In my experience, the helium-oxygen equipment is so rarely indicated that it is always put away and it is not easily accessible in emergencies. Lack of familiarity leads to operator confusion and error.

Movable or fragile FBs can disintegrate with traumatic handling or cough and thus require special care. Suprising objects have been aspirated—from Christmas tree ornaments to peanuts—from children and adults. No foreign body aspiration is routine; patients who have aspirated may present with a FB lodged in the larynx, pharynx, trachea, or bronchus. With a highly placed FB, cricoid pressure may be harmful. Laryngeal or subglottic pressure can cause a fragile FB to break into fragments that could lacerate tissues or that could be pushed to a more inaccessable level of the airway. The use of positive- pressure ventilation or HFJV could also be dangerous. A well-tailored plan for removal of such FBs involves preoxygenation, sedation with narcotics and sedatives, and endoscopy without prior ventilation after intravenous anesthesia and succinyl choline. If repeated endoscopy is necessary because the obstructing object or secretion plug comes out in piecemeal fashion, gentle mask ventilation between passes of the rigid scope or side-arm ventilation via the bronchoscope should be performed. Time for exhalation between breaths must be allowed in order to reduce distal air trapping. No matter how well the procedure goes, the postoperative care plan should involve a chest radiograph to ensure that the obstruction is resolving and that no pneumothorax is present.

If the patient is in no distress but endoscopy is indicated to prevent later complications (FB only partly obstructing or at risk to advance to a lower, more obstructing position, or FB obstruction resulting in progressive atelectasis), time should be devoted to preoperative assessment, planning and communication with the endoscopist. It is essential to avoid time lost through miscommunication. A misstep that involves either endoscopist or anesthesiologist during an airway maneuver could be critical.

Elective and Operative Bronchoscopy

Elective procedures allow time for a more adequate preoperative evaluation. The anesthesiologist should discuss the plan with the surgeon and operating room team before surgery so that all team members have the same plan in mind. Although OR circulating nurses and technicians set up the equipment, the anesthesiologist must be certain that ventilation equipment and adaptors are present and checked prior to the procedure. The endoscopist expects the anesthesiologist to manage ventilation, whether the ventilating bronchoscope or a jet system is used. Consequently, only the anesthesiologist will be attentive to details such as the presence of an adaptor that allows the anesthesia circle or a jet system to attach to the endoscope. The patient must be NPO. Gastric acid prophylaxis or stomach emptying maneuvers may be instituted. It is almost always possible to get a good history, complete a physical examination and review the chest x-rays and computerized tomography (CT) scan, if necessary. The anesthetist or anesthesiologist should see the films and radiologist's report if there is any question of airway compression or deformity that could complicate ventilation during the procedure. Merely noting the American Society of Anesthesiologists' (ASA) classification of physical status is insufficient when patients have complex medical problems as the anesthetic should be tailored to meet each patient's needs.

Anesthetic Techniques

Two techniques are commonly used: intravenous and inhalational. The tendency to use intravenous sedative-narcotic combinations prior to anesthesia and topical anesthetics during anesthesia is widespread. This practice may be appropriate because the relatively "light" techniques are otherwise associated with an incidence of recall that is purported to be as high as 4%.[13] Thus the technique is characterized by whether the induction is intravenous or inhalational and whether relaxants are used. The physical status of the patient, reason for endoscopy, and needs of the endoscopist should be considered in designing the anesthetic. Brief bronchoscopy in a debilitated patient with neuromuscular disease or a history of cerebrovascular accident (CVA), for example, might better be managed with minimal intravenous sedation and monitored anesthesia care. A young, fit patient who is to have bronchoscopic lung lavage should have an anesthetic that preserves respiratory effort and coughing to promote movement of the lavage fluid and secretions out to the suction area. On the other hand, a patient with a fragile FB in the trachea should be completely paralyzed and apneic during FB removal, so that movement does not complicate the endoscopist's difficult task.

During the procedure, care must be taken to avoid trauma to the eyes, face, lips, and teeth. Eyes should be lubricated, closed, and padded for bronchoscopy under general anesthesia. Dental guards or rubber dams are used to protect the teeth. Following demonstration of a satisfactory airway and depth of anesthesia the table should be swiveled 30 to 90 degrees to the side for bronchoscopy so that the endoscopist can have unobstructed access to the patient's airway but the anesthesiologist can readily reach it with a mask or other equipment at any time.

Local Analgesia or MAC

Rigid bronchoscopy is more uncomfortable for the "awake" patent than "awake intubation," because extreme neck extension must be maintained throughout the procedure. On account of the discomfort associated with position and trauma, together with the fact that FFB is better tolerated in awake patients, MAC is rarely requested for rigid bronchoscopy. Nevertheless, large numbers of patients who were awake and sedated have had rigid endoscopy. Good patient rapport together with regional or topical anesthesia and sedation are essential to the sucess of rigid bronchoscopy under local anesthesia or MAC. All of the local agents have been used for topical analgesia at one time or another. Metered dose inhalers, aerosols, or measured volumes of topical agent are recommended to prevent drug overdose. Transmucosal absorption is high (tracheal lidocaine injection achieves blood levels comparable with levels achieved following direct intravenous injection) so that lower concentrations than those recommended for nerve blocks should be used. The benzocaine-tetracaine mixture that was widely promoted for topical airway anesthesia in the 1970s is associated with worrisome plasma levels of benzocaine and tetracaine unless it is used sparingly.

Otolaryngologists once routinely anesthetized the oral cavity perorally under direct or mirror laryngoscopy with internal laryngeal and glossopharyngeal nerve blocks using tonsillar needles and direct application of agent or topical pledgets. Transtracheal or transcricoid topical injections and superior laryngeal nerve blocks are the most useful upper airway blocks used for bronchoscopy. Topical anesthesia and sedation are usually effective for managing the discomfort of the oral cavity and deeper pharynx. For more superficial analgesia of the oral cavity viscous or nebulized lidocaine is equally effective. Laryngeal and tracheal anesthesia requires bilateral laryngeal nerve blocks and topical mucosal anesthesia. Narcotic and sedative agents combine to potentiate these topical and nerve blocking approaches by reducing anxiety and decreasing the gag and cough reflexes.

The *superior laryngeal nerve block* anesthetizes both motor and sensory branches to the larynx as well as the inferior part of the epiglottis. Two to three milliliters of 1 or 2% lidocaine are injected just below the upper horn of the thyroid cartilage in an inferomesiad direction away from the carotid artery with a small gauge, 1.5-inch needle. The operator feels a palpable click or pop as the needle perforates the thyrohyoid membrane, thus gaining access to the interior branches of the superior laryngeal nerve. Motor function of the cords is not greatly affected as these are mostly controlled by the recurrent laryngeal nerve. Indeed, recurrant nerve integrity is desirable if an effective cough and partial glottic closure are to be preserved after endoscopy.

Topical anesthesia of the trachea is initiated by *transtracheal* or *transcricoid* injection of local anesthetic. For this procedure, a small skin wheal is raised over the cricothyroid membrane with a subcutaneous needle. Then, as the patient exhales, a 22-gauge, 1.5-inch needle attatched to a syringe whose volume is greater than the anesthetic solution is advanced in the midline in a caudal direction until air can be aspirated. The local anesthetic solution is then rapidly injected and the needle removed just as the patient inhales in order to cough. Shallow placement and rapid withdrawal of the needle ensures that tracheal laceration will not occur. Minor submucosal hemorrage is almost always evident to the bronchoscopist. The patient's need to inhale before coughing ensures that the drug is drawn further into the trachea. This block can be supplemented by reinjection or by a direct translaryngeal topical spray. Such laryngotracheal anesthesia (LTA) injection under direct visualization is part of a sequence of stimuli that some clinicians use to test the adequacy of topical analgesia and sedation before rigid bronchoscopy. The anesthetist can also predict that the endoscopist should have no difficulty finding the larynx with a rigid bronchoscope if the anesthetist can easily visualize the larynx for an LTA spray. When the anesthetist has difficulty with this maneuver, the endoscopist usually does also. Thus, the LTA can play an important role in the technique. Aerosol therapy from a face mask or mouth piece is a very effective, noninvasive technique for topical analgesia, but the aerosol requires higher doses of topical agent because most is swallowed from the orophargnx. Direct topical instillation of anesthetic solution or spray to the mucosa during the procedure via the bronchoscope is also widely practiced.

Local anesthetic agents most commonly used in the airway for topical and regional analgesia are listed in Table 17-3, together with recommended concentrations and dosage. In recent years tetracaine and benzocaine have fallen into disuse, largely because of toxicity associated with these agents given topically in unmetered doses. Safe practice dictates that a dosage maximum be drawn up into labeled syringes for use and that the lowest concentration necessary be used. For direct injection in the trachea, we use no higher concentration than a 1% solution of lidocaine. Good labeling practice is important for topical anesthesia of the airway because unlabeled syringes of irrigation solution are commonly on the field and easy to confuse, especially when large volumes of irrigating solution are needed for secretion lavage. For the same reasons, the common OR nursing practice of placing sterile, unlabeled bowls of irrigation, local anesthetic, and specimen preservative solutions from which increments are drawn up by syringe should be avoided.

Table 17-3. Local Anesthetic Doses

	Topical		Regional	
Drug	Concentration (%)	Safe Dose	Concentration (%)	Safe Dose
Cocaine	4	150 mg (1.5 mg/kg)	No longer used	For injection
Lidocaine	2–4	200 mg (3 cc/kg)	1–2	500 mg (5–7 cc/kg)
Bupivicaine	Rarely used	Topically	0.25–5	200 mg (3 cc/kg)

Spontaneous Breathing Technique

The patient is premedicated with atropine, an anxiolytic agent, and minimal doses of narcotic (if any). Monitors should include a precordial stethoscope placed over the sternal "notch" where pulse, breath sounds, and laryngeal flow sounds can be appreciated. Increasing concentrations of inhalational agent are added to the inhaled mixture after a "stunning" dose of barbiturate, sedative (midazolam), propofol, or ketamine. Further increments or a tapering infusion can be added to speed transition through the "excitement" phase of induction but the transition from spontaneous to assisted ventilation is made as the patient's depth of anesthesia increases. Care must be taken to avoid large boluses of the intravenous hypnotic agent or narcotic so that apnea, and loss of the respiratory guide to anesthetic depth, does not occur. As the respiratory effort becomes weaker and weaker, the flow of nitrous oxide, if used, is gradually reduced until the patient is anesthetized with the potent volatile agent alone in oxygen and making minimal respiratory effort. Rapid, shallow breaths with little accessory muscle movement and cord motion provide the best initial conditions for passage of the bronchoscope. The concentration of the agent can be lowered during bronchoscopy after laryngotracheal and bronchial stimuli produce a maximal surgical response. The inspired concentration should be increased again for several minutes before removal of the endoscope to avoid laryngospasm. Inspired and expired agent concentration monitoring greatly facilitates this by indicating the rate of uptake and clearance.

Intravenous Technique

Small doses of an anxiolytic agent and atropine are given intravenously. Preoxygenation is more important than during inhalational inductions, as apnea is more likely. Short acting (rapidly redistributed) narcotic agents can be given in larger doses, since apnea is most commonly accepted as part of the intravenous and "balanced" techniques. If it is important to have the patient rapidly return to an awake, self-protected state after bronchoscopy, these drugs should be carefully titrated. Narcotics are effective antitussive agents and, if good postendoscopy coughing is needed, a short-acting agent should be titrated carefully.

After the basal anesthetic has been administered, a hypnotic dose of a potent sedative, ultra-short-acting thiobarbiturate or propofol may be given. Continuous infusion techniques are regaining popularity in the 1990s, especially as a new series of reliable, battery-operated, light-weight infusion pumps that autocalibrate dosage for a preset body mass have become available. The intermediate and long-term nondepolarizing relaxants are used for longer bronchoscopies and "staged" procedures. Succinylcholine by bolus and infusion remains very popular for shorter procedures because it can be titrated on a minute-by-minute basis in a 0.1% to 0.4% solution. Newer, short-acting, nondepolarizing relaxants have become increasingly popular as alternatives to succinlycholine but it remains to be seen whether the cost of these weighs favorably against the low, but real, morbidity of the depolarizing agent.

Intravenous or "balanced" anesthesia has tended to be very "light." Nitrous oxide, narcotics, and hypnotics are not primary cardiovascular depressants, and larger doses of narcotic most commonly used to take patients "deeper" are more likely to cause apnea and delayed emergence following endoscopy. Infusion techniques have provided the most logical method of controlling anesthetic depth. When movement or adverse cardiovascular reflexes are noted, the patient can be rebolused and placed on an increased drip rate. Just as with inhalation techniques, the anesthetist or anesthesiologist must remain alert to operative events so that drug doses will be timed correctly.

Special Issues in Bronchoscopy

Topical Anesthesia—The Lidocaine Controversy

Direct laryngoscopy and translaryngeal spray with topical 2% lidocaine before the bronchoscope is inserted under general anesthesia is often used. Some anesthesiologists argue that the LTA is not worth the time required because nebulized or intravenous lidocaine is equally effective as topical lidocaine in suppressing cough and dysrhythmias during and after bronchoscopy. In practice, the LTA injection not only augments the anesthetic but also ensures that the anesthesiologist has established an adequate depth of anesthesia before relinquishing the patient to the endoscopist. Instrumentation of the airway can cause dramatic reflex responses, whether during placement of an endotracheal tube or an endoscope, but direct laryngoscopy and LTA provide a "reversible" stimulus that fatigues over time and as the topical agent is absorbed. No topical means of administering lidocaine is totally benign. Even aerosolized lidocaine given before flexible bronchoscopy is performed has been shown to increase airway resistance in patients with reactive airway disease. Patients who cough and have laryngospasm during LTA are best managed by the anesthetist before the airway is surrendered to the bronchoscopist. Laryngoscopy for LTA provides an opportunity to place oral dams (tooth guards for uppers and lowers), to lubricate and shield the eyes, and to position the head and shoulders for the bronchoscopist. Direct laryngoscopy prior to bronchoscopy may also warn the anesthesiologist about intubation difficulty and give the endoscopist an impression of how difficult bronchoscope placement will be.

Ventilatory Modalities

Apneic Oxygenation

Frumin and colleagues defined "apneic oxygenation" in the late 1950's.[14] The principle of apneic oxygenation relies upon an open airway, removal of nitrogen from the functional residual capacity (FRC), and a large oxygen tension gradient. A high inspired tension increases the oxygen diffusion gradient between the upper and lower airway four- to five-fold, thus ensuring adequate alveolar oxygen tensions provided the airway and alveoli remain open. Prolonged obstruction by the bronchoscope, suction, lung volume loss, or frank atalectasis disrupts the diffusion gradient to pulmonary capillary blood and establishes conditions where hypoxemia is likely. Fraioli and colleagues established this in the early 1970s for a population of patients who were thought to have a large nitrogen store to body weight ratio due to low lung volumes (functional residual capacity [FRC]), large body mass, or small airway disease.[15] These researchers recommended using an FRC-weight ratio of less than 37cc/kg as a cut off for allowing apnea to last longer than five minutes. All of their patients in the lower FRC/body mass group had PaO_2s that fell to half of baseline by five minutes. Today it is well recognized that conditions that limit the FRC (eg, pregnancy, pneumonia, infancy, morbid obesity, chest wall trauma) are associated with early hypoxemia during apnea. Our uncertainty regarding safe oxygenation is resolved with the widespread use of pulse oximetry.

Duration of apnea should be limited by arterial oxygen saturation and time. For patients who remain well oxygenated, the safety of apnea correlates with carbon dioxide levels. Although the body's buffers can handle some respiratory acid, carbon dioxide accumulation is inevitable and predictable. As a rule of thumb, the arterial pCO_2 rises 6–10 mmHg in the first minute of apnea and at a rate of 3–5 mmHg per minute thereafter in adults with basal oxygen consumption and a normal respiratory quotient. The initial rise is due to equlibration between arterial and venous levels together with metabolic production after tidal exchange ceases. If the patient's oxygen consumption is reduced by anesthetic drugs and the the patient's lungs are hyperventilated prior to apnea, the endoscopist may have 10 to 15 minutes of operating time before carbon dioxide levels rise far enough (30–50 mmHg) to create arrythmias or hypertension in elderly and high risk patients. Metabolic carbon dioxide production will be increased in lightly anesthetized, obese, pediatric, pregnent, or febrile patients. Young, well-oxygenated patients who have no coronary disease, sepsis, or other reason for hypermetabolism are good candidates for apneic oxygenation since they tolerate severe hypercapnea amazingly well. Clinical assessment of the magnitude of hypercapnea is best achieved by intermittent capnometry with tidal ventilation through a closed system.

Ventilating Bronchoscope

If ventilation is managed with a ventilating bronchoscope, it can be used only when the objective lens or eye piece is closed over the scope. Ventilation must be interrupted during suction, biopsy, or passage of angled telescopes through the instrument. In some cases, the term *ventilating* is a misnomer because most of the work is perfomed during apnea in an open system. Even during ventilation there may be a large volume lost around the instrument through the glottis when the endoscope fits loosely. Thus the tidal volume delivered depends upon chest wall compliance and the relationship between the external diameter of the endoscope and the size of the airway. Resistance to exhalation around the bronchoscope acts somewhat like a pressure relief limit, decreasing effective tidal volumes when compliance of the lung-thorax system decreases. The anesthetist can close the airway and compress soft tissue in the neck around the glottis with one hand while ventilating with the other provided this does not make the endoscopist's work harder or compress the carotids. In addition, the anesthetist must be constantly alert to changes in chest wall movement and the position of the bronchoscope. High-pressure inflation or rapid breaths with overly short exhalation times while the instrument is well into distal bronchial segments can cause barotrauma. Most endoscopists withdraw the instrument to or just above the carina periodically so that effective ventilation can be resumed. The pulse oximeter is a good guide to safe apneic periods between breaths. Because the airway is "open," end-tidal carbon dioxide is rarely reliable as an indicator of $PaCO_2$ until mask ventilation is resumed.

Jet Ventilation

Jet systems can be divided between those that are manually triggered by a hand or foot control switch and those with automatic timing. With both systems, the operator should begin with lower driving pressures (~20 psi) and rates. Jet frequency can then be increased manually or automatically after effective ventilation is observed at normal rates. The anesthetist is cautioned to increase the driving pressure only after making certain that other parameters are set properly and the instrument is not obstructed or advanced into a small bronchopulmonary segment. In open systems, delivered tidal volumes increase by a volume entrained from ambient air. The Venturi principle explains this—as the jet injects into the airway, a rapidly expanding, accelerating gas wave front causes a decreased lateral pressure that draws or "entrains" gas from a level above the jetstream down into the airway. The entrainment ratio is a function of the mechanical parameters of the system, driving pressure, and inspiratory time. The entrained volume derives from the ambient gas mixture (usually air) and can be as high as 40% of the total volume delivered. Consequently one should inject an oxygen rich gas mixture through the jet. The anesthesiologist must use chest expansion as a guide in determining whether ventilation is effective. Muscle relaxation is helpful with both high- and low-frequency jet ventilation since changes in lung or chest wall compliance can diminish residual lung volume and alveolar ventilation.

Because an expanding gas flow wavefront and entrained volume follow the direction of the jet, jet injectors can be used with open systems. Distal pressures also pulsate in time with the jet so that the endoscopist may complain of a moving field during Venturi ventilation. When movement is a problem the operator can revert to low-pressure jet oxygenation at a level that does not cause movement (and rarely provides a minute ventilation that is adequate for carbon dioxide removal). The other option is apneic oxygenation; however, without the distending pressure created by jet pulses, lung volume may fall and hypoxemia is even more likely than with low-pressure high-frequency ventilation.

LOW-FREQUENCY JET VENTILATION. Manually triggered devices with high driving pressure applied through a limited orifice deliver low-frequency jet ventilation. Criteria for effective ventilation are the same as those commonly used with the ventilating bronchoscope–chest wall expansion and breath sounds. The devices include a high-pressure gas source with variable pressure reducing valve, a manual or foot-operated pressure switch that initiates and sustains gas flow as long as it is engaged and high-pressure connecting tubing or a jet cannula. An air, helium-oxygen, or nitrous oxide-oxygen blender may be placed proximal to the reducing valve to control gas mixture. Alternatively, a fixed gas mixture such as compressed air or Entanox can be used without a blender. The tubing, reducing valve, and switch should be tested before use. In particular, it is important to make sure that the pressure switch disengages briskly when it is no longer compressed. Since longer inspiratory times allow high driving pressures to overcome the high resistance of a jet cannula and approach equilibration pressures more closely, the jet operator must be careful to observe chest wall motion and bronchoscope position in the airway, and limit the duration of jetting.

HIGH FREQUENCY JET VENTILATION. High frequency jet ventilation (HFJV) requires an automatic switching system. Most of the available units are equiped with an airway pressure cutoff that automatically stops gas flow when a preset pressure, whether measured via an accessory pressure port or at the jet oriface, is exceeded. In practice, the inspiratory:expiratory time ratio (less than 1:2) is set first and the ventilator is tested with low driving pressure at low and high frequencies before it is attached to the bronchoscope. After it is connected to the endoscope, driving pressure is gradually increased at the target frequency (usually 100–150 breaths per minute) until chest wall movement is obvious to the anesthetist with the bronchoscope in proximal or operative position. A "stand-by" mode selecter switch that can allow brief periods of apnea for delicate endoscopic manipulations without disrupting the system setting is a helpful feature. Most high-frequency systems can be set to generate both automatic low-frequency jet ventilation and high frequency modes up to 150 breaths/min.

The rationale for HFJV is the achievement of effective gas exchange and maintenance of lung volume in an open system with limited peak airway pressures. HFJV systems are safer and more versatile than manually triggered devices. Lung volume is variably increased by "auto-PEEP," the gas trapping effect of balancing rapid-rate, positive-pressure gas flow against elastic recoil of the lung and chest wall. The best location for an airway pressure safety cutoff is therefore in the distal trachea or near the tip of the jet endoscope—not just at or above the Venturi oriface. Airway pressures may vary from one area of the lung to another. Because chest wall and lung compliance also varies, different patients have different lung volume-oxygenation effects with the same HFJV settings.

Capnometry is not very useful with jet ventilation because these systems are open, exhaled tidal volumes are small, and gas flows are high. At best one can measure carbon dioxide via a circle system and face mask before, intermittantly during, and after bronchoscopy. Therefore, when one does not notice tidal exchange and chest wall movement at least intermittantly during bronchoscopy, one should limit the duration of the procedure to the 8–10 minutes commonly allowed by apneic oxygenation. Adequate muscle relaxation is important during HFJV, because short inspiratory times limit the peak pressure and hence small changes in lung-thorax compliance can greatly change minute amounts of ventilation.

The Atropine Controversy

Atropine has long been recommended as a means of preventing reflex bradycardia and hypersecretion during endoscopy. It was once thought—and later disproved conclusively—that atropine increased lower esophageal sphincter tone and assisted in preventing aspiration. Because of the secretion drying effect of antisialogogues, it was also feared that atropine would inspissate secretions. Atropine is known to increase dead space in test subjects, and block heart rate change as an indicator of the depth of anesthesia. Turndorf and colleagues have shown that atropine is not a benign drug, as was previously thought. When the drug was given intravenously to anesthetized patients, these investigators documented a significant incidence of supraventricular and ventricular conduction abnormalities and dysrrhythmias. The onset and duration of action of atropine renders it less effective if given as an intramuscular premedicant more than an hour before anesthetic induction. In addition, many patients complain endlessly of dry mouth and thirst both preoperatively and postoperatively. The incidence of a low-key postoperative cholinergic syndrome that frightens the parents of children given atropine preoperatively or intraoperatively is rather high. Glycopyrrolate lasts longer after injection and tends to be a stronger antisialogogue than atropine at equivalent doses and may have fewer central side effects. An older drug, scopolamine, administered via transdermal patches, has recently been popularized. Transdermal scopolamine provides controlled doses that supress motion sickness with few central side effects.

In the thoracic and pulmonary literature, atropine has been emphasized as a means of preventing cholinergic changes in bronchomotor tone that decrease small airway flow, promote air trapping, and increase residual lung volume.[8] High dose anticholinergic therapy has gained wide acceptance as one method of treating reactive airway disease as part of multilevel pharmacologic therapy. Fears that secretion drying and plugging would follow have not been realized. On balance, the risks are outweighed by the benefits of anticholinergic therapy. The drug is now recommended as part of the premedicant routine for airway endoscopy, whether given intravenously, intramuscularly, or by aerosol. This is especially rational in patients with known reactive airway disease who are more likely to have bronchospasm.

Oxygen Concentration

Hypoxemia is noted during and after both flexible fiberoptic and rigid bronchoscopy. Putative mechanisms include V/Q mismatch associated with reflex changes in bronchomotor and vascular tone, airway obstruction, and hypoventilation during bronchoscopy, air trapping and hyperinflation distal to the endoscope, small airway edema due to direct trauma, and overly enthusiastic suction.[17, 18] Most anesthesiologists tend to use high oxygen tensions during rigid bronchoscopy, although some have argued that the improved oxygenation following use of injector (jet ventilation) bronchoscopes allows the use of 50:50 nitrous oxide-oxygen mixtures.[19] The potential for promoting absorption atalectasis and blocking reflex hypoxic pulmonary vasoconstriction (HPV) is weighed against the advantage of having a full FRC of oxygen and a few hundred mmHg of leeway in the alveolar-to-arterial gradient during a brief procedure. Gross changes in V/Q matching and lung oxygen stores caused by instrumentation and the effects of general anesthesia on HPV suggest that the less dramatic consequences of hyperoxia are of little practical significance. The most likely causes of hypoxemia are a direct consequence of events occurring during bronchoscopy. The pulse oximeter has resolved the practical question of whether lower oxygen tension mixtures cause hypoxemia by providing an early warning indicator before precipitously low tissue levels occur. When high inspired oxygen tensions are provided, arterial desaturation is less common during bronchoscopy. Oxygen therapy is wise for a time after the procedure. It can now be titrated noninvasively and prescribed based on a patient's baseline status and actual hemoglobin saturation. When postendoscopy oxygen therapy is needed, it should be administered via a cold aerosol mask or face tent to promote mucosal humidification and vasoconstriction and to decrease upper airway edema.

Bronchoscopic Laser Surgery

Recent interest has grown in laser resection of endobronchial tumors. This is actually a revisitation of an earlier technique that used hot wire electrocautery, rather than a laser, as the heat source for cutting. Since tissue penetration by a laser beam is a function of the wavelength, the carbon dioxide laser (wavelength: 10,600 nm), is used for superficial work in the airway while the ND-YAG (neodynium-yttrium-aluminum-garnet) laser, (wavelength: 1064 nm), which penetrates deeper and has a longer extinction pathway in water and tissue, can be passed through quartz and fiberoptic filiments. Therefore endobronchial laser work can be performed through the rigid bronchoscope or the flexible instrument. With either laser, the energy transmitted is a function of the driving power (Wtts/cm^2) and the length of time (usually measured in milliseconds) the laser beam is applied to tissue. The laser can be aimed in a very precise manner. A tightly focused beam provides either continuous or intermittant cutting effect. For maximum focal effect, the target should not move during laser resection. Whatever the mode of ventilation used for laser work in the airway, apnea during ignition shortens the operating time by allowing more efficient use of the laser. For this reason, we use a high-frequency jet ventilator that can be placed in standby mode intermittantly during the actual laser work. The pulse oximeter provides a monitor of the safe end-point for apneic periods.

A carbon dioxide laser applied directly through the rigid instrument is most commonly used for endobronchial masses in a manner similar to the hot wire or radiofrequency cautery. Obstructing lesions are "cored" and extruding masses are cut away from the tracheal mucosa in pieces. The rigid instrument is used under general anesthesia for very precise laser application in a stationary field. These conditions allow improved suction and retrieval of tumor fragments. Respiratory timing is important becaue ventilation during procedures with either lasers or the guided wire cautery can potentially inject tumor debris and products of combustion into the airway. Any procedure involving cautery can cause airway fires in an air-oxygen or nitrous-oxygen enriched gas mixture. The procedure provides the three critical requirements for fire: a heat source, combustable material, and an oxygen source. Various authors have recommended that either helium or nitrogen (compressed air) as opposed to nitrous oxide in oxygen be blended in the anesthetic gas mixture during laser endobronchial resection as these are inert gases while nitrous oxide supports combustion (Table 17-4). We use an air blender with the lowest inspired oxygen tension that maintains a safe arterial oxygen saturation.

The ND-YAG laser is occasionally used with a flexible bronchoscope through an endotracheal tube or rigid bronchoscope.[20,21] General anesthesia with an intravenous agent and muscle relaxant is recommended. Various approaches to limiting the inspired oxygen tension and risk of combustion have been recommended. Some practitioners use a jet system; others, the ventilating bronchoscope. If the system is used with a tracheal tube, it is important to ensure that the bronchoscope is beyond the tube for fear that tube ignition rather than tissue cautery may occur. The procedure for airway tumors is usually prolonged, since many patients have high-grade airway obstruction to begin with and a large volume of tumor to debulk. As a result, timing of laser pulses with a fixed part of the ventilatory cycle (exhalation) or in sequence with the jet injector may be helpful. This will allow more precise application of the laser beam and cancel tissue movement. Recent investigations of various laser settings and tube options for otolaryngologic (ENT) laser work has clarified the safety and settings necessary for prevention of tube ignition and airway fires.[22] Nevertheless, the risk is omnipresent as all of the elements necessary for combustion are brought together during these procedures. Every time a laser case is planned, the anesthetist would do well to review the airway fire protocol before starting. Table 17-5 summarizes complications reported following laser bronchoscopy (see also Table 17-4).

Table 17-4. Treatment of Airway Fires

Steps	Measures	Rationale
1	Stop ventilation	Smother fire
2	Stop gas flow	Smother
3	Remove tube and scope	Remove combustibles
4	Mask ventilate, intubate if necessary	Reoxygenate after fire is smothered
5	Rigid bronchoscopy	Survey injury
6	Debride tissue	Clear airway
7	Reintubate	Prevent upper airway edema and obstruction
8	Monitor and ventilate 24–36 h, obtain chest x-rays and arterial blood gases	Check other injuries
9	Use a fexible fiberoptic bronchoscope to view the lower airways and a laryngoscope to view the upper larynx after 24 h	Survey local injury

Table 17-5. Complications of ND-YAG Laser Therapy*

Complication	Incidence (Pooled Data)	Percent in Series Reported
Mortality	5/119	0–5
Myocardial Infarct	3/119	2–4.5
Pneumonia	2/119	0–2
Cardiovascular accident	1/119	0–1
Tracheo-esophageal (T-E) Fistula	1/119	0–1
Hemorrhage	2/119	0–2
Hypotension	6/119	2–18
Hypertension	8/119	0–35
Dysrhythmia	14/119	2–55
Ventilator dependence	1/119	0–2

* Data from references 20, 23, and 24 listed in References.

Postbronchoscopy Management

Although bronchoscopy does not leave a surgical scar, recovery may be complicated by secondary insults. Table 17-6 lists some of the complications associated with bronchoscopy and summarizes their presentation and management.

Patients who have had rigid bronchoscopy for diagnostic reasons may demonstrate clinical deterioration following the procedure. For example, the obstructing lesion continues to cause the same blockage but distal atalectasis, hypoxemia, and patient symptoms, especially dyspnea and cough, are worse. Upper and lower airway trauma, a new insult caused by the endoscope, may cause progressive stridor, lower airway obstruction due to bleeding or edema, pneumothorax, pneumomediastinum, bronchospasm, pain, or increased irritation and cough. Cool-mist oxygen supplement, symptomatic therapy, and postbronchoscopy monitoring should be provided for a variable period, depending on the duration of the procedure and magnitude of the insult. Patients who do not demonstrate upper airway edema in the first hour after surgery rarely require further watching. An upright chest film and follow-up examination should rule out pneumothorax. Cough, unless necessary for secretion management, responds well to narcotic antitussive therapy. Hoarseness may persist; if symptomatic therapy lasting hours to two days does not resolve the problem, follow-up indirect laryngoscopy or ENT consultation is appropriate. Bronchospasm may require acute broncholytic therapy interventions, but rarely necessitates a significant, long-term change in drug support.

The chest film sometimes only shows regional lung volume imbalance as a clue that postoperative atalectasis is evolving. Unexpected volume loss in one area or bibasilarly is an indication for follow-up films and chest physiotherapy. A new or fleeting infiltrate associated with fever may be the only evidence of pulmonary aspiration. As in other settings, pulmonary aspiration can be a syndrome that ranges from a limited pneumonic process to cardiovascular collapse and severe, noncardiogenic pulmonary edema. Depending on the severity of the presentation, expectant monitoring, supplemental oxygen therapy, and chest physiotherapy may be all that is required. Observation is important when aspiration is suspected because cardiorespiratory intensive care may be indicated within minutes to hours.

Airway Tears

A rare, but potentially catastrophic, complication is pharyngeal or esophageal perforation. Clinical findings may include dysphagia, signs of sepsis, a mediastinal crunch, delayed empyema, crepitus in the neck or suprasternal and suprascapular areas, or mediastinal and pharyngeal abscess. Empyema and abscess occur days to weeks postendoscopy, not uncommonly both patient and physician are confused by the symptoms, and definitive therapy is delayed.

Therapeutic bronchoscopy usually involves additional maneuvers that prolong the

Table 17-6. Bronchoscopy Complications: Clinical Presentation and Management

Complication	Clinical Presentation	Management
Laryngeal edema	Hoarseness, sore throat, stridor, obstruction	Cool mist, elevation, racemic epinephrine, then reintubation
Atelectasis	Hypoxemia, x-ray	Chest PT, intubate, CPAP and IPPB
Bronchospasm	Dyspnea, wheezing, long exhalation, cough, hypercapnea, hypoxemia	Humidify, oxygenate, bronchodilator therapy, chest PT, rule out pneumothorax and coronary heart failure, support ventilation
Bronchitis, pneumonia	Persistent cough, fever, infiltrate	Culture, antibiotic treatment, nosocomial epidemiology
Laryngeal erosion/polyp	Persistent symptoms, follow-up ENT exam	Above + voice rest, ENT consult, polypectomy or cord injection
Cartilage injury	Above + voice, swallowing dysfunction	Follow-up exams, surgical manipulation, injection
Aspiration	Benign leading to ARDS and shock	Expectant monitoring leading to maximal cardiorespiratory support
Pneumothorax	Pain, cough, dyspnea	Observe or chest tube
Perforation (pharynx, larynx, trachea)	Late infection/abscess, mediastinal crunch, air/widening on x-ray	Early recognition, antibiotics and drainage, secure airway
Sepsis, bacteremia	Fever leading to acute episode in OR or early recovery	Cardiorespiratory support, antibiotic therapy, C&S
Airway bleeding	Direct vision, blood return in tube, hemoptysis, hypoxemia, x-ray infiltrate	Observe and suction, intubate, tamponade with EBT or OTT, surgical cautery or open thoracotomy

procedure and undoubtedly add to the list of possible complications. The physical trauma associated with repeated suction and lavage is more likely to promote small airway injury with submucosal or frank hemmorhage, edema, and obstruction. Sometimes, in spite of the fact that significant large airway obstruction has been removed by therapeutic maneuvers, time may be required for reexpansion of atalectatic lung segments. One may even see worsening atalectasis after either rigid or flexible bronchoscopy for removal of secretion plugging. Clinical deterioration can be significant. Positive pressure ventilation or effective chest physiotherapy reverses the process. The prudent clinician keeps unstable patients intubated and awaits physical or x-ray confirmation that atalectasis is improved before proceeding with extubation.

Airway Bleeding

Airway bleeding following biopsy or trauma to an abnormally vascular structure is not uncommon. Most airway bleeding stops within a few hours of biopsy. Significant hypoxemia or progressive infiltrate with hemoptysis is a strong indication for continued monitoring or a follow-up fiberoptic procedure. Whether bleeding ensues from fiberoptic or rigid endoscopy, the patient should be intubated. Constant return of blood into the breathing system of the ventilator suggests that the magnitude of bleeding is significant enough to drain into lower airways and cause serious ventilation-perfusion abnormalities. When continued observation demonstrates bleeding that drains into dependent airways, pulmonary decompensation follows unless the patient is placed with the bleeding site in a dependent position and intermittant suction or lavage continued until the bleeding stops. This works well if ventilation can be maintained while suction is located near the bleeding site. I have seen a 6mm fiberoptic instrument with a large >2mm suction channel kept in place for control of bleeding for several hours in an awake, coagulopathic adult who was maintained in the lateral position for several hours until bleeding stopped.

Very rarely, the bleeding may be so significant that a double-lumen endobronchial tube is required to tamponade the affected lung while a decision about open thoracotomy is considered. A simple, but less ideal, alternative is to place a single-lumen tube into the dry side with its cuff inflated against the bleeding bronchus to protect and ventilate normal lung. If tamponade is effective, the bleeding side should be placed uppermost, so that V/Q matching is best and blood drains proximally through the nonventilated lumen of an endobronchial tube or into the mouth around a single-lumen endobronchial tube. In this situation, repeat bronchoscopy may be very difficult because bleeding obscures the field.

Patients with preexistent coagulopathy are at high risk for traumatic airway bleeding. If coagulopathy has not been corrected before endoscopy, it should be treated immediately after recognition of bleeding. For example, it may be reasonable to manage the chronically thrombocytopenic individual who has no bleeding history without prebronchoscopy transfusion. Platelets should be available for early transfusion in case of difficulty, however.

Flexible Fiberoptic Bronchoscopy

History

A number of clinicians had the idea of applying flexible instruments for evaluation of the upper and lower airway at approximately the same time. Shortly after the first reported use of a flexible endoscope for difficult tracheal intubation by Murphy in 1967, Ikeda and colleagues introduced a specific flexible fiberoptic bronchoscope into thoracic surgery.[23,24] The instrument was promoted among surgeons as a means of getting a better view of distal airway divisions. Indeed, endoscopists reported routine visualization down to the fifth generation.[25] Within four years the instrument was widely embraced by pulmonologists and internists as a nonoperative medical means of evaluating the airway and performing specific therapeutic maneuvers.[26] Preferential choice of flexible instruments for both diagnostic and therapeutic uses spread to critical care physicians,[27] anesthesiologists,[28] otolaryngologists,[29] and pediatricians.[30] Various types of local, general, and regional anesthetics were widely used.

Within the decade, awake, transnasal bronchoscopy became the outpatient technique of choice for evaluating patients with chronic cough, persistant atalectasis, and hemoptysis long before such patients were referred to thoracic surgeons.[31–33] Indeed, many clinicians were using the FFB instead of the rigid instrument for first attempt at FB removal from the bronchi and trachea.[34] Use of the FFB for diagnosis and therapy in place of the rigid instrument was widespread in Japan by 1979.[35] This trend has continued throughout the world. Clinicians agree that use of the flexible instrument under sedation and topical anesthesia is associated with less direct trauma, discomfort, and risk than rigid bronchoscopy under general anesthesia.[36]

New problems were raised for the anesthesiologist by fiberoptic equipment. The major problem with a rigid system was management of effective spontaneous or controlled ventilation through an open bronchoscope system. Historically, the fiberoptic instrument was first inserted through the open tube as had various open bronchoscopes and rigid telescopes in times past. When larger instruments were passed through endotracheal tubes, a critical issue was available airway area. Relative obstruction during both inspiration and exhalation became important—especially during long procedures. Cardiorespiratory problems associated with bronchoscopy were well described in several series in the literature of each specialty.

Indications

The FFB has evolved in form and design so that it is now almost as versatile as the rigid instrument. Indications (summarized in Table 17-7) for FFB are largely the same as for the rigid instrument, excluding therapeutic manipulations that require the large internal diameter of a rigid instrument like stenting open the compressed upper or lower airway, removal of large foreign bodies, management of massive hemoptysis, or extraction of large clots or plugs in the airways. The FFB was used to treat carcinoma obstructing the trachea shortly following reports of the use of laser resection of obstructing gastric cancer with flexible fiberoptic gastroscopes.[37] Smaller diameter instruments (<4 mm) are now widely used by anesthesiologists for tracheal or endobronchial intubation.[38] It is increasingly common to see the thin and ultrathin instruments replacing the small rigid instrument as the first choice for evaluation of airway problems in newborns and small infants.[38, 39] The flexible instrument has been used as an emergency airway for HFJV through the suction channel. Indeed, situations in which rigid endoscopy is superior to flexible bronchoscopy are so few that surgical and anesthesia training programs have difficulty obtaining enough open tube procedures for teaching the technique. It is likely that this trend towards flexible fiberoptic instrumentation will continue since both risks associated with FFB and costs of using the FFB are lower in a number of settings.

Table 17-7. Indications for Flexible versus Rigid Bronchoscopy

Diagnostic or Therapeutic Indication	*R**	*F**	*B**
Cough		+	
Hemotysis			+
Persistent wheezing		+	
Refractory atelectasis		+	
Unresolved pneumonia		+	
Transbronchial biopsy		+	
Preop tumor workup		+	
Follow-up abnormal chest film		+	
Acute aspiration			+
Acute inhalation injury		+	
Foreign body			+
Laryngeal evaluation (Recurrent nerve)		+	
Reassess postoperative site		+	
Diaphragm paralysis		+	
Tracheoesophageal fistula		+	
Tracheal assessment on ventilator		+	
Selective bronchography			
Closure bronchopleural fistula†			+
Resection tracheal lesions			+
Difficult intubation			+
Extrinsic tracheobronchial obstruction	+		
Placement endobronchial tubes/ blockers		+	

* R-rigid instrument; F-flexible fiberoptic instrument; B-both.
† See reference 40 in reference list.

Equipment

Many anesthesiologists now perform fiberoptic bronchoscopy either alone or together with the thoracic surgeon during and after surgery whether for endobronchial intubation, safe one-lung anesthesia, and therapeutic lavage, or for prevention of post-operative complications. It is important for the thoracic anesthesiologist to have a working knowledge of the instrument.[40–43] All flexible fiberoptic instruments have certain features in common, although the outer diameter, flexion controls, suction or injection ports, light sources, and add-on lens-camara systems vary considerably. The light bundles, flexion controls, and accessory channels must all pass through one flexible, waterproof, tube that is both flexible and relatively sturdy. The proximal end of the instrument must allow room for all of these channels. Light-source bundles and accessory channels can enter from the side, but the eye or camera must have a central lens mounting system, the objective lens, that is directly accessible. All the systems are tied in from the operator's "optical head" and taken off so that the tube can be freely rotated along its main axis. Axial rotation is essential so that all planes will become available to the viewer. The optical or "control" head is, thus, usually held in one hand by the operator while he or she manipulates the shaft of the tube directly. All the bundles and channels are tied in a main shaft as they pass down to the distal tip, which is inserted into the airway. This combined conduit or shaft is commonly called the "insertion tube" and the distal end, the "working tip." Light is transmitted from a remote source through one or more dedicated bundles along the insertion tube to the working tip, where it is reflected off from the remote surface. An optical bundle in the working tip picks up this illuminated image and passes it along the insertion tube to the optical head. The operator's eye or video then picks up the image. The tip is angled by two cables carried in opposite conduits but restrained by joints in the wall of the working tip. Manipulating a lever at the control head flexes the tip to a variable extent as the cable is pulled. The working tip is directed towards the direction of pull on the control lever. The operator directs the FFB by flexing the tip while rotating the shaft of the instrument from the control head with one hand and either advancing or withdrawing the insertion cord and tip with the other.

Image Quality versus Other Features

The power of an adjustable objective lens at the optical head and the lens at the working tip of fiberoptic instruments are important in determining the size and field of view of the image. Nevertheless, image quality is more a function of the diameter of the instrument. A stronger light source can drive more light to the distant surface, but the number and size of the optical fiber array in each bundle determine the amount of light that ultimately reaches the surface and the intensity and discrimination that is transmitted back to the observer and the control head. This poses a design limitation for any system. Field depth and image resolution are limited by the overlap, diameter, and geometric array of tiny fiberoptic strands packed into each bundle. Large fibers with no "overlap" transmit a grainy image with many black spots between image points. More advanced construction and design place many more small optical pixels in the field and provide enough overlap redundancy that the image can be brighter and have better resolution.

The clinical requirement for a large suction channel and cable conduits that allow the tip to flex according to the operator's needs must be weighed against image quality. Very large instruments such as gastroscopes and colonoscopes can have several accessory channels for simultaneous air insufflation and biopsy forceps manipulation and as many as four angulation cables for tip deflection in two planes simultaneously. Standard bronchoscope design, in contrast, sacrifices two tip deflection controls for optical quality and a suction-biopsy channel.

The ultrathins, the smallest instruments now in use, sacrifice either flexion controls or the suction channel to optic quality to achieve the 1.5–3-mm external diameter range needed for infants. A flexible 1.2-mm light wand in the ultrathin range can be used via 2.5–3.0 mm endotracheal tubes in premature infants who are being ventilated. This instrument can decrease the need for chest x-rays and rigid bronchoscopy in this high-risk population. Clearly diagnosis is all that can be supported by such small endoscopes, and any prolonged therapeutic maneuver in premature infants requires an open tube instrument that, itself, doubles as an airway.

Working with Flexible Endoscopes

Flexible fibers will bend and fiberoptic bundles can twist slightly but cannot be acutely stretched, bitten, or kinked without snapping and failing as light conduits. Broken fibers fail to conduct light and appear as a pattern of black dots on the projected image. Fracture of the covering surrounding a fiber bundle allows external fluid to be drawn along the fibers by capillary action. When fluids reach the interface between fibers and the lens system optical discrimination is ruined and images appear distorted and blurred. Repair of either problem requires dissassembly of the delicate bundle system, which is a time-consuming, costly process. Consequently, a bite block should always be used for oral bronchoscopy when patients are not paralyzed. Frequent inspection of the system and "leak testing" of the outer case identifies problems before the cost of repair approaches the cost of a new instrument.

Operating Principles

Several operating principles follow from instrument design. First, the instrument flexes. As a consequence, the operator must control insertion and withdrawal from a position that is as close as possible to the working tip. The instrument will flex and kink rather than advance when attempts are made to insert it from a remote location such as the control head. Because of limited space within the insertion cord of the instrument, there is room only for two flexion cables that operate to bend the tip in opposite directions in only one plane. Thus the operator must rotate the instrument in order to flex it in more than one plane. Rotation is achieved with the control head. Usually the operator uses the dominant hand on the control head and advances or withdraws the insertion shaft with the nondominant hand. A series of flexion, rotation maneuvers is required to advance the instrument around corners and navigate the airway. All rotation and flexion is managed from the control head; the nondominant hand allows the shaft to rotate passively as the eye's point of reference maintains alignment along the central axis.

Because the FFB can be rotated 360° (usually up to 180° in either direction) so that the tip can be deflected in any plane and small diameter instruments often have a small angle of view with a short focal length, it is not difficult to understand why the operator can become lost in the airway. One must pursue a methodical approach, recognizing each structure from upper to lower airway on either side. There is no way to know the location of the tip of the endoscope from surface anatomy, insertion depth, or position of the control head because of the FFB's flexibility and the insertion cord's tendency to spiral. The operator must coordinate hands and eye (or video picture) so that the instrument is advanced to the appropriate location. No amount of operator movement or "body English" makes up for the need to rotate, flex, advance, or withdraw the tip. The instrument follows a desired course after an appropriate sequence of trial and error manipulations. Although some maneuvers are typically "cook book," both normal and pathologic anatomy may vary dramatically among individuals.

Video Bronchoscopy

As video technology applied to diagnostic medicine has exploded in recent years, this technique has been applied to bronchoscopy. Video bronchoscopy has been driven by interest in improved documentation to prevent repeat diagnostic procedures, improve interphysician communication, promote operator convenience, to clarify medicolegal concerns, to increase teaching potential, and to facilitate universal blood and body secretion precautions. Image size can be increased, if resolution and available light allow, and both video and photographic records of the findings can be made. Image resolution with several systems is now excellent. The operator can document anatomic findings, physiologic events over time, response to therapy or diagnostic biopsy, and the safety of the procedure in still or video format. Some patients find the video demonstration of their pathology educational and physicians often use the photographic record for teaching their patients as well as to demonstrate pathology to fellow clinicians. Considerable time can be saved when multiple operators wish to appreciate the anatomy simultaneously. In particular, the anesthesiologist can study the investigations of the surgeon and vice versa. A recent argument used for medical camera systems is that the more remote the operator's eye, the less likely he or she is to have bodily secretions deposited on the face or in the eyes.

Anesthesiologists should be conversant with the increasing types of video attachments that are used in the operating room for laparoscopic, arthroscopic, bronchoscopic, and thoracoscopic procedures. Most attachments are part of integrated systems purchased from the endoscope manufacturer that provide an on-line, large-screen monitor display of the field as well as a simultaneous videocassette recording. High-intensity light sources are essential for effective image amplification. Basic elements include a video camera, endoscope adaptor, camera control box, videocassette recorder, video monitor, and light source with appropriate cables. Since four of these require wall current, a four- or five-outlet, fused recepticle that meets operating room safety specifications is needed. Many manufacturers market carts that combine mounting brackets with switched electrical outlets for their equipment. Such systems range from $15,000 for bare essentials to $50,000 with a complete monitor cart and photography set up. It is important to test the endoscope with the chosen system before attempting a procedure. An inappropriate set up can complicate and delay the procedure regardless of the success of the anesthetic technique or the skill of the anesthesiologist and surgeon. Color balance, image resolution, power, and field attitude adjustment of the camera must be completed before the FFB is inserted into an airway. The wrong conclusions can be drawn from the same anatomic findings if the color adjustment is off. When in doubt about the accuracy of the image, the camera should be disconnected and the operator should immediately obtain a view that's not electronically distorted.

The essential part of a video system that is unique to each manufacturer is the endoscope camera adaptor. The problem of video adaptor incompatability is most likely to involve the anesthesiologist who works with a surgeon who uses several bronchoscopes for specific purposes. Just as with ventilating adaptors, it is important to test each system to be used in advance.

The camera control head adaptor may incorporate a special photography or amplification lens system and electrical contacts that trigger high intensity light source flashes for still photographs. All capabilities are not needed for every endoscopy, especially if a video record of the findings is made. Given appropriate connectors, one endoscope system may adapt to another manufacturer's video setup that is already present in the operating room. This is the case with the Olympus intubating bronchoscope, which has a flat surfaced optical control head that "mates" with video equipment distributed by several manufacturers of cystoscopes, laparascopes, and arthroscopes. The video equipment marketed by the primary manufacturer produces an image that is several times smaller than that produced through some other equipment.

Management Problems in Bronchoscopy

The relative size of the endoscope versus the tracheal airway determined the residual airway when fiberoptic bronchoscopy was first performed via the open tube bronchoscope and later through an endotracheal tube under general anesthesia. Resistance to air flow is a function of the available or residual cross-sectional airway around the endoscope, the length of the obstruction, the turbulance of airflow, and the gas viscosity.[27] Gas viscosity can be manipulated to good effect both in and out of the operating room by substituting helium for nitrous oxide or air in oxygen.[36] Most anesthesia machines are not equipped with helium tank fittings for two reasons: (1) helium is costly and (2) helium is not in widespread use despite many years of advocacy by some anesthesiologists. Consequently helium tanks and a blender must be used when helium is used. Turbulent flow is determined by complex variables that relate to the shape and diameter of the system connectors, velocity of flow, and angulation of flow pathways. Most significant is the cross-sectional area available for gas flow.

Safe Endotracheal Tube Size

One of the best diagrams that illustrates the effect of outer diameter of bronchoscope on effective airway through standard-sized endotracheal tubes was published by Lindholm et al.[27] If a large, 6-mm bronchoscope is passed through an 8.0-mm ID tracheal tube, the equivalent airway is that of a 5-mm tube. A 5-mm bronchoscope leaves approximately the same airway when passed through the typical 7.0-mm tracheal tube used for small women and teenagers. Many centers use a 5.7-mm endoscope which can be used with 7.5-mm and 8-mm endotracheal tubes.

Airway obstruction increases the resistance to lung inflation. It can be overcome by increased inspiratory pressure in most cases. Peak pressure increases during bronchoscopy can be minimized with a ventilatory pattern that allows increased time for flow equilibration and gas distribution. Also, a helium oxygen mixture reduces gas viscosity and improves inspiratory flow to obstructed areas. Obstruction to inspiration is both a general phenomenon of the airway through which the bronchoscope has been passed and a localized problem in the distal airway into which the tip of the bronchoscope has been introduced. Obstruction of smaller, distal lung units will occur during bronchoscopic examination and treatment of bronchopulmonary segments no matter how large the airway through which the endoscope is passed. Therefore, the anesthetist should attempt to manipulate ventilatory flow patterns and times as well as choose the largest tracheal tube possible.

Increased pressure is required to inflate the lungs when the airway is partially obstructed by a bronchoscope, but exhalation depends on passive chest wall and lung recoil. Air trapping or "auto-PEEP" is generated during bronchoscopy. Lindholm and colleagues predict a 20–30-cm positive end-expiratory pressure

(PEEP) equivalent when a 5.7-mm endoscope is passed through 7.5-8-mm endotracheal tubes. Approximate "auto-PEEP" can be measured through the suction lumen of the endoscope. Arterial blood gasses can either show improvement during this period or deterioration, depending upon the cardiorespiratory effects of air trapping and of inspiratory obstruction. A ventilatory pattern that allows adequate time for exhalation will minimize the "auto-PEEP" effect. Similar effects are predicted if the newer 3.5-3.7mm endoscopes are used through 5mm ID endotracheal tubes in children.

As a rule of thumb, one should control ventilation and use an endotracheal tube with an internal diamenter at least two sizes larger than the endoscope. As the radius of the effective airway increases in proportion to the square of the relative diameters, it is obvious that a difference between the inner diameter of the tracheal tube and the outer diameter of the FFB of three millimeters allows more than twice the effective airway than a clearance of two millimeters. The typical tracheal tube (5-mm ID) used for a 2 year old allows less effective ventilation around a 4-mm intubation bronchoscope than the adult can gain around a 6-mm endoscope through a 7-mm ID tracheal tube. Consequently, the airway differential is more critical during pediatric bronchoscopy.

Effective spontaneous ventilation cannot be maintained with only 1–2-mm clearance around the endoscope. With controlled ventilation both inhalation and exhalation are much easier for the clinician with the newly popularized, large suction channel, adult 5-mm bronchoscopes passed via 7 and 8-mm endotracheal tubes. The 4-mm "intubating" bronchoscopes manufactured by Olympus, Pentax, and others provide a margin of ventilatory safety that will permit spontaneous breathing through an endotracheal tube in the adult size range (7–8-mm ID). Cooperative patients do well if they are able to breathe slowly and deeply, since the resistance is also related to flow. Patients who are not undergoing general anesthesia are much more comfortable when they breathe through their own airway around a bronchoscope than through an endotracheal tube, because the average adult trachea is most narrow at the level of the cords but opens to at least 12–15mm internal diameter in the trachea. The natural airway has a shorter segment of narrowing than a tracheal tube and provides less resistance around a 5–6 mm bronchoscope. Anesthetized patients should always have ventilation assisted or controlled with long expiratory times to avoid air trapping. As with the progressive development of smaller "adult" instruments in the 4–5mm range, newer ultrathin instruments offer an advantage for management of infants and small children.

Tube Size and Laser Endoscopy

Fiberoptic bronchoscopy through a rigid endoscope impairs ventilation more at any equivalent internal diameter than through an endotracheal tube, because the tracheal tube can be cut short and has a cuff. A shortened 8-mm ID tracheal tube (typically cut to 25 cm) offers less resistance than a standard 8-mm × 40 cm adult bronchoscope. An imperfect seal around the open instrument tends to decrease air trapping in exhalation; however, this is made up for by inadequate inflation during inspiration. HFJV provides a logical alternative when the endoscopist insists upon using a rigid instrument as the guide for flexible laser bronchoscopy. The anesthesiologist must beware of barotrauma associated with air trapping due to the narrowed exhalation pathway.

Awake Transnasal Bronchoscopy

Transnasal endoscopy has several advantages over peroral endoscopy, including less distortion of the upper airway, a more direct route to the larynx from the posterior nasopharynx, and no risk that the bronchoscope will be bitten by an agitated or insufficiently topicalized patient. The disadvantages are that the nasopharynx is smaller and provides new opportunities for bleeding, trauma, and infection. Today the vast majority of fiberoptic bronchoscopies are performed via the transnasal route on awake, sedated patients with topical anesthesia.

Once the endoscopist has negotiated the turn from the nasopharynx to pharynx, the epiglottis and larynx are immediately in view with very little instrument angulation. Occasionally the tongue needs to be protruded or the jaw lifted in obtunded patients who are supine. Even though larger diameter instruments provide a wider and deeper field of vision, they are not as well tolerated as smaller instruments. Topical anesthesia of the nasopharynx requires prolonged contact time with relatively high concentrations of local anesthetic. The time giving sedatives and narcotics for conscious sedation in increments intravenously is well spent, as topical anesthesia is achieved. Topical vasoconstriction is also helpful. Cocaine, a logical choice for its combined vasoconstricting and local anesthetic properties, can be applied rather simply with long cotton swabs that are left in mucosal contact for 5 or 10 minutes. Because of the low therapeutic index and high abuse potential of cocaine, many clinicians now use a mixture of 1–2% lidocaine and 0.125% phenylephrine. Alternatively, a topical vasoconstrictor such as oxymetazoline hydrochloride (Afrin), 0.25-5%, can be used. Administration of the vasoconstrictor is followed by a topical metered spray or aerosol inhalation of lidocaine solution, application of soaked pledgets, or viscous lidocaine injection.

Since the naris takes an upward course, the would-be endoscopist tends to push swabs or pledgets upward into the narrowist part of the nasal cavity. As with insertion of nasal airways and nasogastric tubes, this is incorrect and uncomfortable. Blind topical anesthesia should begin in the anterior naris and gradually advance in a caudal direction contacting the inferior turbinate and nasal septum along the floor of the nasopharynx. When a straight pledget advances no further, it should be left in place for contact at the site where the bronchoscope or endotracheal tube will most likely lodge as it begins to turn more caudal along the posterior pharynx behind the palate. Additional local anesthetic/vasoconstrictor solution can be dripped along the stick pledgets into the posterior nasopharynx and pharynx if the patient is supine or in the sitting position with the neck extended. The posterolateral nasopharynx, where irregular patches of adenoid tissue are found, presents the typical site for submucous dissection. For this reason, the wary endoscopist should perform nasopharyngoscopy, following the open air column into the pharynx, before attempting to pass tracheal tubes or soft "dilating" airways through the nasopharynx. Secretions are easily managed by lavage and suction with soft catheters or by having the patient swallow. Blood clots are difficult to aspirate and tend to adhere to the tip of the endoscope. For this reason and because the pharynx is better opened when upright, a sitting or semifowler's position is preferred.

Fiberoptic Endoscopy Under General Anesthesia

The majority of thoracic patients having fiberoptic bronchoscopy under general anesthesia are either having a "screening" bronchoscopy as part of another thoracic procedure (eg, mediastinoscopy, staging mediastinotomy, or thoracotomy) or bronchoscopy for perianesthetic indications (eg, endobronchial tube placement or secretion management) (Table

17-8). Intraoperative concerns are the same as those listed under rigid bronchoscopy; hypoxemia, inadequate ventilation (hypercapnea), dysrhythmias, bronchospasm, reflex changes in V/Q matching, direct trauma, positioning trauma, and barotrauma (pneumothorax) may occur.

The anesthetic plan must allow close ventilatory monitoring, cardiovascular reflex control, and effective ventilation. Any patient with significant tracheal or vascular compression should have preoperative bronchoscopy performed when awake and in a position that minimizes airway compression and vascular compromise. A dynamic assessment of airway function with position change and respiratory maneuvers can be made at bronchoscopy. If there is significant compromise, safe tracheal or bronchial intubation can be performed over the endoscope. Awake intubation also allows the patient with superior vena cava syndrome to maintain maximal venous return in the sitting position and minimize airway edema during or after the procedure.

As noted earlier, the smallest diameter endoscope that can be used should be passed via the endotracheal tube with the largest acceptable internal diameter. The tracheal tube should be cut short so that it presents less resistance to ventilation. The anesthetist should be certain that the tube tip is well above the carina to allow the endoscopist an unobstructed view. An appropriately sized swivel adaptor with a sealing bronchoscopy port is required to allow ventilation around the endoscope during bronchoscopy. These adaptors are available from several manufacturers (Portex, Bodai, etc.), but the endoscope fit must be sufficiently exact to allow positive-pressure ventilation without a large leak around the instrument. The perforated tip of a surgical glove, a saline-soaked gauze sponge, or petroleum-impregnated gauze have been used to seal the adaptor effectively if one of the ready-made variety is unavailable.

Table 17-8. Perianesthetic Indications for Flexible Bronchoscopy

Indication	Most Important	Useful
Assessment of obstruction	+	
Document laryngeal function		+
Endobronchial intubation	+	
Intraoperative suction		+
Evaluate surgical site		+
Rule out aspiration		+
Evaluate postop atelectasis		+
Document intubation injury	+	

General anesthesia is commonly maintained with a potent volatile agent by inhalation of 100% oxygen. Choice of muscle relaxant is determined by the duration of the procedure and need for other surgical procedures during the same anesthetic period. Anesthesia for the first endoscopies was managed with an ultrashort-acting barbiturate and succinylcholine by continuous infusion. Succinylcholine remains an excellent choice for shorter bronchoscopies today, provided the dose and duration are limited, because it is provides such close, reversible control over respiratory muscle activity.

Patients who do not tolerate the cardiovascular depression of inhalation anesthesia at levels sufficient for ablation of potentially deleterious sympathetic reflexes may be managed with a "balanced" technique using small doses of narcotic, a potent tranquilizer or hypnotic that promotes amnesia, and a combination of topical and intravenous lidocaine. An evanescently metabolized beta blocker, esmalol, has recently become available. This drug, which can be titrated by intravenous drip infusion, used in combination with either nitroglycerine or nitroprusside provides an effective way to manage patients with hypertension or a significant risk of coronary ischemia. Invasive hemodynamic monitoring is rarely indicated.

Although oximetry provides certain knowledge of oxygenation and allows us to titrate oxygen administration to arterial content, we prefer to use a high inspired oxygen tension that permits longer periods of interrupted or abnormally distributed ventilation and suction before hypoxemia becomes a problem. Ventilation is normally controlled by hand during endoscopy. Such close hand control allows the best "feel" for airway resistance, compliance, and adequacy of exhalation. The newer generation of anesthesia machines that allows continuous monitoring of airway pressures, exhaled carbon dioxide and agent concentrations, and exhalation flow patterns can be most useful during endoscopy. A graphic display provides on-line feedback for the anesthesiologist and can allow coordination of the procedure with the endoscopist and better fulfillment of the patient's ventilatory needs.

Jet Ventilation for Fiberoptic Bronchoscopy

Some centers use HFJV via the suction-access port of the bronchoscope. Jet ventilation or HFJV can be used in an open system or a monitored circle system that can provide a high oxygen tension for entrained gas together with intermittant tidal carbon dioxide analysis.[45] Jet ventilation works best with 5- and 6-mm bronchoscopes because the tip of thinner endoscopes or flexible jet injection catheters tends to whip around during jet ventilation like the end of a high-pressure fire hose. Endotracheal tubes designed for jet ventilation (Mallinckrodt, Hi-Lo Jet) allow the endoscopist to monitor distal tracheal pressures during bronchoscopy and to jet outside the instrument. This avoids jet catheter whip and allows the suction-access port of the bronchoscope to be used for its intended purpose. In addition, the use of such tubes is more likely to prevent barotrauma from local application of high jet pressures as the endoscope is directed into a smaller, distal airway. Alternatively, the Carden tube, a short segment of endotracheal tube, can be placed below the cords so that only the tip of a small-diameter jet catheter and the tube to the pilot baloon pass translaryngeally. The Carden tube can be used for both laryngoscopy and fiberoptic bronchoscopy. The tube segment secures the tip of the jet catheter so that the catheter and the vocal apparatus do not move during jet ventilation from the proximal trachea.

Tracheal Suction

A significant problem during bronchoscopy is excessive tracheal suction. As noted earlier, airway obstruction caused by the endoscope passing through a tracheal tube may be significant and contribute to inadequate tidal volumes or residual "auto-PEEP." Larger bronchoscopes (eg, newer "therapeutic" models with suction channels larger than 2-mm) can suction at dramatic rates.[46] The unwary endoscopist not infrequently leaves a finger over the two-way suction bypass adaptor, providing constant suction throughout the procedure. The anesthesiologist should note failed return of exhaust gas in the ventilatory system or markedly diminished carbon dioxide flows in exhalation during suction before inadequate lung volumes cause hypoxemia as noted by pulse oximetry. Arterial desaturation during endoscopy is an indication for the endoscopist to withdraw the endoscope to a proximal position and discontine suction while effective ventilation is assured and the problem resolves. Since pneumothorax during bronchoscopy with any ventilation mode is always a risk on account of residual distal pressures generated during exhalation (auto-PEEP), the anesthetist must monitor symmetry of breath sounds and chest expansion when desaturation is noted.

Postoperative Care

Management of patients following FFB is similar to that following rigid endoscopy, except that the risk of direct airway or neck trauma is reduced. The problems are summarized in Table 17-6. If the patient has not had general anesthesia, only an hour or so will be required to ensure that laryngeal edema, airway bleeding or pneumothorax are not significant problems. After general anesthesia for outpatient procedures, the monitoring period should last one to four hours. Monitoring after general, regional, or topical anesthesia in the hospitalized patient may last longer on account of underlying illness. Patients who have had topical analgesia or upper airway blocks should, of course, be kept NPO until all topical or regional anesthesia to the upper airway has resolved. Late problems should be identified and managed during appropriate follow-up visits.

Complications of Airway Endoscopy

Prolonged laser bronchoscopic resection is the most traumatic endoscopic procedure. Studies show a low mortality despite a high incidence of morbidity (see Table 17-5) with oxygen desaturation, bronchospasm, and circulatory disturbance.[47–49] In particular, cardiorespiratory disturbances associated with laser bronchoscopy must be significant, because the incidence of supraventricular and ventricular dysrhythmia is so high. Published reports do not clarify the cause of dysrrhythmias, but it is likely that ventilatory disturbance plays the major role. The mortality and major morbidity rates are 5-10 times greater than data reported in series of fiberoptic and rigid bronchoscopy. In contrast with laser bronchoscopic tumor resection, a small series of rigid endoscopies under intravenous general anesthesia reported no deaths and the most common complication was myalgia following succinylcholine administration. Other problems included hypercapnea following the procedure and laryngospasm after removal of the rigid bronchoscope.[50] Mortality related to fiberoptic bronchoscopy in prospective and retrospective series totaling 74,306 procedures from 1974–1981 was approximately 0.02%, while a postal survey of pulmonologists in Great Britain reported a mortality of 0.04% from 40,000 endoscopies in 1982.[51] Major morbidity of fiberoptic procedures reported in the series noted above ranged from 0.3% to 1.7%. Overall, the major and minor complication rates in both fiberoptic and rigid endoscopy are surprisingly low in view of the common comorbidity presented by pulmonary patients, most of whom are older and have other medical problems.

Increased risk should be expected from complex patients with partially obstructing airway tumors who undergo prolonged procedures under general anesthesia during which ventilation is disrupted, hypoxemia is common, and exposure to smoke and tumor debris is ongoing. Considering that death due to airway obstruction is the alternative to laser resection of tumors and masses, significant risks are justified. In light of the potential benefit, most preoperative problems that increase anesthetic risk and cannot be improved before endoscopic resection are only relative contraindications.

Thoracoscopy

History

Jacobaueus described thoracoscopy as a means of evaluating the pleura and for lysis of pleural adhesions during the therapy of tuberculosis early in this century in the German and, later, English literature.[52] Although diagnostic thoracoscopy[53] and a few special therapeutic applications of the thorascope[54] were well described in the United States by the 1970s, thoracoscopy was performed in only a few medical centers. This procedure was most commonly performed under local or regional anesthesia with intravenous sedation, as noted by Curling in the early 1980s.[55] Applications were largely diagnostic, and included low-risk staging of patients for resectability of lung tumors.[56,57] Some clinicians pioneered operative thoracoscopy as less risky and invasive than open procedures for high risk-patients.[58] Thoracoscopy did not become popular in thoracic surgery until recent interest in less invasive procedures grew with the revival of laparoscopic surgery.[59] Along with laparoscopic surgery has come new technology and increased use of the high-resolution, large-screen video display of the procedure. The result is a rapid development of newer approaches to surgical diseases of the chest,[60] together with the formation of new societies and journals devoted to surgical endoscopy (eg, the journals, *Surgical Laparoscopy and Endoscopy* and *The Japanese Society for Surgical Laparoscopy and Endoscopy*) and increased scientific reporting of applications for the procedure. Thoracic surgeons throughout the United States are retraining in thoracoscopy through a series of refresher courses and workshops. It is anticipated that thoracoscopy will be increasingly utilized in the 1990s—with the result that anesthesia techniques will be refined as our experience increases.

Applications

As a diagnostic instrument, the thoracoscope provides the best "closed" examination possible of the parietal and visceral pleurae, peripheral parenchymal disease, pleural effusions, and pleural or chest wall masses (see Table 17-9). Various systems have been used for evaluation of infections, masses, degenerative parenchymal disease (blebs and cysts), and bronchopleural fistulae. The recent revival of interest in endoscopic procedures has led innovative thoracic procedures including laser or cryocauterization of emphysematous blebs,[61,62] control of malignant and other effusions (pleurodesis),[63] lung biopsy,[64] partial and segmental lung resection, and chest wall work.[65]

Table 17-9. Applications for Thoracoscopy

Pleural examination (parietal and visceral)
Drainage of loculated effusions
Chemical, surgical, photo-pleurodesis
Biopsy (chest wall and pleurae)
Bronchopeural fistula of pneumothorax (chemical or laser ablation)
Lung biopsy ("closed")
Photocautery or resection of blebs or lung cysts
Resection of masses (pleural, pulmonary, chest wall)
Lung resection (wedge, partial, or segmental)
Laser, cryo-, or electocautery of pleural/pulmonary bleeders

Equipment

At first, thoracic endoscopists used other small-diameter equipment (eg, rigid cystoscopes and bronchoscopes) for thoracoscopy. With the advent of fiberoptic technology and high-intensity, "cold" light sources, the rigid thoracoscope evolved from an open-tube instrument into a thinner Storz telescope with better resolution. The rigid, fiberoptic thoracoscope could be passed via another instrument or allow visualization of manipulating instruments advanced through a second incision in the chest wall. Flexible fiberoptic endoscopes were later passed through an open tube trochar without an obturator or a rigid laparoscope. Flexible fiberoptic technology truly made all areas of the pleural cavity accessible to the surgical endoscopist.

Lewis et al,[65] who advocated a single incision technique in the 1970s, placed a chest tube through the same incision for postoperative drainage. Swierenga et al, have used one or more trochar incisions for thoracoscope, biopsy forceps, grasping forceps, and controlled operative pneumothorax. Krasna and others have used several incisions and laparascopic video equipment with a rigid fiberoptic laparascope. Dual video monitor displays with a high-resolution camera and powerful cold light source provide a readily accessible, wide-angle display of the field such as that obtained during laparoscopy and thoracoscopy. Like laparoscopy and unlike arthroscopy or cystoscopy, the conductive medium is air or carbon dioxide, controlled through the valved, tube laparoscope. The viewer observes the procedure as various trochars are inserted that allow use of grasping forceps and performance of surgical procedures through the 10–12 mm tube laparoscope. A new stapling device (US Surgical [Norwalk, CT]) allows placement of dual staple lines across a lung segment on either side of a cutting blade for pulmonary resection.

Photocoagulation with a ND-YAG laser through a bronchoscope or other light conduit passed through the rigid thoracoscope has been repeatedly reported since the 1970s. More recently the carbon monoxide laser has been shown to penetrate the lungs' surface less deeply. This laser, which has a wavelength of 5400 nanometers as compared to the ND-YAG at 1060 nm, provides a shorter extinction pathway and a lower probability of causing deep damage to lung parenchyma. The carbon monoxide laser may be more suitable than other medical lasers for photocautery of the peripheral blebs that frequently cause spontaneous pneumothorax.

Anesthetic Implications

Both general and regional or local anesthesia with sedation have been used for thoracoscopy. Advantages of the "awake" technique that have been cited include less cardiovascular stress and barotrauma. Reduced barotrauma, despite pleural or lung resection, is attributed to lower airway pressures and the preservation of spontaneous ventilation. Cough can be limited by appropriate use of topical pleural anesthesia and intravenous antitussive agents (narcotics). Many groups also use an antisialogogue and potent tranquilizer or hypnotic agent to limit unpleasant recall. Regional blocks commonly used for thoracoscopy include rib blocks, intrapleural block, and stellate ganglion block (to decrease the sympathetic response to pleuropulmonary manipulation). Rib and intrapleural blocks assist the thoracoscopist by providing comfort during initial insertion of the instrument and decreasing pleuritic pain associated with the pneumothorax and pleural stimuli. The total dose of anesthetic may become a problem when several chest wall entry sites are planned. The anesthesiologist should remember that intercostal and intrapleural blocks are associated with rapid intravascular uptake and high blood levels of agent. One should limit the dosing accordingly.

Diagnostic work causes little insult other than that due to the partial pneumothorax. Narcotics should be titrated carefully because their respiratory depressant properties can act synergistically with the surgical pneumothorax needed for thoracoscopy. Pulmonary function and oxygenation may improve after lysis of adhesions or drainage of loculated effusions, particularly when involved lung segments or effusions are large. In any event, noninvasive cardiorespiratory monitoring is standard, as in any other procedure where local anesthetic toxicity, oversedation, hypoventilation and hypercapnea, hypoxemia, tension pneumothorax, and hypotension are significant possibilities.

More extensive therapeutic work involves several trochar penetration sites and, as we have seen with video laparoscopic resection of abdominal organs, may take longer than conventional open surgery. This is especially the case during the "learning" period of the thoracoscopist. Under general anesthesia, it is possible to place an endobronchial tube and selectively ventilate each lung as for open chest cases. While other positions have been used for thoracoscopy, depending upon the site of the pathology, the lateral position is preferred for wider access to the lung and apical regions. Many thoracic surgeons prefer general anesthesia for these reasons. Anesthetic techiques are the same as those used for lateral thoracotomy. The procedure is "less invasive" because a large lateral incision that impairs chest wall function postoperatively is not made. Potential intraoperative problems due to redistribution of V/Q matching, traction on pleuropulmonary and mediastinal structures, impaired venous return to the heart, reduced cardiac output, dysrhythmias, hypotension, deletarious sympathetic reflexes, ineffective ventilation, airway bleeding, secretion plugging, etc. These problems are the same as the potential complications of thoracotomy. Consequently, the same level of invasive and noninvasive respiratory monitoring may be required as for thoracotomy. The magnitude of the procedure planned and the patient's underlying condition or comorbid diseases must define the anesthetic approach. One can not assume that operative challenge to the anesthesiologist is lower because thoracoscopic procedures result in less postoperative pain and cause less postoperative decrease in pulmonary capacity.

Complications

Complications reported after thoracoscopy follow a predictable pattern; they include intraoperative hypoxemia or hypercapnea, bleeding, pneumothorax, infection, and late problems related to anesthesia.[66] Like laparoscopic procedures, late problems are less dramatic than those during the procedure, probably because patients have little pain or other physiologic stress following closed procedures. Compared with open procedures, mortality and morbidity are quite low. Page reported one death from myocardial infarction and a 9% incidence of pulmonary infections after 121 procedures performed under general anesthesia (17% of his patients had subsequent thoracotomy). Neither Norre and Bellone nor Rusch and Mountain reported any morbidity in their series, which comprised a total of 66 patients who had general or regional anesthesia. At present, the majority of operative thoracoscopic procedures are reported as case reports; more time is necessary for the accumulation of a significant series of patients using modern operative technique. Although it is likely that the same decrements in lung volume, lung capacity, and chest wall compliance are not seen after thoracoscopic surgery as after limited thoracotomy, no prospective or retrospective study has proven this assertion.

Postoperative Care

Once significant pneumothorax, bronchopleural fistula, bleeding, and secretion plugging of small or intermediate airways have been ruled out, thoracoscopy patients seem less likely than thoracotomy patients to experience postoperative complications. Although a significant percentage of young, relatively fit patients experience transient atelectasis and other pulmonary complications after thoracotomy, few patients appear to have difficulty once effects of anesthesia have passed. Postoperative pain relief is necessary if a chest tube is left in place or a major visceral lesion has been created, but the pain is an order of magnitude less than that after thoracotomy. Rib blocks and intrapleural infusion or intermittant injections are good choices for pain control if the pleural cavity is drained. Otherwise, intermittant intramuscular injections or low-dose patient-controlled analgesia ordinarily suffice.

Several of the authors cited above have reported that patients who are not acceptable risks for thoracotomy have undergone various thoracoscopic procedures in their care without morbidity. Indeed, Rusch and Mountain have suggested that thoracoscopy is a safer alternative for open lung biopsy in the critically ill, immunocompromised patient with diffuse lung infiltrates. The accumulated experience with diagnostic thoracoscopy extends over the past 80 years; however, the actual incidence of complications and a statistically significant data base regarding operative thoracoscopy awaits an accumulation of experience with more major procedures. In the meantime, anesthesiologists should be prepared to treat and monitor high-risk patients who have had thoracoscopic surgery just as they would those who have had more invasive procedures.

Conclusion

Endoscopic techniques of airway assessment have been in clinical use since before the turn of the century. Innovations in the last 30 years have made bronchoscopy and thoracoscopy more widely applical to clinical problems than ever before. A resurgence of interest in surgical endoscopy has been fueled by the public's interest in surgery with less pain. Newer innovations such as video endoscopy, improved anesthetic monitoring, surgical instruments that can pass through small-diameter tubes into body cavities and resect or cauterize tissue, and small-diameter fiberoptic instruments that give good visual resolution have made this new trend possible.

Whether some of the newer approaches to endobronchial or peripheral pleural and pulmonary disease will stand the test of time is not known. It seems likely that the continued trend to "cross-fertilize" airway endoscopy and surgery with techniques and equipment that were designed for the larger number of patients with gastroenterologic or urinary problems will combine with the drive towards less invasive surgery to perpetuate newer bronchoscopic and thoracoscopic procedures. What is clear is that some of the lessons learned by anesthesiologists in dealing with the shared airway in the past will continue to apply in future. In particular, it should be obvious that, although less invasive procedures may result in less physiologic stress after surgery, the newer approaches still involve an invasive operative experience. Anesthesiologists must be prepared for a myriad of cardiorespiratory problems when "band-aid" surgery is performed in the chest or airway. Most problems can be predicted from the patients' underlying problems and the surgical trespass. It is important to remember that the application of newer equipment and techniques to former problems may facilitate a surgical solution, but will likely present anesthesiologists with many of the problems they are accustomed to in addition to new challenges posed by the technology itself.

References

1. Mushin WW, Rendell-Baker L. Endoscopy. In: Origins of thoracic anaesthesia. Park Ridge, IL: Wood Library-Museum of Anesthesiology. 1991, 115.
2. Jacobaueus HC. The practical importance of thoracoscopy in surgery of the chest. Surg Gynecol Obstet 1922;34:280.
3. Raj PP, Forester J, Watson TD, et al. Techniques for fiberoptic laryngoscopy in anesthesia. Anesth Analg 1974;53:708.
4. Vale R. Selective bronchial blocking in a small child. Br J Anaesth 1969;41:452.

5. Watson CB, Bowe EA, Burke. One-lung anesthesia for pediatric thoracic surgery: a new use of the fiberoptic bronchoscope. Anesthesiology 1983; 56:314.
6. Glover W, Chavis TV, Daniel TM, et al. Fibrin glue application through the flexible fiberoptic bronchoscope: closure of bronchopleural fistulas. J Thorac Cardiovasc Surg 1987;93:470.
7. Torre M, Belloni P. ND:YAG laser pleurodesis through thoracoscopy: new curative therapy in spontaneous pneumothorax. Ann Thorac Surg 1989;47:887.
8. Krasna M, Nazem A. Thoracoscopic lung resection: use of a new endoscopic linear stapler. Surg Laparosc Endosc 1991;1:248.
9. Sanders RD. Two ventilating attachments for bronchoscopes. Del Med J 1967;39:170.
10. Sjostrand U. High-frequency positive-pressure ventilation (HFPPV): review. Crit Care Med 1980;8:345.
11. Klain M, Smith RB. High-frequency percutaneous transtracheal jet ventilation. Crit Care Med 1977; 5:280.
12. Benumof JL. Anesthesia for special elective diagnostic procedures. In: Anesthesia for thoracic surgery. Philadelphia: WB Saunders, 1987;326.
13. Feneck R. Anesthesia for diagnostic thoracic surgical procedures. In: Balliere's clinical anaesthesiology. Vol. 1, 1987:25.
14. Frumin J, Epstein R, Cohen G. Apenic oxygenation in man. Anesthesiology 1959;20:789.
15. Fraoli RL, Sheffer LA, Steffenson JL. Pulmonary and cardiovascular effect of apneic oxygenation in man. Anesthesiology 1973;38:588.
16. Neuhaus A. Markowitz D. Rotman HH, et al. The effects of fiberoptic bronchoscopy with and without atropine premedication of pulmonary function in humans. Ann Thorac Surg 1978;25:393.
17. Lukomsky GI, Ovchinnikov AA, Bilal A. Complications of bronchoscopy: comparison of rigid bronchoscopy under general anesthesia and flexible fiberoptic bronchoscopy under topical anesthesia. Chest 1981;79:316.
18. Lindholm CE, Ollman B, Snyder JV, et al. Cardiorespiratory effects of flexible fiberoptic bronchoscopy in critically ill patients. Chest 1978;74:362.
19. Carden E, Schwesinger WB. The use of nitrous oxide during ventilation with the open bronchoscope. Anesthesiology 1973;33:784.
20. George PJM, Garrett CPO, Nixon C, et al. Laser treatment for tracheobronchial tumors: local or general anaesthesia? Thorax 1987;42:656.
21. Blomquist S, Algotsson L, Karlsson SE. Anaesthesia for resection of tumours in the trachea and central bronchi using the ND-YAG laser technique. Acta Anaesthesiol Scand 1990;34:506.
22. Sosis MG, Heller S. A comparison of special endotracheal tubes for use with the CO_2 laser. Anesthesiology 1988;69:A251.
23. Murphy P. A fiberoptic endoscope used for nasal intubation. Anaesthesia 1967;22:498.
24. Ikeda S. Yanai N, Ishikawa S. Flexible bronchofiberscope. Keio Med 1968;17:1.
25. Oho K, Amamiya R. Practical fiberoptic bronchoscopy. Tokyo, Japan: Igaku-Shoin, 1980:109.
26. Sackner MA, Wanner A, Landa J. Applications of bronchofiberoscopy. Chest 1962;62(Suppl):705.
27. Lindholm CE, Ollman B, Snyder J, et al. Flexible fiberoptic bronchoscopy in critical care medicine. Crit Care Med 1974;2;250.
28. Taylor P, Towey R. The broncho-fiberscope as an aid to endotracheal intubation. Br J Anaesth 1972; 44:611.
29. Davidson TM, Bone RC, Nahum AM. Endotracheal intubation with the flexible fiberoptic bronchoscope. Ear Nose Throat J 1975;54:346.
30. Wood RE, Fink RJ. Applications of flexible bronchoscopes in infants and children. Chest 1978;73:737.
31. Harrel JH. Transnasal approach for fiberoptic bronchoscopy. Chest 1978;73(Suppl):704.
32. Landis JF. Indications for bronchoscopy. Chest 1978;73(Suppl):686.
33. Ellis JH. Transbronchial lung biopsy via the fiberoptic bronchoscope. Chest 1975;68:524.
34. Cunanan OS. The flexible fiberoptic bronchoscope in foreign body removal: experience in 300 cases. Chest 1978;73:725.
35. Oho K, Nadajima H, Kato H, et al. Present status of bronchoscopy in Japan. Jpn J Chest Dis 1979;38:35.
36. Lukomsky GI, Ovachinnikov AA, Bilal A. Complications of bronchoscopy: comparison of rigid bronchoscopy under topical anesthesia. Chest 1981; 79:316.
37. Laforet EG, Berger RL, Vaughan CW. Carcinoma obstructing the trachea: treatment by laser resection. N Eng Med 1976;294:914.
38. Watson CB. Fiberoptic bronchoscopy in thoracic anaesthesia. In: Balliere's clinical anaesthesiology. Vol. 1, 1987:33.
39. Bloch EC, Filston HCI. A thin fiberoptic bronchoscope as an aid to occlusion of the fistula in infants with tracheoesophageal fistula. Anesth Analg 1988; 67:791.

40. Glover W, Chavis TV, Daniel TM, et al. Fibrin glue application through the flexible fiberoptic bronchoscope: closure of bronchopleural fistulas. J Thorac Cardiovasc Surg 1987;93:470.
41. Smith G, Hirsh N, Ehrenwerth J. Sight and sound: can double-lumen endotracheal tubes be placed accurately without fiberoptic bronchoscopy? Anesth Analg 1986;65:S170.
42. Spielman F. Which procedural skills should be learned by anesthesia residents? Anesthesiology 1988;69:S798.
43. Watson CB. Problems with endobronchial intubation: a case for fiberoptic postitioning. Anesthesiology Rev 1986;13:52.
44. Pingleton SK, Bone CR, Ruth WC. Helium-oxygen mixtures during bronchoscopy. Crit Care Med 1978;8:50.
45. Satyanaray T, Capan L, Ramanathan S, et al. Bronchofiberscoptic jet ventilation. Anesth Analg 1980; 59:350.
46. Lampton LM. Bronchoscopy: caution! JAMA 1978; 73:138.
47. Brutinel WM, McDougall JC, Vortese DA. Bronchoscopic therapy with neodymium-yttrium-aluminum-garnet laser during intravenous anesthesia. Chest 1983;84:518.
48. Hannowell LH, Martin WR, Savelle JE, et al. Complications of general anesthesia for ND:YAG laser resection of endobronchial tumors. Chest 1991; 99:72.
49. Schiffman PL, Wilhelm J, Parisi RA. Arterial oxygen saturation during ND:YAG laser photoresection of endobronchial tumors under local anesthesia. Use of intermittent supplemental oxygen with pulse oximetry guidance. Chest 1986;94:1300.
50. Godden DJ, Willey RF, Ferfussion RJ, et al. Rigid bronchoscopy under intravenous general anesthesia with oxygen Venturi ventilation. Thorax 1982; 37:532.
51. Simpson FG, Arnold AG, Purvis A, et al. Postal survey of bronchoscopic practice by physicians in the United Kingdom. Thorax 1986;41:311.
52. Jacobaueus HC. The cauterization of adhesions in artificial pneumothorax therapy of tuberculosis. Am Rev Tuber 1922;6:871.
53. Decamp PT, Moseley PW, Scott ML, et al. Diagnostic thoracoscopy. Ann Thorac Surg 1973;16:70.
54. Bloomberg AE. Thoracoscopy in perspective. Surg Gynecol Obstet 1978:147:433.
55. Curling PE. Anesthesia for thoracic diagnostic procedures. In: Kaplan JA, ed. Thoracic anesthesia. New York, Churchill Livingstone:1983:339
56. Miller JI, Hatcher CR. Thoracoscopy: a useful tool in the diagnosis of thoracic disease. Ann Thorac Surg 1978;26:68.
57. Page RD, Jeffrey RR, Donnelly RJ. Thoracoscopy: a review of 121 consecutive surgical procedures. Ann Thorac Surg 1989;48:66.
58. Swierenga J, Wagenaar JPM, Bergstein RGM. The value of thoracoscopy in the diagnosis and treatment of disease affecting the pleura and lung. Pneumonology 1974;151:11.
59. Krasna M, Flowers JL. Diagnostic thoracoscopy in a patient with a pleural mass. Surg Laparosc Endosc 1991;1:94.
60. Krasna M, Nazem A. Thoracoscopic lung resection: Use of a new endoscopic linear stapler. Surg Laparosc Endosc 1991;1:248.
61. Wakabayashi A, Brenner M, Wilson AF, et al. Thoracoscopic treatment of spontaneous pneumothorax using CO_2 laser. Ann Thorac Surg 1991; 50:36.
62. Rusch VW, Torre M, Belloni P. op.cit(ref 7) Mountain C. Thoracoscopy under regional anesthesia for the diagnosis and management of pleural diseases. Am J Surg 1987;154:274.
63. Bonniot JP, Homasson JP, Rodem SL, et al. Pleural and lung cryobiopsies during thoracoscopy. Chest 1989;95:492.
64. Boutin C. Thoracoscopy in malignant mesothelioma. Pneumologie 1989;43:61.
65. Lewis RJ, Kunderman PJ, Sisler GE, et al. Direct diagnostic thoracoscopy. Ann Thor Surg 1976; 21:536.
66. Viskum K. Contraindications and complications to thoracoscopy. Pneumologie 1989;43:55.

CHAPTER

18

Mediastinoscopy, Mediastinal Mass, and Superior Vena Cava Syndrome

Steven M. Neustein
Robert Koorn
James B. Eisenkraft

Mediastinoscopy was first described by Carlens[1] in 1959 as a method for inspection and biopsy of the superior mediastinum. This technique is commonly performed to establish a diagnosis and determine the resectability of a tumor. The advantage of performing mediastinoscopy is that information is acquired that would otherwise only be obtainable by thoracotomy. Anesthetic management may be associated with severe life-threatening complications related to either the surgery or the underlying pathophysiology. Thorough evaluation of the patient can reduce the risk associated with the administration of anesthesia for mediastinoscopy, however.

Anatomy of the Mediastinum

Bordered anteriorly by the sternum and posteriorly by the thoracic vertebrae, the mediastinum is bounded by pleural sacs, the thoracic inlet, and the diaphragm. It is divided into three compartments: anterosuperior, middle, and posterior (Fig. 18-1). The anterosuperior compartment, which is located anterior and superior to the heart, contains the thymus gland, substernal extensions of the thyroid and parathyroid glands, the aortic arch and its branches, the innominate veins, lymphatics, and lymph nodes and loose areolar tissue. The middle mediastinum, which is posterior and inferior to the anterior compartment, includes the heart, pericardium, trachea and main bronchi, pulmonary hilum, phrenic and vagus nerves, and lymph nodes. The border of the posterior mediastinum is formed by the margins of the thoracic vertebrae as seen on lateral projection; it contains the esophagus, descending aorta, azygos and hemiazygos veins, thoracic duct, vagus nerve, sympathetic chains, and lymph nodes.

Mediastinal Tumors

Pathology

Mediastinal tumors can be classified according to their location within the mediastinum (Table 18-1). In adults, neurogenic tumors, thymomas, and developmental cysts account for 60% of all lesions.[2] Neurogenic tumors are the

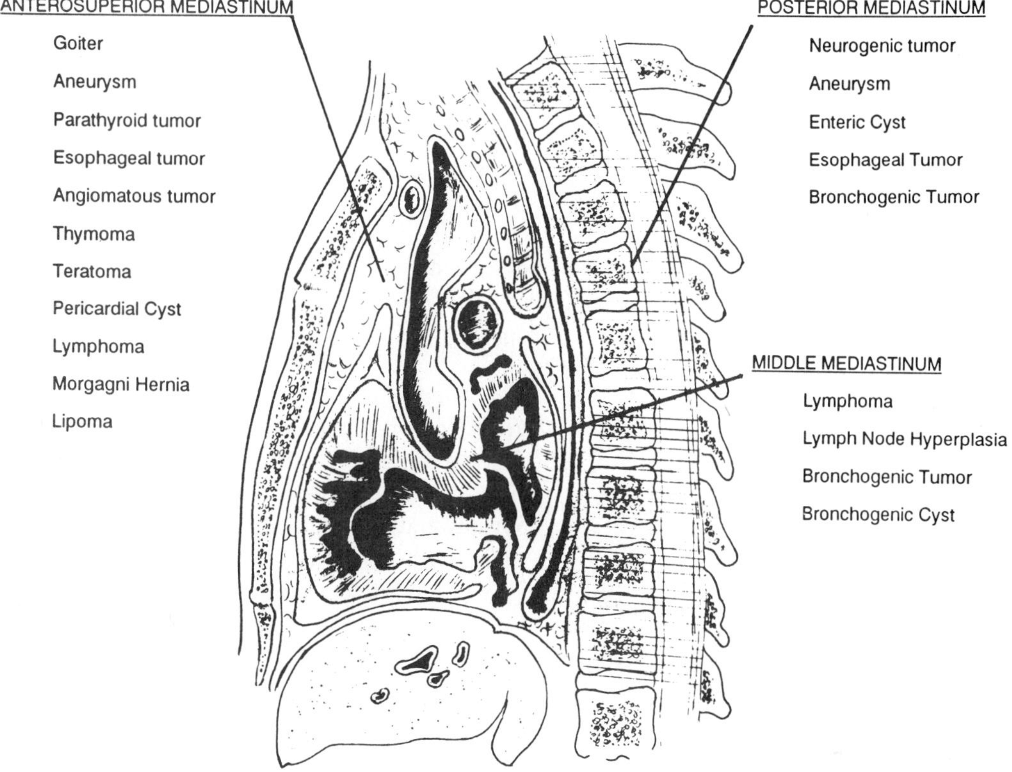

Figure 18-1. Anatomy of the mediastinum showing the location of commonly occurring mediastinal tumors. (Used with permission from Glenn WWL, ed. Thoracic and cardiovascular surgery. Norwalk, CT: Appleton-Century-Crofts, 1983:*182*.)

most common primary lesion of the mediastinum (20%–35% of all lesions),[3,4] and usually occur in the posterior mediastinum. Thymomas are the second most common type (20% of mediastinal neoplasms in adults).[5] Thymomas most often occur in the anterior mediastinum, have a 50% malignancy rate, and a 50% association rate with myasthenia gravis.[6] Lymphomas and germ cell tumors, such as teratoma and seminoma together, make up 25% of lesions. Lymphoid tumors most often occur in the anterior or middle mediastinum. Teratomas, whether benign or malignant, often extend below the sternum, and present as anterior mediastinal masses. Mesenchymal tumors, developmental cysts, vascular masses, diaphragmatic hernias in the middle mediastinum, and esophageal lesions in the posterior mediastinum are included in the remaining 15%.

Ninety percent of lymph node masses in the middle mediastinum result from metastatic spread of malignancies. Other masses in this region are vascular (aneurysms), esophageal (achalasia, diverticuli) or cystic lesions (bronchogenic, pericardial). Masses in the posterior mediastinum are usually of neurogenic origin

Table 18-1. Mass Lesions of the Mediastinum

Superior mediastinum
Goiter
Parathyroid adenoma
Myxoma
Lymphoma
Aortic aneurysm
Zencker's diverticulum
Middle mediastinum
Bronchogenic cyst
Lymphoma
Plasma cell myeloma
Metastatic carcinoma
Aortic aneurysm
Bronchogenic cyst
Pericardial cyst
Tuberculous nodes
Anterior mediastinum
Thymoma
Teratoma
Goiter
Parathyroid adenoma
Lymphoma
Lipoma
Fibroma
Lymphangioma
Hemangioma
Chondroma
Rhabdomyosarcoma
Posterior mediastinum
Neurilemmoma
Neurofibroma
Ganglioneuroma
Sympathicoblastoma
Fibrosarcoma
Lymphoma
Goiter
Xanthofibroma
Chondroma
Myxoma
Paraganglioma
Aortic aneurysm
Diaphragmatic hernia (Bochdalek)
Esophageal duplication cysts

(neurofibromas, schwannomas, and benign ganglioneuromas).

Mediastinal mass lesions in children are usually bronchial cysts, teratomas, or lymphomas. These lesions are usually malignant in older children but benign in children less than two years of age. Airway obstruction, which often develops during anesthesia, is a risk with these lesions.[7] Of the malignant tumors, the majority are either Hodgkin's or non-Hodgkin's lymphomas involving the anterior and middle mediastinum.[8] Almost 50% of patients with such lymphomas present with a mediastinal mass at the time of their initial examination.[9–11] As in adults, tumors of neurogenic origin are most commonly found in the posterior mediastinum.

Signs and Symptoms

Most mediastinal masses are asymptomatic and are discovered incidentally on routine chest x-rays (Table 18-2). Ninety percent of the lesions in asymptomatic patients are benign. Symptomatic mediastinal masses are usually malignant. Large masses with extensive involvement tend to produce more severe symptoms.[12] The most common symptoms are cough (40%), chest pain (40%), dyspnea (20%), and dysphagia (20%).[13] Other symptoms include weight loss (24%), fever (24%), superior vena cava syndrome (16%), tracheal deviation (12%), Horner's syndrome (7%), spinal cord compression (5%), cyanosis (3%), and mediastinal widening (3%).[6] The phrenic nerve may be involved occasionally. Mediastinal tumors are frequently associated with systemic syndromes which include myasthenia gravis (thymoma), pure red cell aplasia (thymoma), Cushing's syndrome (thymoma; carcinoid), gynecomastia (certain germ cell tumors), hypertension (pheochromocytoma, ganglioneuroma), and hypercalcemia (lymphoma, parathyroid adenoma).

Involvement of the Cardiovascular System by Mediastinal Mass Lesions

Superior Vena Cava Syndrome

The superior vena cava (SVC) syndrome is caused by obstruction of venous drainage

Table 18-2. Signs and Symptoms of Mediastinal Mass Lesions

Symptoms
- Airway
  - Cough
  - Cyanosis
  - Dyspnea
  - Orthopnea
- Cardiovascular
  - Fatigue
  - Faintness
  - Headache
  - Dyspnea and orthopnea
  - Cough

Signs
- Airway
  - Decreased breath sounds
  - Wheezing
  - Stridor
  - Cyanosis
- Cardiovascular
  - Neck or facial edema
  - Jugular distension
  - Papilledema
  - Pulsus paradoxus
  - Exaggerated changes in blood pressure associated with changes in posture

through the superior vena cava. This condition, which develops slowly, is due to malignant disease in 97% of cases.[14,15] Benign causes include intrathoracic thyroid goiter, primary SVC thrombosis, SVC thrombosis induced by centrally placed catheters, pericardial constriction, idiopathic sclerosing mediastinitis, and tuberculosis. SVC syndrome is more frequently associated with right-sided mediastinal lesions that usually occur below the level of the azygos vein, and it commonly occurs with bronchogenic carcinoma.[16]

The vena cava is prone to obstruction for two reasons: because intravascular pressure is low and because the vein is contained within rigid structures (Fig. 18-2). Obstruction results in increased venous pressure, causing dilatation of veins of the neck and upper part of the thorax; edema and plethora of the face, neck, and upper part of the trunk; conjunctival edema; and central nervous system symptoms such as headache, visual abnormality, and altered states of consciousness.[17] Venous distension is greatest in the recumbent position, and the veins usually do not collapse when the patient is upright.

The symptoms most commonly associated with SVC syndrome are dyspnea (83%), cough (70%), and orthopnea (64%).[18] These symptoms may be from airway impingement by engorged veins or tumor. Facial and periorbital edema occur early, whereas central nervous system changes reflect a more rapidly progressive course. Upper airway edema, and possibly airway obstruction, can develop. Venous congestion may make blind instrumentation of the nasopharyngeal and laryngotracheal regions dangerous because of possible bleeding.[19,20]

Compression of the Pulmonary Artery

Unlike the aorta, which is protected against external compression within the chest by a high intravascular pressure, the pulmonary artery is vulnerable to the compressive effects of space-occupying lesions.[21,22] The pulmonary artery may be compressed by lymphoma or benign tumors. Compression of either the pulmonary trunk or one of the main pulmonary arteries can produce sudden hypoxemia, hypotension, and cardiac arrest.[23]

Involvement of the Respiratory System by Mediastinal Mass Lesions

Infants with benign masses often present with airway obstruction,[24–26] but this condition may also occur in adults. Most patients with severe respiratory symptoms have significant narrowing of the trachea, which can be demonstrated radiographically in some cases. These symptoms may be worsened or alleviated with posture, depending where gravity is pulling the mass in relation to the other structures in the

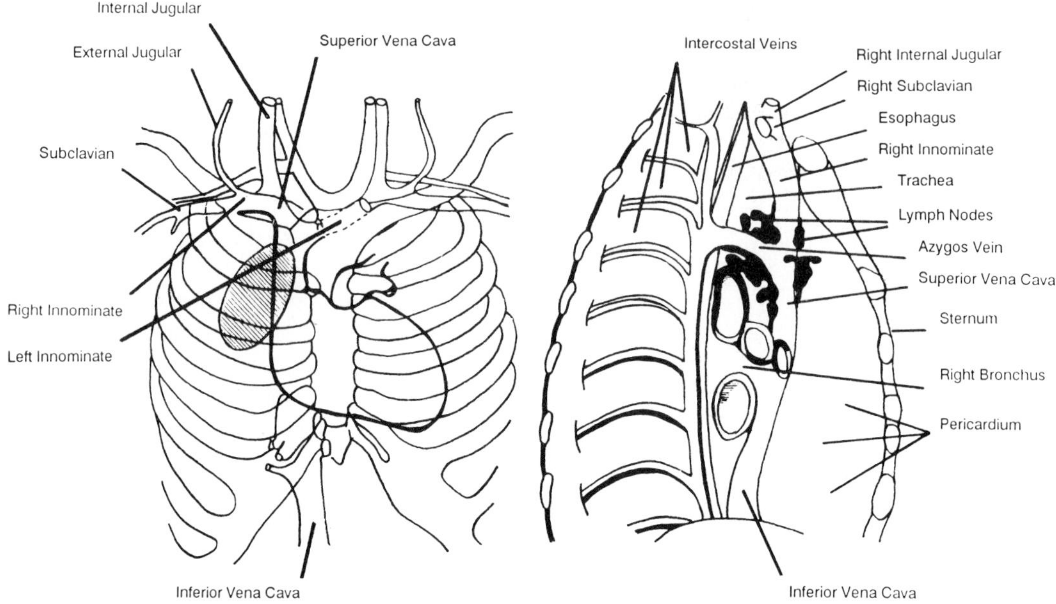

Figure 18-2. Schematic representation of the frontal (left) and sagittal (right) sections of the thorax, which shows (1) the relationship of the azygous vein to the superior vena cava (SVC), (2) the coalescence of the innominates to form the SVC at the right second rib, and (3) the encasement of the SVC by nodal structures. The shaded areas indicate the classical site of obstruction. (Used with permission from Lokich JJ, et al. Superior vena cava syndrome. JAMA 1975;231:58.)

chest. Symptoms are often exacerbated in the supine position. Infants and small children may develop airway obstruction earlier than adults, because small decreases in airway diameter produce relatively larger decreases in area and greater increases in airway resistance.

Bronchospasm, rhonchi, and wheezing have been reported in patients with mediastinal masses. Wheezing can also be caused by the obstruction of the trachea or main bronchi.

Diagnosis of Mediastinal Mass Lesions

The mediastinum can be studied noninvasively by conventional radiography, computed tomography (CT), magnetic resonance imaging (MRI), or radionuclide scanning. Except in rare instances, such as the radiographic demonstration of teeth in a teratoma, or the visualization of functioning thyroid tissue on radionuclide scan, an accurate diagnosis cannot be made noninvasively but requires pathologic examination of mediastinal tissue. Suprasternal mediastinoscopy allows visualization and biopsy of lymph nodes and other masses in the superior portion of the anterior mediastinum. Anterior mediastinotomy in the left second intercostal space permits examination in the subaortic fossa. Advantages these procedures have over sternotomy and mediastinal exploration include lower morbidity and mortality rates and faster recuperation.

Treatment of Mediastinal Mass Lesions

The most effective treatment of SVC syndrome is radiation,[27] which may be administered in combination with chemotherapy, depending on the underlying pathology. In rapidly progressive cases, anticoagulants are often used to prevent clotting in compressed veins. Fibrinolytics have also been administered in conjunction with radiotherapy.[28] Steroids have been shown to be beneficial, possibly by increasing the threshold for edema formation.[29]

Many tumors, especially lymphomas, are extremely radiosensitive and shrink significantly following a single treatment.[2,5] Radiation therapy reduces the effects of pressure on the respiratory tract, heart, and pulmonary artery. Some tumors may also respond well to chemotherapy or surgery.[2,30,31]

Preoperative Evaluation of the Patient with Mediastinal Mass Lesions

A detailed history and clinical examination are important. They may reveal cardiovascular or respiratory involvement and occasionally the presence of non metastatic syndromes such as myasthenia or Eaton-Lambert syndrome. It should be determined whether respiratory symptoms are present; if so, their relationship to posture should be identified. Wheezing at rest, with exercise, or after a change in posture indicates the possibility of major airway obstruction and should not be assumed to be bronchospasm, even in the immunologically compromised patient with obvious respiratory infection. A systolic murmur of recent onset probably originates from the pulmonary artery, which is much more compressible than the aorta. Evidence of SVC obstruction should be sought.

Posteroanterior and lateral chest radiographs should be obtained within a week of surgery, as mediastinal masses can enlarge rapidly. Fluoroscopy and barium swallow are occasionally needed to delineate the middle mediastinum and especially to distinguish between normal thymus and abnormal anterior mediastinal masses.[32] These radiological techniques only provide a two-dimensional view of the tracheobronchial tree, however, and significant compression may not be diagnosed.[7] The penetrated lateral chest x-ray has been recommended for detecting tracheobronchial obstruction,[33] but the predictive yield is poor. Multiple specialized studies may be required including tomograms, computerized tomography and thoracic inlet views.

The CT scan provides a very accurate estimate of the size of a mediastinal mass and the degree of tracheal compression.[34,35] CT scans also show subclinical airway compression in 50% of children with mediastinal masses.[36] MRI is even better for distinguishing between mediastinal masses and the cardiovascular system and offers improved visualization of posterior masses that have intraspinal extension. CT scanning, however, is still better for the study of intrathoracic calcifications and bronchial abnormalities.[37]

The amount of tracheal compression seen on CT scan suggests the potential for airway difficulty during anesthesia. In a study of 50 children with mediastinal masses, the five patients who developed complete or near complete airway obstruction during induction or emergence from anesthesia had over 50% decreases in tracheal cross-sectional areas as measured by CT scan.[7] Although not predictive of survival, the size of a mediastinal mass has been shown to correlate with the duration of remission following initial treatment.[38]

Pulmonary function tests are extremely valuable, particularly when lung pathology coexists. Maximal inspiratory and expiratory flow-volume curves obtained in the upright and supine positions provide an evaluation of functional impairment and help to distinguish fixed from variable obstructive intrathoracic lesions.[30] An intrathoracic mass usually reduces both inspiratory and expiratory flows (Fig. 18-3).[39] A disproportionate decrease in maximal expiratory flow may result from tracheomalacia.

Flexible fiberoptic bronchoscopy under topical anesthesia is a useful method for evaluation of dynamic airway obstruction.[40,41] It allows assessment of the function of the entire airway and the response to changes in intrathoracic pressure when the patient moves from the supine to sitting to semi-prone positions. Ultrasonography and echocardiography have also been used in these patients to study myocardial contractility and the degree of tumor involvement of the heart and great vessels.[42,43]

In addition, the patient may have systemic disease as a result of the administration of chemotherapeutic agents. Doxorubicin may lead to a dose-related cardiomyopathy. An acute form of this condition, which occurs in 10% of patients receiving doxorubicin, is characterized by cardiac conduction abnormalities, left-axis deviation, premature ventricular contractions, supraventricular tachyarrhythmias, and an ECG showing nonspecific ST-T wave changes and decreased QRS voltage.[44] Most of these changes usually resolve within one or two months of discontinuation of doxorubicin treatment.[44] Cardiomyopathy may also develop slowly, with a slow onset of symptoms followed by rapidly progressive heart failure.[44] It is unusual for a cardiomyopathy to develop if the total doxorubicin dose is less than 500 mg/m^2.[44] A preoperative echocardiogram or nuclear scan for the evaluation of cardiac function should be performed in patients who have been treated with doxorubicin.

Figure 18-3. Flow-volume loop for a patient with a normal airway and a patient with an intrathoracic mass. (Used with permission from Pullerits J, Holzman R. Anaesthesia for patients with mediastinal masses. Can J Anaesth 1989;36:681.)

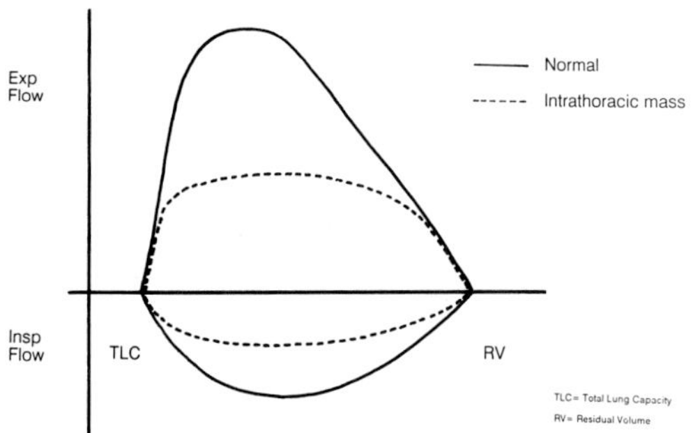

Bleomycin in combination with high inspired concentrations of oxygen may lead to postoperative respiratory failure that can be fatal.[45] The presence of pulmonary toxicity is initially manifested by cough, dyspnea, and basilar rales, which can then take either a mild or severe course. In the mild form, exertional dyspnea and a normal resting PaO_2 are evident. The severe form is characterized by resting hypoxemia and the appearance on chest radiograph of interstitial pneumonia and fibrosis.[46] The alveolar-arterial gradient for oxygen may be increased, and the diffusing capacity may be reduced. The risk for the postoperative development of adult respiratory distress syndrome is greater.[46] It has been hypothesized that exposure to an increased FIO_2 may lead to the formation of superoxide and other free radicals. Although this may be responsible,[44] there are data to the contrary.[47] Interstitial fluid may accumulate in the lungs as a result of impaired lymphatic drainage secondary to the fibrotic changes. Patients over of 70 years of age who have received radiation therapy and more than 400 units of bleomycin have been found to be at increased risk of toxicity.[44] Myelotoxicity, which results in immunosuppression and thrombocytopenia, is a side effect of most antineoplastic drugs. Patients with mediastinal tumors are commonly treated with radiation, which may cause pneumonitis, pericarditis, bleeding, myelitis, and tracheoesophageal fistula.[44]

Other abnormalities frequently accompanying malignant tumors include hypercalcemia, uric acid nephropathy, hyponatremia (especially with small cell carcinoma of the lung), nausea and vomiting, anorexia and cachexia, tumor-induced hypoglycemia, and intracranial metastases.

A flow chart describing the preoperative evaluation of a patient with an anterior mediastinal mass is shown in Figure 18-4.

Mediastinoscopy: General Considerations

Indications

Mediastinoscopy is usually performed to make a diagnosis and to help determine if a tumor is resectable.

Figure 18-4. Flow chart describing the preoperative evaluation of the patient with an anterior mediastinal mass. A plus sign (+) indicates positive finding; a minus sign (−) indicates a negative result. (Used with permission from Neumann G, et al. The anesthetic management of patients with an anterior mediastinal mass. Anesthesiology 1984;60:144.)

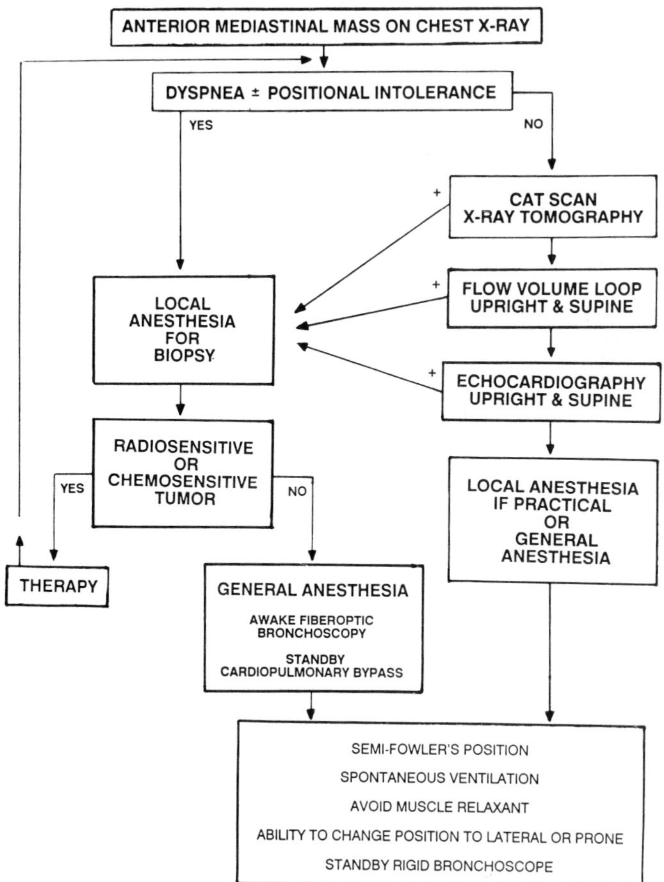

Contraindications

Contraindications include inoperability, involvement of the recurrent laryngeal nerve, aneurysm of the ascending aorta, and anterior mediastinal masses.[48] A repeat mediastinoscopy is technically more difficult because scar tissue that forms after the first mediastinoscopy obscures the plane of dissection. A previous mediastinoscopy is no longer considered an absolute contraindication. Some authors feel that the only absolute contraindication to mediastinoscopy is a patient who is not a candidate for general anesthesia.[49] Tumors of the thymus and anterior mediastinum are not accessible via mediastinoscopy because they are anterior to the great vessels; they are usually approached via an anterior mediastinotomy with an incision in the second intercostal space.

Relative contraindications to mediastinoscopy include upper airway pathology, SVC obstruction, thoracic inlet obstruction, and cerebral vascular insufficiency. The latter condition may be exacerbated by innominate artery compression during mediastinoscopy (Table 18-3).

Surgical Technique

With the neck extended, a transverse incision is made just above the suprasternal notch. Blunt dissection is used to expose the trachea. The patient's head is rotated to the left, and the mediastinoscope is placed in the space between the anterior surface of the trachea and the posterior border of the suprasternal notch. The mediastinoscope is advanced distally in a path created by blunt dissection. The subcarinal region is accessible if no adhesions or anatomical abnormalities are present (Fig. 18-5). The mediastinal structures can then be examined, including the superior mediastinal lymph nodes that are located posterior to the aortic arch. Tissue should be aspirated before biopsy to reduce the risk of hemorrhage, because blood vessels may be distended from the mediastinal mass and such vessels may mimic masses. The presence of contralateral nodes that are positive is an absolute contraindication to lung resection. If only the ipsilateral nodes are involved, however, a thoracotomy may be performed. This individual decision depends on the expected resectability of the tumor.

Table 18-3. Relative and Absolute Contraindications to Mediastinoscopy

Relative
Superior vena cava syndrome
Previous mediastinoscopies
Obstruction and distortion of the upper airway
Impaired cerebral circulation
Myasthenic syndrome
Absolute
Inoperability
Coagulopathy
Ascending aortic aneurysm

Mediastinoscopy: Anesthetic Considerations

Premedication

Premedication should not be given to patients known to have tracheobronchial compromise, because sedation may precipitate cardiopulmonary insufficiency. An antisialagogue may be helpful if the intubation is expected to be difficult.

Choice of Anesthetic Technique

Mediastinoscopy can be performed under either local or general anesthesia, but general anesthesia is the preferred technique.

Local Anesthesia

Although the mediastinum has extensive autonomic innervation there are very few pain fi-

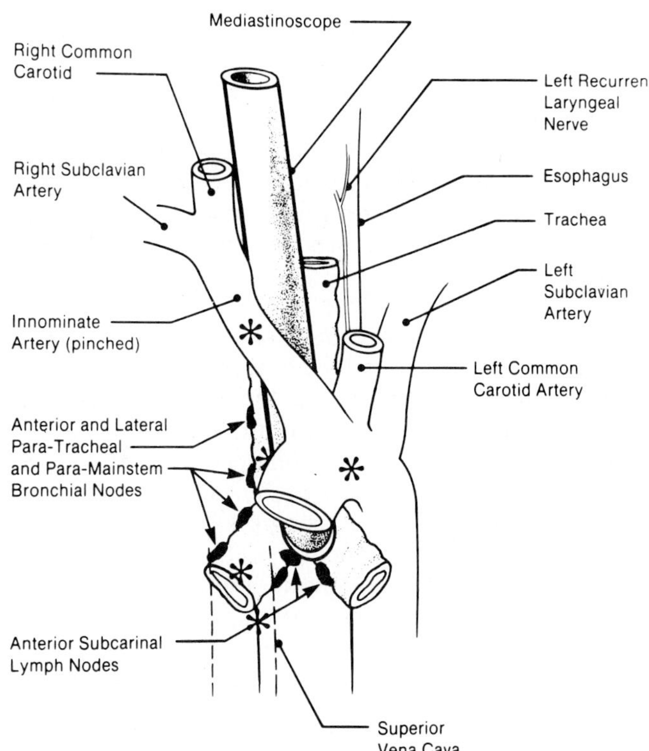

Figure 18-5. Schematic diagram, which shows the placement of a mediastinoscope into the superior mediastinum. The mediastinoscope passes in front of the trachea but behind the thoracic aorta. This location of the mediastinoscope allows for sampling of anterior and lateral paramainstem bronchial lymph nodes, anterior subcarinal lymph nodes, and anterior and lateral paratracheal lymph nodes. Anatomical structures that can be compressed by the mediastinoscope (see areas marked by large asterisk) and can cause major complications are the thoracic aorta (rupture, reflex bradycardia), innominate artery (cerebral vascular symptoms caused by decreased right carotid blood flow, and loss of right radial pulse caused by decreased right subclavian flow), trachea (inability to ventilate), and vena cava (risk of hemorrhage with superior vena cava syndrome). (Reprinted, with permission, from Benumof J, Anesthesia for thoracic surgery. Philadelphia: WB Saunders, 1987:336.)

bers, making mediastinoscopy possible under local anesthesia. In the past, general anesthesia was considered too risky, and local anesthesia was the method of choice.[50] Mediastinoscopy was safely performed under local anesthesia as reported in two series published by Ward and Morton in 1966 and 1971, respectively.[49, 51] The skin, subcutaneous tissue, strap muscles, and posterior aspects of the clavicle were infiltrated with 10 mL of 1% lidocaine. An intratracheal injection of 2 mL of 1% lidocaine was also administered via cricothyroid puncture for suppression of the cough reflex.

The use of local anesthesia presents problems, however. The additional pressure created by the presence of the mediastinoscope in the mediastinum is likely to lead to airway obstruction in patients who already have airway compromise. The combination of sedation and the supine position may not be tolerated. Venous air embolism and pneumomediastinum are also more likely under local anesthesia because of the negative inspiratory pressure created by spontaneous inspiration. General anesthesia has therefore become the anesthetic of choice. This has been made possible by a better understanding of the pathophysiology of mediastinal masses and the routine use of invasive monitoring. General anesthesia gives the surgeon greater flexibility in the dissection. Control of the airway is also of great benefit if a major complication such as massive hemorrhage occurs.[51] Local anesthesia may be considered when cerebrovascular disease is present, so that cerebral function can be monitored continuously while the patient is awake.

General Anesthesia

In recent years, preoperative radiation treatment has been recommended before general anesthesia to decrease the pressure exerted on the respiratory tract, heart, and pulmonary artery.[31, 40, 52] Many tumors, especially lymphomas, are extremely radiosensitive and shrink following a single treatment which reduces the incidence of perioperative complications.[2, 5] A flow-volume loop before and after radiation treatment is shown in Figure 18-6. Unfortunately, it may be difficult to make a diagnosis of tumor cell type following radiation

Figure 18-6. Flow-volume loop before radiation therapy (A) and after radiation therapy (B) in upright and supine positions. In A the reduction in vital capacity and expiratory flow rates is marked, and the expiratory flow rate reaches a plateau, which is indicative of an intrathoracic airway obstruction. In B the expiratory flow rates and vital capacity are improved, showing minimal change in the supine position. (Used with permission from Neumann G, et al. The anesthetic management of patients with an anterior mediastinal mass. Anesthesiology 1984;60:144.)

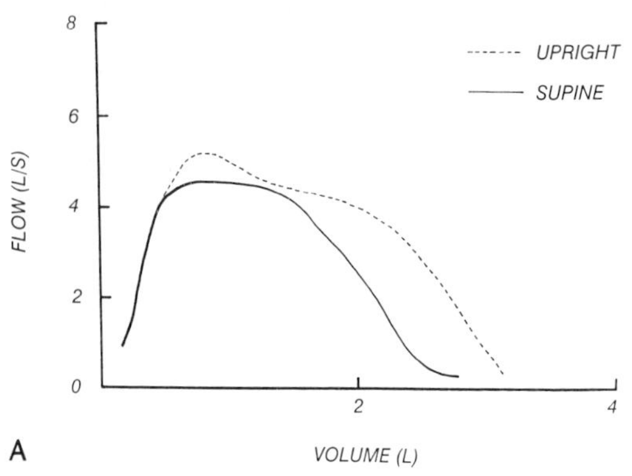

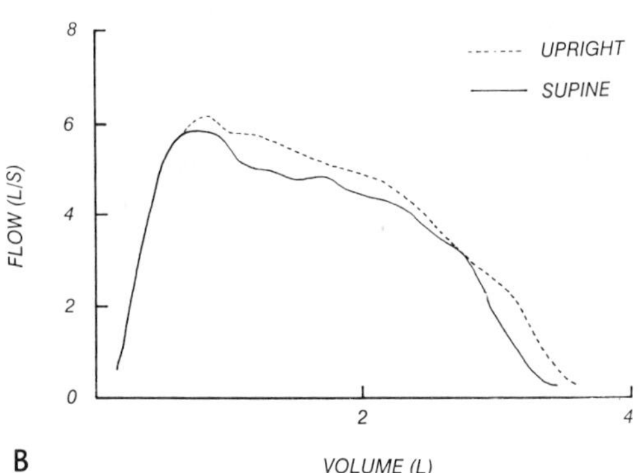

therapy; this is needed to establish which chemotherapeutic agents should be used.[53,54] Even with limitation of radiation to the central area of the mediastinal mass, scattering may be enough to obscure the tissue diagnosis. Anesthesiologists may therefore have to provide general anesthesia to patients who cannot tolerate local anesthesia but in whom tissue diagnosis is required before treatment is initiated.

In a retrospective study performed by Ferrari and Bedford,[53] seven of 44 pediatric patients (16%) with anterior mediastinal masses undergoing general anesthesia developed potentially life-threatening airway compromise one or more times in the perioperative period. Five of these patients had symptoms preoperatively. These authors recommended having a pediatric bronchoscopist available and being prepared to perform unusual maneuvers such as advancing the endotracheal tube into the mainstem bronchus or changing the posture of the patient. Although the authors concluded that it was safe to administer general anesthesia to pediatric patients with anterior mediastinal masses, others have drawn the opposite conclusion.[55–57]

A large-bore intravenous catheter should be inserted prior to the induction of anesthesia, and blood should be immediately available. If the patient has SVC syndrome, venous access should be in a lower extremity. Increased venous pressures may cause excessive bleeding from puncture sites in the upper extremities. In addition, the administration of medications and anesthetic drugs in an upper extremity may have a delayed onset as a result of delayed venous return to the heart. This may lead to overdosage if the anesthesiologist administers additional anesthetic because of an apparent lack of drug effect. SVC syndrome symptomatology can be acutely exacerbated by rapid infusion of crystalloids due to additional edema formation. Although administration of diuretics may initially relieve the edema, the subsequent decrease in preload could further worsen venous return and produce hypotension.

A patient with a mass compressing the pulmonary artery may be asymptomatic when awake, yet develop severe hypoxemia during anesthetic induction or even under mild sedation.[58] A history of syncope during a forced Valsalva maneuver, such as occurs with a bowel movement, may herald this anesthetic complication. A combination of assuming the supine position, which produces additional pressure on the heart and pulmonary artery; a reduction in chest wall tone under general anesthesia; and the use of positive-pressure ventilation, which reduces venous return, can result in a fatal reduction in pulmonary blood flow.[59,60] Very large lymphomas have been associated with arrhythmias under anesthesia from either pericardial or myocardial involvement.[61] Cardiac compression by a thymoma may cause cardiac tamponade.[43]

Superficial diagnostic procedures such as cervical node biopsy are best performed under local anesthesia, and if necessary, with the patient sitting up. If anesthesia or sedation is then required, it is recommended that extracorporeal bypass be immediately available. The patient's groin should be prepped, draped, and the cannulation equipment should be in the sterile field in case cardiopulmonary bypass is urgently needed.[62]

Although preoperative evaluation of the airway is important, the severity of preoperative respiratory symptoms may not correlate with respiratory compromise during anesthesia. Asymptomatic patients have also developed severe airway obstruction during anesthesia.[63–65] Tracheal or bronchial obstruction may occur during any phase of anesthesia: induction, intubation, positioning, maintenance, or recovery.[8] Successful treatment of airway obstruction may require special maneuvers, such as advancing the endotracheal tube to the carina or into a main bronchus.[66]

The administration of muscle relaxants to patients with preexisting respiratory compromise may cause complete airway obstruction and is best avoided until complete control of the airway has been obtained. If the airway is severely compromised, the trachea should be intubated prior to the induction of anesthesia. Intubation may have to be performed with the patient in the sitting position, making laryngoscopy with a rigid laryngoscope very difficult. In addition, blind instrumentation of the nasal and oral passages may cause hemorrhage in patients with SVC syndrome. Thus, the use of awake fiberoptic laryngoscopy has been recommended to accomplish endotracheal intubation in such patients.[39] After securing the airway, anesthesia is induced and the patient is paralyzed. Lidocaine is often administered intravenously or sprayed on the cords directly to prevent coughing. Coughing can be completely prevented by the administration of muscle relaxants.

An inhalation induction is often performed in patients with even slight airway compromise. Ventilation may have to be gently assisted until an endotracheal tube is placed. Succinylcholine may be administered if the vocal cords are easily visualized and there is no evidence of airway obstruction. The surgeon should be prepared to perform rigid bronchoscopy, and a long anode tube should be available because intubation with a conventional polyvinylchloride tube may not relieve an obstruction completely. In one report a 4.5-mm diameter rigid bronchoscope was needed to maintain airway patency in an 11-year-old boy.[19]

Intubation may occasionally appear to cause obstruction, which is usually partial, and involves one of the main bronchi.[67] The obstruction may result from the loss of both muscle tone and negative inspiratory pressure produced by muscle relaxation in patients with narrowed airways. In these cases obstruction may be relieved by return to spontaneous respiration. Intubation of a distorted or compressed trachea may cause total obstruction if the orifice of the tube is against the tracheal wall. If the tube is kinked by a narrowed section or sharp angle, obstruction can also occur. This obstruction may only be relieved by passing either a long thin anode tube or a rigid bronchoscope distal to the stenotic region or by placing the patient in the lateral position to relieve the pressure on the trachea from the mediastinal mass.[68,69]

Maintaining spontaneous ventilation during anesthesia may be associated with less hemodynamic instability in those patients with obstructed venous return. This requires a deep anesthetic to prevent coughing, however, and awakening from anesthesia is slower. An alternative technique involves the use of intermittent positive-pressure ventilation (IPPV). Sudden increases in airway pressure or changes in the capnogram tracing are early signs of airway compression. Muscle relaxants prevent coughing and venous engorgement that occur from straining and movement, and they also permit the use of less anesthesia and allow for a more rapid recovery. In addition, IPPV reduces the likelihood of venous air embolism as compared with spontaneous ventilation, in which air is more likely to be entrained by the negative inspiratory pressure. Air embolism is still a risk, however, if the patient is positioned in the head-up position to minimize venous engorgement and edema formation. The patient can be placed in the sitting position and extubated following adequate recovery from anesthesia.

The use of IPPV also has certain disadvantages. Positive-pressure ventilation reduces venous return, especially in the presence of SVCS syndrome, causing reduced cardiac output and blood pressure. Wrapping of the legs prior to induction may be a useful technique to decrease venous pooling. IPPV may also decrease the diameter of already narrowed airways and worsen ventilation.[70] In addition, myasthenic syndrome may be present, in which case the effects of both the depolarizing and nondepolarizing muscle relaxants are altered.

Respiratory difficulty occurring during recovery may require reintubation.[53] High negative pressures created by inspiration against a closed glottis or an obstructing tongue may lead to a collapse of a weakened trachea in the early postoperative period.[71] Following surgery, there may be more airway edema, as a result of decreased venous return from positive-pressure ventilation and the intravenous administration of fluids. Continued intubation postoperatively is occasionally needed until radiotherapy, chemotherapy, or high-dose steroids have been administered.

Complications

The mortality rate associated with mediastinoscopy is low (0.1%),[72] and the overall complication rate has been reported to range from 1.5% to 3.0%[73–75] Serious complications that usually require aggressive management do occur. The complication rate is substantially higher (23%) in repeat mediastinoscopy.[76]

Hemorrhage is the most common complication and is the greatest cause of morbidity in most series.[77] Vascular masses, such as a thoracic aortic aneurysm, can be accidentally perforated during mediastinoscopy, resulting in sudden and catastrophic bleeding.[73] Bleeding may be successfully controlled by packing, but if this fails a thoracotomy may be necessary. The administration of fluids and blood and pharmacological therapy may be required to support the circulation. If hemorrhage results from a tear in the superior vena cava, fluid replacement and drug administration into cannulas placed in the upper extremities will be lost from the vascular space. Under these circumstances, intravenous treatment should be via the lower extremities. If such access has not been obtained preoperatively, the surgeon may need to tamponade the bleeding while the anesthesiologist obtains the needed venous access in a lower extremity.

A pneumothorax may develop intraoperatively, in which case immediate chest tube drainage may be necessary.[78] A pneumothorax may cause increased peak inspiratory pressures, tracheal shift, distant breath sounds, hypotension, and even cyanosis. Usually, the pneumothorax is not diagnosed until the postoperative period. All patients should be monitored for this complication during recovery, and a chest radiograph should be taken in the immediate postoperative period.

Recurrent laryngeal nerve injury, which is permanent in approximately 50% of patients, may occur. The left recurrent laryngeal nerve is more prone to injury during mediastinoscopy. If such an injury is suspected, the vocal cords should be examined following extubation. If there is bilateral nerve damage, the vocal cords may be immobile or in the midline position and airway obstruction could occur.

The mediastinoscope often compresses the innominate artery, causing hypoperfusion of the right subclavian and right carotid arteries. This condition can be detected by palpation of the right radial pulse or by a continuous pressure tracing from an arterial catheter placed in the right radial artery. The mediastinoscope should be repositioned if the right radial pressure decreases significantly. This is especially important in patients with a history of cerebral vascular insufficiency. Compression of the right carotid artery during mediastinoscopy has been implicated as a cause of reversible postoperative hemiparesis. It is also important to avoid excessive extension of the neck when the patient is positioned. Using the left arm for invasive or noninvasive blood pressure monitoring and evaluation of the right radial artery by palpation or finger plethysmography has been recommended.[79] Neither of these methods is as sensitive as invasive monitoring of right radial artery pressure, however.

A vasovagal reaction to stretching of the vagus, trachea, or great vessels may cause bradycardia, arrhythmias, and hypotension. Repositioning of the mediastinoscope usually alleviates this response. If the bradycardia persists, however, atropine may be required.

Mediastinoscopy exposes the pulmonary veins to atmospheric air, and a risk of venous air embolism exists, as discussed earlier. In the presence of open mediastinal veins in a patient under local anesthesia, air can be entrained into the pulmonary circulation as negative intrathoracic pressures develop during spontaneous inspiration. Placing the patient in the semi-upright position increases the risk further. Controlled positive-pressure ventilation minimizes the risk. Transesophageal echocardiography (TEE) is a very sensitive and specific monitor for air embolism.[80] TEE can also assist in the management of patients with tumor involvement of the heart, pericardium, or pulmonary outflow tract.[43,59]

Summary

The presence of a mediastinal tumor greatly increases the risk associated with administering anesthesia. A thorough understanding of the underlying pathophysiology and a high index of preoperative suspicion for cardiorespiratory compromise is essential to planning the most appropriate anesthetic management.

References

1. Carlens E. Mediastinoscopy: a method of inspection and tissue biopsy in the superior mediastinum. Chest 1959;36:343.
2. Silverman, NA, Sabiston DC Jr. Mediastinal masses. Surg Clin North Am 1980;60:757.
3. Heimburger IL, Battersby JS. Primary mediastinal tumors of childhood. J Thorac Cardiovasc Surg 1969;50:385.
4. Haller JA Jr, Mazur DO, Morgan WW Jr. Diagnosis and management of mediastinal masses in children. J Thorac Cardiovasc Surg 1969;58:385.
5. Wychulis AR, Payne WS, Clagett OT. Surgical treatment of mediastinal tumors. A 40-year experience. J Thorac Cardiovasc Surg 1971;62:379.
6. Hardy JD, Ewing HP. The Mediastinum. In: Glenn WWL, ed. Thoracic and cardiovascular surgery. Norwalk, Appleton-Century-Crofts, 1983:181.
7. Azizkhan RG, Dudgeon DL, Buck Jr, et al. Life-threatening airway obstruction as a complication to the management of mediastinal masses in children. J Pediatr Surg 1985;20:816.
8. King RM, Telander RL, Smithson WA, et al. Primary mediastinal tumors in children. J Pediatr Surg 1982;17:512.
9. Mandell GA, Lantiere R, Goodman LR. Tracheobronchial compression in Hodgkin's lymphoma in children. Am J Radiol 1982;139:1167.
10. Cosset JM, Henry-Amar M, Carde P, et al. The prognostic significance of large mediastinal masses in the treatment of disease: the experience of the Institut Gustave-Roussy. Hematol Oncol 1984;2:33.
11. Ryoo MC, Kagan AR, Wollin M, et al. Observations on the treatment of mediastinal masses in Hodgkin's disease emphasizing site of failure. Am J Clin Oncol 1987;10:185.
12. Koss MN, Hocholzer L, Nichols PW, et al. Primary non-Hodgkin's lymphoma and pseudolymphoma of lung: a study of 1621 patients. Hum Pathol 1983;14:1024.
13. Adkins RB Jr, Maples MD, Hainsworth JD. Primary malignant mediastinal tumors. Ann Thorac Surg 1984;38:648.
14. Schechter MM. The superior vena caval syndrome. Am J Med Sci 1954;227:46.
15. Sheppard KC. Patient management in critical care: care of the patient with superior vena cava syndrome. Heart Lung 1986;15:636.
16. Roswit B, Kaplan G, Jacobson HG. The superior vena cava obstruction syndrome in bronchogenic carcinoma. Radiology 1953;61:722.
17. Urschel HC, Paulson DL. Superior vena caval canal obstruction. Chest 1966;49:155.
18. Lochridge SK, Knibbe WP, Doty DB. Obstruction of the superior vena cava. Surgery 1979;85:14.

19. Bittar D. Respiratory obstruction associated with induction of general anesthesia in a patient with mediastinal Hodgkin's disease. Anesth Analg 1975;54:399.
20. Tonnesen A, Davis F. Superior vena caval syndrome and bronchial obstruction during anesthesia. Anesthesiology 1976;45:91.
21. Dalby AJ, Forman R. Acquired pulmonary stenosis. S Afr Med J 1979;55:218.
22. Shields JJ, Cho KJ, Geisinger KR. Pulmonary artery constriction by mediastinal lymphoma simulating pulmonary embolus. Am J Roent 1980;135:147.
23. Levin H, Bursztein S, Heifetz M. Cardiac arrest in a child with a mediastinal mass. Anesth Analg 1985; 64:1129.
24. Pokorny WJ, Sherman JO. Mediastinal masses in infants and children. J Thorac Cardiovasc Surg 1974;68:698.
25. Whittaker LD, Lynn HB. Mediastinal tumors and cysts in the pediatric patient. Surg Clin North Am 1973;53:893.
26. Haller JA, Shermeta DW, Donahoo JS, et al. Life-threatening respiratory distress from mediastinal masses in infants. Ann Thorac Surg 1975;19:364.
27. Rubin P, Green J, Holzwasser G. Superior vena caval syndrome. Radiology 1963;81:388.
28. Salsali M, Clifton EE. Superior vena cava obstruction with carcinoma of the lung. Surg Gynecol Obstet 1965;121:783.
29. Green J, Rubin P, Holzwasser G. The experimental production of superior vena caval obstruction. Radiology 1963;81:406.
30. Prakash UBS, Abel MD, Hubmayr RD. Mediastinal mass and tracheal obstruction during general anesthesia. Mayo Clin Proc 1988;63:1004.
31. Neuman G, Weingarten A, Abramowitz R, et al. The anesthetic management of patients with an anterior mediastinal mass. Anesthesiology 1984;60:144.
32. Smergel EM, Wolfson BJ. Chest masses in children: the plain film revisited. J Thorac Imaging 1986;1:59.
33. Shaw EA. Mediastinal tumors causing airway obstruction; incidence and diagnosis in children. Anaesthesia 1983;38:66. Letter.
34. Parish JM, Rosenow EC III, Muhm JR. Mediastinal masses: clues to interpretation of radiological studies. Postgrad Med 1984;76:173.
35. Griscom NT. Computed tomographic determination of tracheal dimensions in children and adolescents. Radiology 1982;145:361.
36. Kirks DR, Fram EK, Volk P, et al. Tracheal compression by mediastinal masses in children: CT evaluation. Am J Radiol 1983;141:647.
37. Siegel MJ, Nadel SN, Glazer HS, et al. Mediastinal lesions in children: comparison of CT and MR. Radiology 1986;160:241.
38. Roskos RR, Evans RC, Gilchrist GS, et al. Prognostic significance of mediastinal masses in childhood Hodgkin's disease. Cancer Treat Rev 1982;66:961.
39. Pullerits J, Holzman R. Anaesthesia for patients with mediastinal masses. Can J Anaesth 1989;36:681.
40. Younker D, Clark R, Coveler L. Fiberoptic endobronchial intubation for resection of an anterior mediastinal mass. Anesthesiology 1989;70:144.
41. Shapiro HM, Sanford TJ, Schaldach AL. Fiberoptic stylet laryngoscope and sitting position for tracheal intubation in acute superior vena caval syndrome. Anesth Analg 1984;63:161.
42. Claus D, Coppens JP. Sonography of mediastinal masses in infants and children. Ann Radiol (Paris) 1984;27:150.
43. Canedo MI, Otken L, Stefadouros MA. Echocardiographic features of cardiac compression by a thymoma simulating cardiac tamponade and obstruction of the superior vena cava. Br Heart J 1977;39:1038.
44. Stoelting RK. Pharmacology and physiology in anesthetic practice. Philadelphia: JB Lippincott, 1987:490.
45. Goldiner P, Carlon GC, Cvitkovic E, et al. Factors influencing postoperative morbidity and mortality in patients treated with bleomycin. BMJ 1987;1:1664.
46. Luna MA, Bedrossain CW, Lichtiger B, et al. Interstitial pneumonitis associated with bleomycin therapy. Am J Clin Pathol 1972;58:501.
47. La Mantia KR, Glick JH, Marshall BE. Supplemental oxygen does not cause respiratory failure in bleomycin-treated surgical patients. Anesthesiology 1984;60:65.
48. Welsh LW, Welsh JJ. Mediastinoscopy: application for hilar adenopathy. Laryngoscope 1973;83:576.
49. Ward PH, Stephenson SE Jr, Harris PF. Exploration of the mediastinum under local anesthesia. Ann Otol Rhin Laryngol 1966;75:368.
50. Harken DE, Black H, Clauss R, et al. A simple cervicomediastinal exploration for tissue diagnosis of intrathoracic disease. With comments on the recognition of inoperable carcinoma of the lung. N Eng J Med 1954;251:1041.
51. Morton JR, Guinn Ga. Mediastinoscopy using local anesthesia. Am J Surg 1971;122:696.
52. Marshall M, Trump D. Acquired extrinsic pulmonic stenosis caused by mediastinal tumors. Cancer 1982;49:1496.

53. Ferrari LR, Bedford RF. General anesthesia prior to treatment of anterior mediastinal masses in pediatric cancer patients. Anesthesiology 1990;72:991.
54. Loeffler JS, Leopold KA, Recht A, et al. Emergency prebiopsy radiation for mediastinal masses: impact on subsequent pathological diagnosis and outcome. J Clin Oncol 1986;4:716.
55. Tinker TD, Crane DL. Safety of anesthesia for patients with anterior mediastinal masses: I. Anesthesiology 1990;73:1060.
56. Zornow MH, Benumof JL. Safety of anesthesia for patients with anterior mediastinal masses: II. Anesthesiology 1990;73:1061.
57. Greengrass R. Anesthesia and mediastinal masses. Can J Anaesth 1990;37:596.
58. Hall KD, Friedman M. Extracorporeal oxygenation for induction of anesthesia in a patient with an intrathoracic tumor. Anesthesiology 1975; 42:493.
59. Keon TP. Death on induction of anesthesia for cervical node biopsy. Anesthesiology 1981; 55:471.
60. Halpern S, Chatten J, Meadown AT, et al. Anterior mediastinal masses: anesthesia hazards and other problems. J Pediatr 1983;102:407.
61. Fassoulaki A. Anaesthesia for mediastinoscopy. Anaesthesia 1978; 34:75.
62. Vaughn RS. Anaesthesia for mediastinoscopy. Anaesthesia 1987;33:195.
63. John RE, Narang VPS. A boy with anterior mediastinal mass. Anaesthesia 1988;43:864.
64. Bray RJ, Fernandes FJ. Mediastinal tumour airway obstruction in anesthetized children. Anaesthesia 1982;37:571.
65. de Soto H. Direct laryngoscopy as an aid to relieve airway obstruction in a patient with a mediastinal mass. Anesthesiology 1987;67:116.
66. Todres ID, Reppert SM, Walker PF, et al. Management of critical airway obstruction in a child with a mediastinal tumor. Anesthesiology 1976; 45:100.
67. Piro AJ, Weiss DR, Hellman S. Mediastinal Hodgkin's disease: a possible danger for intubation anesthesia. Int J Radiat Oncol Bio Phys 1976;1:415.
68. Amaha K, Okutsu Y, Nakamuru Y. Major airway obstruction by mediastinal tumour. A case report. Br J Anaesth 1973;45:1082.
69. Shambaugh BE, Seed R, Korn A. Airway obstruction in substernal goiter. Clinical and therapeutic implications. J Chro Dis 1973;26:737.
70. Sibert KS, Biondi JW, Hirsch NP. Spontaneous respiration during thoracotomy in a patient with a mediastinal mass. Anesth Analg 1987; 66:904.
71. Prosnitz LR, Curtis AM, Knowlton AH, et al. Subdiaphragmatic Hodgkin's disease: significance of large mediastinal masses. Int J Radiot Oncol Bio Phys 1980; 6:809.
71. Gordon RA. Anesthetic management of patients with airway problems. Int Anesthesiol Clin 1972; 10:37.
72. Ashbaugh DG. Mediastinoscopy. Arch Surg 1970; 100:568.
73. Roberts JT, Gissen AJ. Management of complications encountered during anesthesia for mediastinoscopy. Anesth Rev 1979;6:31.
74. Weissberg D, Herczed E. Perforation of thoracic aortic aneurysm—a complication of mediastinoscopy. Chest 1980;78:119.
75. Lee CM, Grossman LB. Laceration of left pulmonary artery during mediastinoscopy. Anesth Analg 1979;56:226.
76. Vueghs JM, Schurink GA, Vaes L, et al. Anesthesia in repeat mediastinoscopy: a retrospective study of 101 patients. J Cardiothorac Vasc Anesth 1992;6:193.
77. Provost PE, Oliver P, Schwaber JR. Mediastinoscopy. Surg Clin North Am 1973;53:327.
78. Furgang FA, Saidman LJ. Bilateral tension pneumothorax associated with mediastinoscopy. J Thorac Cardiovasc Surg 1972;63:329.
79. Petty C. Right radial artery pressure during mediastinoscopy. Anesth Analg 1979;58:428.
80. Cucchiara RF, Nugent M, Seward JB, et al. Air embolism in upright neurosurgical patients: detection and localization by two-dimensional transesophageal echocardiography. Anesthesiology 1984;60:353.

CHAPTER

19

Anesthetic Management of Bullae Resection

Edmond Cohen

Bullae are air-containing, thin-wall cavities within the lung parenchyma that result from the destruction of alveolar tissue.[1,2] These giant air-containing cysts arise from a relatively small volume of lung tissue and expand to many times the volume of their original lung parenchymal source because of trapping of inspired air. Bullae are usually large enough to be seen on a plain chest x-ray, and a computed tomography (CT) scan confirms the presence of an area that lacks lung markings (Fig. 19-1). The cavity walls are composed of connective tissue septa, visceral pleura, and compressed lung parenchyma as a result of the cavity expansion.[3] The cause of most cases of giant bullous emphysema is unknown. Histologic studies show no pathogenic changes. Visceroparietal adhesions are usually absent and allow the bullae to expand. In most cases the cysts have some communication with the bronchial tree; otherwise the gas within them would be absorbed and the walls would then collapse. Because the communication with the bronchial tree is present, a pneumothorax that results from rupture of either a single air-containing cyst, or bulla, or from small, widespread multiple cysts, is likely to develop tension.

Isolated cysts are usually congenital, whereas the acquired cysts are multiple. Cysts are bronchogenic, postinfective (most often following staphylococcal pneumonia), or as a result of a degenerative emphysematous disease.[4–6] The congenital or infantile form, in which a single lobe is practically replaced by multiple air-filled cysts (vanishing lobe), is rare and usually presents in infancy.[7] Cysts that occur during infancy are valvular in nature and are manifested by respiratory distress and reluctance to feed.

Air cysts, which have their own epithelial margins, may be associated with chronic obstructive lung disease (COPD) or may be found in the absence of pulmonary pathology. In contrast to the usual diffuse changes in most forms of emphysema, bullous emphysema is an exaggerated local anatomical condition. Bullae can be considered a zone of an end-stage emphysematous destruction of lung parenchyma. They generally enlarge with age due to a one-way valvular mechanism; an increasing amount of air trapping occurs within the cavity. Ting et al.[8] studied the mechanical properties of the bullae in human lung preparation. Analysis of the pressure-volume relationship of a thick-walled lung cyst showed little elastic resistance

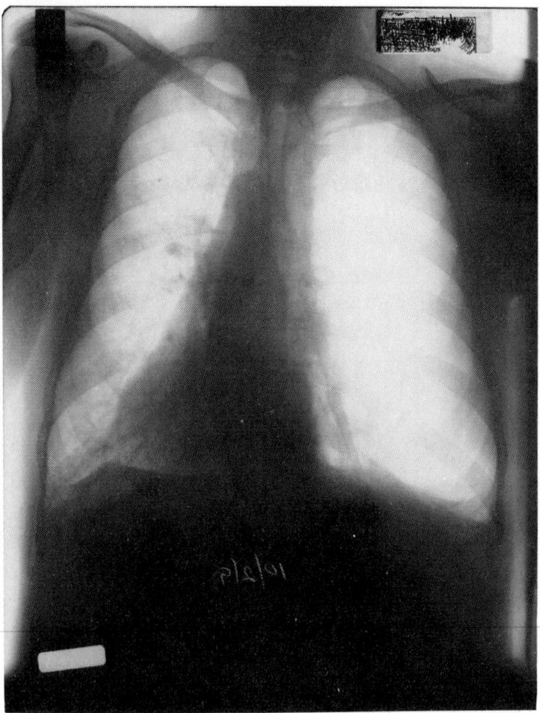

Figure 19-1. A chest x-ray showing a giant air-filled cyst occupying most of the right hemithorax. (From: Gothard JWW. Anesthesia for thoracic surgery. 2nd ed. Oxford: Blackwell Scientific Publications, 1993:176.)

(Fig. 19-2). This type of cyst increases in volume during inspiration, however, since the bullae opening can inflate but not deflate when compressed during inflation. A positive intra-cystic pressure develops. This valvelike effect maintains the bullae in a state of inflation or may lead to the cyst rupture, causing pneumothorax.

In contrast, the thin-walled lung cyst (Fig. 19-3) has the mechanical characteristics of a paper bag (ie, it can be ballooned up to its maximal volume with little pressure). These mechanical characteristics explain the prevalence distribution of the tidal volume into the cyst. When the compliance for both the lung and a bulla reached equal values, the volume of the bulla fails to increase further, but the bulla does develop an intracystic pressure greater than that of the surrounding lung. This explains the various degrees of compression of the surrounding lung caused by bullae.

Indications for Bullectomy*

The key concept underlying indication for surgery is the presence of significant compression of the surrounding nonbullous lung tissue by the expanding bullae. The underlying problem is mechanical and amenable to surgical resection of one or more bullae. Although emphysema may involve all of the lung tissue, elimination of the bullous cystic areas allows the compressed tissue to expand and function in gas exchange and alleviates dyspnea. Indications for bullectomy in the patients with COPD include intolerable shortness of breath despite full medical regime, incapacitating dyspnea and oxygen dependency, rapidly enlarging

* Based on Kirschner PA. The surgeon view. In: Cohen E, Kirschner PA, Benumof JL: Simultaneous bilateral bullectomy for bullous emphysema with severe pulmonary insufficiency. J Cardiothorac Vasc Anesth 1990;4:119.

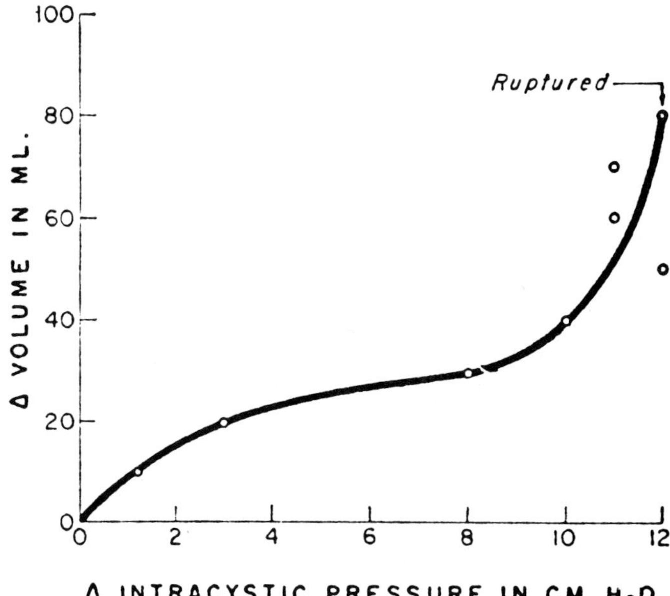

Figure 19-2. The pressure-volume curve of a thick-walled lung cyst (congenital). The characteristics of this curve show little elastic resistance. This type of cyst increases in volume during inspiration, however, since the bullae opening can inflate but not deflate when compressed during inflation; a positive intracystic pressure develops. This valvelike effect maintains the bullae in a state of inflation or leads to rupture of the cyst with pneumothorax. (Used with permission from Ting et al.[8])

Figure 19-3. The pressure-volume curve of a thin-walled cyst and its adjacent lung. When the compliance for both the lung and a bullae reach equal values, the bullae fail to increase further volume but develop an intracystic pressure greater than that of the surrounding lung. This explains the various degrees of compression of the surrounding lung caused by the bullae. (Used with permission from Ting et al.[8])

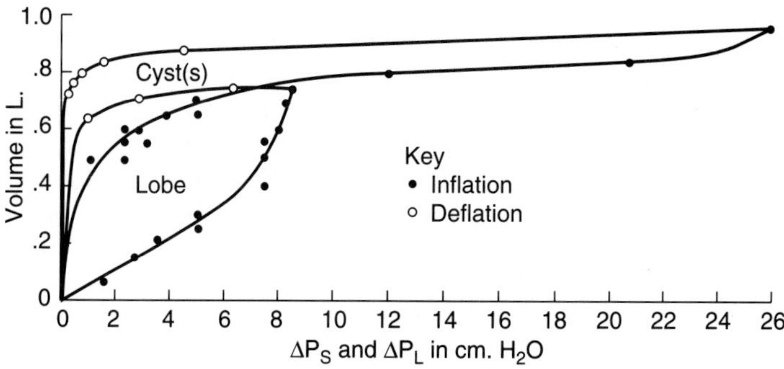

bullae, or the repeated incidence of pneumothorax.

Compression can be graphically documented in three ways: first,

1. Simple inspiration-expiration chest x-rays, which demonstrate the air trapping on expiration with almost no change in the diaphragm position. The large, lucent bullae remain expanded.
2. Visualization of the pulmonary circulation by angiogram, which shows a crowding of the vessels due to compression of the nonbullous lung tissue, indicating the effects of pressure thereon by the tense bullae.
3. Radioisotope studies, which demonstrate the functional impairment if the compress area has adequate perfusion but significantly compromised ventilation.

Potgieter et al. elected to use the bronchogram to asses compression in the belief that the anatomical status of the bronchi may be more informative than the vascular pattern.[9] Those patients who presented with a bronchiectasis on the bronchogram were excluded from having surgical resection, most likely because these patients must have some associated pulmonary fibrosis that prevents adequate reexpansion without benefit from surgery.

Regardless of the degree of pulmonary insufficiency, if a pulmonary parenchymal compression can be evident, the indication for surgical correction is clear-cut. Surgical resection eliminates cystic bullous areas while sparing nonbullous lung tissue. The nonbullous lung tissue will function better in a state of normal volume than when it is markedly compressed.[10–13] A bullectomy is often sufficient to achieve the goal. An anatomical segmental resection, or even a complete lobectomy, may rarely be needed. It should be clearly emphasized that lobectomy most likely implies not removal of functional lung parenchyma but to a nonexistent lobe. This lobe is a nonfunctional part of the lung because the entire lobe has been transformed into bullae.

Unilateral bullectomy is the most common procedure. Until a few years ago, bilateral bullectomy was performed in stages, one site at the time, using conventional posterolateral incisions. Only a unilateral operation was often required because of a significant improvement after one side, usually the worst, was operated upon. Now, with increasing experience, bilateral bullectomy can be carry out simultaneously through a sternal split. Pleural abrasion, which fosters visceroparietal adhesion, has become an integral part of a bullectomy.

Surgical Outcome

A few long-term, follow-up studies of patients who underwent bullectomy are present in the literature. Hughes et al. reported a four-year follow-up in 11 patients, both smokers and ex-smokers, who had undergone bullectomy.[14] All lung function variables declined at a greater rate in those patients who continued to smoke. In ex-smokers, no significant decline or an improvement was noted.

Potgieter et al. reported the surgical outcome of 21 patients with bolus emphysema.[9] Four of six patients with preoperative hypercapnia survived and showed improvement after the surgery. The remaining 15 patients improved symptomatically following surgery with increased forced expiratory volume in 1 second (FEV_1) and vital capacity. In this study five of six patients with an FEV_1 of less than 1 liter showed a postoperative increase of more than 0.3 of a liter, and nine of 13 patients with FEV_1 of more than 1 liter had an change of more than 0.3 liter in FEV_1 (Fig. 19-4). In all patients, positive response to surgical removal of bullae could be predicted if the contribution caused by

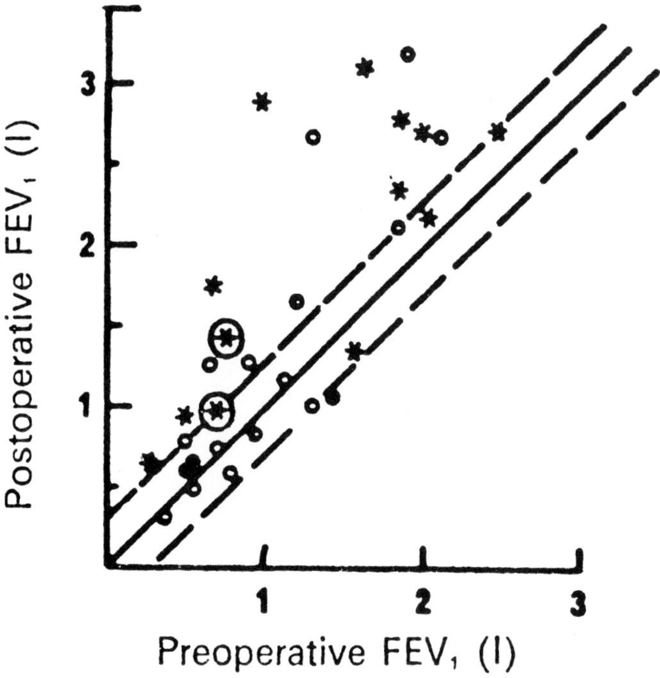

Figure 19-4. Pre- and postoperative FEV_1 of 13 patients from Potgieter et al.[9] (•) and from 18 patients from Pride et al.[29](*) - = line of identity, — = ±0.31 ○ = bronchiectasis on preoperative bronchogram. (Used with permission from Potgieter et al.[9])

the bullae as opposed to that caused by associated obstructive lung disease were possible to determine. As predicted, in these patients with preoperative compressed lung, the best results were obtained subsequent to reexpansion.

Laros et al. reported on 27 emphysematous patients who underwent unilateral (10 patients) or bilateral (17 patients) bullectomy.[15] In all patients, the bullae occupied over 50% of the hemithorax. Bullectomy significantly decreased dyspnea and enable the patients to preform their daily activities. The mean survival postresection time was greater than seven years.

Takashi and colleagues reported experiences with 12 patients who had simultaneous bilateral resection of bullous emphysema by median sternotomy.[16] Drawings of admission chest x-ray films showing the age, sex, and the grade of dyspnea (from I, the mildest stage, to IV the most severe form) of the patients are shown in Figure 19-5. The researchers' criteria for selection for surgery were (1) The bullous lesion occupied more than one-third of the thoracic cavity; (2) the patient experienced a relatively severe degree of shortness of breath; and (3) monitoring of the cyst revealed progressive increases in size. A full lung expansion occurred in all 12 patients. All patients showed reduction in the severity of the dyspnea (Fig. 19-6) associated with marked increase in vital capacity and FEV_1.

The prognosis after surgery depends on several factors, including (1) the patient age, (2) patient smoking history, (3) status of the non-

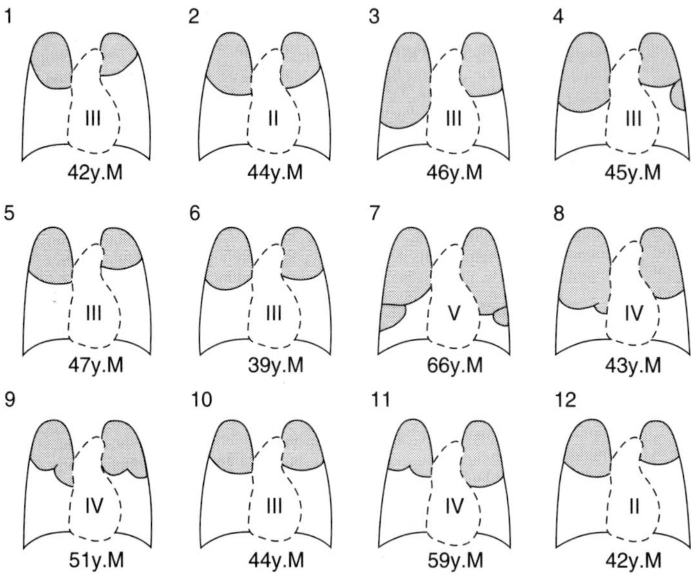

Figure 19-5. Drawings of admission chest x-ray films showing the age, sex, and the grade of dyspnea of 12 patients. The hatched area represents the emphysematous bullous lesions. The roman numerals indicate the grade of dyspnea and range from I (mildest form) to IV (most severe form).

bullous lung or the degree of diffuse emphysema present, (4) cardiac status either secondary to the bullous emphysema (eg, cor pulmonale) or unrelated disease (eg, coronary artery disease, valvular pathology), (5) degree of bronchiectasis, (6) degree of pulmonary infection and bronchitis, and (7) postoperative complications.

Despite all these variables and associate pathology, some patients have shown remarkable improvement that lasted for years after the surgery.[17–19]

Anesthetic Management

The anesthetic management of patients with bullae who are scheduled for bullectomy or have coincidental bullae and are undergoing unrelated surgery is challenging. Most of these patients have severe generalized chronic lung disease with little or no ventilatory reserve. Such patients often present with hypoxemia, hypercarbia, polycythemia, cor pulmonale, and are at increase risk for pneumothorax.

Several important issues should be considered during the anesthetic management of a bullectomy.

During anesthesia, the bullae can further expand as a result of the application of positive-pressure ventilation, because in most cases, the bullae communicate with the bronchial tree. The overinflation produces further compression of the surrounding lung tissue or mediastinal shift, which leads to kinking of the vena cava and hypotension analogous to a tension pneumothorax.

LaPlace's law states that the pressure within a bulla equals two times the value of the bulla

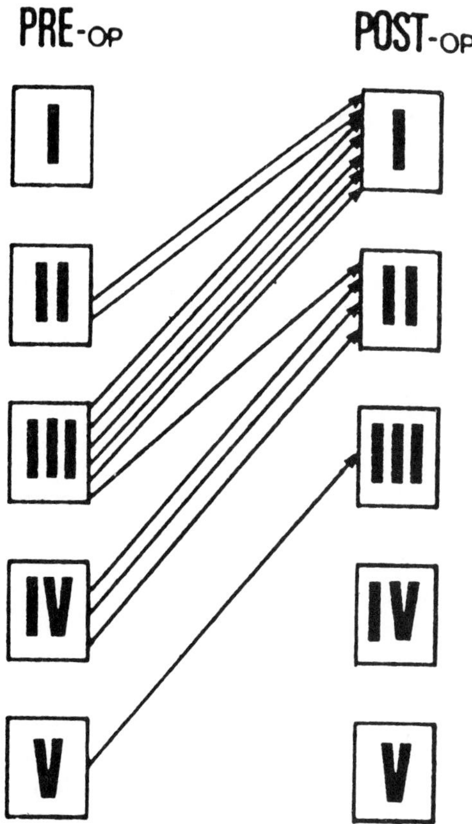

Figure 19-6. The postoperative improvement of subjective symptoms of dyspnea. The roman numerals indicate the grade of dyspnea and range from I (mildest form) to IV (most severe form) (Used with permission from Potgieter et al.[9])

wall tension divided by its radius (the distending pressure [P] inside the bullae is given as P = 2T/R, where T is the surface tension and R is the radius). A larger bulla with a greater radius has a lower internal pressure, and therefore, offers lower resistance to applied positive-pressure ventilation. Because of the low resistance, a large bulla tends to increase in size, since most of the applied tidal volume is delivered to the communicating bullae during positive-pressure ventilation.[20] When a significant portion of the tidal volume enters the bulla cavity, alveolar dead space ventilation is greatly increased. If this wasted ventilation is not compensated by an increase in minute ventilation, hypercarbia, acidosis, and hypoxemia follow. This complication is more likely to occur in a patient with an open chest, where the bulla is no longer confined by the integrity of the chest wall.

Noncommunicating bullae rapidly enlarge during nitrous oxide anesthesia because transfer of nitrous oxide from the blood into air-filled bullae may be 34 times greater than the rate at which nitrogen is removed.[21] The use of nitrous oxide in a patient with bullous disease should be avoided, and a high inspired oxygen concentration should be maintained. This is particularly true in a patient with poor communication with the bronchial tree.

Most importantly, expansion of the bullae and a buildup in pressure with overdistension of the bullae can result in rupture and a pneumothorax. This can be life-threatening in a patient with marginal gas exchange. Pneumothorax can be detected by further diminution in breath sounds on the affected side in addition to tachycardia, hypotension, and increased peak airway pressure. Hemodynamic instability is secondary to the impairment of venous return and decline in cardiac output.

Endotracheal Intubation: Spontaneous Breathing versus Paralysis

During general anesthesia for patients with bullous disease, excessive positive-pressure ventilation should be avoided. This can be achieved by inducing the patients to reach a depth of anesthesia that permits endotracheal intubation without paralysis while they spontaneously breathe inhaled anesthetic. Awake intubation with topical anesthesia is an alternative method to avoid positive-pressure ventilation. If paralysis is used, gentle manual ventilation should be applied to limit the peak airway pressure between 10–12 cm H_2O. With manual ventilation, sufficient time for expiration reduces air trapping within the bullae. Expiratory retard prevents airway collapse and can maintain patency of bullae, thereby reducing air trapping. Negative end-expiratory pressure should be avoided because it invariably produces proximal airway collapse and air trapping.[22] In addition, a slow inspiratory flow rate reduces peak airway pressure and decreases the risk of barotrauma.

Reports of both intubation techniques for bullae resection are in the literature. Cote[7], and Isenhower[20] accomplished the intubation in spontaneously breathing patients, and Benumof[23] and Caseby[22] reported intubation following paralysis. Insertion of a double lumen tube during spontaneous respiration to reduce excessive positive pressure into the diseased lung is indispensable for unilateral bullae. In that case, combining spontaneous breathing with immediate postintubation isolation may be the method of choice to protect the diseased lung from excessive pressure. If intubation is being performed in a paralyzed patient, rapid relaxation with the use of succinylcholine is desirable. This avoids any prolonged period of forced positive-pressure ventilation before intubation and lung isolation for unilateral bullae or until sternal split in case of bilateral bullae resection.

The surgeon should be gloved and gowned, and the patient should be prepared and draped to facilitate immediate decompression of any pneumothorax occurring during the induction of anesthesia. The pneumothorax can be promptly decompressed by the insertion of a chest tube. Such insertion may, however, create a large bronchopleural fistula that diverts most of the tidal volume into the tube. High-frequency ventilation with low tidal volumes and a low peak airway pressure has been successfully used to avoid rupture of the bullae from excessive pressure.[24,25] If a sternal split is planned, it should be performed as rapidly as possible after the induction of anesthesia.

Single-Lumen Tubes versus Double-Lumen Endobronchial Tubes

Resection of bilateral bullae may not be an absolute indication for the use of a double-lumen endobronchial tube, however. Resection of unilateral bullae should be performed using a double-lumen tube. For resection of bilateral bullae, a double-lumen tube allows differential treatment of the lung to maximize gas exchange and to increase capability to treat the ruptured bullae. A single-lumen tube can also be used.[7–9] Using a single-lumen tube for resection of bilateral bullae carries the risk of bilateral pneumothorax during induction with cardiorespiratory collapse.

ADVANTAGES OF DOUBLE-LUMEN TUBES.† In the great majority of thoracic surgery cases, the use of double-lumen tube has very low risk and potentially high benefits. If the vocal cords can be seen, the simple insertion of the double-lumen tube should be no more traumatic than insertion of a single-lumen tube. If a fiberoptic bronchoscope is used, the double-lumen tube can be located in the correct position with great precision. Post double-lumen tube intubation complications are relatively rare. Intubation with a double-lumen tube compared with a single-lumen tube may be more difficult and time-consuming because of the need to ensure proper placement, but excluding malpositioning, it should have little added risk.

† Based on commentary by JL Benumof. In: Cohen E, Kirschner PA, Benumof JL: Simultaneous bilateral bullectomy for bullous emphysema with severe pulmonary insufficiency. J Cardiothrac Vasc Anesth 1990;4:119.

Using a double-lumen tube has several benefits. This tube affords complete control of each lung independent of the other and allows treatment of each lung in any manner desired. The two lungs may be treated with any combination or permutation of intermittent positive-pressure ventilation (IPPV), IPPV plus positive end-expiratory pressure (PEEP), large tidal volume ventilation, sighing, high-frequency ventilation (HFV), induction of complete atelectasis, continuous positive airway pressure (CPAP), suctioning, and other medical therapy (saline lavage, administration of vasoconstrictors, etc). It is a misconception to think that insertion of a double-lumen tube necessarily implies one-lung ventilation. Ventilation of both lungs is also possible (eg, two-lung IPPV with any desired tidal volume either to both lungs or to one lung. Consequently, the fact that both lungs are diseased should have nothing to do with the choice of a double-lumen versus a single-lumen tube.

A double-lumen tube is essential where the risk of rupture of giant bullae during the induction and initial phases of general anesthesia is significant. The occurrence of bilateral rupture of bullae with a closed chest has never been reported, so it is reasonable to argue that rupture, if it occurred, would be unilateral. A double-lumen tube would permit the cessation of ventilation of the ruptured side and thereby minimize the tension of the pneumothorax in that hemithorax. This would allow continued careful ventilation of the unaffected side until the pneumothorax could be decompressed by needle aspiration, chest tube insertion, or thoracotomy. With a single-lumen tube, differential treatment is difficult.

In addition, double-lumen tube permits one-lung ventilation, thereby facilitating surgical exposure. If it is feared that a relatively large tidal volume delivered to the ventilated lung may cause barotrauma, however, $PaCO_2$ can be maintained by decreasing the tidal volume and increasing the respiratory rate. If one-lung ventilation lowers PaO_2 excessively, then hypoxemia can be easily reversed in two ways: (1) with application of CPAP to the nonventilated lung or (2) by ventilating the operative lung with a small, rapid tidal volume. Similarly, if one-lung ventilation causes an increase in pulmonary vascular resistance because of nonventilated operative lung hypoxic pulmonary vasoconstriction, the resistance may be decreased by small tidal volume ventilation or CPAP applied to the operative lung.

Suture or staple lines can be selectively tested for airleaks against a known high pressure at any time without increasing lung volume on the nonresected side. A double-lumen tube permits selective lung suctioning, which may be very important in managing these severely diseased lungs, or can be used postoperatively for differential lung ventilation.

DISADVANTAGES OF DOUBLE-LUMEN TUBES. Several problems may be associated with use of a double-lumen tube. One-lung ventilation implies delivering the entire tidal volume into one lung, which may result in barotrauma. Reduction of tidal volume to reduce peak airway pressure can result in accumulation of CO_2. During one-lung ventilation the transpulmonary shunt through the nonventilated lung may result in hypoxemia, as reported by Benumof.[23] In a case of bilateral bullectomy using a double-lumen tube, one-lung ventilation resulted in hypoxemia (PaO_2, = 52 mmHg) and necessitated application of CPAP to the nonventilated lung, which increased PaO_2 to 132 mmHg. This degree of hypoxemia was expected because the patient depended on an extensively diseased lung and had marginal ability to maintain adequate gas exchange. One-lung ventilation can cause an increase in pulmonary vascular resistance because of hypoxic pulmonary vasoconstriction (HPV). Presumably, HPV reduces the degree of shunt to the nonventilated lung.[28,29] Such an increase in pulmonary vascular resistance can be significant in a patient with associated cardiac disease or cor pulmonale.

Case Presentation‡

A 59-year-old, oxygen-dependent man with severe, giant, bullous emphysema was admitted for pulmonary angiography and possible pulmonary (bullae) resection. His extensive bilateral bullae had been followed for many years, and his emphysematous symptomatology had become progressively more severe and symptomatic in the past 20 years. During this time the man experienced increasing exertional dyspnea associated with reduced exercise tolerance to the point that he was forced to retire from work at the age of 49. He also had a 30-year history of heavy smoking.

At 53 years of age, the man sustained an acute myocardial infarction. Coronary angiography showed total occlusion of the left anterior descending artery, 30% occlusion of the circumflex artery, and moderately impaired left ventricular function with apical akinesia. His ejection fraction was estimated to be 40%. Because of his severe pulmonary disease, he was not considered to be a suitable candidate for coronary artery bypass grafting. Recovery was complicated by congestive heart failure and repeated episodes of ventricular tachycardia. After discharge, his recovery was complicated by congestive heart failure and repeated episodes of ventricular tachycardia. After discharge, his exercise tolerance was further reduced. He now required continuous supplemental nasal oxygen. Occasionally he was excessively short of breath following consumption of a large meal. During the year prior to this admission, he was hospitalized twice for respiratory failure secondary to pulmonary infection.

Medication at the time of admission included digoxin, 0.125 mg once daily; procainamide, 250 mg three times daily; transdermal nitroglycerin, 5 mg once daily; sublingual nitroglycerin, 0.4 mg as required; nifedipine, 10 mg twice daily; isosorbide dinitrate, 10 mg three times daily; furosemide, 40 mg once daily; dipyridamole, 25 mg twice daily; beclomethasone, 2 puffs three times a day; and albuterol, 2 puffs three times a day. Despite this drug regimen, dyspnea at rest increased further, confining him to a bed-and-chair existence with continuous oxygen therapy.

On admission, the 78-kg man was dyspneic and tachypneic at rest despite continuous oxygen supplementation. He was unable to complete an average sentence because of severe shortness of breath and had perioral and peripheral nailbed cyanosis. He was afebrile, with a pulse of 75 beats/min and a respiratory rate of 28 breaths/min. Blood pressure was 130/85 mmHg with no pulsus paradoxus. Anterior-posterior diameter of the chest was increased, with significant intercostal retractions during inspiration. There were no breath sounds over the middle and upper lung fields, both anterior and posterior; distant breath sounds and diffuse inspiratory rates were heard at both bases. Heart sounds were distant, but no murmur or gallop were heard. The jugular veins were distended. Peripheral pulses were intact bilaterally without peripheral edema.

Results of an arterial blood gas analysis obtained during oxygen administration at 3 L/min via nasal prongs were pH, 7.4; $PaCO_2$, 38 mmHg; PaO_2, 46 mmHg; and base excess, +0.1. Blood chemistry was normal, except for a

‡From Cohen E, Kirschner PA, Benumof JL. Simultaneous bilateral bullectomy for bullous emphysema with severe pulmonary insufficiency. J Cardiothorac Vasc Anesth 1990;4:119.

slightly elevated bilirubin of 1.3 mg/dL. Prothrombin time was 13.5/11.5 seconds and partial thromboplastin time was 52.4/43.8 seconds. The hematocrit was 54.8% and hemoglobin concentration was 18.9 g/L. The electrocardiogram showed normal sinus rhythm, an occasional premature ventricular complex, a nonspecific T wave abnormality, and evidence of bilateral atrial enlargement.

Chest roentgenograms (Fig. 19-7) showed bilateral giant bullae occupying the middle and upper thirds of the lung fields. Vascular crowding and increased lung markings were observed at the bases. The expiration film showed air trapping in the bullae with no change in their volume, whereas the nonbullous basal portions of the lungs were empty of air. Pulmonary angiography (Fig. 19-8) showed absent vasculature in the bullous areas. Extreme crowding and depression of the pulmonary arteries were apparent in the basal portions of the lungs, indicating compression of lung tissue.

The results of two pulmonary function tests (PFTs), spirometry and plethysmography, are shown in Figure 19-9. The forced vital capacity (FVC) markedly decreased to 40% of the predicted value, the forced expiratory volume in 1 second (FEV_1) was 25% of the predicted value, and the forced mid-expiratory flow rate ($FEF_{25\%-75\%}$) was only 10% of the predicted value. Severe hyperinflation was evidenced by a residual volume (RV) of 169% of the predicted value and an increased ratio of RV to total lung capacity (TLC) of 72%.

In view of the severity of the progressive dyspnea and confinement to bed, and despite the man's compromised cardiac status, he was scheduled for bilateral bullectomy via median sternotomy. On the morning of surgery he received his usual medications and 10 mg of oral

Figure 19-7. Preoperative chest radiograph during (A) inspiration and (B) expiration. Huge bilateral bullae occupy the upper 90% of both lung fields. The absent of diaphragmatic motion, air trapping in bullae, and the compression of functional lung tissue inferiorly are evident.

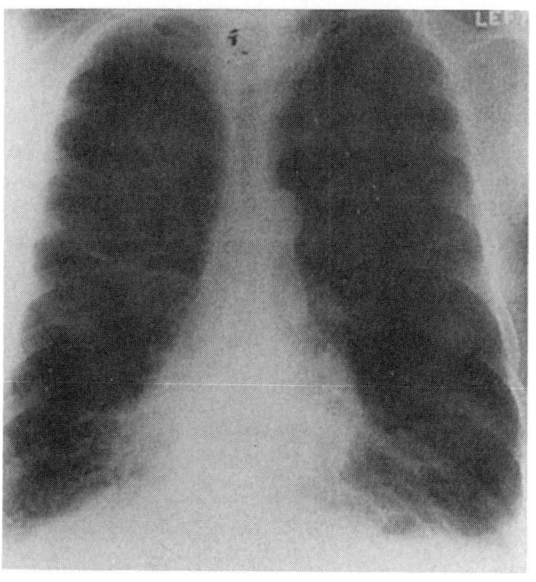

A

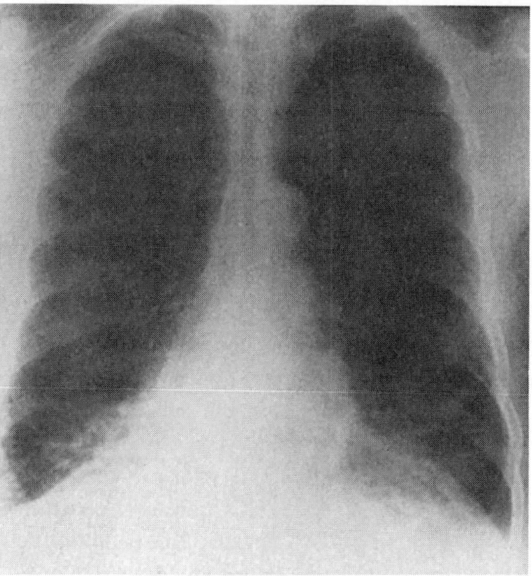

B

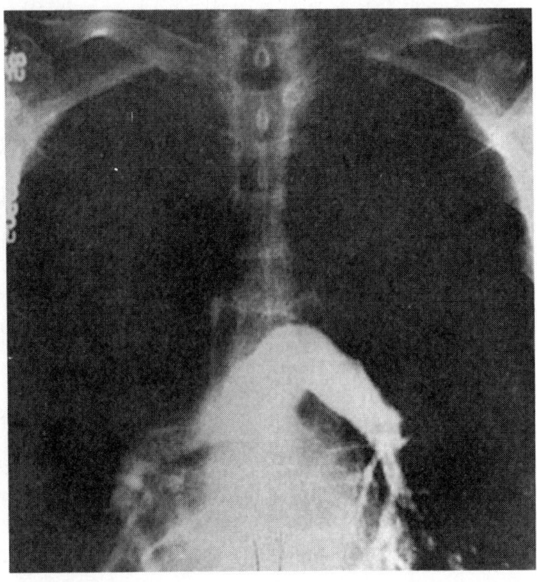

Figure 19-8. Pulmonary angiogram showing marked depression and basal crowding of the pulmonary vasculature and absent circulation in the bullae.

diazepam. Upon arrival in the operating room, a V_5 electrocardiogram lead and a pulse oximeter were placed. A 20-gauge radial artery catheter and a 7.5F Oximetrix pulmonary arterial catheter (Abbott Critical Care Systems, Mountain View, CA) were inserted via the right internal jugular vein for continuous monitoring of arterial oxygen level and mixed venous oxygen saturation (SvO_2). Esophageal temperature, airway pressure was also monitored. Tidal volume measurements were checked by spirometry.

Before the induction of anesthesia, the patient was prepared and draped, and the surgeon was fully gloved and gowned, ready to perform an immediate sternal split. This precaution was taken in the event of pneumothorax or other untoward event developing during induction of anesthesia because of pulmonary overinflation. Hemodynamic and gas exchange measurements were performed before the induction of anesthesia and during the remainder of

Figure 19-9. Preoperative pulmonary function tests and lung volume. Note the increase in RV due to the giant bullae, with associated severe reduction of all the functional parameters. The $FEF_{25\%-75\%}$ was reduced to 10% of its predicted values.

		ACTUAL	PRED	% PRED
SPIROMETRY				
FVC	(L)	1.94	4.81	40
FEV1	(L)	0.85	3.39	25
FEV1/FVC		0.44	0.71	62
FEV 0.5	(L)	0.63		
FEV 3	(L)	1.37		
FEF25–75	(L/S)	0.32	3.21	10
PEAK FLOW	(L/S)	4.11		
FEF 50	(L)	0.43		
FEF50/FVC		0.22		
FEF 75	(L/S)	0.30		
FEF75/FVC		0.15		
MVV	(L/M)	38.40	110.27	35
PLETHYSMOGRAPHY				
SLOW VC	(L)	1.94	4.81	40
FRC	(L)	5.70		
ERV	(L)	0.75		
RV	(L)	4.95	2.93	169
TLC	(L)	6.89	7.74	89
RV/TLC		0.72		

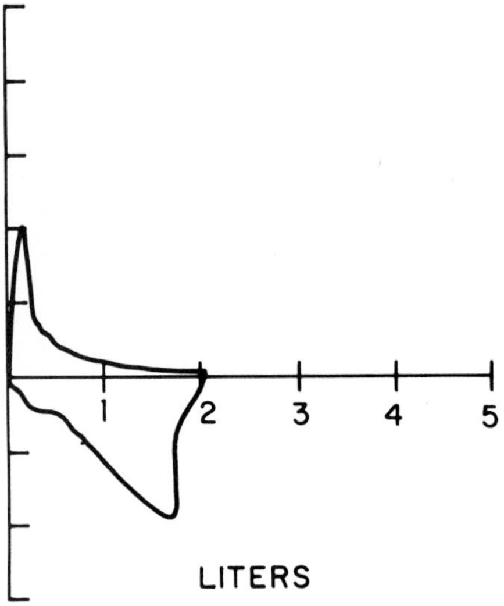

the procedure; these measurements are reported in Table 19-1.

After preoxygenation, anesthesia was induced with the intravenous administration of fentanyl, 500 μg, and thiopental, 125 mg. Intubation was facilitated with the intravenous administration of succinylcholine, 100 mg. Before intubation, ventilation was controlled manually by gentle compression of the anesthesia bag to allow a peak positive inspiratory pressure of between 12 and 15 cm H_2O. A delivered tidal volume of between 200 and 220 mL was measured by the spirometer at the expiratory limb. The trachea was intubated with an 8-mm, single-lumen endotracheal tube. Anesthesia was maintained with isoflurane, oxygen, and fentanyl, and divided doses of metubine were used for relaxation. Following intubation, a slight decrease in blood pressure from 140/80 to 115/80 mmHg was noted, and PaO_2 increased to 283 mmHg (Table 20-1). SvO_2 increased from 67% (preinduction) to 88% (postinduction).

The sternum was split and sternal retractors were placed within 10 minutes. First the right pleural cavity was opened; extensive bullous emphysema, which occupied most of the upper and middle lobes of the lung, bulged into the incision. The right lower lobe was relatively normal in spite of being compressed and displaced inferiorly. In contrast, the right upper and middle lobes were markedly emphysematous. The bullae were delivered out of the chest (Fig. 19-10) and removed using a TIA stapler. Following excision of the right bullae, PaO_2 increased further to 427 mmHg. Hemodynamic values remained essentially unchanged, whereas SvO_2 increased to 96%. An increased tidal volume of 300 mL was manually delivered with a peak airway pressure of 15 cm H_2O. Respiratory rate was adjusted to maintain $PaCO_2$ at 45 cm H_2O.

The left pleura was opened and again giant bullous disease involving the entire upper lobe was delivered into the field and surgically removed. The deflated specimen of the resected bullae is shown in Figure 19-11. Because no clear demarcation between normal lung and bullous disease was identifiable in either lung, surgical judgment was used to determine the extent of diseased lung to be removed. Not all of the bullous areas could be resected because they blended almost imperceptibly into relatively normal lung.

After the bullous regions were removed, a bilateral pleural abrasion was performed. Following the left bullectomy, hemodynamic values and gas exchange stabilized; the SvO_2 was 90%. The patient was mechanically ventilated with a tidal volume of 500 mL and a peak airway pressure between 15 and 18 cm H_2O. Before closure of the chest, bilateral chest tubes were placed. Both lungs were reexpanded with a peak airway pressure of 40 cm H_2O to confirm the absence of air leaks.

The patient was then transferred to the intensive care unit and was extubated that evening. He was hemodynamically stable and had satisfactory arterial blood gas values. He remained in the intensive care unit overnight and was then transferred to the ward. Postoperative chest x-rays showed good expansion of the previously compressed lungs (Fig. 19-12).

The patient made a remarkably good recovery following surgery. Arterial blood gas analysis obtained while the patient breathed room air showed a pH of 7.43, a $PaCO_2$ of 52 mmHg, and a PaO_2 of 64 mmHg. After discharge on the eighth postoperative day he improved objectively, was able to walk up and down the corridor without difficulty, and carried out his daily activities without the need for oxygen.

Two months later, blood gas analysis showed a pH of 7.39, a $PaCO_2$ of 33 mmHg, a PaO_2 of 62 mmHg, and a SaO_2 of 91%. Comparison of the preoperative pulmonary function tests with those performed 2 months and 1 year post-

Table 19-1. Hemodynamics and Oxygenation During Bullectomy*

Time (AM) of Event	8:10 Preinduction: O_2—Cannula	8:30 Preinduction: O_2—Mask	9:00 Postinduction: Intubated	9:15 Postresection: R/Bullae	9:30 Postresection: L/Bullae	10:00 Chest Closed	10:40 ICU
pH	7.45	7.42	7.34	7.39	7.41	7.46	7.43
$PaCO_2$(mm Hg)	39	43	55	47	42	37	40
PaO_2 (mm Hg)	47	142	283	427	352	329	197
SaO_2(%)	84	98	99.6	99.8	99.7	99.7	99
BE (mEq/L)	4	3.7	4.3	4.3	3	3	3
Hb (g)	16.9	—	—	—	—	16	16
HR (beats/min)	90	88	—	100	90	—	90
BP (mm Hg)	140/55	130/60	115/60	110/60	130/70	130/65	128/80
Temp (C°)	—	—	35.3	35.3	35.4	35.3	35.2
MAP (mm Hg)	83	80	70	76	90	88	91
CO (L/min)	5.9	5.4	4.9	5.8	4.6	4.5	5.0
PCWP (mm Hg)	16	13	15	20	16	18	18
MPAP (mm Hg)	39	47	42	40	33	31	30
CVP (mm Hg)	3	3	8	3	2	3	3
SvO_2 (%)	67	83	88	96	90	85	80
PIP (cm H_2O)	—	—	12	15	19	18	18
TV (mL)	—	—	200†	300†	300†	520‡	520‡
SVR ($dyne \cdot s \cdot cm^{-5}$)	1084	1140	1012	1006	1530	1550	1408
PVR ($dyne \cdot s \cdot cm^{-5}$)	311	503	440	775	295	231	192

* Abbreviations: ICU, intensive care unit; BE, base excess; Hb, hemoglobin; HR, heart rate; BP, blood pressure; Temp, temperature; MAP, mean arterial pressure; CO, cardiac output; PCWP, pulmonary capillary wedge pressure; MPAP, mean pulmonary arterial pressure; CVP, central venous pressure; PIP, peak inspiratory pressure; TV, tidal volume; SVR, systemic vascular resistance; PVR, pulmonary vascular resistance.

† Manual ventilation.

‡ Mechanical variation.

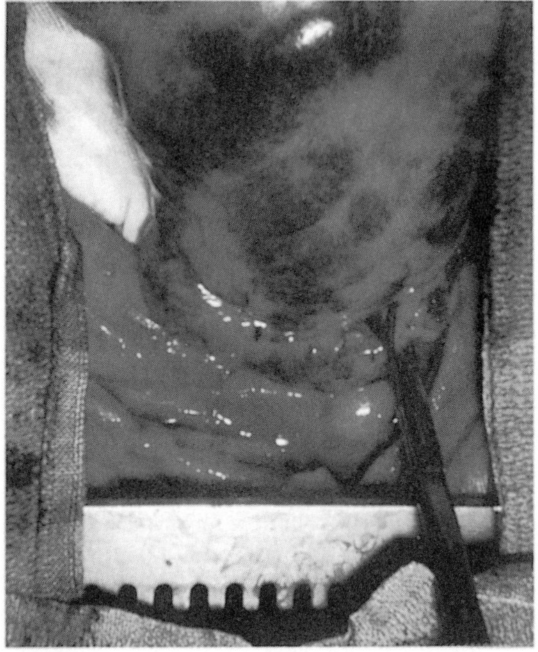

Figure 19-10. Operative view showing bullae bulging through the incision and compressing the underlying lung parenchyma inferiorly.

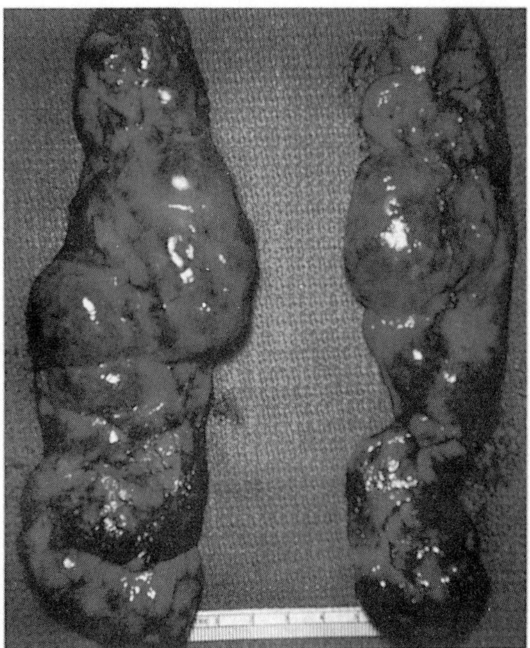

Figure 19-11. Photograph of the resected surgical specimens. Note that the bullae have deflated.

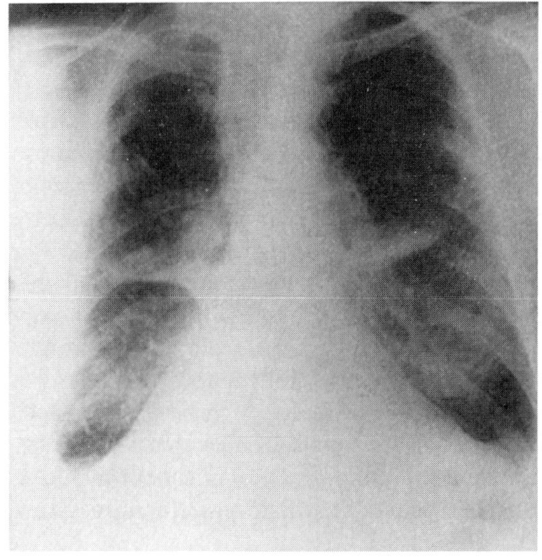

Figure 19-12. Postoperative chest radiograph showing expansion of previously compressed but now more functional lung tissue and only small residual apical bullae.

operatively is shown in Table 19-2. FVC increased from 40% to 88%, FEV_1 from 25% to 62%, and maximum voluntary ventilation from 35% to 71% of the predicted values. Two years after surgery, the patient was doing well with remarkable improvement in exercise capacity. He no longer needed supplemental oxygen. Apart from the significant objective improvement in pulmonary function tests, the patient now lives a normal life without restriction, has traveled abroad, and has resumed sexual activity with his wife, which he was unable to enjoy before surgery.

Discussion of Case Report

The patient had extensive bilateral bullous emphysema occupying most of both lung fields,

Table 19-2. Pulmonary Function Tests (PFTs)*

	Preoperative			2-mo Postoperative		1 yr Postoperative	
	Actual	Pred	% Pred	Actual	% Pred	Actual	% Pred
FVC (L)	1.94	4.81	40	4.18	87	4.19	88
FEV_1 (L)	0.85	3.39	25	2.13	62	1.92	57
FEV_1/FVC	0.44	0.7	62	0.51	72	0.46	65
$FEF_{25\%-75\%}$ (L/s)	0.32	3.21	10	0.86	26	0.71	22
$FEF_{50\%}$ (L/s)	0.43	4.96	8	1.05	21	0.87	17
$FEF_{75\%}$ (L/s)	0.30	1.95	15	0.35	17	0.35	17
PEF (L)	4.11	8.4	48	5.07	60	4.98	60
MVV (L/min)	38	110	35	79	71	80	71

* Abbreviations: FVC, forced vital capacity; FEV_1, forced expiratory volume in 1 second; FEF, forced expiratory flow rate; PEF, peak expiratory flow rate; MVV, maximum voluntary ventilation; Pred, predicted value.

which resulted in total disability, oxygen dependency, and extremely poor pulmonary performance. His PFTs were consistent with severe lung restriction and markedly reduced ventilatory ability. Interpretation of the pulmonary function tests supports the lack of change in the size of bullae on radiographs taken at full inspiration and full expiration, which also suggests that the bullae were not ventilated. The reduced FEV_1/FVC ratio indicated severe expiratory obstruction secondary to air trapping by large noncommunicating compartments (bullae). The increased functional residual capacity (FRC) was the result of severe hyperinflation and increased RV from the presence of enlarged noncommunicating compartments.

In addition, the patient had associated cardiac disease with two previous myocardial infarctions, moderately compromised left ventricular function, and coronary artery disease. He was obviously a high-risk patient and was unable to tolerate any hemodynamic insult. Because both lungs were equally diseased, it was decided that a single-lumen tube would be the best choice during anesthesia.

Because of the severe degree of hypoxemia, his cardiac status, and the fact that "bucking" during awake endotracheal intubation might increase the risk of bulla rupture and pneumothorax, intubation was performed under general anesthesia. Bronchospasm induced by awake intubation is common in patients with sensitive airways, and necessitates the application of positive pressure to maintain ventilation. Much of the tidal volume is displaced into the low-resistance area of bullae. Generous doses of fentanyl and thiopental were given to prevent bucking or bronchospasm and to maintain cardiovascular stability. Nitrous oxide was avoided, and manual ventilation was carried out with peak airway pressures of 12 cm H_2O and a tidal volume of 200 mL. Increased alveolar ventilation was achieved by increasing the respiratory rate.

Following the resection of the right bullae, PaO_2 was significantly increased to 427 mmHg. A tidal volume of 300 mL was then deliverable with peak airway pressure of 15 cm H_2O. SvO_2 increased to 90%. Since cardiac output was not significantly increased, the rise in SvO_2 was secondary to the increase in arterial saturation and oxygen delivery. When bilateral bullectomy was completed, the patient was mechanically ventilated with a peak airway pressure of 18 cm H_2O, delivering a tidal volume of 520 mL. This improvement in lung compliance was caused by the expansion of normal lung parenchyma that were previously compressed.

Postoperatively, bilateral lung expansion was associated with improved arterial blood gas levels. Pride et al. studied the effect of bulla removal on thoracic gas volumes and PFTs.[29] These researchers found that the most consistent changes in pulmonary function were an increase in PaO_2 and reduction in FRC measured by body plethysmography (reduced RV). The significant improvement in maximum voluntary ventilation and FVC occurred when the tidal volume was no longer directed into the air-trapping bullae but instead actively participated in the gas exchange.

In summary, careful anesthetic management and close cooperation between the surgeon and the anesthesiologist are needed to guide this type of patient through surgery successfully. In this case, the surgery added quality to the life of this man, providing him with the ability to live almost normally and to carry out his daily activities without being oxygen-dependent and disabled.

References

1. Forman S, Weill H, Duker GR, et al. Bullous disease of the lung. Ann Intern Med 1968;69:757.
2. Leape LL, Longino LA. Infantile lobar emphysema. Pediatrics 1964;34:246.
3. Morgan MD, Edward CW, Morris HR. Origin and behavior of emphysematous bullae. Thorax 1990; 44:533.
4. Normadale JP. Bullous cystic lung disease. Anaesthesia 1985;40:1182.
5. Richards DW. Pulmonary emphysema: etiologic factors and clinical forms. Ann Intern Med 1960; 53:1105.
6. Laurenzi GA, Turino GM, Fishman AP. Bullous disease of the lung. Am J Med 1962;32:361.
7. Cote CF. The anesthetic management of congenital lobar emphysema. Anesthesiology 1978;49:296.
8. Ting EY, Klopstoclz R, Lyons HA. Mechanical properties of pulmonary cysts and bullae. Am Rev Respir Dis 1963;87:538.
9. Potgieter PD, Benatar SR, Hewitson RP, et al. Surgical treatment of bullous lung disease. Thorax 1981;36:885.
10. Peters RM. Indications for operative treatment of bullous emphysema. Ann Thorac Surg 1983;35:479.
11. Stone DJ, Schwartz A, Feltman JA. Bullous emphysema. A long-term study of the natural history and the effects of therapy. Am Rev Respir Dis 1960; 82:493.
12. Halkier E, Rasmussen E, Vejlsted H, et al. Surgical improvement of respiratory insufficiency. A study of patients with giant lung cysts or localized bullous emphysema. Scand J Thorac Cardiovasc Surg 1977;12:75.
13. Kinnear WJ, Tattersfield AE. Emphysematous bullae. Surgery is best for large bullae and moderately impaired lung function. (Editorial.) BMJ 1990;300:308.
14. Hughes JA, Macarthur AM, Hutchinson DCS, et al. Long-term changes in lung function after surgical treatment of bullous emphysema in smokers and ex-smokers. Thorax 1984;39:140.
15. Laros CD, Gelissen HJ, Bergstein PG, et al. Bullectomy for giant bullae in emphysema. J Thorac Cardiovasc Surg 1986;91:63.
16. Takashi I, Natanabe Y, Fukatani G. Simultaneous bilateral operations for bullous emphysema by median sternotomy. J Thorac Cardiovasc Surg 1981; 81:732.
17. Lucido JL, Murphy P, Sweet HC. Resection for localized air trapping pulmonary disease. J Thorac Cardiovasc Surg 1963;45:112.
18. Ikeda M, Uno A, Yamane Y, et al. Median sternotomy with bilateral bullous resection for unilateral spontaneous pneumothorax, with special reference to operating indications. J Thorac Cardiovasc Surg 1988;96:615.
19. Connolly JE, Wilson A. The current status of surgery for bullous emphysema. J Thorac Cardiovasc Surg 1989;97:351.
20. Isenhower N, Cucchiara RF. Anesthesia for vanishing lung syndrome. Anesth Analg 1976;55:750.
21. Eger EI, Saidman LJ: Hazards of nitrous oxide anesthesia in bowel obstruction and pneumothorax. Anesthesiology 1965;26:61.
22. Caseby NG. Anesthesia for the patient with coincidental giant lung bulla. A case report. Can J Anaesth 1981;28:272.
23. Benumof JL. Sequential one-lung ventilation for bilateral bullectomy. Anesthesiology 1987;67: 268.

24. Kan AF, Oh TE. Anaesthesia for bullectomy. Use of propofol, high-frequency jet ventilation and extradural blockade. Anaesthesia 1992;47:480.
25. McCarthy G, Coppel DL, Gibbons JR. High-frequency jet ventilation for bilateral bullectomy. Anaesthesia 1987;42:411.
26. Tinker J, Vandam L, Cohn LH. Tension lung cyst as a complication of postoperative ventilation therapy. Chest 1973;64:518.
27. Mudge BJ, Kilaru P, Pandit UA, et al. Anesthetic management for resection of a giant emphysematous bulla in a patient with bilateral bullous disease. Anesthesiol Rev 1982;9:34.
28. Benumof JL. One-lung ventilation and hypoxic pulmonary vasoconstriction: implications for anesthetic management. Anesth Analg 1985;64:821.
29. Pride NB, Barter CE, Hugh-Jones P. The ventilation of bullae and the effect of their removal on thoracic gas volumes and tests of overall pulmonary function. Am Rev Respir Dis 1973;107:83.

CHAPTER

20

Tracheal Resection and Reconstruction

Elizabeth C. Behringer
Roger S. Wilson

Anesthetic management of the individual requiring surgical resection of a portion of the large airways continues to challenge the skills of even the most experienced anesthetist. The large airways, including the trachea, carina, and the major bronchi, can harbor a myriad of pathologic conditions that necessitate surgical resection and reconstruction.[1-3] The patient who presents for airway surgery is often complex medically. Existing disease states frequently contribute to the development of lesions of the large airways. Thus it is imperative to tailor the anesthetic management for tracheal reconstruction to each patient. A specific preoperative, intraoperative, and postoperative plan should be developed, taking into account the past medical history and active medical issues of the patient. The extent and location of the large airway pathology and the planned surgical approach should also be considered.

The goals of this chapter are to review the etiology of large airway lesions; preoperative evaluation, including pulmonary function testing and methods of radiologic evaluation; and the anesthetic management for tracheal resection and reconstruction, including monitoring and patient positioning. Specific anesthetic considerations for reconstruction of the proximal and distal trachea and carina are discussed. Postoperative care of the patient, posttracheal resection, and reconstruction are outlined.[4-8]

Historical Overview

Prior to 1960 the management of patients with tracheal lesions was extremely conservative. Extrathoracic lesions required permanent tracheostomy, while distal lesions were managed by serial dilations or rarely limited resections.[4] Subsequent advances in diagnosis, medical management, anesthetic and surgical techniques, and postoperative intensive care has allowed the successful primary resection and reanastomosis of a wide variety of complex large airway lesions.

A variety of anesthetic techniques have been described, which take several different approaches. The first approach involves placement of a standard size, uncut orotracheal tube proximal to the lesion following the induction of general anesthesia.[9,10] Eventually the tube is positioned distal to the lesion by the surgeon. This method, albeit simple, has several disadvantages. It is feasible in only minor stenotic lesions. A standard size endotracheal tube may disrupt a critical stenosis or polypoid mass. The bleeding, airway edema, and dislodged tissue that ensues may result in further airway obstruction. It is difficult to reanastomose the trachea using this technique, because the endotracheal tube remains in the surgical field throughout the course of the operation.

A second approach uses intermittent jet ventilation through a small gauge orotracheal tube or catheter positioned in the distal trachea or mainstem bronchus.[11–17] With the tube or catheter in the open distal trachea, oxygenation is maintained by the Venturi effect. Ventilation is adequately maintained using this technique, especially in cases involving minor stenotic lesions. It is technically easier to perform the tracheal reanastomosis with only a small catheter present in the surgical field. This approach has several important disadvantages, however. Blood and secretions often obstruct the catheter or distal airways. The catheter can be easily displaced. High-pressure injectors are fraught with technical difficulties including pneumothoraces, and ventilation may not be adequate when the catheter is passed through a tight stenosis and exhalation around the catheter is minimal.

The third approach involves the use of high-frequency positive-pressure ventilation (HFPPV), which has previously been described.[18–25] Adequate oxygenation and ventilation in cases of proximal, distal, tracheal, or carinal resection have been reported. Small tidal volumes of 50–200 mL are used with rates of 60–150 breaths per minute and positive inspiratory pressures of 40 psi. HFPPV has several advantages, including uninterrupted ventilation, minimal lung and mediastinal movement, minimal obstruction from blood and secretions, and continuous positive airway pressure decreasing the risk of atelectasis.

Cardiopulmonary bypass has also been used for distal tracheal and carinal reconstruction.[26,27] The need for endobronchial intubation is eliminated. However, systemic anticoagulation in the face of lung retraction predisposes patients to intrapulmonary hemorrhage and potential intraoperative death. Improved anesthetic and surgical techniques have essentially eliminated this approach.

The remaining technique for airway management during tracheal resection involves insertion of a cuffed tube into the open trachea or mainstem bronchus distal to the area of resection.[4,8,28–34] This technique is used most often for resection and reconstruction of the trachea or carina at the Massachusetts General Hospital. In the past 25 years more than 600 tracheal and carinal reconstructions have been performed on adults and children. The details of this technique will be described in depth shortly.

Etiology of Tracheal Lesions

Tracheal lesions arise from a diverse array of pathologic causes (Table 20-1). Postintubation injuries, trauma, primary and secondary tumors, congenital anomalies, vascular lesions, infectious agents, and certain connective tissue diseases may lead to substantial tracheal pathology. Knowledge of the existing tracheal pathology is vital to a smooth, successful anesthetic. An understanding of the etiology of the tracheal lesion allows the anesthesiologist to anticipate its potential location, extent, and anatomy. This information invariably dictates the anesthetic regimen as well as the surgical approach.

Postintubation injury was the leading cause of tracheal stenosis encountered by Grillo et al.[35] In his series of 416 patients undergoing primary tracheal resection and reconstruction for tracheal stenosis, 279 patients (67%) had postintubation injuries (Table 20-2). Tracheal lesions may occur primarily from "traumatic" intubation or secondary to an endotracheal tube cuff or tracheostomy.[36] Postintubation in-

Table 20-1. Etiology of Tracheal Lesions*

Congenital lesions
Tracheal agenesis/atresia
Congenital stenosis
Congenital chondromalacia
Neoplastic lesions
Primary neoplasms
Squamous cell carcinoma
Adenoid cystic carcinoma (cylindroma)
Carcinoid adenoma
Carcinosarcoma-chondrosarcoma
Secondary neoplasms
Bronchogenic carcinoma
Esophageal carcinoma
Tracheal carcinoma
Breast carcinoma
Head/neck carcinoma
Postintubation injuries
Laryngeal stenosis
Cuff injury
Ulceration/fistula
Granuloma formation
Posttracheostomy injury
Cuff lesions
Stoma lesions
Trauma
Penetrating
Blunt injuries
Cervical
Intrathoracic
Infection

* Used with permission from Wilson.[7]

Table 20-2. Tracheal Resection and Primary Reconstruction (1962–1982)*

Type of Lesion	Patients
Postintubation	279
Primary tumors	56
Adenoid cystic	18
Squamous	19
Other	19
Secondary tumors	30
Other	51
Total	416
Staged reconstruction	21

* Used with permission from Grillo.[35]

juries may be apparent throughout the adult trachea as illustrated in Figure 20-1.[1]

Two hundred and sixty-three of the 279 postintubation injury patients (94%) had primarily stenotic lesions, and six patients (2.2%) had tracheomalacia alone. Ten patients (3.6%) had lesions that were a combination of both tracheomalacia and stenosis. The locations of the postintubation injuries varied as well. Nine patients sustained injury to their cricoid cartilage, while 31 patients had subglottic laryngeal injury. Twelve patients had a tracheoesophageal fistula, and one patient had a tracheoinnominate artery fistula.

Several factors can predispose an intubated patient to significant tracheal mucosal injury and the risk of development of tracheal stenosis. Prolonged hypotension, which reduces blood flow to the tracheal mucosa, or concur-

Figure 20-1. The most frequent types and locations of injuries in the adult trachea after intubation and tracheostomy. Reproduced with permission. (Used with permission from Grillo.[1])

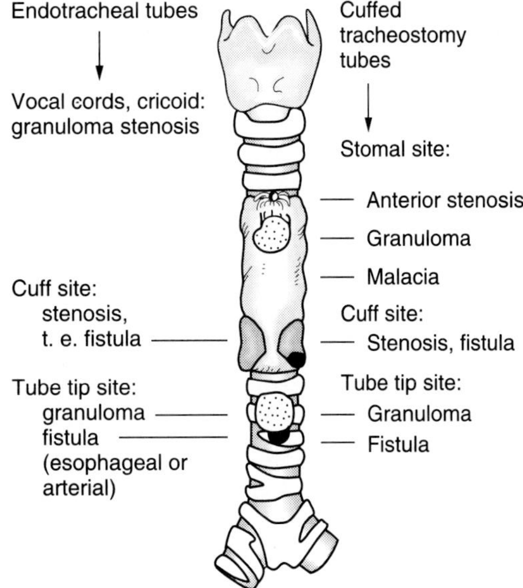

rent infection may result in tracheal injury. In addition, persistent elevation in endotracheal tube or tracheostomy cuff pressures may predispose to tracheal damage by impeding mucosal blood flow.[37] High cuff pressures are entirely avoidable by the judicious choice of the appropriate size of endotracheal tube or tracheostomy tube and the frequent monitoring of cuff pressures in all intubated patients. Cuff pressures are measured manometrically and are maintained below 25 mm Hg whenever possible.[37] Certainly, the risk of tracheal injury increases with the length of time the patient remains intubated. Persistent hypotension, concurrent infection, or elevated cuff pressures may elicit tracheal damage within a relatively short period of time, however.

Neoplasms are the second major indication for primary tracheal resection and reconstruction.[35] Fifty-six patients with primary tracheal tumors, or 13.5% of the total patient population, underwent resection with reconstruction in Grillo's study of 416 patients. The pathology was varied. Nineteen patients had squamous cell carcinomas, and 18 had cystic adenomas or cylindromas. The remaining 19 patients had a variety of rare tumors. Carcinoid adenomas, carcinosarcomas, pseudosarcomas, mucoepidermoid carcinomas, squamous papillomas, fibromas, hemangiomas, chondromas, and chondrosarcomas are examples of the rare primary tracheal tumors requiring resection. In another study of 198 patients with primary tracheal tumors recently reported by Grillo et al,[38] 147 tumors were excised (74%). Seventy patients had squamous cell carcinoma (36%), 80 had adenoid cystic carcinoma (40%), and the remaining 48 patients (24%) had a variety of lesions. Squamous cell carcinoma and adenoid cystic carcinoma were the most common primary tracheal tumors in several other series.[39, 40]

Squamous cell and adenoid cystic carcinomas are amenable to aggressive surgical therapy and are potentially curable when detected early.

Squamous cell carcinoma of the trachea may present as discrete exophytic lesions or ulcerating lesions.[41] Grillo suggests that squamous cell carcinoma of the trachea metastasizes first to regional tracheal lymph nodes and then by direct extension into mediastinal structures.[41] Adenoid cystic carcinomas are slow-growing tumors with two distinct patterns of spread. They may infiltrate the submucosa of the airway for longer distances than apparent on gross examination. Highly malignant lesions may spread by direct invasion of the lungs and pleura prior to diagnosis. The greatest opportunity for surgical cure is during the initial surgical effort by ensuring wide resections at the margins.[42]

Several pathological varieties of secondary tumors of the trachea exist. In Grillo's series of 416 tracheal reconstructions, 30 patients (7.2%) had secondary tumors of the trachea.[35] Metastatic cancers or mediastinal tumors of the trachea composed this group. Thyroid, esophageal, bronchogenic, and breast cancers can invade the trachea; thymomas, lymphomas, and carcinomas of the head and neck may be secondary neoplasms of the trachea as well. In Grillo's study, thyroid tumors occurred most frequently in this group. Such cancers may cause extrinsic compression of the trachea or cause symptoms of upper airway obstruction by direct invasion of the trachea. Thyroid carcinomas were the most amenable to palliation and cure. Other secondary tumors of the trachea were not amenable to therapy because of the advanced nature of the underlying malignancy.

Trauma to the tracheobronchial tree may result from blunt or penetrating injuries. Failure to recognize acute airway injuries and provide an adequate airway may result in death or eventual laryngotracheal stenosis[43]. Mathisen and Grillo reported a series of 10 patients with acute laryngotracheal injuries in 1987.[44] Blunt trauma to the trachea and larynx occurred in 50% of patients with acute laryngotracheal injuries. Penetrating injuries such as gunshot or stab wounds affected 40% of these patients. Traumatic attempts at intubation composed the remaining 10% of acute laryngotracheal injuries. Blunt trauma to the head, neck, and chest were the most common associated injuries in patients with laryngotracheal injury. The laryngotracheal junction, the most frequent site of injury, occurred in six patients. Sudden deceleration injuries resulted in injury to the posterior membranous wall of the trachea involving the carina in two patients. All patients in this series underwent successful definitive primary repair of their airway injuries. All 10 patients maintained an excellent airway postoperatively.

It is critical to remember that the failure to identify acute laryngotracheal injury can result in progressive airway obstruction as cicatrization occurs and stenosis develops.[45] This group of patients may present for the management of delayed traumatic laryngotracheal stenosis. Mathisen and Grillo reported a series of 17 patients treated for this condition.[44] Blunt trauma to the airway from motor vehicle accidents, the most common mechanism of injury, occurred in 11 patients. "Clothesline" injuries were seen in five patients. One patient had sustained a penetrating injury to the airway. The laryngotracheal junction and the upper third of the trachea were injured most frequently. Injury at this level was sustained by 11 patients. The middle or lower third of the trachea was involved in three patients.

Associated injury to the esophagus was found in five patients. Three of these patients had tracheoesophageal fistulas, and the esophagus of one patient ended in a proximal blind pouch.[44] Vocal cord paralysis was a significant associated injury in 14 patients. Bilateral vocal cord paralysis occurred in seven patients, and the seven remaining patients had evidence of unilateral vocal cord paralysis. Seven patients were found to have inadequate laryngeal airways. It is critical to provide an adequate, secure laryngeal airway prior to the attempted repair of a tracheal stenosis. Procedures such as laryngofissure lysis of adhesions, vocal cord lateralization, cricoarytenoid arthrodesis, and arytenoidectomy were used to provide a satisfactory laryngeal airway.[44] Subsequently, all 17 patients underwent resection of the stenotic segment of trachea with primary repair. As a result, 16 patients had good airways with no limitation of physical activity. Ten patients had excellent voice quality; six patients had functional, albeit husky, voices.

Cicala and colleagues recently reviewed the initial evaluation and management of upper airway injuries in a trauma population.[46] Forty-six cases of upper airway injury admitted to a large, metropolitan, university-affiliated trauma center were reviewed retrospectively over a four-year period. Twenty-six cases of upper airway injury were the result of penetrating trauma; 17 injuries were due to gunshot wounds, and 9 were due to knife wounds. The remaining 20 patients sustained blunt trauma to their upper airway. Motor vehicle accidents, the leading cause of this trauma, occurred in 13 patients. Diagnostic findings were varied, as illustrated in Table 20-3. The location of the injury was the larynx in 13 cases, the trachea in 24 cases, the cricoid cartilage in 5 cases, and multiple sites in 4 cases. The overall mortality rate in this series was 24%, and this rate did not vary according to patient age or mechanism of injury. Appropriate initial airway management depends on the rapid accurate diagnosis of the extent and location of the upper airway injury.

A series of 80 patients with inflammatory stenoses of the subglottic larynx and the upper trachea was recently reported by Grillo et al. These patients were treated with single-stage laryngotracheal resection and reconstruction.[43]

Table 20-3. Diagnostic Findings in Patients with Airway Injuries*

	Stab Wound (n = 9)	Gunshot Wound (n = 17)	Blunt Trauma (n = 20)
Radiographic soft tissue air	3 (33%)	9 (53%)	10 (50%)
Subcutaneous emphysema†	3 (33%)	4 (24%)	8 (40%)
Airway open into wound	5 (56%)	4 (24%)	1 (5%)
Computerized tomography	0	1 (6%)	4 (20%)
Bronchoscopy	1 (11%)	1 (6%)	1 (5%)
Pneumothorax	0	2 (12%)	0
Sudden loss of airway	0	0	2 (10%)
Autopsy	0	0	1 (5%)

*Used with permission from Cicala.[46]
† All patients with subcutaneous emphysema also had soft tissue air present on radiography.

Fifty originated from postintubation injuries, 7 from trauma, 19 from idiopathic causes, and 4 from miscellaneous causes. One postoperative death occurred. Long-term results were excellent in 18 patients, good in 48 patients, satisfactory in 8 patients, and failed in 2 patients.

A variety of relatively rare diseases may cause tracheal stenosis. Infectious diseases such as typhoid, diphtheria, syphilis, or tuberculosis may lead to this condition.[41] Systemic lupus erythematosis, Wegener's granulomatosis, fibrosing mediastinitis, and amyloidosis may involve the trachea as well.[41] Idiopathic tracheal stenosis occurs rarely in previously healthy patients without an antecedent history of intubation, tracheal trauma, or infection.[41]

Congenital lesions of the trachea have been infrequently described.[41] Significant anomalies of the major airways, such as tracheal agenesis or atresia, are often fatal at birth. Congenital tracheoesophageal fistulas, a more common anomaly, are rarely associated with tracheal stenosis. Several patterns of congenital tracheal stenosis have been described. Weblike diaphragms can be found in the neonatal or pediatric trachea. The level of the trachea just below the cricoid is the most common site of these webs. Intralaryngeal webs have been described. Webs tend to involve only a minute segment of trachea.[41] Cantrell and Guild discussed the three principal kinds of congenital tracheal stenoses.[47] Generalized hypoplasia of the trachea in the newborn to 1 to 3 mm from the level of the cricoid cartilage to just above the carina may occur. A funnel-shaped narrowing of the trachea resulting in a tight stenosis just above the carina may be evident. Finally, segmental stenoses of various lengths may occur throughout the trachea. (Fig. 20-2). Coexisting bronchial anomalies can be found. A right upper lobe bronchus may arise from the trachea above the stenotic segment.

Several congenital vascular anomalies are associated with congenital tracheal stenosis or compression. An aberrant left pulmonary artery may lead to an associated congenital stenosis.[48] The tracheal rings are often completely circular.[49] A competent airway is obtained through repair of both the pulmonary artery sling and the tracheal stenosis.[7]

Vascular ring or sling malformations may compress the neonatal trachea and esophagus, thus resulting in respiratory difficulty. No associated tracheal anomaly exists. Thus, repair of the vascular sling or ring most often relieves the respiratory distress. An anomalous innominate artery, aberrant subclavian artery, double aortic arch, anomalous left common carotid artery or right aortic arch with patent ductus arteriosus, or ligamentun arteriosum may lead to tracheal

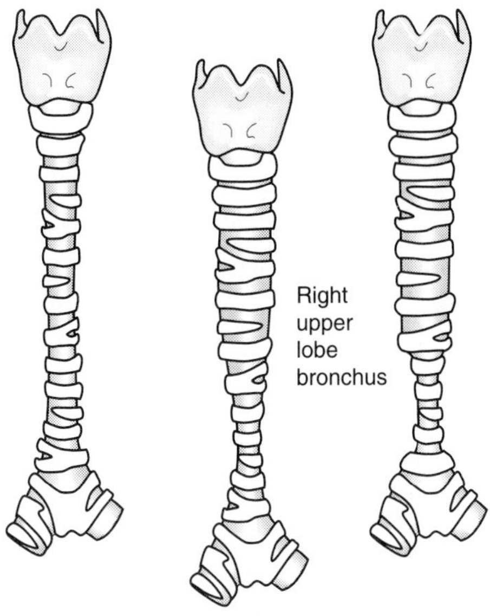

Figure 20-2. Congenital tracheal stenosis. Type I. Left: Generalized hypoplasia of the trachea. The airway is of normal caliber at the level of the cricoid cartilage and also in the main bronchi. Type II. Center: Funnel-like narrowing. The trachea is of normal caliber immediately below the cricoid cartilage but funnels to its narrowest point most frequently just above the carina. Type III. Right: Segmental stenosis. This may be accompanied by bronchial anomalies. The segmental stenosis may vary in length and be at varying levels. Type III is most commonly seen. (Used with permission from Cantrell.[47])

compression.[50–52] Congenital tracheomalacia or congenital tracheobronchomegaly (Maunier-Kuhn disease) are rare causes of airway collapse.[41]

Several varieties of congenital tumors and cysts resulting in laryngotracheal narrowing heve been described.[52] Congenital subglottic hemangiomas, laryngeal lymphangiomas or cystic hygromas, congenital cysts, and laryngoceles may cause severe upper airway narrowing. Squamous papillomata of the trachea and invasive papillary carcinoma of the trachea reportedly cause tracheal obstruction in children.[53] Grillo and Zannini reported a series of 52 patients from age 7 weeks to 15 years with obstructive tracheal disease.[53] Six patients had congenital lesions, and 46 had acquired tracheal lesions. Thirty-two patients were treated nonoperatively with conservative methods including observation, irradiation, cryotherapy, tracheostomy, or T-tube. Twenty patients aged 5 to 15 years underwent tracheal resection and reconstruction (Table 20-4). Three patients had congenital stenosis, while 17 had acquired lesions. Postintubation tracheal stenosis, the most common cause of all juvenile tracheal lesions presenting for primary repair, occurred in nine patients. Two patients had a posttraumatic stenosis, four patients had primary tracheal tumors, one patient had idiopathic tracheal stenosis, and one patient had a postintubation tracheoesophageal fistula. Two patients required carinal resection. Two patients died, and two patients developed stenoses postoperatively. One restenosis was repaired subsequently, so 17 patients had good results.

Preoperative Evaluation

Thorough preoperative diagnostic evaluation of patients with obstructive lesions of the air-

Table 20-4. Tracheal Resection and Primary Reconstruction in Children*,†

		Results		
	No.	Good	Failure	Death
Congenital stenosis	3	2	–	1
Primary tumor	4	4	–	–
Posttraumatic stenosis	2	2	–	–
Idiopathic Stenosis	1	–	1	–
Postintubation				
Stenosis	9	8	–	1
TEF	1	1	–	–
TOTAL	20			

* One Congenital patient needed reoperation for stenosis. One posttraumatic and the idiopathic patient had prior operative failures elsewhere.
† Used with permission from Grillo.[53]

way is essential. Diagnostic evaluation entails a detailed history and physical examination, pulmonary function studies, roentgenographic studies, and bronchoscopy. The diagnostic regimen is often dictated by the severity and urgency of airway compromise. For example, in life-threatening situations in which there is a high index of suspicion as to the nature of the tracheal pathology, bronchoscopy may be the primary method of diagnosis in addition to the detailed history and physical examination. On the contrary, the patient presenting for elective repair warrants a detailed evaluation.[54]

History and Physical Examination

A detailed history can be revealing in several areas. The physician should seek etiologies likely to produce airway compromise. A patient with an antecedent history of endotracheal intubation or tracheostomy should be considered to have an organic lesion until proven otherwise.

The signs and symptoms of large airway obstruction are affected by several factors. The anatomic location of the lesion, the severity of airway obstruction, and the presence of preexisting cardiopulmonary disease are important variables to consider. Clinical symptoms of airway obstruction include dyspnea, especially with effort, and wheezing, which may present as frank stridor. Persistent cough, hoarseness, and difficulty in clearing secretions are other common symptoms. Complete airway obstruction may occur from the inability to clear secretions due to an underlying organic lesion. Adult patients become symptomatic when the cross-sectional diameter of the airway is reduced to 5–6 mm or roughly 50% of normal.[7] Extremely active adults may have symptoms with a milder degree of airway obstruction. Stridor at rest is indicative of severe airway narrowing (4 mm or less). Patients with stridor have extremely tenuous airways. Because such patients deserve close monitoring, they warrant preoperative admission to an intensive care unit. Vocal cord or recurrent laryngeal nerve pathology is indicated by hoarseness. Direct or indirect laryngeal examination is necessary.

The symptoms described above, albeit straightforward but nonspecific, are frequently misdiagnosed. Several patients, especially those with tracheal tumors, have been diagnosed as having asthma. An alternative diagnosis is entertained only when the "asthma" is unresponsive to conventional medical therapy, which often unfortunately includes the use of corticosteroids.

To review, a detailed history is essential in the patient with a known or suspected tracheal lesion. Salient points of the history include a history of smoking, prior intubation, or tracheostomy. A precise evaluation of the patient's exercise tolerance is warranted, including any recent onset of hoarseness or stridor, inability to tolerate the supine position, persistent cough, or inability to clear secretions. The severity of preexisting cardiopulmonary disease may limit the patient's exercise tolerance. Tracheal lesions may present at an advanced stage in this case.

A careful physical examination entails a detailed examination of the airway. The trachea should be palpated for extrathoracic compression or deviation. Audible stridor, either at rest or with a maximal expiratory effort with an open mouth, is often elicited. Auscultation of the chest may reveal diffuse inspiratory and expiratory wheezing, which is difficult to differentiate from bronchospasm. Auscultation of the upper cervical airway may reveal high-pitched inspiratory and expiratory sounds characteristic of air flow obstruction. It is obvious that any difficulties in airway management should be anticipated in the patient with a tracheal lesion. The size and difficulty of the mask airway should be anticipated.

The range of motion of the neck is an essential component of the physical examination. The patient should be able to tolerate both hyperextension and hyperflexion comfortably. Several disease states are associated with instability of the cervical spine (Table 20-5).[55] If the cervical spine is in question, it should be evaluated radiographically prior to surgery in nonurgent cases. The type and function of the in situ tracheal appliance is important to ascertain preoperatively;[37] the patient may have a cuffed or cuffless tracheostomy tube in situ or a T-tube. The location of the tracheal appliance in relationship to the lesion is also important. The patient's tolerance to decannulation should be determined. The stoma should be patent and stable, and the patient should give a history of a relatively stable airway if decannulated. The existing tracheal appliance may then be removed and replaced with a cuffed Tovell or Anode tube just prior to the induction of general anesthesia.

Table 20-5. Syndromes Associated With Odontoid Hypoplasia and Conditions Associated With Atlantoaxial Subluxation*

Morquio's syndrome
Klippel-Feil syndrome
Down's syndrome
Spondyloepiphyseal dysplasia
Dysproportionate dwarfism
Congenital scoliosis
Osteogenesis imperfecta
Neurofibromatosis
Conditions Associated With Atlantoaxial Subluxation
Congenital
Down's syndrome
Odontoid anomalies
Muccopolysaccharidoses
Acquired
Rheumatoid arthritis
Still's disease
Ankylosing spondylitis
Psoriatic arthritis
Enteropathic arthritis—Crohn's disease
—ulcerative colitis
Reiter's syndrome
Trauma—odontoid fracture
—ligamentous disruption

* Used with permission from Crosby.[55]

Diagnostic Studies

Pulmonary Function Tests

Standard spirometry may demonstrate reduction in measured air flow during inspiration and expiration, but this technique is of limited value in the diagnosis of obstructive airway lesions. The maximal expiratory or inspiratory flow is characteristically affected to a far greater degree than is the forced expiratory volume in 1 second (FEV_1). The ratio of peak expiratory flow to FEV_1 is a useful index of obstruction. A ratio of 10:1 or more is suggestive of airway obstruction.

The flow-volume loop is a very reliable and specific test in the diagnosis of upper airway obstruction, however (Fig. 20-3).[54,56] During a forced expiration from total lung capacity, the maximal flow achieved during the first 25% of the vital capacity depends on effort alone. In general, circumferential stenoses, such as those produced by cuff lesions, are fixed in origin. Pedunculated tumors and tracheomalacia produce a variety of intermittent obstructions. In the case of fixed airway obstruction, the peak expiratory flow is markedly reduced, producing a characteristic plateau. With fixed intrathoracic or extrathoracic lesions, the inspiratory flow has the same characteristic plateau. In the case of a variable obstruction, the maximal cutoff of inspiratory or expiratory flow depends on the location of the lesion. Extrathoracic or cervical lesions produce a plateau during inspiration, with minimal effect on expiratory flow. Variable trathoracic lesions tend to demonstrate alterations in the expiratory flow curve with minimal or no effect on inspiration (Fig. 20-4).

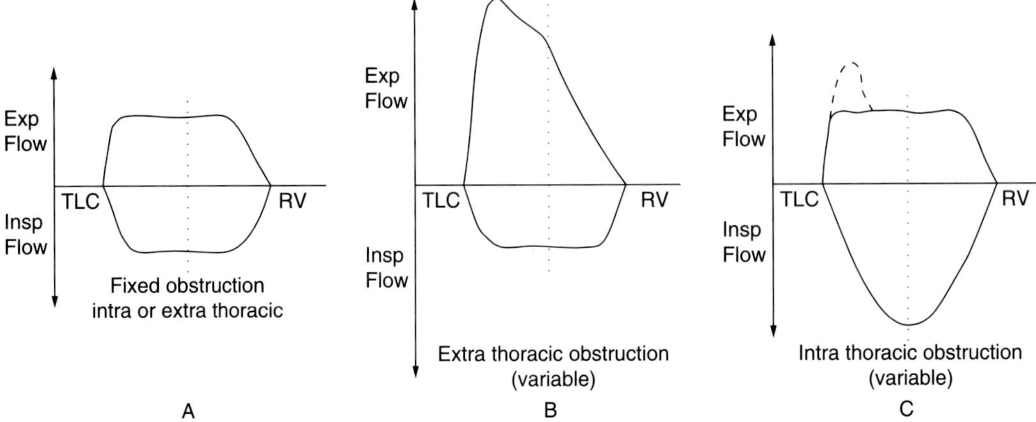

Figure 20-3. Maximal inspiratory and expiratory flow-volume curves in fixed obstruction (A), extrathoracic variable obstruction (B) and intrathoracic variable obstruction (C). The dashed line represents a flow transient that occasionally is observed just before the plateau in intrathoracic obstruction. See text for full description. (Used with permission from Kryger.[54])

Figure 20-4 A: Effect of the phase of respiration on an extrathoracic variable obstruction. Direction of airflow is indicated by the long thin arrows. During forced expiration the intratracheal pressure (P_{tr}) is greater than the pressure around the airway (P_{atm} = atmospheric pressure), resulting in a decrease of the obstruction. During forced inspiration when the pressure around the airway exceeds the intratracheal pressure the obstruction is increased.
B: Effect of the phase of respiration on an intrathoracic variable obstruction. Direction of airflow is indicated by the long thin arrows. During forced expiration the pressure acting around the airway (P_{pf} = pleural pressure) may be greater than the intratracheal pressure (P_{tr}), resulting in an increase in the obstruction. During forced inspiration the intratracheal pressure is greater than the pleural pressure thus decreasing the obstruction. (Used with permission from Kryger.[54])

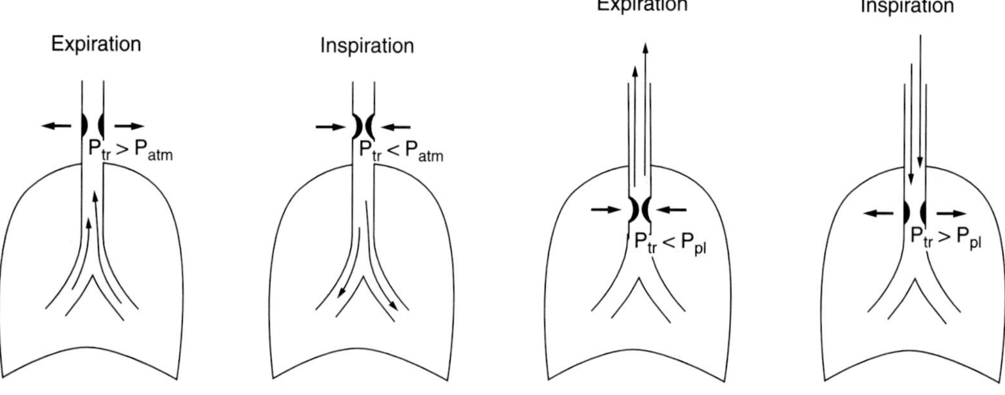

The functional impairment of the tracheal lesion may be estimated by using a restricted orifice in the patient's mouthpiece as the patient undergoes the flow-volume study. As the size of the mouthpiece is gradually reduced with the use of restrictive orifices of different sizes, this limited-size mouthpiece begins to have additional effects on the flow-volume loop. It is assumed that the intrinsic lesion has reduced the trachea to the cross-sectional diameter of the mouthpiece. As previously stated, the cross-sectional diameter of the airway must be reduced to 5 to 6 mm before the signs and symptoms of airway obstruction become clinically evident. The peak expiratory flow rate decreases to approximately 80% of normal when the airway diameter is reduced to 10 mm.

Radiologic Evaluation

Radiologic studies are useful in demonstrating the extent and the location of tracheal pathology.[57–59] The posteroanterior and lateral chest roentgenogram are standard. A lateral neck film shows the larynx and the cervical trachea. Supplemental oblique views may be obtained to view the entire trachea. Even nondiagnostic plain films are helpful in that surrounding structures, such as the spine, mediastinum, and lungs, are visualized. Plain films not only aid in planning other radiographic studies, but they are important in the interpretation of tomograms and computed tomography scans.[57]

Fluoroscopy is another useful diagnostic tool. Fluoroscopy of the larynx allows the physician to observe the motion of the vocal cords. Fluoroscopic views of the trachea with the patient in the oblique position outline the trachea and eliminate any superimposed bony structures.[58] This diagnostic technique is also helpful in the demonstration of airway malacia.

Tomography of the larynx and trachea is useful in the investigation of laryngeal tumors or the site and extent of tracheal stenosis. Tomograms of the larynx are obtained in the anteroposterior (AP) and lateral views, and tomograms of the trachea are obtained in the AP, lateral, and oblique positions.[57] These studies help to define the exact position of the lesion.

A barium study of the esophagus is another useful study. Once completely distended with barium, the hypopharynx may be assessed for symmetry, distensibility, and masses. The barium-filled, well-distended esophagus details the relationship between the thoracic trachea and the surrounding lymphatic and vascular structures.[57]

Other specialized radiologic studies to evaluate the larynx and trachea include angiography to diagnose and define the vascular supply to presumed vascular tumors, xeroradiography, and contrast laryngotracheography.[57]

Computed tomography (CT) scans of the neck and chest can evaluate mediastinal and laryngeal structures and the extent of the tracheal stenosis. Tracheal deviation may be visualized as well. Ideally, the optimal radiologic examinations are obtained without the presence of a tracheostomy or endotracheal tube. Thus airway compromise may occur shortly following decannulation. It is mandatory that decannulation during radiographic evaluation be closely supervised by medical personnel trained and properly equipped to reinstitute tracheal intubation.

Magnetic resonance imaging (MRI) to date has been inferior to CT for the depiction of tracheobronchial disorders because of limited spatial resolution and signal to noise. MRI has the ability to image directly in oblique planes, however, which is advantageous in displaying the relationship of masses to the central bronchi.[60, 61]

Laboratory Studies

The laboratory studies obtained in the patient presenting for tracheal resection and reconstruction should consider the patient's underlying medical history. Assessment of any cardiopulmonary dysfunction is especially important. The patient may require echocardiography, gated blood pool scanning, or Persantine thallium scanning in addition to the admission electrocardiogram to evaluate a history of cardiac dysfunction. The value of pulmonary function testing has been discussed elsewhere. A room air arterial blood gas is often obtained preoperatively to serve as a guideline of baseline oxygenation and ventilation. A preoperative hematocrit is especially useful in the patient with a presumed vascular tumor with the potential for significant blood loss. Based on the studies previously discussed, the preoperative workup should localize the nature, location, and the extent of the trachea requiring reconstruction. The preoperative assessment from the anesthesiologist's vantage point should consider several factors, including degree of airway limitation; presence of preexisting disease, especially of the heart and lungs; and anticipated postoperative problems. The patient should be evaluated with the understanding that intraoperative difficulties associated with the airway, as well as potential problems during induction, may expose the individual to undue stress from hypoxia, hypercarbia, or cardiovascular instability. Thus the general approach to the anesthetic technique used and possible alternatives to be relied on during the procedure must be based on these factors in addition to the anticipated surgical approach.

Anesthetic Management

Several approaches to the problems of airway obstruction and the maintenance of anesthesia during surgery for tracheal reconstruction have been described.[3,4,6,8,13,62] The primary method described in this chapter is the one employed by Grillo and colleagues for several hundred patients who have undergone tracheal resection and reconstruction at the Massachusetts General Hospital since 1962.[1–3,63–66] It should be remembered that approximately one-third to one-half of the adult trachea can be resected and a primary reanastomosis performed.

The goals of anesthetic management for the patient presenting for tracheal resection are several. The primary goal is the maintenance of an adequate airway from the time of anesthetic induction through the postoperative period. An adequate airway not only allows for adequate oxygenation and ventilation but ensures that secretions and blood may be cleared easily. Maintenance of the airway implies a thorough evaluation of the potential difficulties involved in masking, laryngoscopy, and intubation. The airway should not be jeopardized due to inattention to the basics of airway management. Airway maintenance also implies a thorough understanding of the nature and the extent of the tracheal lesion and a detailed knowledge of the surgical approach.

Given this information, it should be recognized that the airway may become particularly tenuous at several stages of the operation. This may occur during the induction of general anesthesia in the patient with significant tracheal narrowing. This condition may be compounded by inexpert airway management and the addition of anesthetic drugs that depress airway reflexes and muscle tone. The airway may also be tenuous during the resection, when it may become obstructed with secretions and blood; rarely, the distal trachea may be lost and withdraw into the mediastinum. In addition, the airway may be tenuous during the immediate postoperative period due to patient positioning, significant airway edema from multiple airway manipulations, and edema at the site of the anastomosis. Thus the traditional approach to the anesthetic management of the patient includes oxygen and inhaled volatile agents. Fixed agents, which diminish airway tone and respiratory drive, are avoided. In general, muscle relaxants should not be given because of their obvious effects on muscle tone, potential residual blockade despite adequate reversal, and the loss of the ability of the patient to breathe spontaneously. It is particularly important to maintain the potential for spontaneous ventilation in the patient whose airway is constantly in a precarious state.

Premedication

The patient's airway anatomy and the degree of anxiety expressed during the preoperative assessment govern the approach to premedication. The preoperative visit by the anesthesiologist involved in the patient's care also serves to establish a rapport that helps diminish the need for sedative and analgesic premedication.[67,68] A skillful, instructive, and understanding visit from the anesthesiologist to discuss the anesthetic plan and risks ensures an informed, cooperative, and calm patient.

Patients with significant tracheal narrowing, less than 5 to 6 mm in diameter, as determined by history, symptoms, pulmonary function tests, radiologic studies, or previous bronchoscopy, should not receive preoperative sedation. The obvious concern when faced with airway obstruction is to avoid oversedation and central respiratory depression. Opiates cause respiratory depression and have an antisialogogue effect. In addition to having anxiolytic effects, benzodiazepines are potential sedatives. Atropine and other agents that may produce drying of secretions should also be avoided. In addition, inspissated mucus plugs may form and impact in the already narrow portion of the airway, which can lead to near total airway obstruction. When in doubt, all premedication should be withheld until the patient arrives in the operating room and is under the close supervision of the anesthesiologist and surgeon. It is often prudent to have the anesthesiologist and surgeon transport the patient with a critical airway lesion from the intensive care unit to the operating room with appropriate transport monitoring.

In those patients in whom airway obstruction is minimal or in whom airway obstruction exists but has been adequately bypassed by either an endotracheal tube, tracheostomy tube, or a T-tube, the use of premedication is governed by the patient's needs and the conditions compatible with safe induction of anesthesia.

Equipment

Several pieces of specialized equipment must be readily available and functional prior to induction of anesthesia. An anesthesia machine capable of delivering high flows of oxygen (ie, up to 20 L/min) must be used. High oxygen flows are used routinely during rigid bronchoscopy. Once inserted into the trachea, the rigid ventilating bronchoscope requires high flows of oxygen in order to oxygenate and ventilate the patient adequately.

Masks and oral airways must be individualized for the patient undergoing an inhalation induction. Masks straps must be placed behind the patient's occiput, ready for immediate use if warranted. Appropriate equipment must be provided to facilitate laryngoscopy and topicalization of the airway. The choice of a laryngoscope blade is not as important as the user's ability to use a given blade with facility. A long bronchial sprayer, with 4% lidocaine, is useful for the topicalization of the pharynx and the tracheal mucous membranes.

Perhaps the most important equipment to be kept readily available is a variety of endotracheal tubes. In general, the tube size is selected when the airway is visualized during rigid bronchoscopy. Tube size and type also depend on the location of the lesion and the planned surgical approach. For patients with a proximal tracheal lesion, a set of uncut red rubber tubes ranging in size from 20–30F should be available. A set of uncut polyvinylchloride tubes ranging from size 4.0–8.0 mm can be used instead. The optimal size to ensure an adequate airway, provide for suctioning of secretions and allow sufficient room for surgical manipulation and suturing of the airway is 28F tube. Reusable red rubber endotracheal tubes, which remain stiff and relatively inflexible during a prolonged procedure and multiple manipulations, are used for their rigidity and ability to pass more easily through a stenotic trachea. Polyvinyl chloride tubes ranging in size from 4 to 8 mm ID in both the cuffed and uncuffed variety should be available for the patient who requires postoperative intubation. In such a situation, it is important to avoid placing the cuff on the anastomotic site.

Patients with an indwelling uncuffed tracheostomy tube require placement of a cuffed tube prior to the induction of anesthesia. In patients who are known to tolerate decannulation easily, the tracheostomy tube should be removed and an unsterile, cuffed, flexible, armored Tovell or Anode tube inserted. Sizes ranging from 20–34F should be available. A complete set of sterile Tovell tubes for endotracheal and endobronchial intubation from the field should be on hand. A set of sterile tubing and connectors that can be passed to the anesthesiologist from the surgical field must be available. This is connected to the anesthesia circuit to facilitate ventilation during reconstruction.

Single-lumen endobronchial tubes are often used during a distal tracheal or carinal resection. We use Wilson tubes, which are constructed by joining standard red rubber endotracheal tubes with the cuff end cut off to the proximal end of a Tovell endotracheal tube using a metal connector. Sizes ranging from 20–30F are available (Fig. 20-5). Another useful piece of special equipment is a high-frequency jet ventilator. This ventilator is capable of rates of 60–120 breaths/min with variable inspiratory: expiratory ratios and pressure settings. High-frequency jet ventilation is used during tracheal reconstruction on rare occasion.

Monitoring

The approach for monitoring the otherwise uncomplicated patient presenting for tracheal reconstruction includes use of an electrocardiograph, blood pressure cuff, esophageal stethoscope, pulse oximeter, end-tidal carbon dioxide monitor, and a radial artery catheter. Standards of monitoring during anesthesia are well established,[68] and several monitoring techniques deserve special mention. A pulse oximeter is especially helpful during an airway procedure in which the risk of desaturation and hypoxemia is always present. An end-tidal carbon dioxide monitor is useful during induction and intraoperatively especially during sponta-

Figure 20-5. Endotracheal tubes used for tracheal resection. Top—Wilson tube; middle—Tovell tube or Anode, bottom—uncut red rubber Rusch tube.

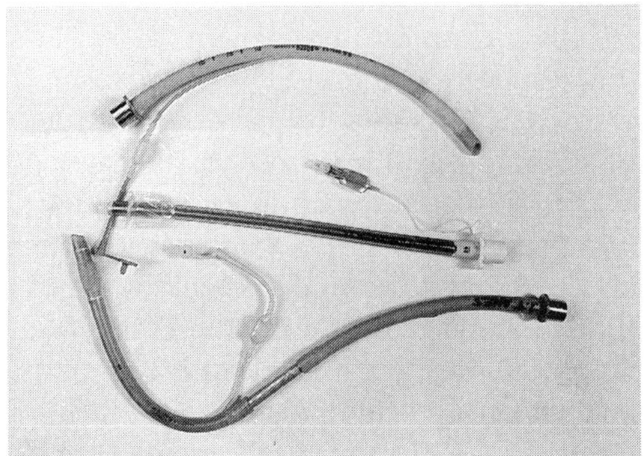

neous ventilation. Following intubation, the placement of an esophageal stethoscope not only provides useful information pertaining to breath sounds, heart tones, rhythm, but is also a foreign body that guides the surgeon in helping to identify the esophagus in the surgical field.

The arterial catheter is useful for instantaneous monitoring of blood pressure during the intra- and postoperative periods. It facilitates sampling of arterial blood to follow the efficiency of gas exchange as well as essential electrolytes, glucose, and hematocrit. The selection of the site of cannulation is governed not only by the availability of appropriate vessels but also by the fact that the right radial artery is often lost owing to compression or the occasional deliberate sacrifice of the innominate artery, which crosses the trachea and hence the operative field anteriorly from left to right. Thus, the left radial artery is preferred. In addition, when the approach is via a right thoracotomy and surgical exposure dictates that the right arm be prepared and moved into the surgical field, the left radial, left brachial, left axillary, dorsalis pedis, or femoral arteries are generally used.

In general, the use of central venous or pulmonary artery catheters is dictated by a history of significant cardiopulmonary disease. Difficulties in interpreting the waveforms may be encountered intraoperatively with the chest open, but useful in formation can be provided during the postoperative period. The cardiac output and stroke volume may be monitored consistently during both the intraoperative and postoperative periods with a pulmonary artery catheter, if needed. In most cases, the intraoperative blood loss and fluid requirements are minimal and in capable surgical hands a straightforward repair can be completed in a few hours. If central access is warranted the location of the catheter must be carefully considered. If the surgical approach is via a cervical collar incision or a mediansternotomy, then the neck and clavicles are prepared and moved into the field. Thus, the internal jugular and subclavian approaches to central venous access are forbidden. In these circumstances, central venous access is best accomplished through the antecubital vein or the femoral vein.

Induction and Bronchoscopic Examination

In preparation for the induction of general anesthesia, the patient is placed on the operating room table in the position most comfortable for breathing. Ideally for the anesthesiologist, this is the supine position. However, a patient with a particularly critical airway or extrinsic compression of the trachea may prefer to sit upright. Thus the anesthesiologist must be prepared to induce anesthesia in this position. It is needless to reiterate the importance of having one's equipment perfectly organized and reachable in these circumstances. A stand may be helpful. The previously mentioned monitors are applied to the patient in preparation for the induction. A deflated "thyroid bag" is placed beneath the patient's shoulders, and care is taken to pad all pressure points, especially the elbows. Prior to the induction of anesthesia all medical personnel involved in the airway management of the patient should be present. This includes surgeons, anesthesiologists, and nursing staff. The equipment needed for rigid bronchoscopy should be set up and ready to go.

At this point the induction of anesthesia may begin. In patients in whom airway obstruction is of minor significance, owing to either a good natural airway or the presence of an intratracheal appliance, anesthesia may be induced with thiopental or a similar intravenous induction agent such as propofol. When airway conditions are consistent with a high degree of obstruction, it is desirable to use a gentle, controlled inhalational induction with a volatile anesthetic. First the patient is denitrogenated with oxygen via a mask for an appropriate period of time, and then a volatile anesthetic gas is gradually introduced into the inspired oxygen. Relaxants should be avoided, and reliance should be placed on spontaneous ventilation and assisted breaths whenever possible, since the ability to intubate the larynx and provide an airway is not always guaranteed. In many cases in which airway obstruction is severe, it is impossible to provide adequate gas flow through a limited orifice with a mask and positive-pressure ventilation. During spontaneous ventilation, however, even in the anesthetized state, the patient is able to breathe adequately.

Anesthesia is induced until it is judged that the patient will tolerate direct laryngoscopy. Laryngoscopy is then performed and at this time topical anesthesia, generally with 4% lidocaine, is applied to the oral pharynx and glottis with a bronchial sprayer. The mask is reapplied, the volatile anesthetic-oxygen mixture readministered, and it is determined whether the patient has responded unfavorably to this procedure. If conventional signs, including tachycardia, hypertension, tearing, or any other manifestations of light anesthesia are evident, then the induction is continued for an adequate period of time. When conditions again are favorable, a second laryngoscopy is undertaken and an attempt is made to topicalize the trachea by inserting the tracheal spray immediately below the cords. When an adequate depth of anesthesia is present, bronchoscopy may be undertaken.

During bronchoscopy, it is critical for the anesthesiologist to inspect the status of the airway visually with regard to the nature and the extent of the lesion. This is important in terms of appreciating the difficulty of endotracheal tube placement and selection of the appropriate size tube. There are several potential problems which must be considered at this time. Lesions involving the upper one-third of the trachea, especially those in the subglottic region, pose special problems with placement owing to cuff position. A lesion that is located high in the airway does not allow the tube to pass because of its limited orifice, and the cuff does not pass below the cords. This results in the inability to attain a complete airway seal. Selection of a tube that is small enough to pass through the lesion poses additional problems. The decreased internal diameter of the tube may lead to potential airway obstruction with secretions and blood during the operative procedure. This is especially true when the 20–24F tubes are used.

Lesions located in the middle and lower two-thirds of the trachea have a special set of problems. The endotracheal tube may need to pass through the lesion itself to maintain oxygenation and ventilation until the trachea is transected. If the airway measures more than 5 mm, an endotracheal tube is generally passed to a point above the stricture in lesions of the lower two-thirds of the trachea. It may also be passed through the stricture in lesions of the upper one-third of the trachea as previously described.

The lesion may require dilatation at the time of bronchoscopy to provide an adequate airway. Tracheal dilatation must be considered with great caution. The risks of significant airway damage, bleeding, or perforation into adjacent structures such as the esophagus or the great vessels are real. Grillo dilates strictures if the airway measures less than 5 mm in diameter.[3,62] Tracheal dilatation is accomplished under direct vision with several rigid pediatric ventilating bronchoscopes. Bronchoscopes of graded size are exchanged and passed through the trachea in succession. Care should be taken, because dilators passed through a large bronchoscope may easily perforate the tracheobronchial wall, especially if the stricture is in the distal trachea.

Airway tumors must be handled with great caution. Direct trauma to the tumor may occur with the passage of the endotracheal tube. The tube may dislodge a piece of the tumor leading to near complete airway obstruction and the potential for serious hemorrhage into the airway. In general, strictures of the anterior tracheal wall or stomal strictures are easy to manage. The mobile posterior membranous wall of the trachea usually allow passage of an endotracheal tube or sufficient gas flow beyond the lesion should the tube be positioned above it.

Once bronchoscopy is completed, endotracheal intubation with the appropriate size tube is performed. This procedure is done in the usual fashion by using the sniffing position and direct laryngoscopy. As the tube is advanced down the airway, the area of stricture can often be appreciated. Once the tube is believed to be in the appropriate position, the chest is auscultated in standard fashion to ensure bilateral lung ventilation. A flexible pediatric fiberoptic bronchoscope may be used to confirm the adequacy and location of endotracheal tube placement. Subsequently, the tube is secured, the eyes taped, and an esophageal stethoscope passed. At this time it is important to pass an orogastric tube to empty the stomach of gas as well as fluid. Once this maneuver is completed, the orogastric tube is usually removed. Anesthesia is maintained with a volatile anesthetic-oxygen combination. In patients with normal pulmonary function and minimal airway obstruction, nitrous oxide may supplement the oxygen-volatile anesthetic mixture. The patient is allowed to breathe spontaneously. If controlled ventilation of the patient is chosen, this is generally accomplished manually. Given the degree of airway obstruction and the multiple manipulations of the airway during the operative procedure, it is best to keep in contact with the airway compliance at all times.

Positioning

As shown in Figure 20-6, several approaches are used depending upon the extent and location of the tracheal lesion. For most lesions located in the upper half of the trachea, an anterior collar incision is used with or without a vertical partial sternal split. For this incision, the patient is positioned supine with a thyroid bag or bolster placed under the shoulders and the head on a supporting doughnut. The back of the table is elevated approximately 10 to 15 degrees to position the cervical and sternal areas parallel to the floor when the head is fully extended. The arms are either tucked in at the sides or the left arm is extended on an arm board at a 45 degree angle to the trunk. Exploration of the lesion is done through the anterior collar incision, and the sternum is divided at a later time if this is deemed necessary for surgical exposure.

Lesions of the lower half of the trachea are approached through a right posterior lateral thoracotomy incision in the fourth interspace or in the bed of the fourth rib. The position for this incision is standard left lateral decubitus with the right arm draped and prepared so that it can be moved into the field for easier access to the neck. In this position, a thoracotomy can be done and a collar incision added to free the trachea if a laryngeal release procedure is needed. In special cases of extensive or unusual lesions involving a greater area of the trachea, a vertical incision can be extended into the right and left fourth intercostal spaces from the sternal incision (Fig. 20-7).

Specific Anesthetic Considerations

Reconstruction of the Upper Trachea

Lesions of the upper half of the trachea are approached surgically as shown in Figure 20-7. A low, short collar incision is made across the

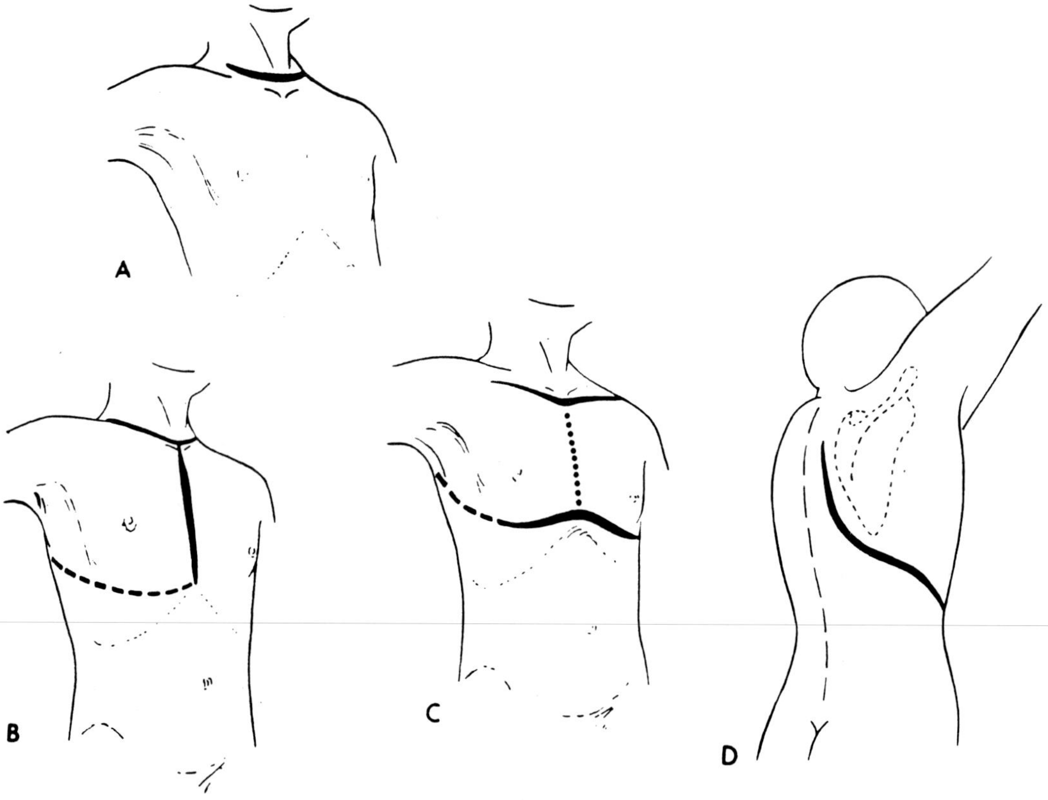

Figure 20-6. Incisions for tracheal resection. A: Standard collar incision for the majority of benign strictures and neoplastic lesions of the upper trachea. B: Sternotomy extension: the dotted line shows an extension that may be carried through the fourth interspace to provide total exposure of the trachea from cricoid to carina. C: Technique for raising a large bipedicle flap for total exposure and use in cases in which mediastinal tracheostomy is required. D: Posterolateral thoracotomy, carried through the bed of the fourth rib or the fourth interspace for exposure of the lower half of the trachea. (Used with permission from Grillo.[41])

neck and a T-incision is extended vertically over the sternum. Anterior dissection of the trachea is carried from the cricoid cartilage to the carina. Care is taken not to injure the innominate artery or other structures adjacent to the trachea. Dissection around the back of the trachea is done at a point inferior to the lesion. If the patient has not been intubated through the stricture, caution must be undertaken during this dissection. It is possible to produce progressive, eventually complete, airway obstruction with release of the external supporting structure of the trachea.

During this portion of the cervical procedure, anesthesia is maintained through the previously placed oral endotracheal tube. At the point at which it is anticipated that the trachea will be divided, nitrous oxide, if present, is eliminated from the anesthetic gas mixture. At this time anesthesia is maintained with oxygen and

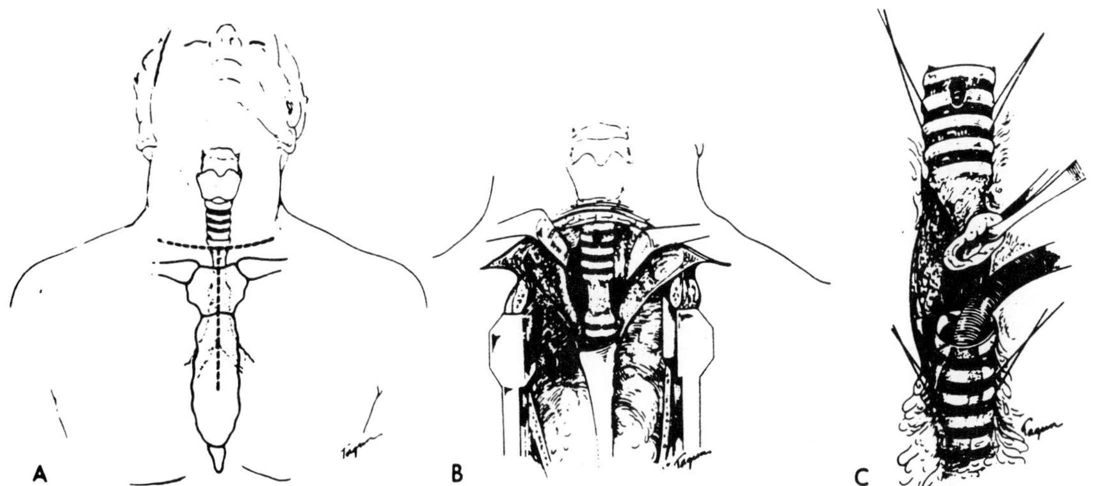

Figure 20-7. Reconstruction of the upper trachea. A: Collar incision and extension for upper sternotomy. B: Dissection is carried down to isolate the damaged segment. C: Circumferential dissection is carried out immediately beneath the level of pathology. Traction sutures are in place and the distal airway intubated via the operating field. (Used with permission from Grillo.[41])

a volatile anesthetic alone. Next a tape is placed around the trachea below the lesion, and lateral traction sutures are placed through the full thickness of the tracheal wall in the midline on either side at a point no more than 2 cm below the point of division of the trachea. It is important to anticipate the placement of these sutures so that the cuff of the endotracheal tube may be deflated to prevent it from being injured by the suture needle. The trachea is then transected below the lesion, as demonstrated in Figure 20-7. The distal trachea is intubated across the operative field with a flexible armored Tovell tube. The sterile connecting equipment, consisting of corrugated tubing and a Y-piece, are passed to the anesthesiologist for connection to the anesthesia circuit. The ability to ventilate the lungs is then assessed by manual ventilation with positive pressure. The surgical dissection continues to free and excise the tracheal lesion.

Once the adequacy of the tracheal lumen and extent of the tracheal resection has been determined, an attempt is made to approximate the two free ends of the trachea. This is accomplished by use of the traction sutures. The surgeon is assisted by the anesthesiologist, who tilts the patient's head from above, thus flexing the neck. When it is possible to reanastomose the tracheal ends directly, intermittent sutures are placed through the trachea. Anesthesia is maintained through the Tovell tube in the distal trachea. In cases where it is not possible to bring the ends together owing to undue tension, a laryngeal release procedure is performed. Once all sutures have been placed, the distal Tovell tube is removed. The oral endotracheal tube, which has remained in the proximal portion of the trachea, is advanced through the anastomosis into the distal trachea under direct vision. Care must be taken not to pass the tube too far distally in the trachea, because subsequent flexion of the neck for surgical foreshortening of the trachea potentiates right mainstem bronchial intubation. Before this exchange, the airway is suctioned to remove any aspirated blood or secretions. Anesthesia is then administered through the oral endotracheal tube as the sutures are tied down to produce an airtight anastomosis. The anastomosis is checked for leaks by giving a sustained breath at 30 mm Hg pressure. After all sutures have been placed, the patient's neck is flexed and the head supported in the position shown in Figure 20-8. The incision is then closed. A retention suture is placed from the chin to the sternum to maintain neck flexion and to decrease anastomotic tension.

Figure 20-8. Details of anastomotic technique. A: Original endotracheal tube positioned in the upper trachea with the distal trachea intubated. Once all sutures are in place, the endotracheal tube is advanced and the sutures are tied in serial fashion. B: With cervical flexion, the maximum amount of approximation is obtained. (Used with permission from Grillo.[41])

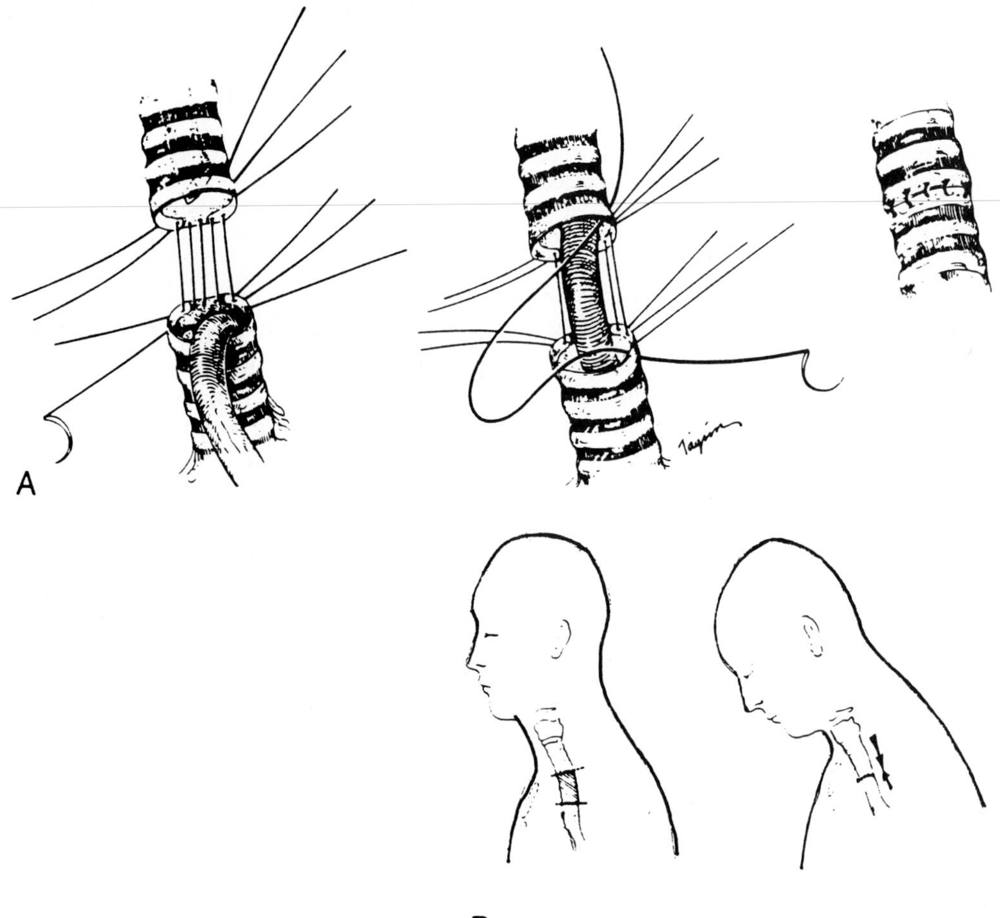

At the completion of the operation, the patient should be breathing spontaneously. Extubation should be anticipated under awake conditions. It is prudent to allow the patient to awaken fully, supporting the head and neck during the excitement phase to avoid excessive motion. The purpose of this maneuver is to avoid undue tension on the anastomosis. It is possible to extubate the patient under moderately deep anesthesia if certain conditions are fulfilled. If the mask airway or laryngoscopy was difficult, the patient should be allowed to awaken fully before extubation is attempted. Therefore, it is generally preferable to attempt extubation in the operating room, where the quality of airway patency may be evaluated quickly. Under such controlled circumstances, reintubation or diagnostic bronchoscopy can be done more easily and safely than in the recovery room or the intensive care unit. If reintubation is required because of unexpected airway or laryngeal pathology or edema, this is best achieved with care using a flexible fiberoptic bronchoscope. An endotracheal tube is passed orally or nasally over the bronchoscope under direct vision. Care is taken to position the tube either well above or below the anastomotic site. If the anastomotic site is high in the trachea, the use of a cuffless endotracheal tube is particularly helpful. It is best to avoid cuff pressure on the suture line.

Remember that a common reason for respiratory decompensation in the immediate postoperative period is upper airway edema. In general, this requires the stenting effect of the endotracheal tube in order for the patient to breathe adequately. If reintubation is attempted bronchoscopically, then excessive tension on the suture line is avoided. The chin sutures may be left in situ and the neck kept in strict flexion. Fortunately, given the techniques described, reintubation is an infrequent event. Once the airway and ventilation are judged to be adequate, the patient may be transported safely with supplemental oxygen and the appropriate monitoring to the intensive care unit.

Reconstruction of the Lower Trachea and Carina

The surgical approach and technique for the management of lower tracheal and carinal lesions is unique in several respects (Figs. 20-9 and 20-10). A right posterior lateral thoracotomy incision is preferred.[69] There are several important anesthetic concerns when dealing with the resection of the lower trachea or carina. These include anesthetic requirements and postoperative pain management, tube selection and positioning, and maintenance of adequate oxygenation and ventilation.

The general principles concerning airway management and the induction and maintenance of anesthesia are similar to those described for the upper trachea. The location and impact on pulmonary function of the lateral thoracotomy incision is well described.[71] This is particularly pertinent in the patient with an airway lesion. The goal at the end of the procedure is to have the patient extubated and comfortable with an adequate airway. Given these guidelines it is helpful to provide epidural anesthesia and immediate postoperative analgesia.[72,73] Currently, a thoracic epidural catheter is placed prior to the induction of anesthesia. Once the patient is turned into the lateral thoracotomy position, the epidural is bolused with a suitable solution such as 2% xylocaine or 0.1% marcaine with 10 μg/mL of fentanyl. The marcaine-fentanyl mixture may be run as a continuous epidural infusion in the intraoperative and postoperative periods.[74]

During the thoracotomy and surgical resection of the trachea, positive-pressure ventilation is used. It is preferable to maintain the patient's ability to ventilate spontaneously in

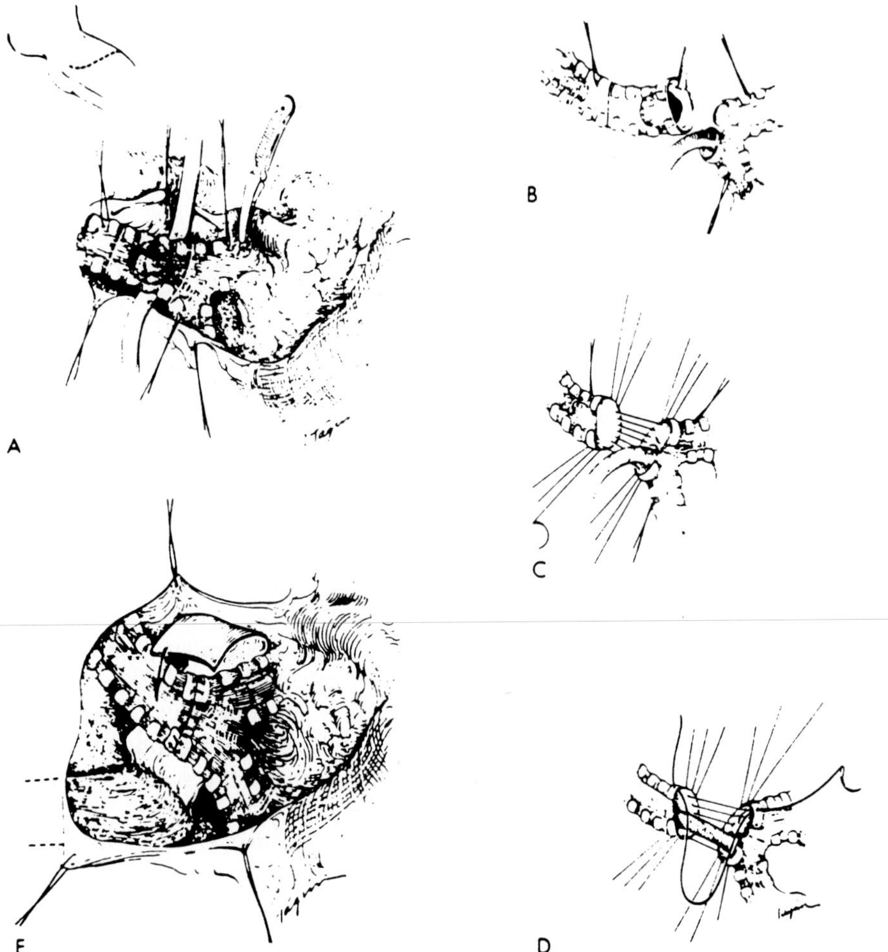

Figure 20-9. Transthoracic approach. A: The lesion in the distal trachea has been isolated and the right pulmonary artery is shown to be clamped, although this is not done routinely. B: The trachea has been divided above the carina and the left main bronchus intubated. C: Anastomotic sutures are placed by a procedure similar to that used in the upper trachea. D: The endotracheal tube has been advanced through the anastomosis and the remaining sutures appropriately placed. E: Anastomosis completed with a pedicle pleural flap secured for additional support. (Used with permission from Grillo.[41])

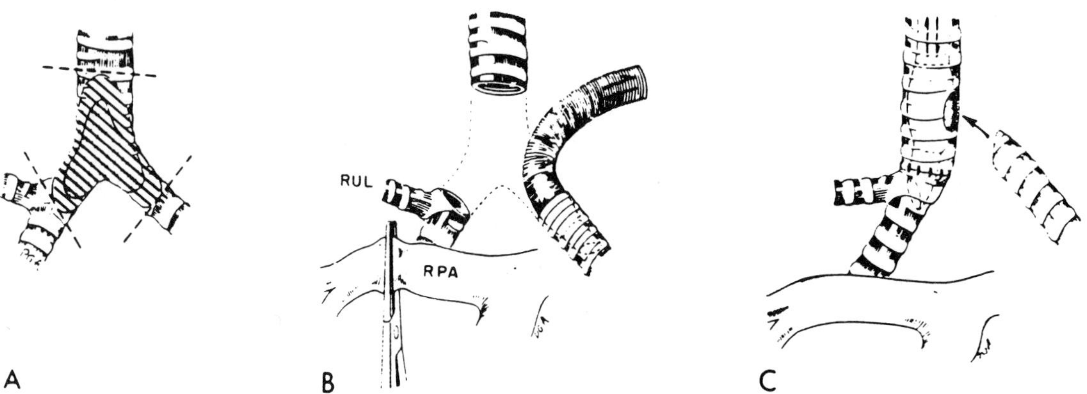

Figure 20-10. Resection and reconstruction of the carina. A: Tumor position is outlined by the stippled area. B: With the tube positioned in the left main bronchus, the right lung is mobilized and the stump of the right mainstem bronchus sutured into the trachea. C: The left main bronchus is anastomosed in end-to-side fashion into the trachea. (Used with permission from Grillo.[41])

the circumstances enumerated previously. The potential for spontaneous ventilation is important during periods of discontinuity of the airway when positive-pressure ventilation is not feasible. Muscle relaxants of intermediate action should be used in cases of mild airway narrowing. In cases requiring their use, they should be reversed fully as soon as possible.

When dealing with lesions of the lower trachea or carina, it is advantageous to have a tube that is long enough to enter either mainstem bronchus. For this purpose, an armored Tovell tube connected proximally to an uncut red rubber tube (Wilson tube) is used to provide both flexibility at the distal end and adequate length for bronchial intubation. This tube is generally passed with the aid of a stylet. It is positioned according to the anatomical location and extent of the lesion with the aid of a flexible fiberoptic bronchoscope (Fig. 20-5). Resection involving the distal trachea and carina is carried out with the endotracheal tube in a position proximal to the lesion. Surgical exposure and resection is much the same as previously described for upper tracheal lesions. Once the trachea is divided, the distal tracheal stump not infrequently is too short to hold the endotracheal tube and cuff. It is not convenient or possible to ventilate both lungs adequately under these circumstances. In most cases, the left mainstem bronchus is intubated through the operative field. Thus anesthesia and ventilation are carried out entirely via the left lung while the diseased segment is excised. Rarely, oxygenation and ventilation are inadequate during this period of one-lung ventilation. In addition, the endobronchial tube may need to be removed so frequently to provide surgical exposure that oxygenation and ventilation cannot be maintained satisfactorily.

In this circumstance, the anesthesiologist should be aware and well versed in the several alternative methods to provide satisfactory oxygenation and ventilation. It is theoretically possible to eliminate perfusion to the right lung temporarily with pulmonary artery clamping. This procedure, which is often technically very difficult, entails the potential hazard of injury to the right pulmonary artery. A second alternative technique that provides adequate oxygenation and ventilation includes the use of a second endobronchial tube and anesthesia machine. A second tube is advanced into the right mainstem bronchus, preferably in the bronchus intermedius. A second anesthesia machine and sterile tubes are used to maintain continuous positive airway pressure (CPAP) (approximately 5 cm water) with oxygen to the nondependent lung. Several other methods for the administration of CPAP that do not require the use of a second anesthesia machine have been described. These require another oxygen source.[75–77] Ventilation is carried out in the dependent left lung. This technique has several obvious disadvantages. The need for a second anesthesiologist and anesthesia machine are evident. The second endobronchial tube in the right mainstem bronchus may make the surgical access to perform the anastomosis quite difficult.

A third alternative includes the use of high-frequency positive-pressure ventilation (HFPPV) to the right lung. This may afford excellent oxygenation and ventilation to the patient. The need for the second anesthesiologist and anesthesia machine is eliminated. Interference with completion of the anastomosis is less as well. A small sterile catheter is placed into the right mainstem bronchus from the surgical field, and the proximal end is passed underneath the drapes to the anesthesiologist. The HFPPV ventilator is set to maintain adequate inflation of the right lung and arterial oxygen saturation as noted by pulse oximetry and arterial blood gas values. This method of HFPPV may be used in other ways as well. A catheter may be placed in the left mainstem bronchus in lieu of a larger endobronchial catheter. Oxygenation and ventilation of the left lung is provided. On rare occasions, a bifid catheter may be used to ventilation both lungs if ventilation and oxygenation are insufficient with one-lung ventilation alone.

With lesions of the distal trachea not involving the carina, anastomosis and tube positioning are carried out in much the same manner as for lesions of the upper trachea (Fig. 20-11). Once the anastomosis is complete, it is prudent to withdraw the endotracheal tube back into the proximal trachea so that ventilation occurs through the area of anastomosis. Position of the tube is confirmed with the aid of a flexible fiberoptic bronchoscope.

In resections involving the carina in which end-to-end and end-to-side anastomosis between the trachea and right and left mainstem bronchi must be carried out, a variety of tube manipulations and combinations of the previously considered techniques must be undertaken (Fig. 20-11). Generally, the right mainstem bronchus is anastomosed to the distal trachea and the left mainstem bronchus reimplanted in an end-to-side fashion into the bronchus intermedius or the distal trachea. Significant periods of one-lung anesthesia are not uncommon during such procedures. The need to insufflate the second lung is dictated by the level of arterial oxygenation.

Once all the anastomoses have been completed and the adequacy of ventilation is assured, the surgical wounds are closed in a standard fashion. The patient should resume spontaneous ventilation at this point. When a right thoracotomy has been used for surgical dissection, the decision as to whether to extubate the airway is of major importance. The potential for inadequacy of ventilation and pulmonary toilet must be balanced against the problems of continued intubation, potential infection, and direct trauma to the suture line. Providing that significant parenchymal lung disease was absent preoperatively, it is generally possible to extubate patients following thoracotomy and major carinal reconstruction uneventfully. Immediate postoperative extubation should be carefully considered in patients who have undergone bilateral thoracotomy. These patients may require endotracheal intubation and mechanical ventilatory support as a result of significant dimunition in pulmonary function. If intubation and mechanical ventilation is required postoperatively, the position of the endotracheal tube is adjusted with the use of a flexible fiberoptic bronchoscope. This ensures that the cuff is positioned either well above or below the suture line. The use of epidural analgesia is especially important in patients with thoracotomy incisions to assist in pain relief, deep breathing, and the coughing and clearing of secretions.

Following thoracotomy, the procedures for extubation are similar to those described for the upper airway approach. An exception is that the patient is returned to the supine position before extubation to facilitate placement of the chin sutures and adequate exposure of the airway. The patient is transported to the recovery room or the intensive care unit once stability of the circulation and adequacy of ventilation is assured. The patient should be monitored during transport.

Thus, the most widely used anesthetic technique includes the use of oxygen, a volatile anesthetic vapor with or without supplemental nitrous oxide. The inhalation agents are the most potent bronchodilators available in the current anesthetic armamentarium. They are ideally suited for patients with reactive airway disease and airway pathology. In addition, inhalation agents allow for a smooth, controlled mask induction, maintaining spontaneous respirations as outlined previously. Halothane, which is less pungent than isoflurane or enflurane, has been used almost exclusively as an induction and maintenance agent. Isoflurane and enflurane have now surpassed halothane as the authors' induction and maintenance agent of choice for several reasons. The potential for hepatic toxicity is avoided. Isoflurane and enflurane are less arrhythmogenic, and this is particularly important in patients who may receive drugs such as theophylline, aminophylline, epinephrine or β_2-agonists with arrhythmogenic potential. Patients undergoing tracheal resection and reconstruction are prone to hypercarbia and respiratory acidemia, which may potentiate arrhythmias as well. Our current practice in cases with significant tracheal pathology is to induce the patient with a combination of oxygen and either isoflurane or enflurane by mask. Halothane is reserved for patients with extremely tenuous airways in whom the pungent nature of isoflurane and enflurane is a concern. As discussed previously, epidural anesthesia has proved to be a helpful adjunct in cases where the right thoracotomy approach is used. Muscle relaxants are eschewed in the majority of cases for the reasons given earlier.

On occasion, we are presented with a patient with significant ventricular dysfunction and a tracheal lesion. The most common etiology of this combination is the postmyocardial infarction patient with significant left ventricular dysfunction who presents with a cuff related stenosis. Monitoring of these patients may include the use of a pulmonary artery catheter as discussed. In addition, the anesthetic goals must include preservation of cardiovascular function and airway maintenance. In such cases, the use of vecuronium or atracurium in combination with a short-acting narcotic such as alfentanil may be used. Nitrous oxide may be used when appropriate. Alternatively, a constant infusion of propofol may be helpful to avoid intraoperative awareness.[78] As stated previously, the muscle relaxant must be fully reversed in anticipation of extubation.

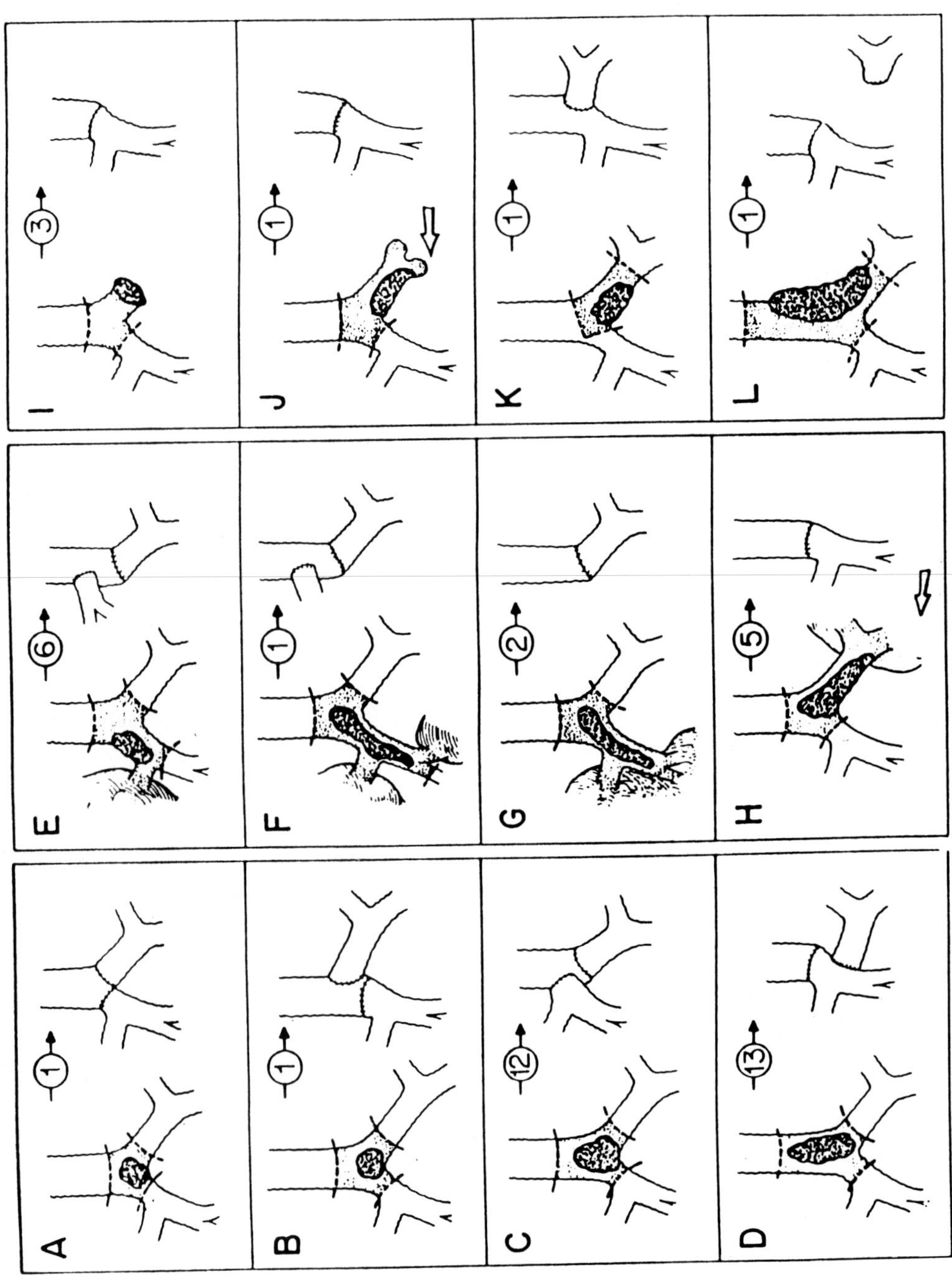
A
1
B
1
C
12
D
13
E
6
F
1
G
2
H
5
I
3
J
1
K
1
L
1

Postoperative Care

Patients are admitted postoperatively to the intensive care unit. Monitoring includes electrocardiogram, pulse oximetry, and arterial pressure. A radiograph of the chest is obtained shortly after arrival to ensure that a pneumothorax is not present. Sufficient oxygen is administered with a high flow humidified system via a face mask to provide adequate arterial oxygenation and thinning of secretions. The head is maintained in the flexed position with the use of several firm pillows placed behind the occiput and the anterior chest.

Chest physical therapy and routine nursing procedures are dictated by the nature of the other underlying diseases and the ability to effectively maintain gas exchange and pulmonary toilet. Blind nasotracheal suctioning is undertaken with caution in those patients whose cough is inadequate to clear secretions. This is best accomplished by physicians, nurses, or chest physical therapists well versed in this procedure. Potential complications include perforation of the anastomotic site, tracheal and glottic irritation with subsequent edema and airway obstruction, or vomiting, and aspiration. In cases where copious secretions are a significant concern, frequent flexible fiberoptic bronchoscopy can be a useful adjunct to pulmonary toilet. This is particularly pertinent in cases of carinal resection. Secretions tend to pool in major bronchi without being propelled by the normal mechanisms of mucociliary clearance. The need for emergency reintubation secondary to hemorrhage, airway obstruction, or dehiscence of the anastomosis has occurred only rarely.

In cases of inadequate ventilation and deterioration of oxygenation, endotracheal intubation is necessary. This procedure is undertaken with caution, generally with the aid of topicalization and judicious sedation. The tube is placed either nasally or orally with direct visualization of the larynx. This must be accomplished with the patient maintaining the flexed position without producing undue tension on the suture line. Flexible fiberoptic bronchoscopy in experienced hands is an extremely useful aid. Following intubation, the need for ventilation is reassessed following aggressive pulmonary toilet. Therapy is directed at minimizing both positive pressure on the airway and the time needed for intubation. The latter is especially true in cases where the endotracheal tube passes through the anastomosis, such as high tracheal reconstructions. The potential for dehiscence in the early stage of recovery is real. When prolonged intubation is anticipated, elective tracheostomy is seriously considered. The hazards of tracheostomy are dictated by the patient's body habitus, the location of the anastomosis,

Figure 20-11. Modes of carinal resection and reconstruction used. *Circled number* is number of patients. *Open arrows* indicate side of approach when not conventionally right sided. A: Limited resection permits carinal restitution. B: Technique used in initial carinal resection; technique in A: would now be used. C: More extensive resection. D: Greater length of trachea. Technique of Barclay and coworkers. E: Involvement of right main bronchus and right upper lobe bronchus requires right upper lobectomy. F: Middle lobe also removed. Right lower lobe bronchus may be anastomosed to left main bronchus. G: Right carinal pneumonectomy. H: Left carinal pneumonectomy. I: Resection of carina after previous left pneumonectomy. J: Resection of carina with extra long stump. K: Wedge removal of left main bronchus from the right. L: Tracheocarinal resection with long segment of left main bronchus. Exclusion of remaining left lung from the right. Left pneumonectomy also through bilateral thoracotomy. (Used with permission from Grillo.[38])

and the ability to safely dissect and position the tracheostomy tube following the reconstructive surgery.

Upper airway obstruction secondary to laryngeal edema is an infrequent complication. It has occurred most commonly when there has been a high anastomosis or previous history of laryngeal disease. Prophylactic measures should be undertaken to avoid laryngeal edema if the patient has a history of cord paralysis, if episodes of laryngeal edema occur, or if the trachea is anastomosed directly to the larynx at the level of the cricoid cartilage. Therapy includes the use of high humidity and the inhalation of topical steroids and racemic epinephrine. Racemic epinephrine, 0.5 mL of a 1:200 dilution in 2.5 mL of normal saline, is administered via nebulizer every 4 hours as needed. Dexamethasone may be inhaled or given parenterally. This regimen is continued for a minimum of 24 hours or longer if laryngeal edema, evidenced by stridor and hoarseness, persists.

Methods to control pain postoperatively have been well described in the literature.[79] Efficient control of postoperative pain is mandatory in the patient post tracheal resection. The method of pain control depends in part on the site of the surgical incision and the patient's preoperative pulmonary dysfunction and pain threshold. Successful modalities of pain control in patients after resection of an upper airway lesion via the cervical collar incision include parenteral or intramuscular narcotics or patient-controlled analgesia (PCA).[79] Patients recovering from the effects of a thoracotomy incision may achieve pain control with a variety of methods. These include epidural analgesia,[72–74] intrapleural analgesia,[80] intrathoracic intercostal nerve blocks,[81,82] or PCA.[79]

Patients should be kept in the intensive care unit at least overnight until it is deemed safe to return to the general surgical floor. This is dictated by the ability to discontinue cardiovascular monitoring, the need for frequent assessment of pulmonary status, and the level of nursing care.

Conclusion

As stated in this chapter, patients with lesions of the large airways present for surgical repair infrequently. Such operations are performed regularly at only a few major institutions. Surgery of the airways is performed frequently at the Massachusetts General Hospital. The evaluation and anesthetic management of the patient presenting for airway surgery detailed are those developed during the last 30 years in this institution. In summary, the ability to deliver a safe anesthetic depends upon the anesthesiologist's knowledge of the anticipated surgical procedure, the etiology, and the location and extent of the lesion. The anesthesiologist must also be aware of the potential complications of this fascinating and challenging problem and have a thorough understanding of the patient's other medical problems. This allows the anesthesiologist to devise a smooth, successful anesthetic technique.

References

1. Grillo HC. The management of tracheal stenosis following assisted respiration. J Thorac Cardiovasc Surg 1969;57:521.
2. Grillo HC. Reconstruction of the trachea. Experience in 100 consecutive cases. Thorax 1973;28:667.
3. Grillo HC. Circumferential resection and reconstruction of the mediastinal and cervical trachea. Ann Surg 1965;162:374.
4. Geffin B, Bland J, Grillo HC. Anesthetic management of tracheal resection and reconstruction. Anesth Analg 1969;48:884.
5. Ellis RH, Hinds CJ, Gadd LT. Management of anes-

thesia during tracheal resection. Anaesthesia 1976; 31:1076.
6. Lee P, English ICW. Management of anesthesia during tracheal resection. Anaesthesia 1974;29:305.
7. Wilson RS. Tracheostomy and tracheal reconstruction. In: Kaplan J, ed. Thoracic anesthesia. New York: Churchill Livingstone, 1991:421.
8. Young-Beyer P, Wilson RS. Anesthetic management for tracheal resection and reconstruction. J Cardiothorac Anesth 1988;2:821.
9. Belsey R. Resection and reconstruction of the intrathoracic trachea. Br J Surg 1950;38:200.
10. Kamvyssi-Dea S, Kritikon P, Exarhos N, et al. Anaesthetic management of reconstruction of the lower part of the trachea. Br J Anaesth 1975;47:82.
11. Macnaughton FI. Catheter inflation ventilation in tracheal stenosis. Br J Anaesth 1975;47:1225.
12. Baraka A. Oxygen jet ventilation during tracheal reconstruction in patients with tracheal stenosis. Anesth Analg 1977;56:429.
13. Clarkson WB, Davies JR. Anesthesia for carinal resection. Anaesthesia 1978;33:815.
14. Ismail AB. Anaesthesia for tracheal resection. Modified use of the Carlen tube. Can J Anaesth 1979; 26:134.
15. Conacher ID, Paes ML, Morritt GN: Anaesthesia for carbon dioxide laser surgery on the trachea. Br J Anaesth 1985;57:448.
16. Borland LM, Reilly JS, Smith SD. Anesthetic management of tracheal-esophageal fistula with distal tracheal stenosis. Anesthesiology 1987;67:132.
17. Baraka A, Mansour R, Jaoude CA, et al. Entrainment of oxygen and halothane during jet ventilation in patients undergoing excision of tracheal and bronchial tumors. Anesth Analg 1986;65:191.
18. Vourch G, Fischler M, Michon F et al. Manual jet ventilation versus high-frequency jet ventilation during laser resection of tracheo-bronchial stenosis. Br J Anaesth 1983;55:973.
19. Scamman FL, Choi WW. Low-frequency jet ventilation for tracheal resection. Laryngoscope 1986; 96:678.
20. Rogers RC, Gibbons J, Cosgrove J, et al. High-frequency jet ventilation for tracheal surgery. Anaesthesia 1985;40:32.
21. Neuman GG, Asher AS, Stern SB, et al. High-frequency jet ventilation for tracheal resection in a child. Anesth Analg 1984;63:1039.
22. Erikson I, Nilsson LG, Nordstrom S, et al. High-frequency positive-pressure ventilation (HFPPV) during transthoracic resection of tracheal stenosis and during perioperative bronchoscopic examination. Acta Anaesthesiol Scand 1975;19:113.
23. El-Baz N, El-Ganzouri A, Gottschalk W, et al. One-lung high-frequency positive-pressure ventilation for sleeve pneumonectomy: an alternative technique. Anesth Analg 1981;60:683.
24. El-Baz N, Holinger L, El-Ganzouri A, et al. High-frequency positive-pressure ventilation for tracheal reconstruction supported by tracheal T-tube. Anesth Analg 1982;61:796.
25. El-Baz N, Jensik R, Fauer P, et al. One-lung high-frequency ventilation for tracheoplasty and bronchoplasty: a new technique. Ann Thorac Surg 1982; 34:564.
26. Woods F, Neptune W, Palatchi A. Resection of the carina and mainstem bronchi with extracorporeal circulation. N Eng J Med 1961;264:492.
27. Coles JC, Doctor A, Lefcoe M, et al. A method of anesthesia for imminent tracheal obstruction. Surgery 1976;80:379.
28. Theman TE, Kerr JH, Nelems JM, et al. Carinal resection. A report of two cases and a description of the anesthetic technique. J Thorac Cardiovasc Surg 1976;71:314.
29. Dodge TL, Mahaffey JE, Thomas JD. The anesthetic management of a patient with an obstructing intratracheal mass: a case report. Anesth Analg 1977; 56:295.
30. Akdikmen S, Landmesser CM. Anesthesia for surgery of the intrathoracic portion of the trachea. Anesthesiology 1965;26:117.
31. Lippman M, Mok MS. Tracheal cylindrona: anesthetic management. Br J Anaesth 1977;49:383.
32. Abou-Madi MN, Cuadrado L, Domb B, et al. Anaesthesia of tracheal resection: a new way to manage the airway. Can J Anaesth 1979;26:26.
33. Boyan PC, Privitera PA. Resection of stenotic trachea: a case presentation. Anesth Analg 1976; 55:191.
34. Debrand M, Tseuda K, Browning SK, et al. Anesthesia for extensive repair of congenital tracheal stenosis in an infant. Anesth Analg 1979;58:431.
35. Grillo HC, Zannini P, Michelassi F. Complications of tracheal reconstruction. J Thorac Cardiovasc Surg 1986;91:322.
36. Fryer ME, Marshall RD. Tracheal dilatation. Anaesthesia 1976;31:470.
37. Wilson DJ. Airway appliances and management. In: Kacmarek R, Stoller JK, eds. Current respiratory care. Philadelphia: BC Decker, 1988:80.
38. Grillo HC, Mathisen, DJ. Primary tracheal tumors: treatment and results. Ann Thorac Surg 1990;49:69.

39. Hajdu SI, Huvas AG, Goodner JT, et al. Carcinoma of the trachea. Clinicopathologic study of 41 cases. Cancer 1970;25:1448.
40. Houston H, Payne W, Harrison E. Primary cancers of the trachea. Arch Surg 1969;2:123.
41. Grillo HC. Congenital lesions, neoplasms and injuries of the trachea. In: Sabiston DC Jr, Spencer FC, eds. Gibbon's surgery of the chest. 3rd ed. Philadelphia: WB Saunders, 1976.
42. Pearson FG, Thompson DW, Weissberg D, et al. Adenoid cystic carcinoma of the trachea. Experience with 16 patients managed by tracheal resection. Ann Thorac Surg 1974;18:16.
43. Grillo HC, Mathisen DJ, Wain JC. Laryngotracheal resection and reconstruction for subglottic stenosis. Ann Thor Surg 1992;53:54.
44. Mathisen DJ, Grillo HC. Laryngotracheal trauma. Ann Thorac Surg 1987;43:254.
45. Mathisen DJ, Grillo HC. Laryngotracheal trauma—acute and chronic. In: Grillo HC, Eschapasse H, eds. International trends in general thoracic surgery. Volume 2: Major challenges. Philadelphia: WB Saunders, 1987.
46. Cicala RS, Kudsk KA, Butts A, et al. Initial evaluation and management of upper airway injuries in trauma patients. Journ Clin Anesth 1991;3:91.
47. Cantrell JR, Guild HG. Congenital stenosis of the trachea. Am J Surg 1964;108:297.
48. Clarkson PM, Ritter DG, Rahimtoola SHl, et al. Aberrant left pulmonary artery. Am J Dis Child 1967; 113:373.
49. Jacobson JH, Morgan BC, Anderson DH, et al. Aberrant left pulmonary artery. J Thorac Cardiovasc Surg 1960;39:602.
50. Gross RE. The surgery of infancy and childhood. Philadelphia: WB Saunders, 1953.
51. Lincoln JCR, Deverall PB, Stark J, et al. Vascular anomalies compressing the oesophagus and trachea. Thorax 1969;24:295.
52. Maze A, Bloch E. Stridor in pediatric patients. Anesthesiology 1979;50:132.
53. Grillo HC, Zannini P. Management of obstructive tracheal disease in children. J Pediatr Surg 1984; 19:414.
54. Kryger M, Bode F, Antic R, et al. Diagnosis of obstruction of the upper and central airways. Am J Med 1976;61:85.
55. Crosby ET, Liu A. The adult cervical spine: implications for airway management. Can J Anesth 1990; 37:77.
56. Hyatt RE, Black LF. The flow-volume curve: a current perspective. Am Rev Respir Dis 1973;107:191.
57. Momose KJ, Macmillan AS. Roentgenologic investigations of the larynx and trachea. Radiol Clin North Am 1978;16:321.
58. Weber AL, Grillo HC. Tracheal tumors, a radiological, clinical and pathological evaluation of 84 cases. Radiol Clin North Am 1978;16:227.
59. Weber AL, Grillo HC. Tracheal stenosis, an analysis of 151 cases. Radiol Clin North Am 1978;16:291.
60. Gefter WB. Chest applications of magnetic resonance imaging: an update. Radiol Clin North Am 1990;28:573.
61. Naidich DP. CT/MRI correlation in the evaluation of tracheobronchial neoplasia. Radiol Clin North Am 1990;28:555.
62. Grillo HC. Surgical approaches to the trachea. Surg Gynecol Obstet 1969;129:347.
63. Grillo HC. Terminal or mural tracheostomy in the anterior mediastinum. J Thorac Cardiovasc Surg 1966;51:422.
64. Grillo HC Tracheal tumors: surgical management. Ann Thorac Surg 1978;26:112.
65. Grillo HC. Surgical treatment of postintubation tracheal injuries. J Thorac Cardiovasc Surg 1979; 78:860.
66. Grillo HC, Mathisen DD. Surgical management of tracheal strictures. Surg Clin Am 1988;68:511.
67. Egbert LD, Battit GE, Turndorf H, et al. The value of the preoperative visit by an anesthetist. JAMA 1963; 185:553.
68. Leigh JM, Walker J, Janaganathan P. Effect of preanesthetic visit on anxiety. BMJ 1977;2:987.
69. Eichorn JH, Cooper JB, Cullen DJ, et al. Standards for patient monitoring during anesthesia at Harvard Medical School. JAMA 1986;256:1017.
70. Ravitch MM, et al, eds. Current problems in surgery. Chicago: Year Book Medical Publishers, 1970.
71. Cooper JD, Nelems JM, Pearson FG. Extended indication for median sternotomy in patients requiring pulmonary resection. Ann Thorac Surg 1978;26:413.
72. James EC, Kolberg HL, Iwen GW, et al. Epidural analgesia for postthoracotomy patients. J Thorac Cardiovasc Surg 1981;82:898.
73. Logas WG, El-Baz N, El-Ganzouri A, et al. Continuous thoracic epidural analgesia for postoperative pain relief following thoracotomy. A randomized prospective study. Anesthesiology 1987;67:787.
74. Fischer RL, Lubenow TR, Liceaga A, et al. Comparison of continuous epidural infusion of fentanyl-bupivicaine and morphine-bupivicaine in management of postoperative pain. Anesth Analg 1988;67: 559.

75. Cohen E, Eisenkraft JB, Thys C, et al. Oxygenation and hemodynamic changes during one-lung ventilation: effects of $CPAP_{10}$, $PEEP_{10}$ and $CPAP_{10}/PEEP_{10}$. J Cardiothor Anesth 1988;2:34.
76. Cook CE, Wilson RS. Dangers of using an improvised underwater seal for CPAP oxygenation during one-lung ventilation. Anesthesiology 1987;66:707.
77. Scheller MS, Varvel JR. CPAP oxygenation during one-lung ventilation using a Bain circuit. Anesthesiology 1987;66:708.
78. Steegers PA, Backx PJ. Propofol and alfentanil anesthesia during one-lung ventilation. J Cardiothorac Anesth 1990;4:194.
79. Coleman DL. Control of postoperative pain: nonnarcotic and narcotic alternatives and their effect on pulmonary function. Chest 1987;92:520.
80. Symreng T, Gomez MN, Ross N. Intrapleural bupivicaine vs saline after thoracotomy—effects on pain and lung function—a double blind study. J Cardiothorac Anesth 1988;3:144.
81. Woltering EA, Flye MW, Huntley S, et al. Evaluation of bupivicaine nerve blocks in the modification of pain and pulmonary function changes after thoracotomy. Ann Thorac Surg 1980;30:122.
82. Toledo-Pereyra LH, DeMeester TR. Prospective randomized evaluation of intrathoracic intercostal nerve block with bupivicaine on postoperative ventilatory function. Ann Thorac Surg 1979;27:203.

Index